OF WISDOM

Family Medicine
BOARD REVIEW

Fourth Edition

Cynthia M. Waickus, MD, PhD
William A. Schwer, MD
Scott H. Plantz, MD

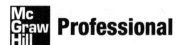 **Professional**

New York   Chicago San Francisco Lisbon London   Madrid Mexico City Milan
New Delhi   San Juan Seoul Singapore   Sydney Toronto

Notice

Medicine is an ever-changing science. As new research and clinical experience broaden our knowledge, changes in treatment and drug therapy are required. The authors and the publisher of this work have checked with sources believed to be reliable in their efforts to provide information that is complete and generally in accord with the standards accepted at the time of publication. However, in view of the possibility of human error or changes in medical sciences, neither the authors nor the publisher nor any other party who has been involved in the preparation or publication of this work warrants that the information contained herein is in every respect accurate or complete, and they disclaim all responsibility for any errors or omissions or for the results obtained from use of the information contained in this work. Readers are encouraged to confirm the information contained herein with other sources. For example and in particular, readers are advised to check the product information sheet included in the package of each drug they plan to administer to be certain that the information contained in this work is accurate and that changes have not been made in the recommended dose or in the contraindications for administration. This recommendation is of particular importance in connection with new or infrequently used drugs.

This book was set in Adobe Garamond by Aptara®, Inc.
The editors were Kirsten Funk and Christine Diedrich.
The production supervisor was Sherri Souffrance.
Project management was provided by Satvinder Kaur, Aptara®, Inc.
The cover designer was Ty Nowicki.
Worldcolor Dubuque was printer and binder.

This book is printed on acid-free paper.

Library of Congress Cataloging-in-Publication Data

Waickus, Cynthia M.
    Family medicine board review / Cynthia M. Waickus, William A. Schwer, Scott H. Plantz. —4th ed.
        p. ; cm. — (Pearls of wisdom)
    Rev. ed. of: Family practice board review / [editor-in-chief] William A. Schwer ; [associate editors] Scott H. Plantz, Gillian Emblad. 3rd ed. c2006.
    Includes bibliographical references.
    Summary: "The chapters presented parallel the core content areas included on the Family Medicine Certification/Recertification Examination. Every attempt has been made to include the most accurate, current information. Nonetheless, medicine is a dynamic field. The half-life of medical information continues to decline, while the addition of new information is exploding at an exponential rate. In this text, we have attempted to condense complex concepts into basic principles. The intent of the text is to maximize your test scores, not to serve as reference source for information"—Provided by publisher.
        ISBN 978-0-07-162551-7 (alk. paper)
        1. Family medicine—Examinations, questions, etc.   I. Schwer, William A. (William Arthur)   II. Plantz, Scott H.
III. Family practice board review.   IV. Title.   V. Series: Pearls of wisdom.
        [DNLM: 1. Family Practice—Examination Questions. WB 18.2 W138f 2010]
        RC58.F332 2010
        610.76—dc22
                                                                                                2010010468

McGraw-Hill books are available at special quantity discounts to use as premiums and sales promotions or for use in corporate training programs. To contact a representative, please e-mail us at bulksales@mcgraw-hill.com.

CONTENTS

EDITORS

Cynthia M. Waickus, MD, PhD
Associate Chair for Educational Programs
Department of Family Medicine
Rush University Medical Center
Chicago, Illinois

William A. Schwer, MD
Professor and Chairman
Department of Family Medicine
Rush University Medical Center
Chicago, Illinois

Scott H. Plantz, MD
Clinical Professor
Chicago Medical School
Mt. Sinai Medical Center
Chicago, Illinois

CONTRIBUTORS

Joel Augustin, MD
Assistant Professor
Department of Family Medicine
Rush University Medical Center
Chicago, Illinois
Rheumatology, Immunology, and Allergy

Robert L. Barkin, MBA, PharmD, FCP, DAAPM
Professor of Anesthesiology, Family Medicine
 and Pharmacology
Rush University Medical Center
Chicago, Illinois
Clinical Pharmacologist
Northshore University Health System
Department of Anesthesiology
Pain Centers at Evanston & Skokie Hospitals
Evanston, Illinois
Clinical Pharmacology and Toxicology

Krystian Bigosinski, MD
Assistant Professor
Department of Family Medicine
Rush University Medical Center
Chicago, Illinois
Orthopedics
Sports Medicine

Maria I. Brown, DO
Assistant Professor
Department of Family Medicine
Rush University Medical Center
Chicago, Illinois
Obstetrics/Gynecology

Brenda K. Fann, MD, FAAFP
Assistant Professor
Department of Family Medicine
Rush University Medical Center
Chicago, Illinois
Program Director
Rush-Copley Family Medicine Residency
 Program
Aurora, Illinois
Hematology and Oncology

Joe Guidi, DO
Residency, Attending Physician
Rush-Copley Family Medicine Residency Program
Chicago, Illinois
Gastrointestinal

Gina Kring, MD
Assistant Professor
Department of Family Medicine
Rush University Medical Center
Chicago, Ilinois
Pulmonary

Lorna H. London, PhD
Rush-Copley Family Medicine Residency Program
Aurora, Illinois
Behavioral Science

Carrie E. Nelson, MD, MS, FAAFP
Assistant Professor
Rush University Medical Center
Chicago, Illinois
Former, Program Director
Rush-Copley Family Medicine Residency Program
Aurora, Illinois
Dermatology

Deepak S. Patel, MD, FAAFP
Assistant Professor
Department of Family Medicine
Rush University Medical Center
Chicago, Illinois
Director of Sports Medicine
Rush-Copley Family Medicine Residency Program
Aurora, Illinois
Orthopedics
Sports Medicine

Scott H. Plantz, MD
Clinical Professor
Chicago Medical School
Mt. Sinai Medical Center
Chicago, Illinois
General Surgery and Trauma

Steven K. Rothschild, MD
Associate Professor
Departments of Family Medicine and
    Preventive Medicine
Rush University Medical Center
Chicago, Illinois
Preventive Medicine and
    Biostatistics

Norman S. Ryan, MD
Assistant Professor
Department of Family Medicine
Rush University Medical Center
Chicago, Illinois
Cardiovascular

Miguel A. Salas, MD, MPH
Clinical Instructor
Department of Family Medicine
Rush University Medical Center
Associate Director
Rush University Family Physicians
Chicago, Illinois
Environmental Medicine

William A. Schwer, MD
Professor and Chairman
Department of Family Medicine
Rush University Medical Center
Chicago, Illinois
Ophthalmology
Radiology

Raj C. Shah, MD
Assistant Professor
Department of Family Medicine
Rush Alzheimer's Disease Center
Rush University Medical Center
Chicago, Illinois
Neurology
Geriatrics

David A. Stewart, MD
Assistant Professor
Department of Family Medicine
Rush University Medical Center
Chicago, Illinois
Ear, Nose, and Throat

Susan Vanderberg-Dent, MD
Associate Dean for Graduate Medical Education
Associate Professor
Department of Family Medicine
Rush University Medical Center
Chicago, Illinois
Pediatrics

Cynthia M. Waickus, MD, PhD
Associate Chair for Educational Programs
Department of Family Medicine
Rush University Medical Center
Chicago, Illinois
Metabolic and Endocrine
Genitourinary

Andrew H. Zalski, MD
Assistant Professor
Department of Family Medicine
Rush University Medical Center
Chicago, Illinois
Infectious Disease

INTRODUCTION

Thank you for your purchase of *Family Medicine Board Review: Pearls of Wisdom, Fourth Edition*. This simple text was originally designed as a study aid to improve performance on family medicine written, recertification, or in-service examinations. Although the original version was intended for family medicine specialists, over the years we have learned that house officers and medical students have also found this unique format useful as a general-purpose study aid, as well as an optimal tool for USMLE preparation. The format, intent, use, and limitations of this review text are discussed below.

The text is written in rapid-fire question/answer format. This way, readers receive immediate feedback; misleading or confusing foils are not presented. This method eliminates the risk of erroneously assimilating an incorrect piece of information. Questions themselves often contain a "pearl" of knowledge intended to reinforce the answer; answers often contain additional information, not necessarily requested in the question, intended to assist in retention of the specific information. These additional hooks are included in a variety of forms, including mnemonics, visual imagery, repetition, and humor. Emphasis has also been placed on distilling trivia and key facts that are easily overlooked, that are quickly forgotten, but that somehow seem to be included on board examinations.

The chapters presented parallel the core content areas included on the Family Medicine Certification/Recertification Examination. Every attempt has been made to include the most accurate, current information. Nonetheless, medicine is a dynamic field. The half-life of medical information continues to decline, while the addition of new information is exploding at an exponential rate. In this text, we have attempted to condense complex concepts into basic principles. The intent of the text is to maximize your test scores, not to serve as reference source for information.

Many questions have answers without extensive explanation. This enhances the ease of reading, as well as the rate of learning. More thorough explanations are often presented in a later question/answer on the same topic. When reading an answer, the reader may think, *"Hmm . . . why is that?"* or, *"Are you sure?"* If this happens to you, go to the literature and verify the information for yourself. Truly assimilating disparate facts into a framework of knowledge absolutely requires further exploration of the topic area. The deliberate acquisition of information to support the contextual framework of a subject optimizes long-term retention of knowledge to a much larger extent than does passive learning. Use this process to your advantage by having ready access to your preferred reference and sources while reviewing the questions.

Family Medicine Board Review is intended to be used, not simply read. It is designed to be an interactive text to measure your knowledge, identify your strengths, and identify those areas that you need to review in greater depth. The text works well for individual study, but it also works well in small group sessions where questions and answers can be "fired" around the room. Try it—it's almost fun.

The text is an ongoing effort and we welcome your comments, suggestions, and criticism. We have attempted to verify the answers in this book, but if your find errors, please let us know. We continuously update and improve this text, and we would greatly appreciate any input with regard to format, organization, content, or presentation or with regard to any specific question. We also are interested in recruiting new contributing authors, if you are interested. Thank you, and we look forward to hearing from you.

Study hard and good luck!

C.M.W., W.A.S., & S.H.P.

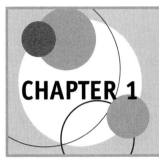

CHAPTER 1 Cardiovascular

Norman S. Ryan, MD

○ **What makes the first heart sound?**
Closure of the mitral and tricuspid valves

○ **What makes the second heart sound?**
Closure of the pulmonary and aortic valves

○ **What makes the third heart sound?**
Deceleration of blood flowing into a noncompliant left ventricle

○ **What makes the fourth heart sound?**
Vibrations of the left ventricular (LV) muscle, the mitral valve, and the LV flow tract during the atrial kick phase

○ **What is a common pathological cause of an S_3?**
Congestive heart failure (CHF)

○ **What are the pathological causes of an S_4?**
Decreased LV compliance due to hypertension is the most common cause. Others include aortic stenosis, subaortic stenosis, coronary artery disease (CAD), myocardiopathy, anemia, and hyperthyroidism.

○ **What is pulsus paradoxus?**
A change in measured systolic blood pressure (BP) of more than 10 mm Hg from expiratory to inspiratory phases

○ **What are the most common causes of pulsus paradoxus?**
Chronic obstructive pulmonary disease (COPD) and asthma

○ **What is the most common cause of superior vena cava obstruction?**
Bronchogenic carcinoma

○ **What murmurs will the Valsalva maneuver increase?**
Only idiopathic hypertrophic subaortic stenosis—all other murmurs are diminished

○   **What effect does the Valsalva maneuver have on the heart?**

The Valsalva maneuver decreases blood return to both the right and left ventricles. All murmurs decrease in intensity except idiopathic hypertrophic subaortic stenosis and mitral valve prolapse (MVP).

○   **Name the 2 primary causes of peripheral cyanosis with a normal arterial oxygen saturation.**

Decreased cardiac output and redistribution (may be secondary to shock, disseminated intravascular coagulation, hypothermia, or vascular obstruction)

○   **Are aortic aneurysms more common in men or women?**

Men (10:1). Other risk factors include hypertension, atherosclerosis, diabetes, hyperlipidemia, smoking, syphilis, Marfan disease, and Ehlers-Danlos disease.

○   **A patient presents with sudden-onset chest and back pain. Further workup reveals an ischemic right leg. What is your diagnosis?**

Suspect an acute aortic dissection when chest or back pain is associated with ischemic or neurologic deficits

○   **What physical findings suggest an acute aortic dissection?**

BP differences between arms and/or legs, cardiac tamponade, and aortic insufficiency murmur

○   **What chest radiographic findings occur with a thoracic aortic aneurysm?**

Change in aortic appearance, mediastinal widening, hump in the aortic arch, pleural effusion (most commonly on the left), and extension of the aortic shadow

○   **A 74-year-old man presents with acute-onset testicular pain. Ecchymosis is present in the groin and scrotal sac. What is the diagnosis?**

A ruptured aortic or iliac artery aneurysm

○   **What radiographic study should be ordered for a patient with an abdominal mass and a suspected ruptured abdominal aortic aneurysm (AAA)?**

None. The patient should go to surgery immediately. About 60% of AAAs occur with calcification and appear on a lateral abdominal radiograph.

○   **What may a radiograph of a patient with an aortic dissection reveal?**

Widening of the superior mediastinum, a hazy or enlarged aortic knob, an irregular aortic contour, separation of the intimal calcification from the outer aortic contour that is greater than 5 mm, a displaced trachea to the right, and cardiomegaly

○   **What is the most common symptom of aortic dissection?**

Interscapular back pain

○   **In which section of the aorta do dissections most often occur?**

Proximal ascending aorta (60%). Twenty percent of aortic dissections are found between the origin of the left subclavian artery and the ligamentum arteriosum in the descending aorta, and 10% are found in the aortic arch or the abdominal aorta. Dissection involves intimal tears propagated by hematoma formation.

○ **What aortic aneurysm diameter is generally considered to be an indication for surgery: (1) in the thorax and (2) in the abdomen?**

Those with nondissecting thoracic aneurysm larger than 7 cm in diameter are candidates for surgery. However, surgery should be considered with smaller aneurysms for those with Marfan syndrome because of a higher incidence of rupture. Nondissecting AAAs larger than 4 cm in diameter should be considered for surgical repair.

○ **Describe the DeBakey classification of aortic dissections.**
- Type I: Dissection of the aortic root, arch, and descending aorta
- Type II: Ascending aorta only
- Type III: Distal aorta only

○ **Describe the Stanford classification of aortic dissections.**
- Stanford Type A: Involve ascending aorta
- Stanford Type B: Do not involve ascending aorta

○ **What dissections can be treated medically?**

Patients with Type B (and DeBakey type III) are eligible for medical rather than surgical treatment. Surgical treatment may be required for those with uncontrollable pain, aortic bleeding, hemodynamic instability, increasing hematoma size, or an impending rupture.

○ **What is the prognosis for an untreated aortic dissection?**

Twenty percent of individuals with untreated aortic dissection die within 24 hours, 60% within 2 weeks, and 90% within 3 months. With surgical treatment, the 10-year survival rate is 40%. Redissection occurs in 25% of these patients within 10 years after the original episode.

○ **What murmur is audible in patients with substantial aortic stenosis?**

A prolonged, harsh, loud (grade 4, 5, or 6) systolic murmur

○ **What peripheral artery is most likely to develop an aneurysm from arteriosclerotic disease?**

The popliteal artery. Other sites include the femoral, carotid, and subclavian arteries.

○ **How long can ST and T changes on an electrocardiogram (ECG) persist after an episode of pain in unstable angina?**

Several hours

○ **What are the classic signs and symptoms of aortic stenosis?**

Left-sided heart failure, angina, and exertional syncope

○ **What is the optimal patient position and maneuver for auscultation of aortic insufficiency?**

Have the patient sit up and lean forward with his or her hands tightly clasped. During patient exhalation, listen at the left sternal border.

○ **What is the most common source of arterial embolisms?**

Embolism from atheromatous plaques from the aorta is the most common source of arterial embolisms. Next most common is atrial thrombi originating in the presence of atrial fibrillation. Other causes include LV thrombi, postanteroapical infarction, valvular heart disease, rheumatic heart disease, and subacute bacterial endocarditis.

○ **Among those with Marfan syndrome, at what age does aortic aneurysm become problematic?**

30s and 40s

○ **Matching:**

1. Quincke pulse   **a.** Uvular pulsation during systole
2. Corrigan pulse   **b.** Head bobbing
3. de Musset sign   **c.** Visible pulsations in nail bed capillaries
4. Müller sign   **d.** Femoral artery murmurs during systole if the artery is compressed proximally and during diastole if the artery is compressed distally
5. Duroziez sign   **e.** Collapsing pulse
6. Pulsus paradoxus   **f.** Decrease in systolic BP of more than 10 mm Hg with inspiration

Answers: (1) c, (2) e, (3) b, (4) a, (5) d, and (6) f

These are all signs pertaining to aortic insufficiency.

○ **What is the most common cause of aortic regurgitation in adults?**

Mild aortic regurgitation frequently develops as a result of a bicuspid aortic valve. A severe aortic regurgitation is induced by rheumatic heart disease, syphilis, endocarditis, trauma, an idiopathic degeneration of the aortic valve, a spontaneous rupture of the valve leaflets, or aortic dissection.

○ **What are the signs and symptoms of acute aortic regurgitation?**

Dyspnea, tachycardia, tachypnea, and chest pain

○ **What is the most common cause of aortic stenosis in patients younger than 50 years? What is the most common cause of aortic stenosis in patients older than 50 years?**

Younger than 50 years: Calcification of congenital bicuspid aortic valves (1% of the population has congenital bicuspid valves)

Older than 50 years: Calcification of degenerating leaflets

○ **What triad of symptoms characterizes aortic stenosis?**

Syncope, angina, and left-sided heart failure. As the disease progresses, systolic BP decreases, and pulse pressure narrows.

○ **What are the clinical findings in a patient with aortic stenosis?**

Angina, dyspnea at exertion, syncope, sustained apical impulse, narrow pulse pressure, pulsus parvus et tardus, systolic ejection crescendo-decrescendo murmur that radiates to the neck, systolic ejection click (not heard in severe cases when the valve is so stenosed that it is immobile), paradoxically split S_1 and soft S_2, and audible S_4

○ **When should surgery be considered for patients with aortic stenosis?**

Only when symptoms are displayed. The risk of morbidity and mortality associated with the replacement of an aortic valve outweighs any benefit of operating on asymptomatic patients.

○ **What is the risk of mortality from surgery to replace the aortic valve for stenosis?**

Remarkably low, even in the elderly: 2% to 5%. The low risk is thought to be due to the dramatic hemodynamic improvement that occurs with release of the increased afterload.

○ **Match the rhythm with the type of supraventricular tachycardia (SVT).**

1. Wolff-Parkinson-White syndrome
2. Multifocal atrial tachycardia
3. Atrial fibrillation
4. Atrial flutter
5. Accelerated junctional tachycardia
6. Unifocal atrial tachycardia
7. Intraartrial reentrant tachycardia
8. Nodal tachycardia

a. Atrioventricular (AV) reciprocating tachycardia
b. Automatic tachycardia
c. Reentrant atrial tachycardia
d. AV reentrant nodal tachycardia

Answers: (1) a, (2) b, (3) c, (4) c, (5) d, (6) b, (7) c, and (8) d

○ **What are the most common causes of multifocal atrial tachycardia?**

COPD, CHF, sepsis, and methylxanthine toxicity

Treat the arrhythmia with magnesium, verapamil, or β-blocking agents.

○ **What is the treatment for multifocal atrial tachycardia?**

- Treat the underlying disorder.
- Administer magnesium sulfate, 2 g over 60 seconds, with supplemental potassium to maintain the serum potassium level above 4 mEq/L.
- Consider verapamil, 10 mg intravenously (IV), as a second treatment.

○ **What are symptoms of atrial flutter?**

Symptoms of flutter depend largely on how fast the ventricles beat. A modest increase in the ventricular rate to less than about 120 beats per minute (bpm) may produce no symptoms. Higher rates cause unpleasant palpitations or chest discomfort. Also, the following are symptoms of atrial flutter:

- A regular, fast pulse
- A feeling of weakness
- Dizziness or faintness
- Shortness of breath
- Chest pain, especially in older adults
- Rarely, BP may decrease, causing shock. This usually occurs only in people having atrial fibrillation or flutter who also have severe heart disease.

○ **How is atrial flutter treated?**

Initiate AV nodal blockade with β-blockers, calcium-channel blockers, or digoxin. If necessary, treat a stable patient with chemical cardioversion by using a class IA agent, such as procainamide or quinidine, after administration of digitalis. If this treatment fails or if the patient is unstable, attempt electrocardioversion at 25 to 50 J.

○ **What are some causes of atrial fibrillation?**

Hypertension, rheumatic heart disease, pneumonia, thyrotoxicosis, ischemic heart, pericarditis, ethanol intoxication, pulmonary embolism, CHF, and COPD

○ **How is atrial fibrillation treated?**

Control heart rate with β-blockade or calcium-channel blocker (such as verapamil or diltiazem) then convert to sinus rhythm with procainamide, quinidine, or verapamil. Digoxin may be considered, although its effect will be delayed. Synchronized cardioversion at 100 to 200 J should be performed in an unstable patient. In a stable patient with atrial fibrillation of unclear duration, anticoagulation should be considered for 2 to 3 weeks before chemical or electrical cardioversion. Watch for hypotension with the administration of negative inotropes.

○ **What drugs should never be used for atrial fibrillation with Wolff-Parkinson-White syndrome?**

Digitalis, verapamil, and phenytoin. Atrial fibrillation with Wolff-Parkinson-White syndrome should be treated with cardioversion or procainamide. SVT with Wolff-Parkinson-White syndrome should be treated with verapamil or adenosine.

○ **What are the classic ECG findings for Wolff-Parkinson-White syndrome?**

A change in the upstroke of QRS, the delta wave

○ **What is the most common arrhythmia associated with Wolff-Parkinson-White syndrome?**

Paroxysmal atrial tachycardia. The patient presents with angina, syncope, and shortness of breath.

○ **Why is verapamil a bad choice to treat ventricular tachycardia?**

Verapamil could increase heart rate and decrease BP without converting the rhythm, resulting in sudden death.

○ **What mechanism most commonly produces SVTs?**

Reentry. Another common cause is abnormal automaticity (ie, ectopic foci).

○ **What is the most common arrhythmia associated with digitalis?**

Premature ventricular contraction (PVC; 60%), ectopic SVT (25%), and AV block (20%)

○ **What is the treatment for SVT caused by digitalis toxicity?**

Stop the digitalis, treat the hypokalemia, and administer magnesium or phenytoin. Provide digoxin-specific antibodies to the unstable patient. Avoid cardioversion.

○ **What is the treatment for stable SVT not caused by digitalis toxicity or Wolff-Parkinson-White syndrome?**

Vagal maneuvers, adenosine, verapamil, or β-blockers to slow rate; quinidine, procainamide, or magnesium to decrease ectopy.

○ **What are the indications for administering digitalis-specific Fab?**
- Ventricular arrhythmias
- Potassium level greater than 5.5 mEq/L
- Unresponsive bradyarrhythmias

Some authors refer to an ingestion of more than 0.3 mg/kg of digitalis as requiring Fab. The number of vials required is 1.33 per milligram ingested. You can use this formula to determine dose on the basis of serum digoxin level, or you can administer 10 vials (40 mg Fab each) if the amount ingested is unknown.

Children and adolescents have an even higher sensitivity to digoxin overdose and may need Fab therapy with ingestion of less than the recommended 0.3 mg/kg.

Remember, in an acute overdose situation, the serum level of digitalis is unreliable for evaluating toxicity. Digitalis levels typically become accurate only after 4 to 6 hours; this is too long to wait for treatment.

○ **You administer digoxin-specific antibody (Fab) to a digoxin-toxic patient with an elevated digoxin level. The digoxin level is measured again after this treatment, and it is much higher than the previous level. Why is this? Did the Fab work?**

Digoxin assay measures free and bound digoxin; the latter increases about 15 times via binding to Fab.

○ **Carotid massage or Valsalva maneuver is useful for slowing supraventricular rhythms. When is carotid massage contraindicated?**

With ventricular arrhythmias, digitalis toxicity, stroke, syncope, or seizures or in those with a carotid bruit

○ **What are some common vagal maneuvers?**

Breath holding, Valsalva maneuver (bearing down as if having a bowel movement), stimulating of the gag reflex, squatting, pressure on the eyeballs, and immersing the face in cold water

○ **Which is more common: premature atrial beats or ventricular beats?**

Premature atrial beats. Palpitations that occur because of premature atrial beats are generally benign and asymptomatic. Reassurance is the only treatment. Less frequent but more serious causes of atrial premature beats include pheochromocytoma and thyrotoxicosis. Random PVCs are also benign but common in the general population. Runs of PVCs or associated symptoms of dyspnea, angina, or syncope require investigation and are most likely related to an underlying heart disease.

○ **What substances increase PVCs?**

Caffeine, ethanol, and tobacco

○ **How much workup should you think about with a patient with the new occurrence of left bundle-branch block (BBB)?**

The major significance of BBB is that it may indicate the presence of previously unknown underlying cardiovascular disease. When BBB is found, therefore, a search for such underlying disease ought to be carried out. Since right BBB often occurs in healthy individuals, while left BBB usually indicates underlying disease, the search for underlying disease generally should be more aggressive with left BBB than with right BBB.

○   **What is the prognostic significance of new left BBB?**

The most common causes of left BBB are as follows:

- CAD
- Hypertensive heart disease
- Cardiomyopathy

Left BBB and coronary heart disease: The Framingham study revealed that during an 18-year period, 89% of individuals who developed left BBB also developed some apparent cardiovascular abnormalities. Also, within a decade of the development of left BBB, 50% of these individuals had died secondary to a cardiovascular cause.

In a series of patients studied in the cardiac catheterization laboratory, patients with left BBB and concomitant left axis deviation were significantly more likely to have organic heart disease, with a sensitivity of 42% and a specificity of 92%.

○   **What is the treatment for left BBB?**

There is no specific treatment for many cases of BBB. Most people with BBB are symptom free and do not need treatment. Nevertheless, you may need to treat the underlying heart condition causing BBB.

In clinical settings of possible MI where left BBB is present (nondiagnostic ECG), the suspicion of AMI should be increased, efforts should be made to obtain previous ECGs, and particular attention should be paid to subtle changes in repolarization, which will lead to more definitive test results.

In older patients in whom the suspicion of acute MI (AMI) is high, reperfusion therapy should be seriously considered because of the high mortality of AMI-left BBB in elderly patients. A highly individualized approach is needed, with careful consideration of the patient's general health activity status and comorbidity. If fibrinolytic therapy is selected, streptokinase has been demonstrated in all studies to have a lower risk of cerebral hemorrhage—the most dreaded complication of therapy, which increases in the elderly population.

In older patients with left BBB in whom the diagnosis of MI is probable but not certain, emergency cardiac catheterization both for diagnosis and to plan management is justified. Achieving immediate reperfusion with a catheter-based intervention in this setting is almost certainly more effective than thrombolytic therapy and avoids the risk of central nervous system hemorrhage.

○   **What is the significance of right BBB?**

Right BBB occurs in medical conditions that affect the right side of the heart or the results of a screening examination for such conditions. These include blood clots to the lung (pulmonary embolus), chronic lung disease, cardiomyopathy, and atrial and ventricular septal defects. However, right BBB also commonly occurs in healthy individuals, and the screening examination results, therefore, often show no medical problems. In these cases, the right BBB has no apparent medical significance and can be seen as a normal variant and safely ignored.

○   **What are the diagnostic criteria for a Q wave?**

More than 0.04 seconds and at least one-fourth the size of the R wave in the same lead. Beware, ECGs can be normal in up to 10% of all AMIs.

○   **Name 2 selective cardioselective β-blockers.**

Metoprolol and atenolol (Remember: "Look MA! I'm cardioselective!").

○ **What effect do β-blockers have on Prinzmetal variant angina?**

They worsen the syndrome by allowing unopposed α-adrenergic stimulation of the coronary arteries.

○ **What is the most common adverse effect of esmolol, labetalol, and bretylium?**

Hypotension

○ **What adverse event can occur with a rapid infusion of procainamide?**

Hypotension. Other adverse events include QRS/QT prolongation, ventricular fibrillation, and torsade de pointes.

○ **What are some adverse effects of lidocaine?**

Drowsiness, nausea, vertigo, confusion, ataxia, tinnitus, muscle twitching, respiratory depression, and psychosis

○ **Patients with abdominal aorta stenosis may complain of impotence. What causes this?**

Decreased blood flow through the hypogastric arteries. Stenosis is caused by luminal narrowing secondary to ulcerating atherosclerotic plaques, thrombi, emboli, or fibrointimal thickening. Stenosis of the abdominal aorta also results in claudication.

○ **What artery is usually affected by arterial occlusive disease in diabetics?**

The popliteal artery. Because of diabetic neuropathy and the potential for the development of a necrotizing infection in a leg with compromised circulation, it is important that patients with diabetes are knowledgeable about pedal hygiene.

○ **What is Budd-Chiari syndrome?**

Thrombosis in the hepatic vein, resulting in abdominal pain, jaundice, and ascites

○ **A mother has rubella in the first trimester of her pregnancy, and her baby is born with a congenital heart disease. The baby probably has which type of heart disease?**

Patent ductus arteriosus

○ **What is the cause of Prinzmetal angina?**

Coronary artery vasospasm with or without fixed stenotic lesions. Prinzmetal angina is more often associated with ST segment elevation than with depression. Calcium-channel blockers are the drugs of choice to treat this condition. β-Blockers are contraindicated in patients who have vasospasm without fixed stenotic lesions.

○ **Eighty percent to 90% of patients who experience sudden nontraumatic cardiac arrest are in what rhythm?**

Ventricular fibrillation. Early defibrillation is the key. In an AMI, the infarction zone becomes electrically unstable. Ventricular fibrillation is most common during initial coronary occlusion or when the coronary arteries begin to reperfuse.

○ **What is the New York Heart Association functional classification of heart disease?**
- Class I: No limitation of physical activity
- Class II: Slight limitation of physical activity
- Class III: Marked limitation of physical activity, comfortable at rest
- Class IV: Unable to engage in physical activity without discomfort

○ **How much does an increase in 1 body mass index (BMI) unit increase the risk of cardiac events in men?**

An increase of 1 BMI unit increases the risk of cardiac events in men by approximately 10%.

○ **What criteria must be met for a patient to qualify for the diagnosis of metabolic syndrome?**

Patients must meet 3 or more of the following:
1. Abdominal obesity (waist circumference greater than 35 inches in female, and 38 inches in males)
2. Triglyceride level higher than 150 mg/dL
3. High-density lipoprotein cholesterol (HDL-C) level lower than 40 mg/dL in men or lower than 50 mg/dL in women
4. Fasting glucose level higher than 110 mg/dL
5. Hypertension: BP greater than 130/85.

○ **Which of the following provide the best indicator of CAD risk: family history of CAD, dyslipidemia, diabetes mellitus, or sedentary lifestyle?**

Family history of CAD

○ **What are the indications for using a radionuclide perfusion imaging test rather than exercise ECG?**
- Complete left BBB
- Electronic ventricular pacing
- Wolff-Parkinson-White syndrome
- Greater than 1 mm ST segment depression at rest
- Inability to exercise at a level high enough to perform stress ECG
- Angina and history of revascularization

○ **When is transesophageal echocardiography (TEE) indicated?**
- To derive information about posterior structures (atria and AV valves)
- To examine prosthetic heart valves
- To examine intracardiac masses: vegetations in endocarditis or thrombi on pacemaker leads
- To monitor patients during surgery
- To detect aortic dissection and severe atherosclerosis of proximal ascending aorta

○ **Which is the most common type of cardiomyopathy?**

Dilated cardiomyopathy (all 4 chambers). This condition is induced by progression of myocarditis, ethanol, doxorubicin, diabetes, pheochromocytoma, thiamine deficiency, thyroid disease, and valve replacement. The other types of cardiomyopathy are hypertrophic and restrictive/obliterative pregnancy.

○ **Which is the most common type of cardiac failure: high or low output?**

Low output failure. Reduced stroke volume, lowered pulse pressure, and peripheral vasoconstriction are all signs of low output failure.

○ **What is the most common cause of low output heart failure in the world?**

Chagas disease. In addition to heart failure, patients present with prolonged fever, hepatosplenomegaly, megaesophagus, megacolon, edema, and lymphadenopathy. This disease is most prevalent in Latin America.

○ **What is the most common cause of low output heart failure in the United States?**

CAD. Other causes include congenital heart disease, cor pulmonale, dilated cardiomyopathy, hypertension, hypertrophic cardiomyopathy, infection, toxins, and valvular heart disease.

○ **What is the most common reason in the United States for hospitalization in patients older than 65 years?**

CHF

○ **What is the prevalence of CHF in the United States among people older than 40 years?**

Overall, approximately 1 in 56 or 1.76% of 4.8 million people in the United States [Source for calculation is the National Heart, Lung and Blood Institute]

- 2%: age 40 to 59 years
- 5%: age 60 to 69 years
- 10%: older than 70 years

○ **Compare the mortality rate from CHF between the sexes.**

Women fare slightly better. The 5-year mortality rate for a woman with CHF is 45%, compared with 60% for men. The majority of deaths from CHF result from ventricular arrhythmias.

○ **What is the life expectancy of a patient with CHF?**

Half of the patients with CHF will be dead within 5 years. An estimated 4.8 million Americans have CHF. Increasing prevalence, hospitalizations, and deaths have made CHF a major chronic condition in the United States. It often is the end stage of cardiac disease. Each year, there are an estimated 400,000 new cases. The annual number of deaths directly from CHF increased from 10,000 in 1968 to 42,000 in 1993, with another 219,000 related to the condition. CHF is the first-listed diagnosis in 875,000 hospitalizations and the most common diagnosis in hospital patients aged 65 years or older. In that age group, one-fifth of all hospitalizations have a primary or secondary diagnosis of heart failure.

○ **Describe the 3 stages of chest radiograph findings in CHF.**

- Stage I: Pulmonary arterial wedge pressure (PAWP) of 12 to 18 mm Hg. Blood flow increases in the upper lung fields (cephalization of pulmonary vessels).
- Stage II: PAWP of 18 to 25 mm Hg. Interstitial edema is evident, with blurred edges of blood vessels and Kerley B lines.
- Stage III: PAWP greater than 25 mm Hg. Fluid exudes into alveoli with the generation of the classic butterfly pattern of perihilar infiltrates.

○ **How much rapid weight gain (1 day) may signal decompensation in a previously compensated CHF patient?**

Typically 2 to 3 pounds of weight gain in a day or 3 to 5 pounds in a week should warrant a call by a patient with CHF to a health care provider to evaluate for possible fluid retention.

○ **What is the target heart rate for a CHF patient receiving beta-blockers?**

There is no target heart rate. There is no proven value to achieving a specific resting heart rate. Low doses of β-blockers are beneficial in CHF, and there appears to be a dose-dependent improvement.

○ **What is the effect of nitrates on preload and afterload?**

Nitrates mostly dilate veins and venules to decrease preload.

○ **Which does hydralazine affect: preload or afterload?**

Afterload

○ **What effect does morphine have on preload and afterload?**

Morphine decreases both preload and afterload.

○ **Does furosemide affect preload or afterload?**

Furosemide decreases preload.

○ **Do prazosin, captopril, and nifedipine affect afterload?**

Yes

○ **When is dobutamine used in CHF?**

When heart failure is not accompanied with severe hypotension. Dobutamine is a potent inotrope with some vasodilation activity.

○ **When is dopamine used in CHF?**

When a patient is in shock. Dopamine is a vasoconstrictor and a positive inotrope.

○ **What is the chief effect of dobutamine?**

Dobutamine increases cardiac contractility. It has only minor effects on peripheral α-receptors. It can increase cardiac output with mild reduction in systemic vascular resistance and BP.

○ **How does dobutamine differ from dopamine?**

Dobutamine decreases afterload with less tendency to cause tachycardia.

○ **What is the most common cause of right ventricular heart failure?**

LV heart failure

○ **Match the sign or symptom with left-sided (L) or right-sided (R) heart failure.**

1. Hypotension
2. Hepatomegaly
3. Orthopnea
4. Cough
5. Dyspnea at exertion
6. Abdominal distension
7. Paroxysmal nocturnal dyspnea

8. Hemoptysis
9. S_3 gallop
10. Early satiety
11. Jugular venous distension
12. Ascites
13. Rales

Answers: (1) L, (2) R, (3) L, (4) L, (5) L, (6) R, (7) L, (8) L, (9) L, (10) R, (11) R, (12) R, and (13) L

○ **What is the rate of restenosis after percutaneous transluminal coronary angioplasty?**

Twenty percent to 30% restenose within 6 months; 40% restenose within the year. Successful dilation occurs in 90% of cases, but because of the high rate of restenosis, this option is less attractive than coronary artery bypass graft (CABG).

○ **What is the restenosis rate of coronary vessels after CABG?**

With use of venous grafts, there is a 50% restenosis rate within 5 to 10 years. When the internal mammary artery is used, there is only a 5% restenosis rate at 10 years. Occlusion of the grafts are caused by incorrect anatomical anastomosis, trauma to the vessel, postoperative adhesions, or atherosclerosis.

○ **How are AMI, angina pectoris, and Prinzmetal angina differentiated?**

The pain is similar but typically differs in radiation, duration, provocation, and palliation. Obtaining an accurate history is the most important tool for diagnosing chest pain.

Angina pectoris is aggravated by exercise, cold, and excitement, but it is relieved by rest and nitroglycerin.

Prinzmetal angina occurs at rest, during normal activity, and generally at night or in the early morning. It lasts longer than angina pectoris.

AMIs produce pain with a greater radius of radiation that may last for hours.

○ **A patient presents to the hospital 1 month after placement of a mechanical prosthetic valve with fever, chills, and leukocytosis. Endocarditis is suspected. Which bacterium is most common?**

Staphylococcus aureus or *S epidermidis*

○ **Which arteries are most commonly involved in giant cell arteritis (chronic inflammation of the large blood vessels)?**

The carotid artery and its branches. Treatment includes high doses of corticosteroids.

○ **Lovastatin and niacin are used to treat hyperlipoproteinemia. Both of these drugs lower triglyceride and low-density lipoprotein cholesterol (LDL-C) levels. Which one raises HDL-C levels?**

Only niacin. Lovastatin has little affect on HDL-C. However, because niacin often produces significant adverse effects, such as gastritis, reactivation of peptic ulcers, gout, hyperglycemia, cutaneous flushing, and scaling skin, lovastatin remains the drug of choice.

○   **What amount of omega-3 oil is recommended by the American Heart Association for the prevention of heart disease?**

Patients with documented coronary heart disease: Consume about 1 g of eicosapentaenoic acid (EPA) and docosahexaenoic acid (DHA) per day, preferably from fatty fish. EPA and DHA in capsule form could be considered in consultation with the physician.

Patients without documented coronary heart disease: Eat a variety of (preferably fatty) fish at least twice a week. Include oils and foods rich in α-linolenic acid (flaxseed, canola, and soybean oils; flaxseed and walnuts).

Patients who need to lower triglyceride levels: 2 to 4 g of EPA and DHA per day provided as capsules under a physician's care.

Patients taking more than 3 g of omega-3 fatty acids from capsules should do so only under a physician's care. High intakes could cause excessive bleeding in some people.

○   **What hypertensive medications should be avoided in patients with diabetes?**

Diuretics and β-blockers. These drugs increase insulin resistance.

○   **What are the most common adverse effects of β-blockers?**

Fatigue will occur early in treatment, followed later by depression.

○   **How do you determine the cuff size for taking BP in adults?**

Arm Circumference Range at Midpoint of Humerus/Thigh

- Adult: 27 to 34 cm, up to 13.38 in
- Large adult: 35 to 44 cm, 13.7 to 17.3 in
- Adult thigh cuff: 45 to 52 cm, 17.7 to 20.4 in

○   **What percentage of hypertension is due to a secondary cause?**

5%. Secondary hypertension should be suspected in patients younger than 35 years, patients with sudden-onset hypertension, and those without a family history for hypertension.

○   **What is the most common cause of secondary hypertension?**

Renal parenchymal disease. In women, the most common cause is oral contraceptives. In patients older than 50 years, secondary hypertension usually can be attributed to renal artery stenosis. Other causes include pheochromocytoma, coarctation of the aorta, drugs (cocaine), hyperthyroidism, aldosteronism, and Cushing syndrome.

○   **What percentage of patients with aortic dissection have hypertension?**

70% to 90%

○   **Is diastolic BP elevation an important independent risk factor for young people?**

Yes. Diastolic BP has been and remains, especially for younger people, an important hypertension number. The higher the diastolic BP, the greater the risk for heart attacks, strokes, and kidney failure. As people age (older than 50 years), diastolic BP begins to decrease, and systolic BP begins to increase and becomes more important.

○ **What is the upper level of normal BP in a diabetic patient, nondiabetic patient, and patient with chronic renal disease?**

For patients with diabetes and/or chronic renal disease, the upper limit is 129/79 mm Hg. For nondiabetic patients, the upper limit is 139/89 mm Hg. A reading of 130/80 mm Hg indicates high BP in diabetes. There is excess morbidity for pressures above 129/79 mm Hg in patients with diabetes or renal disease and at levels above 140/90 mm Hg in nondiabetic patients.

○ **A 55-year-old white man with a BMI of 29 is in the office and has elevated BP. He is taking a low dose of hydrochlorothiazide, and his measured BP is 141/95 mm Hg. What is the next step in medication management for this patient?**

Add a calcium-channel blocker or an angiotensin-converting enzyme (ACE) inhibitor.

○ **What is the risk of a normotensive person aged 55 years of developing hypertension in his or her lifetime?**

90% per Seventh Report of the Joint National Committee on Prevention, Detection, Evaluation, and Treatment of High Blood Pressure

○ **Under what circumstance would you initiate hypertension treatment with combination therapy?**

If BP is 20/10 mm Hg or more, higher than goal, consideration should be given to initiating therapy with a 2-drug combination, 1 of which would usually be a diuretic.

○ **α-Blockers are known to be associated with first-dose syncope. What other hypertension drug can cause this adverse event?**

Captopril and other ACE inhibitors also are associated with first-dose syncope.

○ **What percentage of patients with uncontrolled hypertension have LV hypertrophy (LVH)?**

Approximately 37%. An eccentric type of LVH is the prevalent pattern in patients treated long term. The persistence of LVH depends significantly on BP levels achieved during treatment; the prevalence of LVH is low in patients with optimal BP control, whereas it is elevated (37%) in patients with uncontrolled BP. This is the primary reason that hypertension is a major risk factor for MI, CHF, and sudden death.

○ **What are the adverse effects of thiazide diuretics?**

Hyperglycemia, hyperlipidemia, hyperuricemia, hypokalemia, hypomagnesemia, and hyponatremia

○ **Which drugs should be administered to lower the BP in a patient with thoracic aortic dissection?**

Sodium nitroprusside. A β-blocker should also be used to reduce the rate of rise of LV pressure (dP/dt; propagation speed).

○ **A patient who has a psychiatric history and is taking an monoamine oxidase inhibitor has consumed a 12-pack of beer with a meal of pickled herring and a nicely aged cheese. He now complains of severe headache. At examination, his BP is elevated. A diagnosis of acute hypertension is made secondary to hyperstimulation of the adrenergic receptors. What is the treatment?**

An α- and β-adrenergic antagonist such as labetalol

○ **What is the most common complication of nitroprusside?**

Hypotension. Thiocyanate toxicity accompanied by blurred vision, tinnitus, change in mental status, muscle weakness, and seizures are more prevalent in patients with renal failure or prolonged infusions. Cyanide toxicity is uncommon. However, this type of toxicity may occur with hepatic dysfunction, after prolonged infusions, and in rates greater than 10 mg/kg per minute.

○ **Define hypertensive emergency.**

Elevated diastolic BP higher than 115 mm Hg with associated end-organ dysfunction or damage

○ **How quickly should a patient's BP be lowered in a hypertensive emergency?**

Gradually over 2 to 3 hours to 140 to 160 mm Hg systolic and 90 to 110 mm Hg diastolic. Cerebral hypoperfusion can be prevented by not decreasing BP by more than 25% of the mean arterial pressure.

○ **What drug can be used for almost all hypertensive emergencies?**

Sodium nitroprusside. It assists in relaxing smooth muscle tissue through the production of cyclic guanosine monophosphate. As a result, there is decreased preload and afterload, decreased oxygen demand, and a slightly increased heart rate, with no change in myocardial blood flow, cardiac output, or renal blood flow. The duration of action is 1 to 2 minutes. Sometimes, β-blockade is required to treat rebound tachycardia.

○ **Define hypertensive urgency.**

Dangerously elevated diastolic BP higher than 115 mm Hg without signs of end-organ damage. BP should be reduced gradually over 24 to 48 hours.

○ **Define uncomplicated hypertension.**

Diastolic BP lower than 115 mm Hg without symptoms of end-organ damage. Uncomplicated hypertension does not require short-term treatment.

○ **How much above normal levels does elevated BP increase the risk of stroke?**

Small increases in BP can dramatically increase a person's risk of stroke. In 1 study, for every 10 mm Hg increase in the systolic BP over normal, the risk of stroke increased by 28%. This means that someone with a systolic BP of 170 mm Hg has an 84% greater chance of having a stroke than does someone with a systolic BP of less than 140 mm Hg.

○ **What laboratory findings can be used to confirm a hypertensive emergency?**

- Urinalysis: Red blood cells, red cell casts, and proteinuria
- Ratio of serum urea nitrogen to creatinine: Elevated
- Radiograph: Aortic dissection, pulmonary edema, or coarctation of the aorta
- ECG: LVH and cardiac ischemia

○ **What are the signs and symptoms of hypertensive encephalopathy?**

Nausea, vomiting, headache, lethargy, coma, blindness, nerve palsies, hemiparesis, aphasia, retinal hemorrhage, cotton wool spots, exudates, sausage linking, and papilledema. Treat with labetalol or sodium nitroprusside and lower the mean arterial pressure to approximately 120 mm Hg.

O **Cardiac hypertrophy will most likely displace the point of maximal impulse to which area of the chest?**

The normal apical impulse at the medial to midclavicular line in the fourth or fifth intercostal space will be displaced downward to the sixth intercostal space.

O **What maneuvers will increase hypertrophic cardiomyopathy murmurs?**

Valsalva maneuver, standing, and amyl nitrate

O **What maneuvers will decrease hypertrophic cardiomyopathic murmurs?**

Handgrip, squatting, and leg elevation in the supine patient

O **Livedo reticularis commonly develops on what body parts?**

The legs. Livedo reticularis is a bluish red discoloration of the skin resulting from vasospasm of the arterioles. This condition is worsened by exposure to cold.

O **What is the most common source of acute mesenteric ischemia?**

Arterial embolism (40% to 50%). The source is usually the heart, generally from a mural thrombus. The most common point of obstruction is the superior mesenteric artery.

O **What laboratory results strongly suggest that a patient has mesenteric ischemia?**

Leukocytosis ($>15,000/\mu L$), metabolic acidosis (sometimes with anion gap), hemoconcentration, and elevated phosphate and amylase levels

O **What is the most common cause of cardiac arrest in a uremic patient?**

Hyperkalemia

O **What drug should be used to treat a patient in cardiac arrest secondary to hyperkalemia?**

Calcium chloride—IV acts fastest. Also provide sodium bicarbonate.

O **In an MI, when do creatine kinase (CK) levels begin to increase, and when do they peak?**

CK levels begin to increase at 6 to 8 hours, they peak at 24 to 30, and they stabilize at 48.

O **In an MI, when do LDH-C levels begin to increase, and when do they peak?**

LDH isozyme I (from heart) begins to increase at 12 to 24 hours; it peaks at 48 to 96.

O **Third-degree heart block is often seen in which type of MI?**

Anterior wall AMI

O **Which type of MI is more often associated with thrombosis: transmural or subendocardial?**

Transmural. Thrombolytic therapy increases LV ejection fraction after MI, reduces the development of postinfarction CHF, and can reduce early MI mortality by 25%.

○   **How much aspirin should a patient ingest daily after MI to reduce the incidence of reinfarction?**

75 to 325 mg/day.

○   **What is the most common cause of death during the first few hours of a MI?**

Cardiac dysrhythmias, generally ventricular fibrillation

○   **Which patients with AMI should not receive β-blocker treatment?**

Although β-blockers may be useful in many patients with AMI, some patients have contraindications to the use of this class of drugs. Relative contraindications include heart rate lower than 60 bpm, systolic BP lower than 100 mm Hg, moderate or severe LV failure, shock, PR interval at ECG greater than 0.24 seconds, second- or third-degree heart block, and active asthma/reactive airways disease.

○   **How common are PVCs in patients after MI?**

Ninety percent will have PVCs within the first few weeks. Concern arises if the PVCs are complex, which is the case in 20% to 40% of MI patients. Risk of sudden death in patients after MI with complex PVCs increases 2 to 5 times.

○   **What percentage of the LV myocardium must to be damaged to induce cardiogenic shock?**

40%. Twenty-five percent or more results in heart failure.

○   **What percentage of MIs are clinically unrecognized?**

Approximately 20%

○   **A non-Q-wave MI usually is associated with what?**

Subsequent angina or recurrent infarction. Non-Q-wave MIs also have a lower in-hospital mortality rate than do Q-wave MIs.

○   **Why do T waves invert in an AMI?**

Infarction or ischemia causes a reversal of the sequence of repolarization (ie, endocardial-to-epicardial as opposed to normal epicardial-to-endocardial).

○   **What conduction defects commonly occur in an anterior wall MI?**

The dangerous kind. Damage to the conducting system results in a Mobitz II second- or third-degree AV block.

○   **A patient presents 1 day after discharge for an AMI with a new, harsh systolic murmur along the left sternal border and pulmonary edema. What is the diagnosis?**

Ventricular septal rupture. Diagnosis is confirmed with Swan-Ganz catheterization or ECG. The treatment regimen includes nitroprusside for afterload reduction and possibly an intraaortic balloon pump followed by surgical repair.

○ **When does cardiac rupture usually occur in patients who have had AMIs?**

Fifty percent arise within the first 5 days, and 90% occur within the first 14 days after MI.

○ **Which type of infarct commonly leads to papillary muscle dysfunction?**

Inferior wall MI. Signs and symptoms include a mild transient systolic murmur and pulmonary edema.

○ **A patient presents 2 weeks after AMI with chest pain, fever, and pleuropericarditis. A pleural effusion is detected at radiography. What is the diagnosis?**

Dressler (post-MI) syndrome. This syndrome is caused by an immunologic reaction to myocardial antigens.

○ **What percentage of patients older than 80 years experience chest pain with an AMI?**

Only 50%. Twenty percent experience diaphoresis, stroke, syncope, and/or acute confusion.

○ **What are the most common causes of myocarditis in the United States?**

Viruses. Other causes include postviral myocarditis, an autoimmune response to recent viral infection, bacteria (diphtheria and tuberculosis), fungi, protozoa (Chagas disease), and spirochetes (Lyme disease).

○ **What percentage of patients with mitral stenosis who are not receiving anticoagulants experience systemic emboli?**

25%. Patients with chronic atrial fibrillation or mitral stenosis should receive long-term anticoagulation to prevent atrial mural thrombi.

○ **What are believed to be the most common causes of mitral stenosis?**

Rheumatic fever is a frequent cause, but actual history of rheumatic fever is discovered in only about one-third of mitral stenosis cases. Congenital heart disease due to chordal fusion, mitral annulus calcification in the elderly, or end-stage renal disease are also common causes.

○ **What physical findings may be associated with mitral stenosis?**

Prominent A-wave, early systolic left parasternal lift, loud and snapping S_1, and early diastolic opening snap with a low-pitched middiastolic rumble that crescendos into S_1.

○ **A midsystolic click with a late systolic crescendo murmur is indicative of what cardiac disease?**

MVP

○ **What patient position will enhance the murmur of mitral stenosis?**

Left lateral decubitus

○ **Is MVP more common among men or women?**

Women have a stronger genetic link to the disease. However, only 2% to 5% of the entire population has symptomatic MVP.

○ **What age group typically develops MVP syndrome?**

Patients in their 20s and 30s. Most patients with MVP are asymptomatic. MVP syndrome is symptomatic with chest pain, fatigue, palpitations, postural syncope, and dizziness.

○ **What is the hallmark sign of MVP?**

A midsystolic click, sometimes accompanied by a late systolic murmur. MVP is largely a clinical diagnosis. ECG is performed to assess the degree of prolapse. Other clinical findings include a laterally displaced, diffuse apical pulse; decreased S_1; split S_2; and a holosystolic murmur radiating to the axilla.

○ **What is the most common patient complaint in MVP?**

Fatigue is most frequently stated complaint. Most patients with MVP are asymptomatic with no complaints related to MVP. The reason for fatigue is not understood. Other typical complaints are palpitations, chest pain, anxiety, and migraine headaches. Stroke is a rare complication of MVP. Those who have symptoms commonly report chest discomfort, anxiety, fatigue, and dyspnea, but whether these are actually due to MVP is not certain.

○ **How do the fixed-rate and demand modes of pacemakers differ?**

Fixed-rate mode produces an impulse at a continuous specific rate, regardless of the patient's own cardiac activity. Demand mode detects the patient's electrical activity and triggers only if the heart is not depolarizing.

○ **What is the treatment for ventricular fibrillation in a patient with a pacemaker?**

Defibrillation, but be sure to keep the paddles away from the pacemaker

○ **What is the average life span of a pacemaker?**

7 to 11 years

○ **A 25 -year-old patient presents with splinted breathing and sharp, precordial chest pain that radiates to the back. The pain increases with inspiration and is mildly relieved by placing the patient in a forward sitting position. What might the ECG show?**

The ECG may reveal intermittent SVTs, ST-segment depression in aVR and VI, ST-segment elevation in all other leads, PR depression, and T-wave inversion may arise. The patient probably has pericarditis.

○ **What is the most common cause of pericarditis?**

Idiopathic. Other causes are MI, postviral syndrome, aortic dissection that has ruptured into the pericardium, malignancy, radiation, chest trauma, connective tissue disease, uremia, and drugs, (ie, procainamide or hydralazine).

○ **What physical finding indicates acute pericarditis?**

Pericardial friction rub. The rub is best heard at the left sternal border or apex with the patient in a forward sitting position. Other findings include fever and tachycardia.

○ **Acute pyogenic pericarditis is most commonly caused by what organisms?**

Staphylococcus aureus and *Haemophilus influenzae*

○ **When diagnosing pericardial effusion, how much fluid must be present in the pericardial sac for visualization at cardiac ECG and radiography?**

At least 15 mL for ECG and 250 mL for radiography

○ **What is the appearance of a pericardial effusion on a radiograph?**

A water bottle silhouette

○ **At what volume does pericardial effusion affect the intrapericardial pressure?**

80 to 200 mL. However, the rate of accumulation is more important than the amount of accumulation. If the fluid is accumulated slowly, the pericardium can tolerate up to 2000 mL of fluid.

○ **What are the signs and symptoms of acute pericardial tamponade?**

Triad of hypotension, elevated central venous pressure, and tachycardia. Muffled heart tones may be auscultated.

○ **What ECG result is pathognomonic of pericardial tamponade?**

Total electrical alternans. Pulsus paradoxus is nonspecific. Muffled heart tones are subjective findings and are difficult to hear.

○ **What is the treatment for pericarditis without effusion?**

A 2-week treatment of 650 mg of aspirin every 4 hours, if no contraindications exist. Ibuprofen, indomethacin, or colchicine are other alternatives. The use of corticosteroids is controversial because recurrent pericarditis is common when doses are tapered.

○ **Rheumatic heart disease is the most common cause of stenosis of what 3 heart valves?**

Mitral, aortic (along with congenital bicuspid valve), and tricuspid

○ **What is the most serious consequence of rheumatic fever?**

Carditis. This may be pancardiac inflammation but also can be limited. This may be valvulitis (leading to mitral insufficiency for instance, most commonly) or myocarditis or pericarditis.

○ **What is the 1-year recurrence rate for patients who have been resuscitated from sudden cardiac death?**

30%

○ **Describe the Trendelenburg test for varicose veins.**

Raise the leg above the heart and then quickly lower it. If the leg veins become distended immediately after this test is performed, valvular incompetency is evident.

○ **What is a paradoxical embolus?**

A venous thrombus that goes through a right-to-left intracardiac shunt to the arterial side

○ **Why is a paradoxical embolus able to cause septic end-organ disease?**

An infected venous thrombus can enter the arterial circulation via the right-to-left intracardiac shunt and be sent distally to affect end organs.

○ **Splinter hemorrhages, Osler nodes, Janeway lesions, petechiae, and Roth spots can be indications of what process?**

They are physical signs associated with infective endocarditis.

○ **True/False: Osler nodes are usually nodular and painful.**

True. In contrast, the macular Janeway lesions are painless.

○ **In what other conditions besides infective endocarditis can Osler nodes be found?**

Nonbacterial thrombotic endocarditis, gonococcal infections, and hemolytic anemia

○ **What percentage of patients with infective endocarditis display peripheral manifestations of the disease?**

50%

○ **What is bacterial endocarditis?**

Blood-borne bacteria that attach onto damaged or abnormal heart valves or on the endocardium near anatomic defects

○ **How is bacterial endocarditis diagnosed?**

The diagnosis of infective endocarditis usually is based on a constellation of history, clinical findings, laboratory study results (particularly blood cultures—at least 3 blood cultures from separate sites over a period ranging from a few hours to 1 to 2 days), and evidence of valvular vegetations at ECG.

○ **Who is at high risk for developing endocarditis?**

People with prosthetic heart valves, previous incidents of endocarditis, complex congenital heart disease, IV drug use, and surgically devised systemic pulmonary shunts

○ **What are the risk factors for endocarditis?**

Risk factors include IV drug use, prosthetic valves, acquired valvular heart disease, hypertrophic cardiomyopathy, hemodialysis, peritoneal dialysis, indwelling venous catheters, cardiac surgery, rheumatic heart disease, and uncorrected congenital conditions. It is controversial as to whether MVP with significant regurgitation is a moderate risk factor.

○ **What are the most common organisms associated with endocarditis?**

Streptococcus viridans, *S aureus*, *Enterococcus*, and fungal organisms. *S aureus* is responsible for 75% of disease in IV drug abusers.

○ **Fungi cause what percentage of prosthetic valve infective endocarditis?**

15%

○ **What is more common in the general population: left-sided or right-sided endocarditis?**

Left-sided (aortic and mitral involvement)

○ **What is more common in IV drug abusers; right-sided or left-sided disease?**

Right-sided (60%) is most common.

○ **How is infective endocarditis treated?**

IV antibiotics, typically for 4 to 6 weeks. Close follow-up is necessary, and the patient should have a series of 2 separate negative blood culture results to demonstrate resolution of the condition. If resolution of the infection does not occur promptly, embolization occurs, or fulminant CHF ensues, surgical valve replacement is indicated.

○ **What are the ECG changes associated with pericarditis?**

Concave upward ST elevation in at least 7 leads except V_1 and aVR. PR segment depression also may be present.

○ **Postpericardotomy syndrome, occasionally confused with infectious pericarditis, occurs in what percentage of patients who have undergone pericardotomy?**

10% to 30%

○ **What is the most frequently reported bacterial isolate in patients with myocardial abscesses?**

S aureus

○ **What is the clinical picture of myocardial abscesses?**

Low-grade fevers, chills, leukocytosis, conduction system abnormalities, nonspecific ECG changes, and signs and symptoms of AMI

○ **What is the definitive treatment of an infected atrial myxoma?**

Urgent surgical resection is required because of the risk of embolization or cardiovascular complications, including sudden death.

○ **What is the risk for infection of a transvenous pacemaker during the first 3 years after insertion?**

1% to 6%

○ **What are the risk factors associated with the development of pacemaker infections?**

Risk factors include recent manipulation of the device (particularly generator exchange); temporary pacing before permanent device placement; diabetes mellitus; underlying malignancy; prior treatment with anticoagulants, glucocorticoids, or other immunosuppressive medications; advanced patient age; and operator inexperience.

○ **What are complications of pacemaker insertion?**

Postinsertion hematoma, seroma, or infection

○ **What is a major risk factor for prosthetic vascular graft infection?**

Location. The incidence of infection is 1% to 1.5% for aortoiliac grafts as opposed to 2% to 7% for femoropopliteal arterial grafts.

○ **What is thought to be the cause of prosthetic vascular graft infection?**

Ninety-five percent of the time, contamination at the time of insertion is thought to cause the infection.

○ **What is the clinical presentation of prosthetic vascular graft infection?**

Erythema, skin breakdown, or purulent drainage. Other symptoms may be thrombosis of the graft, fluid around the graft, or pseudoaneurysm formation.

○ **What are complications from arterial catheterization?**

Thrombosis (19%-38%), infection (4%-23%), pseudoaneurysm, and rupture

○ **What is the most frequent cause of mitral stenosis?**

Rheumatic fever. Far less common causes include congenital defect, malignant carcinoid, systemic lupus erythematosus, rheumatoid arthritis, infective endocarditis with a large vegetation, and the mucopolysaccharidoses of the Hunter-Hurley phenotype.

○ **What percentage of patients with rheumatic mitral stenosis are women?**

66%

○ **What percentage of patients with rheumatic heart disease have pure mitral stenosis?**

25%. An additional 40% have combined mitral stenosis and mitral regurgitation.

○ **What is the cross-sectional area of the mitral valve orifice in critical mitral stenosis?**

The cross-sectional area is 1 cm^2 or less. The normal cross-sectional area is between 4 and 6 cm^2. Mild mitral stenosis begins when the valve is reduced to approximately 2 cm^2.

○ **What are the principal symptoms in mitral stenosis?**

Dyspnea is most common. Patients with severe mitral stenosis can experience orthopnea, hemoptysis, chest pain, and frank pulmonary edema, often precipitated by exertion, fever, upper respiratory infection, sexual intercourse, pregnancy, or the onset of rapid atrial fibrillation.

○ **What is Ortner syndrome?**

Hoarseness caused by compression of the left recurrent laryngeal nerve by a greatly dilated left atrium, enlarged tracheobronchial lymph nodes, and dilated pulmonary arteries, occurring in severe, advanced mitral stenosis.

○ **What are the 2 most serious complications of mitral stenosis?**

They are (1) thromboembolism, most often occurring in the setting of atrial fibrillation, and (2) pulmonary edema

○ **What maneuvers can the patient perform to differentiate the opening snap of mitral stenosis from a split S₂ sound?**

Sudden standing widens the A2-opening snap interval, whereas a split S_2 narrows at standing. Progressive narrowing of the A2-OS interval on serial examinations suggests an increase in the severity of mitral stenosis.

○ **What is the most accurate noninvasive technique for quantifying the severity of mitral stenosis?**

Doppler ECG

○ **What is the medical management strategy for rheumatic mitral stenosis?**

1. Aggressive and prompt treatment of anemia and infections
2. Avoidance of strenuous exertion but active participation in symptom-limited physical activity
3. Oral diuretics, sodium restriction, β-blockade, and digoxin use, all to be reserved and used accordingly in symptomatic patients
4. Long-term oral anticoagulation (international normalized ratio [INR] range, 2.0 to 3.0) in patients who have a prior embolic event; left atrial thrombus; or paroxysmal, persistent, or permanent atrial fibrillation, with the addition of low-dose aspirin (50 to 100 mg/d) in patients who have an embolic event or have left atrial thrombus despite oral anticoagulation at a therapeutic INR (or increase the INR range to 3.0). The current guidelines no longer recommend antibiotic prophylaxis for patients with only valvular disease (including mitral stenosis).

○ **What is the asymptomatic period after an attack of rheumatic fever in patients with mitral stenosis?**

In temperate zones, such as the United States and Europe, about 15 to 20 years. In tropical and subtropical areas and in underdeveloped areas, about 6 to 12 years.

○ **What is the indication for mitral valve surgery or balloon valvuloplasty in patients with mitral stenosis?**

Moderate symptoms (class II) or greater in a patient with moderate to severe mitral stenosis (mitral valve orifice size less than 1.0 cm² per square meter body surface area; less than 1.5 to 1.7 cm² mitral valve area in normal-sized adults).

○ **A 28-year-old Hispanic woman is referred to you for evaluation of dyspnea and palpitations. She has a diastolic murmur consistent with mitral stenosis. ECG results show severe, noncalcific mitral stenosis with trivial mitral regurgitation. The mitral valve area is 0.8 cm². ECG reveals atrial fibrillation. What is the most appropriate course of therapy for this patient?**

Open mitral valvotomy (commissurotomy) followed by cardioversion to normal sinus rhythm. This is palliative, obviates the need for anticoagulation for the immediate future, and results in at least 5 to 10 years of symptom-free life for more than half of the patients.

○ **What is the most common cause of mitral regurgitation?**

Rheumatic heart disease. It is more frequent in men than women. Other causes include infective endocarditis, MVP, ischemic heart disease, trauma, systemic lupus erythematosus , scleroderma, hypertrophic cardiomyopathy, dilated cardiomyopathy involving the left ventricle, and idiopathic degenerative calcification of the mitral annulus.

○ **What percentage of patients with CAD who are considered for CABG have mitral regurgitation?**

30%. It is secondary to ischemic papillary muscle dysfunction.

○ **What are the physical findings in patients with chronic mitral regurgitation?**

Harsh, pansystolic murmur heard best at the apex, radiating to the axilla or the base. The murmur is diminished by maneuvers that decrease preload or afterload, such as amyl nitrate inhalation, Valsalva maneuver, or standing, and increases with maneuvers that increase preload or afterload, such as squatting, handgrip, or phenylephrine administration.

○ **What are the most common causes of acute mitral regurgitation?**

AMI with papillary muscle dysfunction (15% of AMI results in acute mitral regurgitation) or papillary muscle rupture (0.3% of AMI), infective endocarditis, chordae tendineae rupture secondary to chest trauma, rheumatic fever, MVP, and hypertrophic cardiomyopathy with rupture of chordae tendineae

○ **What infarct is most commonly associated with acute mitral regurgitation?**

Inferior wall

○ **Which is the best test to assess the detailed anatomy of rheumatic mitral valve disease and determine whether mitral valve replacement is necessary or whether reconstruction is feasible?**

TEE

○ **What is the appropriate medical management of mitral regurgitation?**

Vasodilator therapy with ACE inhibitors is the hallmark of therapy, even in patients who are asymptomatic. Diuretics are used in patients with severe mitral regurgitation. Cardiac glycosides, such as digoxin, are indicated in patients with severe mitral regurgitation and clinical evidence of heart failure. Anticoagulation should be administered to all patients in atrial fibrillation.

○ **A 33-year-old woman comes to you for a physical examination, and you notice a harsh systolic murmur at the apex that is also heard at the base. The murmur increases at standing and Valsalva maneuver and decreases with handgrip. What is the most likely finding at ECG?**

MVP. The murmur of pure mitral regurgitation decreases with Valsalva maneuver and standing and increases with handgrip or squatting.

○ **A 46-year-old man with a history of rheumatic fever at age 12 years is admitted with an AMI. The patient's post-MI course is complicated by CHF. ECG reveals severe mitral regurgitation with rupture of one of the papillary muscles and prolapse of the posterior mitral valve leaflet without apparent calcification. Systolic function seen at ECG is mildly reduced. What is the appropriate course of action in this patient?**

Mitral valve reconstruction and repair of the papillary muscle

○ **What are the indications for surgery in patients with severe, chronic mitral regurgitation?**

Patients with New York Heart Association class II symptoms with end-systolic LV diameter greater than 45 mm at ECG. Asymptomatic patients with severe mitral regurgitation who are younger than 70 years with ejection fractions less than 70% and end-systolic LV diameter greater than 40 mm at ECG who are likely to be candidates for mitral valve repair also should be strongly considered for surgery.

○ **What is the classic triad of symptoms of aortic stenosis?**

Syncope (often exertional), angina, and heart failure

○   **What is the most common cause of aortic stenosis in patients younger than 65 years?**

Calcification of congenitally bicuspid aortic valves (50%), followed by rheumatic heart disease (25%)

○   **What is the most common cause of aortic stenosis in patients older than 65 years?**

Calcific degeneration of the aortic leaflets

○   **Once patients with aortic stenosis become symptomatic, what is their average survival without valve replacement?**

From the onset of syncope or angina, the mean survival is 2 to 3 years. From the onset of CHF, the mean survival is 1.5 years.

○   **How does a heart murmur reflect the severity of aortic stenosis?**

The longer the duration of the murmur and the greater the increase in intensity of the murmur, the more severe the aortic stenosis. The degree of loudness of the murmur is not as important in assessing severity.

○   **What is the best cardiac pharmacologic agent for patients with asymptomatic aortic stenosis?**

Without contraindications, β-blockers are the best agents, as they are the most useful in treating LVH and its sequelae that develop as a result of aortic stenosis.

○   **A 68-year-old woman with severe asymptomatic aortic stenosis suddenly complains of dyspnea and palpitations. At ECG, she is found to be in atrial fibrillation, with a ventricular rate of 130 bpm. What is the most appropriate action to take?**

Immediate direct current cardioversion, followed by a search for previously unrecognized mitral valve disease. Once stabilized, the patient should be referred for cardiac catheterization and aortic valve replacement.

○   **What is the most common sustained tachyarrhythmia in patients with MVP?**

Paroxysmal SVT

○   **What do patients with MVP have in common with patients with recognized inheritable disorders of connective tissue?**

MVP may be inherited as an autosomal dominant phenotype, and a large proportion of patients with MVP have systemic features such as anterior chest deformity, scoliosis, kyphosis, hypermobile joints, and arm span greater than height. In addition, MVP is common in patients with Marfan syndrome, Ehlers-Danlos syndrome, and adult polycystic kidney disease.

○   **What is MVP syndrome?**

A symptom complex consisting of palpitations, chest pain, easy fatigability, exercise intolerance, dyspnea, orthostatic phenomena, and syncope or presyncope in patients with MVP, predominantly related to autonomic dysfunction

○   **What disorders are seen with increased frequency in patients with MVP syndrome?**

Graves disease, asthma, migraine headaches, sleep disorders, fibromyositis, and functional gastrointestinal syndromes

○ **What is the most common cause of isolated severe aortic regurgitation?**

Aortic root dilatation resulting from medial disease. Other common causes include congenital (bicuspid) aortic valve, previous infective endocarditis, and rheumatic heart disease.

○ **A 64-year-old man, 3 weeks after cholecystectomy, has moderate malnutrition. He has been receiving total parenteral nutrition for 10 days, and for the last 4 days has had a fever of 102°F. The patient is noticeably dyspneic with a respiratory rate of 26 breaths per minute and a heart rate of 110 bpm, in sinus rhythm at ECG. Blood cultures grow *Candida albicans*. Chest radiography reveals moderate pulmonary congestion. An S$_3$ gallop is heard at the apex, and a low-pitched decrescendo diastolic murmur is heard at the left sternal border. ECG reveals a 17-mm-diameter vegetation on the noncoronary cusp of the aortic valve, and Doppler ECG reveals severe aortic regurgitation. What is the best course of action for this patient?**

IV amphotericin, IV vasodilators such as nitroprusside, and IV dobutamine followed by urgent AV replacement. Vegetations larger than 10 mm in diameter, particularly fungal, are rarely controlled with pharmacologic therapy alone, and surgery is almost always needed, even if the aortic regurgitation is mild or moderate.

○ **What murmur may be mistaken for mitral stenosis?**

The Austin Flint murmur of severe aortic regurgitation, which occurs from a powerful regurgitant jet from the aorta that is imparted to the anterior leaflet of the mitral valve, limiting the valve's opening

○ **What is the survival after diagnosis of chronic aortic regurgitation?**

The 5-year survival after diagnosis is 75%. The 10-year survival is 50%. Once symptoms begin, without surgical treatment, death occurs within 4 years after the development of angina, 2 years after the development of CHF.

○ **What are the indications for aortic valve replacement in patients with chronic aortic regurgitation?**

LV end-systolic dimension greater than 50 mm, LV ejection fraction (LVEF)₋ less than 50%, and the onset of symptoms of angina or CHF

○ **What is the preferred pharmacologic agent in patients with asymptomatic chronic aortic regurgitation?**

Nifedipine or ACE inhibitors. Both have shown major improvements in LVEF and major reduction in LV end-diastolic volume and mass with significantly lower incidence of the need for aortic valve replacement at 5 years.

○ **What is the most common acquired abnormality that produces clinically significant tricuspid regurgitation?**

Dilatation of the tricuspid annulus related to right ventricular dilatation

○ **What is the most common congenital abnormality producing tricuspid regurgitation?**

Tricuspid valve prolapse. Less common is Ebstein anomaly.

○ **What is the most common cause of tricuspid regurgitation?**

Right-sided heart failure secondary to left-sided heart failure

○ **What is the most common cause of acute tricuspid regurgitation, and what is the preferred management of this situation?**

Tricuspid valve endocarditis, often as a result of IV drug abuse. The preferred management is complete removal of the valve, with immediate or eventual replacement of the valve. Antibiotic therapy usually is futile in preventing valve surgery.

○ **A 38-year-old Hispanic woman with known MVP is scheduled for dental cleaning. Her dentist calls you asking for recommendations for endocarditis prophylaxis. She is not allergic to penicillin. What are your recommendations?**

This patient does not require antibiotic prophylaxis for dental procedures according to the current 2007 American Heart Association guideline for the prevention of infective endocarditis, as MVP is not a considered a cardiac condition at high risk for development of infective endocarditis.

○ **How does the sensitivity of transthoracic ECG compare with TEE in the diagnosis of infective endocarditis?**

Transthoracic ECG has a diagnostic sensitivity of 30% to 40%, whereas TEE has a diagnostic sensitivity between 90% and 100%.

○ **A 55-year-old man who had undergone 4-vessel CABG 3 years ago has mild mitral and tricuspid regurgitation and is scheduled for colonoscopy for rectal bleeding. What recommendations regarding endocarditis prophylaxis would you give the surgeon?**

No antibiotic prophylaxis is needed in this setting.

○ **How much myocardial damage from an AMI is necessary to result in CHF?**

CHF is usually evident clinically if more than 25% of the left ventricle is infarcted.

○ **How much functional loss of LV myocardium is required to result in cardiogenic shock?**

40%

○ **What 3 secondary processes resulting in myocardial deterioration occur after AMI?**
1. Ventricular remodeling, typically following Q-wave infarctions
2. Infarct expansion, occurring most frequently from anteroapical infarctions and resulting in thinning of the LV wall
3. Ventricular dilatation, an early and progressive response to AMI that is an important predictor of increased mortality after MI

○ **What factors play a role in the peak incidence of MI being from 6 AM to noon?**

BP, coronary arterial tone, blood viscosity, circulating catecholamines, and platelet aggregability increase at awakening and assumption of an erect posture.

○ **What is the most common cause of death related to AMI?**

Ventricular fibrillation, occurring within the first hour after symptoms

○ **What percentage of patients with AMI develop cardiogenic shock?**

10%

○ **What percentage of arteries successfully opened with thrombolytic therapy for AMI reocclude?**

Fifteen percent of arteries successfully opened reocclude during the first few days after thrombolytic therapy.

○ **What is the mortality benefit from aspirin alone in AMI with thrombolytic therapy and in subsequent reinfarction?**

Aspirin reduced mortality from AMI by 23% and reduced nonfatal reinfarction by 49%. When used with thrombolytic therapy, there was a 40% to 50% reduction in mortality from AMI.

○ **A 63-year-old man presents to the emergency department with moderate substernal chest pressure and light-headedness for 90 minutes. His BP at admission is 80/40 mm Hg, and his heart rate is 110 bpm and regular. Physical examination reveals jugular venous distension to the angle of the jaw, a right parasternal S_3 gallop, an apical S_4 gallop, and clear lungs at auscultation. ECG reveals a 2-mm ST elevation in leads II, III, and aVF, with reciprocal ST depression in V_1 through V_3. What is the most likely diagnosis, and what is the most appropriate initial therapy?**

Inferior MI with right ventricular infarction. After administration of 75 to 325 mg of aspirin, thrombolytic therapy, and a large IV bolus of saline followed by a moderately high infusion rate of saline are indicated. If the patient remains hypotensive despite adequate IV saline (as measured by the development of lung congestion at auscultation), IV ionotropic agents are indicated.

○ **A 47-year-old woman is admitted to you with substernal chest pressure for 1 hour. Serial ECGs and CK measurements indicate a non-Q-wave anterior wall MI. She has no arrhythmias, no evidence of heart failure, and no recurrent chest pain while in the hospital. You discharge her with metoprolol, aspirin, and clopidogrel on the fifth hospital day after normal results from a predischarge low-level treadmill exercise test. You schedule her for a symptom-limited treadmill test in 2 weeks. Three days after discharge, she reports a 10-minute episode of substernal chest pressure while walking across the room, which was relieved with sublingual nitroglycerin. What should you advise her to do?**

Readmit her to the hospital, administer IV heparin and nitroglycerin, and perform cardiac catheterization with coronary angiography the next morning.

○ **A 70-year-old man is admitted to the hospital with chest pain of 3 hours' duration. ECG demonstrates anterior ST elevation for which he is given aspirin, recombinant tissue plasminogen activator, heparin, and IV nitroglycerin. His symptoms resolve. Results of serum chemistry tests reveal a peak CK level of 1800 U/L and a CK-MB fraction of 15%. He eventually is transferred out of the cardiac care unit, and his hospitalization is uneventful until day 5, when he develops sudden, severe shortness of breath. His BP is 110/75 mm Hg, and his pulse is 125 bpm and regular. Examination reveals a new systolic murmur. What would the most appropriate therapeutic intervention be?**

This patient most likely has rupture of the LV septum and subsequent defect, a not uncommon complication of MI. Stabilization with vasodilators (afterload reduction to decrease LV pressure and the left-to-right shunt), ionotropic agents (to increase cardiac output), diuretics, and intraaortic balloon pump counterpulsation (vasodilatation). This is followed by cardiac catheterization to define the coronary anatomy and then surgical repair.

○ **A 60-year-old patient has an inferior AMI. Three hours after he arrives in the hospital, he develops ventricular fibrillation and undergoes successful defibrillation back to normal sinus rhythm within 30 seconds. He makes a full recovery and has no further post-MI complications. What does his ventricular fibrillation episode indicate with regard to his subsequent risk of sudden death?**

This episode has no bearing on his subsequent risk of sudden death. Ventricular fibrillation in the immediate setting of an AMI has no prognostic significance.

○   **A 65-year-old woman presents to the hospital with sudden crushing chest discomfort and moderate shortness of breath. Her initial ECG reveals 2-mm ST depression in leads V_1 through V_4 with inverted T waves. She has bibasilar rales in the lower half of both lungs at auscultation. Chest radiography reveals moderate pulmonary edema. Results of serial ECGs and tests of CK levels indicate a non-Q-wave MI. With diuretics, her pulmonary edema resolves within 24 hours. What is the most appropriate management strategy at this point?**

Cardiac catheterization with coronary angiography. A non-Q-wave MI that results in pulmonary edema signifies a large amount of myocardium at risk for reinfarction within the next year.

○   **What arrhythmias that occur in patients with AMI require temporary pacing?**

Complete heart block (third-degree AV block); new left BBB; new bifascicular block; marked sinus bradycardia with ischemic pain, hypotension, CHF, frequent PVCs, or syncope despite use of atropine; and Mobitz type II second-degree AV block

○   **A 54-year-old man, admitted 2 days ago with an anterolateral AMI, suddenly develops atrial fibrillation with a ventricular rate of 135 bpm. He subsequently complains of substernal chest discomfort. His BP is 135/70 mm Hg. What is the most appropriate immediate action to be taken?**

Synchronized direct current cardioversion

○   **What percentage of patients with AMI develop paroxysmal atrial fibrillation?**

10% to 15%

○   **A 58-year-old man is admitted with an anteroseptal AMI. He has pulmonary edema clinically, as shown at chest radiography. His BP is 122/76mm Hg, and his heart rate is 122 bpm. Despite 2 doses of 80 mg of IV furosemide, he still has pulmonary edema. A Swan-Ganz pulmonary artery catheter is inserted, and his initial hemodynamics reveal a cardiac output of 3.1 L/min and a pulmonary capillary wedge pressure of 27 mm Hg. What is the most appropriate pharmacologic agent in this setting?**

IV dobutamine, at a dose of 5 to 20 μg/kg per minute

○   **What is hibernating myocardium?**

In cardiology, hibernating myocardium is a state in which some segments of the myocardium exhibit abnormalities of contractile function. These abnormalities can be seen during ECG or ventriculography. The wall of the affected segments is hypokinetic, akinetic, or dyskinetic.

The phenomenon is highly significant clinically because it usually manifests itself in the setting of chronic ischemia, which is potentially reversible by means of revascularization. The regions of myocardium are still viable and can restore its function. There develops a new steady state between myocardial blood flow and myocardial function in which myocardial blood flow is reduced so that function is reduced, too. The clinical situations in which one can expect hibernating myocardium are as follows:

- Chronic stable angina
- Unstable angina
- Silent ischemia
- After AMI

○   **What are the major complications of LV aneurysms?**

LV thrombus formation (with the subsequent risk of thromboembolic events), CHF, and ventricular arrhythmias

○ **What is the significance of pericarditis after AMI?**

Pericarditis occurs in about 12% to 20% of patients with AMI, more likely in Q-wave infarcts than non-Q-wave infarcts. Patients with pericarditis usually have significantly larger infarcts, lower ejection fractions, and a higher incidence of CHF. The presence of pericarditis and/or pericardial effusion after AMI is associated with a higher mortality. The incidence of post-MI development of pericarditis is significantly reduced (5%) in patients treated with fibrinolytic agents.

○ **A previously healthy 65-year-old man is admitted with an inferior AMI. Within several hours, he is hypotensive (BP, 90/60 mm Hg) and oliguric. Insertion of a pulmonary artery catheter reveals the following pressures: PAWP, 3 mm Hg; pulmonary artery pressure, 21/3 mm Hg; and mean right atrial pressure, 11 mm Hg. What is the best treatment for this man?**

Fluids until his PAWP is between 16 and 20 mm Hg

○ **A 60-year-old man with a recent syncopal episode is hospitalized with CHF and chest pain. His BP is 165/85 mm Hg, his pulse is 85 bpm, and there is a grade 3/6 harsh systolic murmur at the apex and aortic area. ECG reveals a disproportionately thickened septum and anterior systolic motion of the mitral valve. What is this patient's diagnosis, and what physical findings would most likely be present?**

Obstructive hypertrophic cardiomyopathy. The murmur typically decreases with handgrip and squatting and increases with Valsalva maneuver, vasodilators, standing, nitroglycerin, diuretics, and digoxin. Mitral regurgitation is frequent as a result of anterior systolic motion of the mitral valve. CHF is present because of diastolic dysfunction, thus an S_4 gallop is common.

○ **A 68-year-old man with diabetes and a 60-pack-year history of smoking presents with sudden, severe substernal chest discomfort, radiating through to the interscapular area. BP is 150/80 mm Hg in the right arm and 135/65 mm Hg in the left arm. He complains of right arm numbness and weakness, and you hear a 2/6 diastolic murmur along the left sternal border. ECG reveals a 1.5-mm ST elevation in the inferior leads. What is the diagnosis?**

Acute proximal thoracic aortic dissection, with involvement of the right coronary artery and brachiocephalic artery, as well as acute aortic regurgitation

○ **In the patient described in the last question, what other life-threatening complication must one look for, both at auscultation and chest radiography?**

Pericardial effusion with cardiac tamponade. Listen for a pericardial rub at auscultation and look for marked cardiomegaly at chest radiography. Pulsus paradoxus greater than 10 mm Hg is virtually diagnostic of cardiac tamponade in this setting.

○ **What chest radiography findings occur with a dissecting thoracic aortic aneurysm?**

Tortuosity of the proximal aorta with an enlarged aortic knob, mediastinal widening, pleural effusion (most common on the left), extension of the aortic shadow, displaced trachea to the right, cardiomegaly, and separation of the intimal calcification that is greater than 5 mm from the outer contour

○ **What is the prognosis for an untreated dissecting aortic aneurysm?**

Twenty-five percent die within 24 hours, 50% die within 1 week, 75% die within 1 month, and 90% die within 3 months. With surgical treatment, the 10-year survival is 50%, and the 5-year survival is 75% to 80%. Redissection occurs in 25% within 10 years after the original dissection.

○ **What are the most common causes of multifocal atrial tachycardia?**

COPD with exacerbation is the most common cause, followed by CHF, sepsis, and methylxanthine toxicity. Treatment consists of treatment of the underlying disorder, as well as the use of verapamil, magnesium, or digoxin for slowing the arrhythmia.

○ **What are the most common causes of atrial fibrillation?**

CAD with myocardial ischemia and hypertensive heart disease are the most common causes. Mitral or aortic valvular heart disease, cor pulmonale, dilated cardiomyopathy, hypertrophic cardiomyopathy (particularly the obstructive type), ethanol intoxication, "holiday heart syndrome," hypo- or hyperthyroidism, pulmonary embolism, sepsis, hypoxia, preexcitation syndrome, and pericarditis are also common causes.

○ **How is atrial fibrillation treated?**

The treatment of atrial fibrillation consists of three major considerations: (1) control of ventricular rate, (2) conversion, if possible or feasible, to sinus rhythm, and (3) prevention of thromboembolic events, particularly cerebrovascular accident. Rate control is best managed with β-adrenergic blockers or calcium-channel blockers (diltiazem or verapamil), or, less desirably, digoxin. Digoxin should be used in patients with poor LV systolic function and those with a contraindication to β-blockers and calcium-channel blockers. Digoxin provides good rate control at rest but often suboptimal rate control during exertion. Conversion to sinus rhythm may be attempted in the stable patient with a duration of symptoms less than 48 hours. Atrial fibrillation is best managed, initially, with antiarrhythmic agents (amiodarone, ibutilide, propafenone, or procainamide). In the unstable patient or the patient with acute ischemia, hypotension, or pulmonary edema, immediate synchronized electrical cardioversion, starting at 200 J, should be performed. If, in the stable patient, cardioversion with antiarrhythmic agents is unsuccessful, synchronized electrical cardioversion should be performed without interruption of antiarrhythmic therapy. Patients with atrial fibrillation of 1 year duration or longer, or those with left atrial size greater than 5.0 cm at ECG, should not undergo cardioversion because of the extremely low success rate. Patients with recent atrial fibrillation for more than 2 days should begin receiving warfarin and anticoagulation to an INR between 2 and 3.5 for at least 3 weeks before any attempt of cardioversion to sinus rhythm because of the significant risk of embolic cerebrovascular accident. Patients with chronic atrial fibrillation should receive lifelong warfarin, unless an absolute contraindication to warfarin exists or the patient cannot reliably take warfarin.

○ **What percentage of patients with atrial fibrillation converted to sinus rhythm will revert back into atrial fibrillation?**

Fifty percent will revert back to atrial fibrillation within 1 year of cardioversion, regardless of medical therapy.

○ **What is the most common mechanism responsible for SVT?**

AV node reentry

○ **What are the common causes of SVT?**

Myocardial ischemia, MI, CHF, pericarditis, rheumatic heart disease, MVP, preexcitation syndrome, COPD, ethanol intoxication, hypoxia, pneumonia, sepsis, and digoxin toxicity

○ **What is the key feature of Mobitz I second-degree AV block (Wenckebach)?**

A progressive prolongation of the PR interval until the atrial impulse is no longer conducted through to the ventricle, resulting in a dropped QRS. It is almost always transient, and atropine and transcutaneous/transvenous pacing are required for the rare instances of symptoms or cardiac instability.

○ **What is the key feature of Mobitz II second-degree AV block?**

A constant PR interval until 1 sinus beat fails to conduct through to the ventricle, resulting in a dropped QRS. Since this rhythm indicates His bundle damage, and 85% of patients with this rhythm eventually develop complete heart block, temporary followed by permanent pacing usually is required.

○ **What is the treatment for Mobitz II second-degree AV block?**

Atropine and transcutaneous/transvenous pacing, if symptomatic.

○ **A 57-year-old man is scheduled for a total colectomy for ulcerative colitis. He has had stable angina for several years and has hypertension. His preoperative ECG reveals normal sinus rhythm, LVH, and first-degree AV block. What is the likelihood of high-degree AV block occurring perioperatively?**

Patients with first-degree AV block have an extremely low incidence of developing high-degree AV block perioperatively or at any other time. Thus, no perioperative temporary pacing is required.

○ **A 26-year-old man presents to your clinic for an insurance physical examination. ECG reveals Wolff-Parkinson-White syndrome. He is asymptomatic and has no history of palpitations or arrhythmia. What is the most appropriate care for this patient?**

No therapy or workup is required at this time, since there is no evidence that the risk of sudden death can be mitigated safely or that individuals with asymptomatic Wolff-Parkinson-White syndrome can be reliably risk stratified with regard to sudden death.

○ **What is the most commonly occurring form of ventricular tachycardia?**

Ventricular tachycardia occurring in patients with healed MI. Other causes include bundle branch reentry ventricular tachycardia, ventricular tachycardia of right ventricular outflow tract origin, idiopathic LV tachycardia, drug-induced ventricular tachycardia (proarrhythmia), and ventricular tachycardia due to right ventricular dysplasia. Rare causes include long QT syndrome and lymphocytic myocarditis.

○ **A 48-year-old man with no history of angina, MI, or other cardiac symptoms is referred to you for evaluation of palpitations. Results of a 24-hour Holter monitor test reveal 4 3-beat runs of ventricular tachycardia without any symptoms. The patient has no risk factors for CAD, is a nonsmoker, and has normal resting ECG results. His ECG results are normal. What is the best management strategy for this patient?**

No therapy or further workup is required. The patient should be reassured that the risk of sudden death is low and that medical therapy will either worsen his arrhythmia or be of no significant benefit.

○ **A 28-year-old man with 2 previous episodes of palpitations and shortness of breath in the last year is brought in to the emergency department by paramedics with severe palpitations, hypotension, and shortness of breath. His BP is 90/55 mm Hg, and his heart rate is 195 bpm. A rhythm strip reveals narrow complex QRS tachycardia. Twelve-lead ECG results reveal what appears to be atrial fibrillation. Synchronized cardioversion is successful in terminating the arrhythmia, and postcardioversion ECG reveals Wolff-Parkinson-White syndrome. What is the most appropriate management strategy for this patient?**

Electrophysiology testing with intracardiac mapping, followed by catheter ablation of the accessory conduction pathway

○ A 67-year-old woman with severe 3-vessel CAD with small distal vessels, deemed inoperable, is brought into the emergency department after a syncopal episode. The paramedics caught the final beats of what looked like wide complex QRS tachycardia on a rhythm strip, and you confirm this at inspection of the tracing. She is now awake, alert, and breathing comfortably. ECG performed 1 month previously revealed a dilated left ventricle with poor systolic function (estimated ejection fraction, ~20%-25%). What is the most appropriate management strategy for this patient?

Empiric therapy with amiodarone

○ What percentage of patients treated with long-term amiodarone for ventricular tachycardia will develop bradycardia that requires permanent pacing?

15%

○ What is appropriate laboratory and imaging surveillance during amiodarone antiarrythmic therapy?

Pulmonary functions baseline should be determined if there is underlying pulmonary disease, and testing should be repeated at 3, 6, and 12 months.

- Chest radiograph: 3, 6, and 12 months—some say every 3 to 6 months
- Thyroid panel: 3 months—some recommend every 6 months
- Liver panel: 3 months
- ECG: 3 months after baseline
- Eye examination: 3, 6, and 12 months
- Complete blood cell count: 3, 6, and 12 months
- Chem-7: 3, 6, and 12 months

○ What are the major adverse effects of amiodarone when used to treat cardiac arrhythmias?

Adverse reactions have been common in virtually all series of patients treated with amiodarone for ventricular arrhythmias with relatively large doses of drug (400 mg/d and higher). They occur in about three-fourths of all patients, causing discontinuation in 7% to 18%.

The most serious reactions (potentially fatal) are related to pulmonary toxicity (interstitial pneumonitis long term or acute respiratory distress syndrome short term) and occur in 10% to 17% in some series of patients with ventricular arrhythmias receiving doses of approximately 400 mg/d.

Exacerbation of arrhythmias is a potential adverse effect.

Gastrointestinal complaints, most commonly nausea, vomiting, constipation, and anorexia, occur in about 25% of patients. Serious liver injury occurs rarely.

Ophthalmic abnormalities, including optic neuropathy and/or optic neuritis, in some cases progressing to permanent blindness, papilledema, corneal degeneration, photosensitivity, eye discomfort, scotoma, lens opacities, and macular degeneration have been reported.

Asymptomatic corneal microdeposits are present in virtually all adult patients who have been receiving amiodarone for more than 6 months. Vision rarely is affected, and drug discontinuation rarely is needed.

Neurologic problems are extremely common, occurring in 20% to 40% of patients, and include malaise and fatigue, tremor and involuntary movements, poor coordination and gait, and peripheral neuropathy. They are rarely a reason to stop therapy and may respond to dose reductions or discontinuation. Serum T4 levels increase by 20% to 40% during the first month of therapy and then gradually decrease toward high normal.

○ **A 63-year-old man with mild CHF and CAD comes to the emergency department with episodes of fainting and an irregular heartbeat. ECG results show rapid, polymorphic ventricular tachycardia with a twist of the QRS complex around the isoelectric baseline. QRS complexes change shape with each beat. BP is 90/64 mm Hg. Laboratory test results reveal normal levels of hemoglobin, hematocrit, magnesium (2.4 mg/dL; normal range, 1.5-2.5 mg/dL), and potassium (3.2 mEq/L; normal range, 3.5-5 mEq/L). Would this patient be best treated with magnesium sulfate or antiarrhythmics?**

Magnesium. Despite the normal magnesium level, a patient with torsade de pointes usually can be treated successfully with magnesium infusion and careful monitoring of magnesium levels to watch for hypermagnesemia.

○ **Among patients with CAD, which patients have been shown to benefit from revascularization with bypass grafting?**

Patients with left main CAD (>50% stenosis) and those with 3-vessel CAD (>70% stenosis) with depressed LV systolic function (<40% LVEF)

○ **What is the first-line pharmacologic therapy for a 40-year-old obese white woman with uncomplicated mild hypertension?**

A low-dose thiazide diuretic, a long-acting ACE inhibitor/angiotensin II receptor blocker (ARB), or a long-acting dihydropyridine calcium-channel blocker

○ **What is the preferred choice of antihypertensive therapy for a 58-year-old white man with severe COPD and mild hypertension?**

Long-acting calcium-channel blockers, such as verapamil or nifedipine. In addition to effectively lowering BP, they also act to oppose muscle contraction in tracheobronchial smooth muscle, inhibiting mast cell degranulation and possibly reinforcing the bronchodilator effect of β-agonists. These agents are particularly useful in patients with a likelihood of pulmonary hypertension.

○ **Which antihypertensive agent(s) have been shown to slow the progression of renal disease in diabetic patients?**

ACE inhibitors and ARBs

○ **Which drugs have been shown to reduce LVH and reduce LV mass?**

Rapid regression of LVH over a few months has been reported with ACE inhibitors, ARBs, the direct renin inhibitor aliskiren, some calcium-channel blockers (particularly diltiazem, verapamil, and amlodipine), and some sympatholytic agents (including methyldopa and α-blockers).

○ **Which agent is more likely to cause bradycardia: verapamil or diltiazem?**

Diltiazem. Diltiazem blocks conduction through both the sinoatrial and AV nodes, whereas verapamil blocks only the AV node.

○ **Which drugs can increase serum digoxin levels?**

Quinidine, procainamide, verapamil, and amiodarone

○ **What pharmacologic agent should be avoided in a patient with paroxysmal atrial fibrillation who is presently in sinus rhythm?**

Dihydropyridine calcium-channel blockers such as nifedipine. They predispose patients to relapse back into atrial fibrillation.

○ **What medications, used to maintain sinus rhythm in a patient who recently has undergone cardioversion from atrial fibrillation, should be avoided in patients with stress-test proven myocardial ischemia?**

Class 1C antiarrhythmics, such as flecainide and propafenone and class 1A agents, such as quinidine and procainamide. They can lead to lethal proarrhythmia in patients with active myocardial ischemia. Amiodarone, an agent that has anti-ischemic properties, is the preferred agent.

○ **Nontraumatic cardiac arrest patients are most likely to be resuscitated successfully from what abnormal rhythm?**

Ventricular fibrillation. Success is time dependent, generally decreasing at a rate of 2% to 10% per minute.

○ **What are the end points in procainamide loading infusion for a patient with unstable ventricular tachycardia?**

Hypotension, QRS widened more than 50% of pretreatment width, arrhythmia suppression, or a total of 17 mg/kg

○ **How many deaths per year in the United States are due to cardiovascular disease?**

A total of 930,000, or 43% of all deaths per year. Two-thirds of sudden deaths due to CAD take place outside the hospital, and most occur within 2 hours after the onset of symptoms.

○ **If a defibrillator is available, what is the immediate treatment for a patient with ventricular fibrillation?**

Unsynchronized countershock at 200 J, then 200 to 300 J, then 360 J

○ **What is the differential diagnosis of pulseless electrical activity?**

- Hypoxia
- Hypovolemia
- Hyperkalemia/hypokalemia
- Hyperthermia
- AMI
- Acidosis
- Tension pneumothorax
- Tamponade (cardiac)
- Thrombosis (pulmonary)
- Tablets (drug overdose)

○ **What is the differential diagnosis of asystole?**

Drug overdose, acidosis, hyperkalemia, hypothermia, hypokalemia, and hypoxia

○ **What is the treatment for unstable SVT?**

Synchronized cardioversion: 100, 200, 300, and then 360 J

○ **A patient in the emergency department suddenly demonstrates ventricular fibrillation on the monitor. The patient is alert and has a pulse. What should you do?**

Check the monitor leads

○ **Inferior wall MIs commonly lead to what 2 types of heart block?**

First-degree AV block and Mobitz Type I (Wenckebach) second-degree AV block. Sinus bradycardia also can occur. Progression to complete AV block is not common. The mechanism for this is damage to autonomic fibers in the atrial septum giving increased vagal tone impairing AV node conduction.

○ **Anterior wall MIs may damage intracardiac conduction directly. This may lead to which type of arrhythmia?**

The dangerous type. A Mobitz II second-degree AV block can suddenly progress to complete AV block.

○ **Which type of drug is contraindicated for the treatment of torsade de pointes?**

Any drug that prolongs repolarization (QT interval). For example, class 1a antiarrhythmics, such as quinidine and procainamide, are contraindicated for treating torsade de pointes. Other drugs that share this effect include tricyclic antidepressants, disopyramide, and phenothiazine.

○ **What is the treatment for torsade de pointes?**

The goal is to accelerate the heart rate and shorten ventricular repolarization.

1. Crank pacemaker to 90 to 120 bpm ("overdrive").
2. Administer isoproterenol.
3. Administer magnesium sulfate, 2 g IV.

Avoid class 1A antiarrhythmics (quinidine, procainamide, and disopyramide), tricyclic antidepressants, and phenothiazine because they will increase or prolong repolarization and thereby exacerbate torsade de pointes.

○ **What are the classic ECG results associated with posterior MI?**

A large R wave in leads V_1 and V_2, ST depression in leads V_1 and V_2, Q waves in the inferior leads, and, occasionally, ST elevation in the inferior leads

○ **Which valve is most commonly injured during blunt trauma?**

The aortic valve

○ **What is the most likely cause of a new systolic murmur and ECG infarct pattern in a patient with chest trauma?**

Ventricular septal defect

○ **What is the most common complication of extracorporeal circulation?**

Stroke occurs in 1% to 2% of patients after open-heart operations. Other postoperative complications are arrhythmias, bleeding, renal failure, and respiratory complications.

○ **What drug is used to reverse heparin after open-heart surgery?**

Protamine

○ **In 90% of the population, the right coronary artery terminates as:**

The posterior descending artery

○ **The left main coronary artery gives rise to which 2 coronary arteries?**

The left anterior descending artery and the left circumflex coronary artery

○ **What is the vessel of preference in CABG?**

The internal mammary artery. This artery has a much higher rate of patency at 10 years than do venous grafts (95% versus 50%). Also, venous grafts tend to be more prone to atherosclerosis.

○ **Which nerve should be located and avoided during pericardiotomy?**

Phrenic nerve. The phrenic nerve runs along the superolateral aspect of the pericardium.

○ **A radial pulse at examination indicates a systolic BP of at least what level?**

80 mm Hg

○ **A femoral pulse at examination indicates a systolic BP of at least what level?**

70 mm Hg

○ **A carotid pulse indicates a systolic BP of at least what level?**

60 mm Hg

○ **In what area of the left ventricle are aneurysms most commonly found?**

Anterolateral left ventricle (80%). LV aneurysms result from transmural infarctions and subsequent replacement of muscle with fibrous tissue. Unlike atherosclerotic aneurysms, these aneurysms progressively enlarge but rarely rupture.

○ **What is the cardiac arrhythmia?**

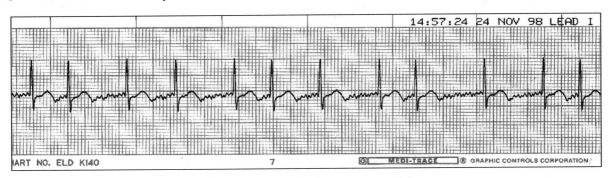

Atrial fibrillation.

○ **What is the cardiac arrhythmia?**

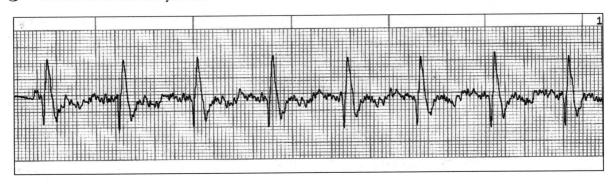

Ventricular paced rhythm with artifact.

○   **What is the cardiac arrhythmia?**

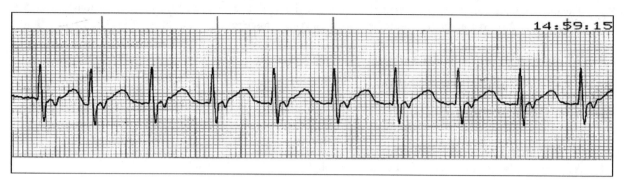

Accelerated junctional rhythm with retrograde P waves.

○   **What is the cardiac rhythm seen below?**

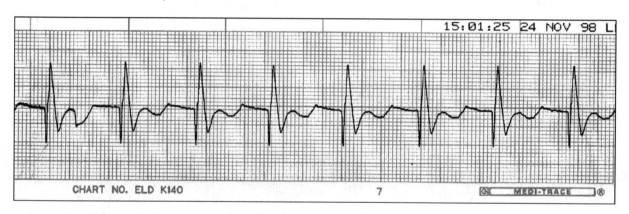

Ventricular pacemaker rhythm.

○   **What is the ECG rhythm abnormality seen below?**

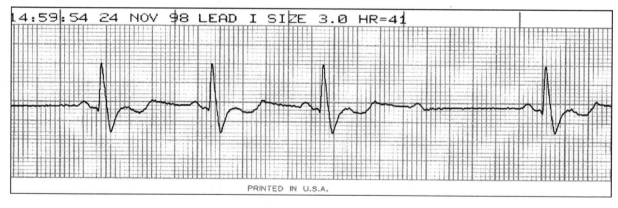

Mobitz II 2nd degree AV block.

○   **What is the ECG rhythm abnormality seen below?**

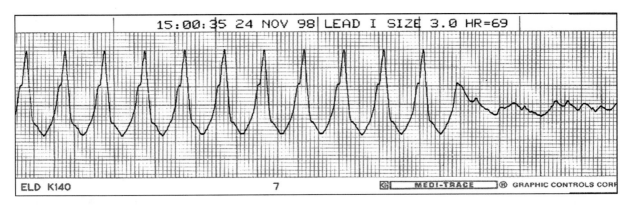

Ventricular tachycardia evolving into ventricular fibrillation.

○   **What is the cardiac arrhythmia below?**

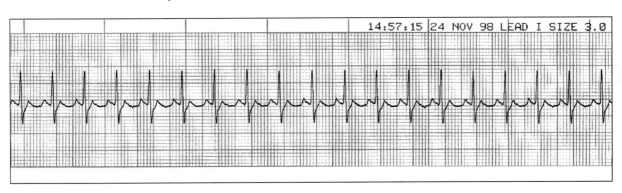

Atrial tachycardia with 2:1 conduction.

○   **What is the abnormality seen in the rhythm below?**

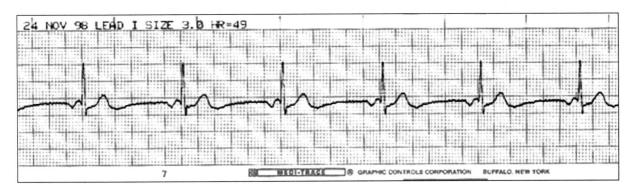

Junctional rhythm.

○ **What is the abnormality in the ECG seen below?**

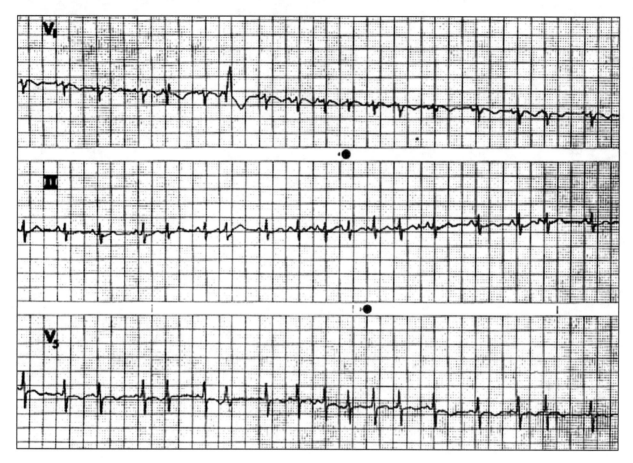

Multifocal atrial tachycardia.

○ **What is the abnormality seen in the rhythm below?**

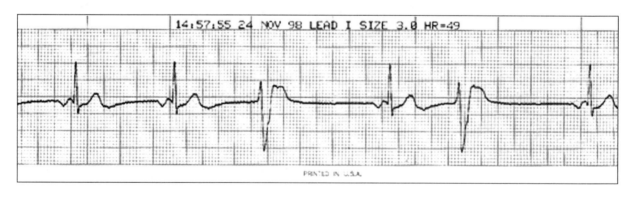

Junctional rhythm with escape ventricular beats.

○ **What is the abnormality seen in the rhythm below?**

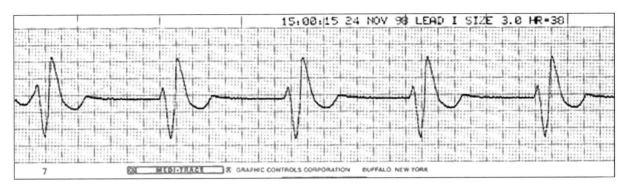

Idioventricular rhythm.

○ **What is the abnormality seen in the rhythm below?**

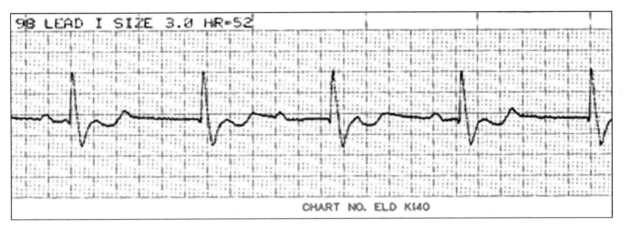

2:1 AV block.

○ **What is the abnormality seen in the rhythm below?**

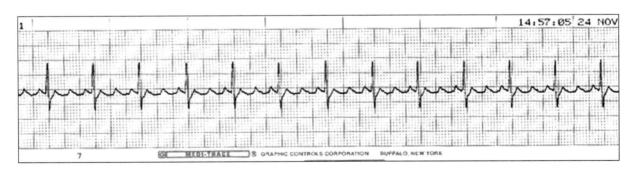

Atrial flutter.

○ **What is the abnormality seen in the rhythm below?**

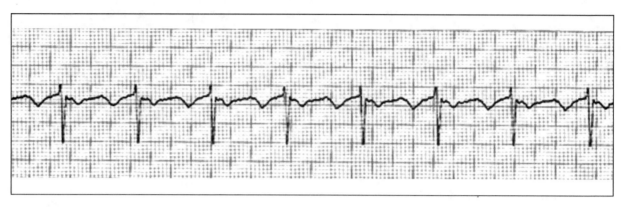

Rhythm strip erroneously mounted upside down. When viewed right-side up, it shows normal sinus rhythm.

○ **What is the rhythm abnormality seen below?**

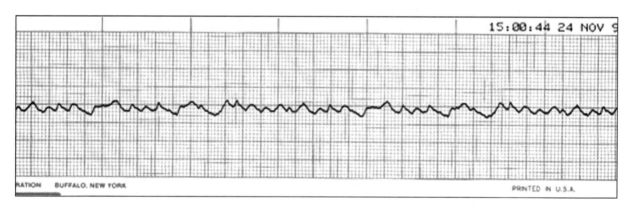

Ventricular fibrillation.

○   **What is the interpretation of this ECG shown below?**

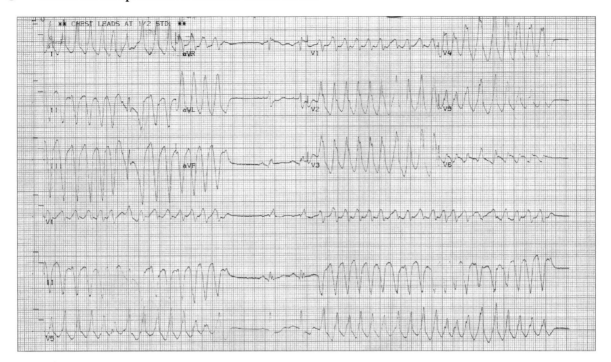

Ventricular tachycardia, most likely originating from the left ventricle.

○   **What is the interpretation of this ECG shown below?**

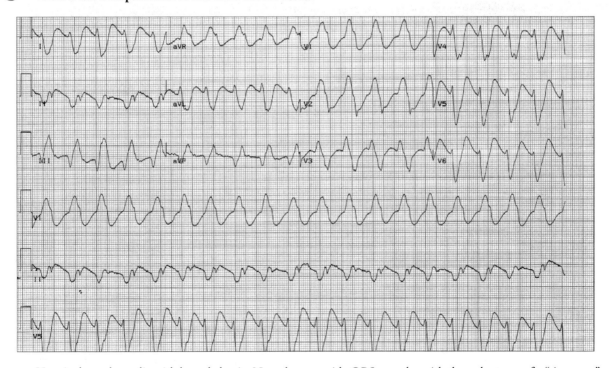

Ventricular tachycardia with hyperkalemia. Note the very wide QRS complex with the early stages of a "sine wave".

○ **What is the interpretation of the ECG shown below?**

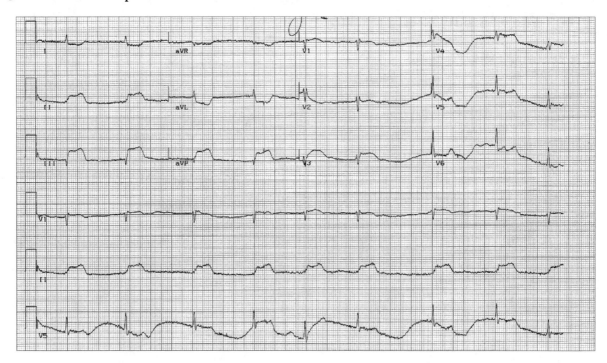

Acute inferior myocardial infaction with posterior wall involvement, atrial fibrillation with slow ventricular rate.

○ **What is the interpretation of the ECG shown below?**

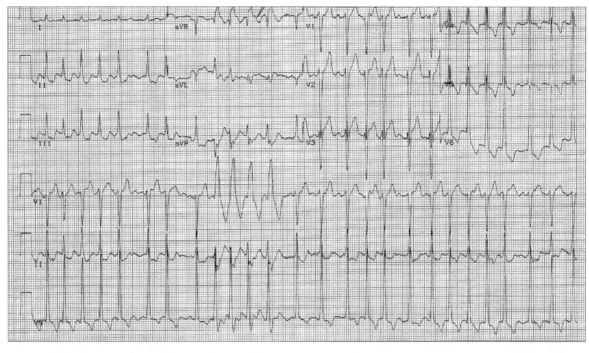

Atrial fibrillation with rapid ventricular rate of 155, LVH, and ischemic-type ST depression in the inferior and lateral leads.

○ **What is the interpretation of the ECG shown below?**

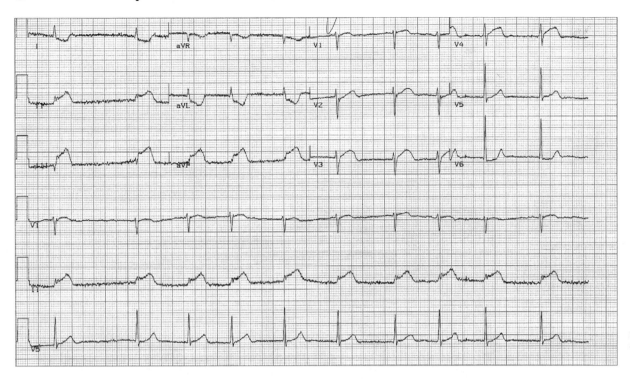

Acute inferior myocardial infaction, atrial fibrillation with slow ventricular rate.

○ **In the above ECG, does this patient absolutely have myocardial ischemia?**

Not necessarily. Patients with supraventricular tachycardia of any type with ST depression can have "ischemic" appearing ST depression without having myocardial ischemia. The ST depression can be as a result of abnormal repolarization that occurs in any tachyarrhythmia. Nonetheless, it would be incorrect to automatically assume that this patient's ST depression is not due to myocardial ischemia.

○ **What is the interpretation of the ECG shown below?**

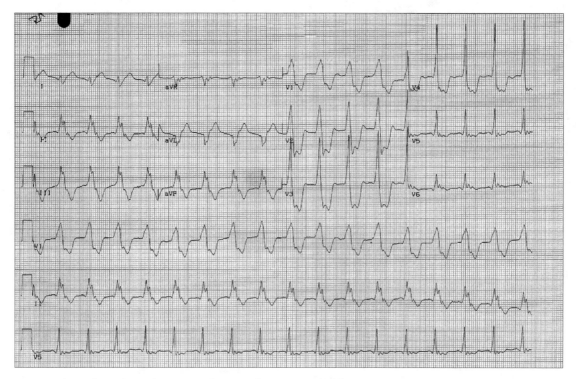

Ventricular tachycardia with a ventricular rate of 103. Note the VA conduction evidenced by the retrograde P waves, which occur in the early part of the ST segment.

○ **What is the abnormality in the M-mode echocardiogram shown below?**

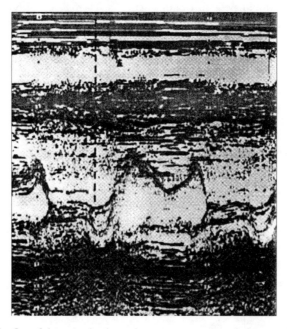

Prolapse of the posterior leaflet of the mitral valve.

○ **What is the abnormality in the echocardiogram shown below?**

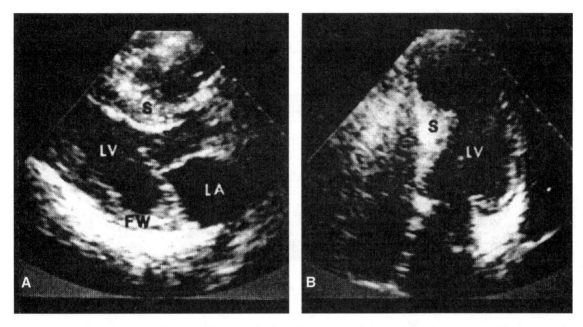

Hypertrophic cardiomyopathy. Note the very thickened septum and anterior systolic motion of the mitral valve.

○ **What is the interpretation of the ECG seen below?**

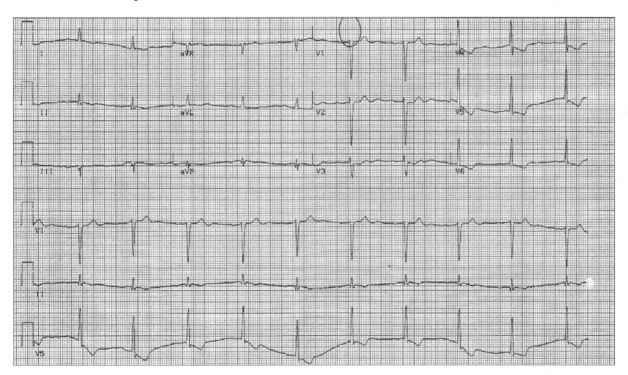

Ectopic atrial rhythm with an old inferior infarction and non-specific ST-T abnormality.

○   **What is the interpretation of the ECG seen below?**

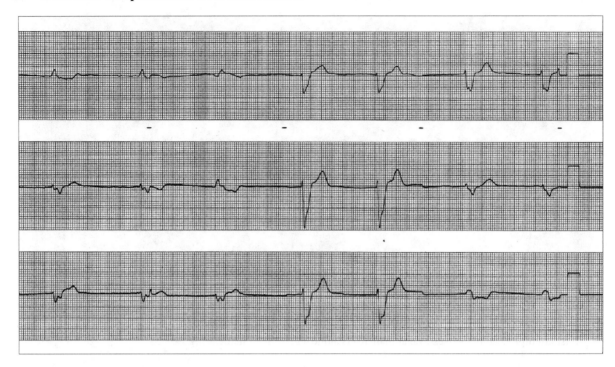

Idioventricular rhythm, rate of 40/min.

○   **What is the interpretation of the ECG seen below?**

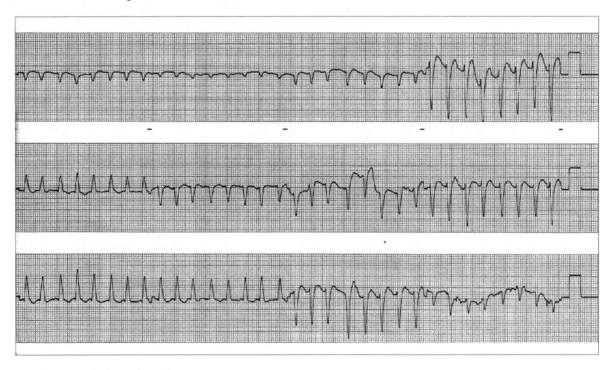

Supraventricular tachycardia.

○ **How do you treat ventricular fibrillation?**

- Defibrillate (360 J monophasic, 150-200 J biphasic) for a single initial defibrillatory shock.
- Resume cardiopulmonary resuscitation immediately after defibrillation without rechecking for a pulse.
- Administer 1 mg of epinephrine IV push every 3 minutes, or vasopresin 40 U IV may replace the first or second dose of epinephrine.
- Continue defibrillation at 360 J (150-200 J).
- Consider other antiarrythmics (amiodarone, lidocaine, magnesium, procainamide).

These are the American Heart Association's guidelines for 2007.

○ **How do you treat pulseless ventricular tachycardia?**

Using the same algorithm as for ventricular fibrillation (see above)

○ **How do you treat pulseless electrical activity?**

Treat the underlying causes first (hypovolemia, hypoxia, hyper/hypokalemia, hypothermia, acidosis, AMI, cardiac tamponade, tension pneumothorax, pulmonary thrombus, tablets). If the cause is unknown, or the treatment unsuccessful, treat with 1 mg of epinephrine IV push every 3 to 5 minutes. If the pulseless electrical activity rate is slow, use atropine 1 mg IV every 3 to 5 minutes to a total dose of .04 mg/kg.

○ **How do you treat stable, narrow complex, paroxysmal SVT?**

First attempt vagal maneuvers; vagal maneuvers alone (eg, Valsalva maneuver, carotid sinus massage) convert up to 25% of SVTs to sinus rhythm. SVT refractory to vagal maneuvers may be treated with nucleoside adenosine (6 mg IV) injected as rapidly as possible into a large proximal vein, followed immediately by a 20-mL saline flush and elevation of the extremity to ensure the drug enters the central circulation before its degradation. If the first dose of adenosine does not convert the rhythm, a second and third dose of 12 mg IV may be administered. If heart function is preserved (ejection fraction >40%), then consider the following drugs in this order of priority: calcium-channel blockers, β-blockers, digoxin, procainamide, amiodarone, and sotalol. If heart function is not preserved (ejection fraction <40%), there is no priority order. Use digoxin, amiodarone, or diltiazem. These are the American Heart Association's guidelines for 2007.

○ **What is an ABI, and why is it significant?**

An ankle brachial index. The ankle systolic pressure (numerator) is compared to the higher of the 2 brachial arterial pressures (denominator). It is used to determine if arterial obstruction is present.

○ **What technical factors can affect the accuracy of the ABI?**

Probe pressure, rapid deflation of the BP cuff, arterial wall calcifications, and probe placement, which should be longitudinal to the vessel and at a 30° to 60° angle to the skin surface

○ **Where do you check the pulse on an unresponsive 1-year-old?**

Apical cardiac impulse

○ **What size BP cuff should be used in a child?**

The widest cuff that fits between the axilla and the antecubital fossa should be used. Most children aged 10 to 11 years will use an adult-sized cuff; somewhat older children may use a large adult cuff.

○ **What cardiovascular defects produce diminished pulses in the lower extremities of a pediatric patient?**

Coarctation of the aorta

○ **What conditions produce cardiac syncope in pediatric patients?**

Aortic stenosis, which does not cause cyanosis, and tetralogy of Fallot, which does cause cyanosis

○ **What are 2 unique clinical findings of tetralogy of Fallot?**

A boot-shaped heart at radiography and exercise intolerance that is relieved by CV

○ **What is the most common cause of aortic regurgitation in children?**

Aortic valve prolapse associated with a congenital ventricular septal defect

○ **What is a serious, life-threatening adult cardiovascular manifestation of Turner syndrome?**

Aortic dissection. It is generally associated with other risk factors, such as hypertension, aortic dilatation, biscuspid aortic valve, or coarctation of the aorta.

○ **What is the leading cause of acquired heart disease in children in the United States?**

Kawasaki disease. Complications include myocarditis, pericarditis, valvular heart disease (mitral or aortic regurgitation), and coronary arteritis.

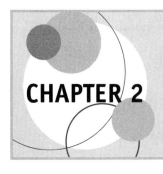

CHAPTER 2 Pulmonary

Gina Kring, MD

○ **What should be suspected if a young, nonsmoking patient has symptoms similar to those associated with emphysema?**

α_1-Antitrypsin deficiency. Without α_1-antitrypsin, excess elastase accumulates, resulting in lung damage. Treatment for this condition is the same as that for emphysema. An α_1-proteinase inhibitor may also may be useful.

○ **List 2 drugs that can cause acute respiratory distress syndrome.**

Heroin and aspirin

○ **A 14-year-old boy was exposed to asbestos for 3 days and has a nonproductive cough and chest pain. Does this boy have asbestosis?**

No. Although a nonproductive cough and pleurisy are symptoms of asbestosis, other signs, such as exertional dyspnea, malaise, clubbed fingers, crackles, cyanosis, pleural effusion, and pulmonary hypertension, should be displayed before making a diagnosis of asbestosis. In addition, asbestosis does not develop until 10 to 15 years after regular exposure to asbestos.

○ **Asbestosis increases the risk of what 2 diseases?**

Lung cancer and malignant mesothelioma. It also causes pneumoconioses that invade the lungs.

○ **What parts of the pulmonary system are affected by asbestosis?**

The pleura and peritoneum

○ **Where does aspiration generally occur as revealed at chest radiography?**

The lower lobe of the right lung. This is the most direct path for foreign bodies into the lung.

○ **Which patients are most at risk for aspiration?**

Those who are neurologically impaired, such as with stroke, seizures, or multiple sclerosis, and persons with alcoholism

○ **What radiographic markings may be observed in a patient with a long history of bronchial asthma?**

Increased bronchial wall markings and flattening of the diaphragm. The bronchial wall markings are caused by epithelial inflammation and thickening of the bronchial walls.

○ **What are the radiographic findings with acute asthma exacerbation?**

- No infiltrates
- Peribronchial cuffing
- Flat diaphragm, hyperinflation

○ **What is the best pulmonary function test for the diagnosis of asthma?**

Spirometry is the reference standard and allows for the most accurate determination of forced expiratory volume in the first second of expiration (FEV_1)/forced vital capacity (FVC). This test is used to determine the amount of air exhaled in 1 minute compared with the total amount of air in the lung that can be expressed. A ratio lower than 80% is diagnostic of asthma. Peak flow meters are helpful in monitoring asthma at home or during an acute exacerbation.

Reversibility of airway constriction is confirmed with either an increase in FEV_1 by 10% or more after administration of a short-acting bronchodilator such as albuterol or levalbuterol.

○ **How can a peak flow meter be used to diagnose asthma?**

Although formal spirometry is still the reference standard, the Global Initiative for Asthma (GINA) guidelines last updated in 2007 by the National Institutes of Health acknowledges that access to spirometry should not limit the ability to diagnose asthma if the patient has clinical symptoms, clinical examination results consistent with asthma, and reversibility of airway demonstrated by an increase of 12% or more above the patient's previously established baseline or 10% or more reversibility with bronchodilator use.

○ **What differential diagnoses need to be explored/excluded before asthma can be diagnosed in children?**

A quick mnemonic for listing differential diagnoses is VITAMIN C&G. Use this mnemonic to spark your brain when you need to expand your differential diagnoses.

Vascular: Congenital heart disease

Infectious: Viral bronchiolitis (croup)

Traumatic: Foreign body aspiration

Autoimmune: Allergic rhinosinusitis

Metabolic: Recurrent gastroesophageal reflux disease (GERD)

Inflammatory: Bronchopulmonary dysplasia (although often treated similarly to asthma), chemical aspiration/ingestion

Neoplasms: Childhood leukemias, lymphomas (luckily rare in childhood)

Congenital: Bronchiectasis, congenital constrictions of the bronchial tree such as laryngotracheomalacia

Genetic: Cystic fibrosis, acute chest syndrome with sickle cell

○ **What differential diagnoses need to be explored/excluded before asthma can be diagnosed in adults?**

Use the VITAMIN C&G mnemonic again.

Vascular: Congestive heart failure (CHF), pulmonary artery hypertension, pulmonary embolism

Infectious: Pneumonia, viral upper respiratory infection, bronchitis

Traumatic: If recent trauma, consider pneumomediastinum

Autoimmune: Lupus erythematosus, sarcoidosis

Metabolic: Noncardiac pleural effusion such as with ascites, medications such as angiotensin-converting enzyme (ACE) inhibitors

Inflammatory: Chemical aspiration, chronic obstructive pulmonary disease (COPD)

Neoplasms: Lung cancer

Congenital: Same as for children but less likely to go undiscovered into adulthood

Genetic: Same as for children but less likely to go undiscovered into adulthood

○ **Is wheezing an integral part of asthma?**

No. Thirty-three percent of children with asthma will have only cough-variant asthma with no wheezing.

○ **A 44-year-old woman with a history of asthma is admitted with shortness of breath and respiratory rate of 28 breaths per minute, but lung examination results reveal no wheezing. What is your diagnosis?**

Do not be fooled by initial examination results without wheezing. If bronchospasm is severe, there may not be enough air movement to produce wheezes. Often after an albuterol nebulizer is administered, the airway will open enough for air movement, and the wheezes will be unmasked.

○ **Which is more effective for relieving an acute exacerbation of bronchial asthma in a conscious patient: nebulized albuterol or albuterol metered-dose inhaler administered via an aerosol chamber?**

They are equally effective. Eight puffs of albuterol with a spacer used correctly are equal to one nebulizer of 2.5 mg in 3 mL of sterile water, usually administered over 5 minutes in the office or emergency department.

○ **What is the correct way to use a spacer?**
- One puff of medication per inhalation
- Shake the metered-dose inhaler and connect to the spacer
- Place spacer with the metered-dose inhaler connected into the mouth
- Push on the metered-dose inhaler to dispense medicine while inhaling
- Hold breath for count of 10 (to allow mist of medication to enter airway)
- Exhale
- Repeat for each puff

○ **List potential complications of inhaled steroids.**

Oral thrush—can be avoided with good oral hygiene (gargling, brushing, and flossing). Esophageal thrush is rare unless the patient is immunocompromised.

○ **Will children who use inhaled corticosteroids have stunted growth?**

Technically, no.

Study results have indicated a possible initial slowing in the growth curve for children treated with inhaled corticosteroids. However, studies performed over longer periods indicate that children treated with inhaled corticosteroids seem to compensate with more growth in height later in childhood. Children with asthma who are not treated adequately with inhaled corticosteroids or who require frequent oral corticosteroids statistically have the most measurable height delay by adulthood.

○ **What are the chances that a child born to 2 asthmatic parents will also have asthma?**

As high as 50%

○ **What extrinsic allergens most commonly affect asthmatic children?**

Dust and dust mites

○ **What extrinsic irritant inhalant most commonly affects asthmatic children?**

Cigarette smoke

○ **List the 10 most common triggers of asthma exacerbations.**

1. Infections (eg, viral upper respiratory infections, chronic sinusitis)
2. Allergens (eg, cat dander, smoking)
3. Exercise
4. Cold air
5. GERD
6. Air pollutants
7. Smoking or secondhand smoke
8. Occupational exposures such as dust, fumes, fine particulates
9. Drugs (eg, aspirin)
10. Emotional stress

○ **Persons with asthma most likely will have a family history of what?**

Asthma, allergies, or atopic dermatitis

○ **What medication allergy is commonly associated with asthma?**

Aspirin allergy often is associated with asthma and with nasal polyps and atopic dermatitis.

○ **What medications should be avoided for a pregnant patient with asthma?**

Epinephrine and parenteral β-adrenergic agonists because of the effects of vasoconstriction on the uteroplacental circulation. However, in a severe asthma attack, the reversibility of short-acting β_2-agonists to open the maternal airway will outweigh the risks to the fetus.

○ **Should inhaled corticosteroids be used during pregnancy?**

Yes. Inhaled corticosteroids are the preferred controller medication in pregnant and nonpregnant adults. Second-line agents can include long-acting β-agonists coupled with inhaled corticosteroids for women whose asthma is not controlled adequately with inhaled corticosteroids alone. In severe cases of asthma, montelukast may be used as second- or third-line agent. Theophylline is reserved for only the most severe cases of asthma during pregnancy.

○ **Does asthma typically improve or worsen during pregnancy?**

During pregnancy, 25% of women have asthma symptoms that improve, 50% of pregnant women have asthma symptoms that stay the same, and 25% of women have asthma symptoms that worsen. Thus, all women should have monitoring of their asthma during pregnancy and may benefit from an asthma action plan. Remember that overall peak flows will decrease during pregnancy because of pressure on the diaphragm, and lung volume will decrease as the uterus enlarges during the third trimester.

○ **What is the normal partial pressure of carbon dioxide (PCO_2) during pregnancy?**

30 to 34 mm Hg from chronic mild hyperventilation, presumably as a result of progesterone

○ **What is the predominant change in the lung volume during pregnancy?**

Decrease in functional residual capacity by as much as 15% to 25%

○ **Why is the incidence of thromboembolism increased during pregnancy?**

Venous stasis from uterine pressure on the inferior vena cava, increase in clotting factors, increased fibrinogen, and decreased fibrinolysis

○ **What are some of the risk factors for thromboembolism during pregnancy?**

Cesarean section, multiparity, bed rest, obesity, increased maternal age, and surgical procedures

○ **What are the predisposing factors for amniotic fluid embolism?**

Older maternal age, multiparity, cesarean section, amniotomy, and insertion of intrauterine fetal monitoring devices

○ **How does amniotic fluid enter maternal circulation?**

Through uterine tears or injury or through endocervical veins

○ **What are the major consequences of amniotic fluid embolism?**

Cardiorespiratory collapse and disseminated intravascular coagulation. Treatment is supportive.

○ **What are the potential mechanisms of cardiorespiratory collapse?**

Mechanical obstruction of pulmonary vasculature, alveolar capillary leak, pulmonary edema from left ventricular failure, anaphylaxis

○ **What is the mortality rate from amniotic fluid embolism?**

About 80%

○ **What is the classic presentation of venous air embolism?**

Sudden hypotension with a mill wheel murmur audible over the precordium

○ **What is the preferred patient position if venous air embolism is suspected?**

Left lateral decubitus and Trendelenburg

○ **What factors increase the risk of aspiration of stomach contents during pregnancy?**

Increased intragastric pressure from the gravid uterus, progesterone-induced relaxation of the lower esophageal sphincter, delayed gastric emptying during labor, and depressed mental status from analgesia

○ **What are some of the common misconceptions about the management of asthma during pregnancy?**

That dyspnea is common during pregnancy and that medications should be used sparingly. Uncontrolled asthma causes more fetal harm than medications do.

○ **Name the anticoagulant that is safe for use during pregnancy.**

Heparin. Warfarin is contraindicated.

○ **What is the most characteristic presentation of bleomycin lung toxicity?**

Pulmonary fibrosis

○ **What is a normal peak expiratory flow rate in adults?**

For men, 550 to 600 L/min; for women, 450 to 500 L/min. However, this varies somewhat with body size and age.

○ **What specific factors influence expected peak flow rates?**

Height and sex influence lung volume and, therefore, peak flow. Note that weight does not factor into expected peak flow.

○ **Sympathomimetic agents are used to treat asthma. What enzyme do they activate?**

Adenyl cyclase

○ **What does ABPA stand for?**

Allergic bronchopulmonary aspergillosis. It also includes non-*Aspergillus* causes of severe allergic bronchopulmonary asthmatic disease.

○ **What treatments are most effective for ABPA?**

For those with high titers of *Aspergillus*, oral itraconazole can be effective. Omalizumab is an injectable medication that is often helpful. Oral corticosteroids are often needed long term, in addition to bronchodilators needed for frequent rescue.

○ **What asthma medication may worsen depression and increase suicidal ideation?**

Montelukast is an excellent medication for patients with allergic or cold air–induced asthma; however, the US Food and Drug Administration released statements in March 2008 raising the possibility of a connection between suicidality and use of montelukast. Studies are still underway. Until then, clinicians are advised to monitor patients using this medication for depression or suicidal thoughts and consider continuing the medication cautiously in those without depressive symptoms.

○ **What effects do increased levels of cyclic adenosine monophosphate (cAMP) have on bronchial smooth muscle and the release of chemical mediators, such as histamine, proteases, platelet activation, and chemotactic factors, from airway mast cells?**

Smooth muscles are relaxed, and release of mediators is decreased. Recall that the effects of cAMP are opposed by cyclic guanosine monophosphate (cGMP). Thus, another treatment approach can be provided by decreasing the levels of cGMP via the use of anticholinergic (antimuscarinic) agents, such as ipratropium bromide.

○ **Right upper lobe cavitation with parenchymal involvement is a classic indicator for what?**

Tuberculosis (TB). Lower lung infiltrates, hilar adenopathy, atelectasis, and pleural effusion also are common.

○ **What is the size of a positive purified protein derivative (PPD?**

PPD of 5 mm or more is recommended to be considered positive in high-risk groups	Immunosuppressed patients (eg, human immunodeficiency virus [HIV], chemotherapy, organ transplant)
	Patients with a high likelihood of infection due to close contact with a confirmed case of TB
	Patients with clinical symptoms of weight loss, night sweats, fevers, chills, hemoptysis, and chest radiographs suspicious for TB or radiographs with changes of milliary or fibrotic old TB
PPD of 10 mm or more is considered positive	Children younger than 4 years
	Moderately immunosuppressed patients such as those undergoing hemodialysis for end-stage renal disease, diabetes mellitus, failure to thrive (body weight less than 10% of ideal body weight)
	High-risk groups such as persons who live in institutions like nursing homes or prisons
	Health care workers
	Immigrants from countries with a high prevalence of TB infection, even if BCG vaccine was administered in the past
PPD of 15 mm or more is considered positive	Healthy individuals at low risk

○ **What is the booster response in TB screening?**

Preemployment TB screening for health care workers often involves asking an individual with an initially negative TB test result to repeat the TB test 1 to 8 weeks later. If the individual then has a 6-mm increase in induration and a PPD reading of 10 mm or more, it is treated as a positive result, thus requiring evaluation for active TB before considering treatment for latent TB infection.

○ **What other test has been approved by the US Food and Drug Administration for TB screening? What are the advantages and disadvantages of this test?**

The QuantiFERON Gold Assay is a serum-based test that relies on serum markers of T-cell–related response to TB. It is a particularly useful way to test patients who received β-human chorionic gonadotropin in the past because it will determine true TB infection and not detect B-cell–mediated BCG vaccination. Its main drawback is cost and lack of widespread availability.

○ **Is it useful to place an anergy panel when testing for TB?**

No. Once common practice, use of an anergy panel with injection of small amounts of antigens such as *Candida* or mumps to use as a controls is no longer recommended when placing PPD in immunosuppressed/anergic patients. Response was too individually varied to warrant continued use.

○ **What are the adverse effects of isoniazid?**

Neuropathy, pyridoxine loss, lupus-like syndrome, anion gap acidosis, and hepatitis

○ **What percentage of TB cases are drug resistant?**

About 15%. The rate depends highly on geographic location.

○ **What are the classic signs and symptoms of TB?**

Night sweats, fever, weight loss, malaise, cough, and a greenish yellow sputum most commonly observed in the mornings

○ **Name some common extrapulmonary TB sites.**

Lymph nodes, bone, gastrointestinal (GI) tract, genitourinary tract, meninges, liver, and pericardium

○ **True/False: Patients younger than 35 years with positive TB skin test results should undergo at least 6 months of isoniazid chemoprophylaxis.**

True. They should undergo a minimum of 4 months of treatment; ideally, they should be treated for 9 months. The preferred regimen is isoniazid and vitamin B6 for 9 months, and the alternative is rifampin.

○ **What are the typical radiographic features of TB pleural effusions?**

They usually are unilateral, small to moderate in size, and more commonly on the right side. Two-thirds of them can be associated with coexisting parenchymal disease that may not be apparent at chest radiography. They commonly are associated with primary disease. The incidence of loculations may be as high as 30%.

○ **What are the characteristic features of a TB pleural effusion?**

Pleural fluid is exudative, with a protein content greater than 0.5 g/L and greater than 90% to 95% lymphocytes; in the acute phase, there may be a polymorphonuclear response.

○ **What is the typical eosinophil count of a TB pleural effusion?**

An eosinophil count greater than 10% usually excludes TB effusion. The eosinophil count in pleural fluid can be elevated after pneumothorax and thoracentesis.

○ **What is the treatment for TB pleural effusion?**

A 9-month course of isoniazid 300 mg and rifampin 600 mg daily. However, because of increasing rates of multidrug resistance, many patients will require treatment with 3 or even 4 anti-TB medications. A therapeutic thoracentesis is recommended only to relieve dyspnea. Corticosteroids can decrease the duration of fever and time required for fluid absorption, but they do not decrease the amount of pleural thickening at 12 months after treatment is initiated. They are, therefore, recommended only for patients who are markedly symptomatic and only after institution of appropriate antimicrobial therapy.

○ **Which β-adrenergic receptors primarily control bronchiolar and arterial smooth muscle tone?**

β_2-adrenergic receptors

○ **Terbutaline is administered subcutaneously for asthma in what dose?**

0.01 mL/kg of 1 mg/mL terbutaline up to 0.25 mL (ie, 0.25 mg), which may be repeated once in 20 to 30 minutes

○ **Is theophylline useful in the emergency management of severe asthma in a pediatric patient?**

No. It has not been shown to affect further bronchodilatation in patients fully treated with β-adrenergic agents. However, theophylline can be used successfully for inpatient management of asthma and may be started in the hospital.

○ **If corticosteroids are prescribed for acute asthma exacerbation, how should prednisone be dosed?**

1 to 2 mg/kg per day in 2 divided doses. Tapering is not necessary if therapy duration is 5 days or fewer. The National Institutes of Health, Global Initiative for Asthma also recently recommended once daily dosing as equally effective in most patients.

○ **What are the risks of long-term oral steroid use?**
- Osteoporosis
- Ulcer
- Prednisone-induced diabetes mellitus
- Adrenal suppression

○ **What effect does preexisting acidosis have on the effectiveness of treatment with β-adrenergic agonists?**

Decreased effectiveness

○ **What is a potentially serious adverse effect of continuous, around-the-clock treatment with albuterol nebulizer?**

Hypokalemia

○ **If one prefers the most simplified algorithm for determining the loading dose of theophylline, what are the appropriate doses for a patient who has not received theophylline recently? A patient who has received theophylline recently?**

- No recent dose: Load with 7 mg/kg theophylline
- Recent dose: Load with 5 mg/kg theophylline

○ **What is the appropriate parenteral dose of methylprednisolone to administer in a pediatric patient with status asthmaticus?**

1 to 2 mg/kg every 6 hours

○ **What is the most common postoperative respiratory complication?**

Atelectasis. Respiratory failure and aspiration pneumonia are other common postoperative complications.

○ **Atelectasis accounts for what percentage of postoperative fevers?**

90%

○ **Why do we care about postoperative atelectasis?**

If it persists for more than 72 hours, pneumonia may develop. Perioperative mortality rates are then 20%. Incentive spirometry is an important therapy for preventing atelectasis.

○ **Chest radiography shows honeycombing, atelectasis, and increased bronchial markings. What is the diagnosis?**

Bronchiectasis, an irreversible dilatation of the bronchi that is generally associated with infection. Bronchography shows dilatations of the bronchial tree, but this method of diagnosis is not recommended for routine use.

○ **Bronchiectasis occurs most frequently in patients with what conditions?**

Cystic fibrosis, immunodeficiencies, lung infections, or foreign body aspirations

○ **Which is the most common type of pathogen in bronchiolitis?**

Respiratory syncytial virus (RSV). It generally affects infants younger than 2 years. Bronchiolitis rarely develops in adults.

○ **What is the treatment for severe bronchiolitis caused by RSV?**

Ribavirin, although nebulized ribavirin is recommended only in the most severe cases. Otherwise, treatment is oxygen and supportive care.

○ **What is the vaccination for RSV and who should receive it?**

Palivizumab is recommended monthly during RSV season (October through April) for children younger than 24 months with a history of congenital heart conditions or preterm birth at less than 35 weeks' gestational age.

○ **What is the most common bacterial cause of cough spread from adults to children?**

Pertussis. Tetanus, diphtheria, and pertussis (Tdap) vaccine for adults every 10 years is the key in preventing the spread of pertussis.

○ **What age group usually gets pertussis?**

Infants younger than 2 years. Adults spread pertussis (whooping cough). Pertussis in adults is a common, persistent, dry barky cough. However, it causes more mortality in infants younger than 2 years than in adults.

○ **What is the treatment for pertussis?**

Erythromycin 4 times daily for 7 to 14 days has the best cure rate. However, its use is often limited by GI adverse effects.

Azithromycin administered once daily for 7 to 14 days also is effective and is much better tolerated.

For patients allergic to macrolide antibiotics, trimethoprim-sulfamethoxazole can be administered twice daily for 14 days with reasonable cure rates.

○ **When would prophylaxis be warranted for contacts of persons infected with pertussis?**

Prophylactic treatment for pertussis should be considered for close household contacts. Prophylactic antibiotic regimens are the same dosing and duration as treatment for pertussis. Revaccination with Tdap would be recommended for individuals 7 years or older, and Dtap would be administered in younger children as long as a minimum of 2 years have passed since the last vaccination.

○ **Where in the United States is coccidioidomycosis most prevalent?**

The Southwest. If the infection is severe, treat the patient with amphotericin B.

○ **Which populations are predisposed to progressive infection with coccidioidomycosis?**

Persons of Filipino decent, African Americans, and Native Americans have a higher incidence of disseminated disease with coccidioidomycosis. Persons with military service in endemic areas are likely to have seropositive test results, although most infections are self-limited.

○ **What is the hallmark symptom of COPD?**

Exertional dyspnea

○ **What parameters should make you consider initiating home oxygen therapy for a patient with COPD?**

Arterial oxygen saturation (SaO_2) of 88% or less, if the patient has a resting partial pressure of oxygen (pO_2) lower than 55 mm Hg or if the patient has a pO_2 lower than 60 mm Hg with evidence of tissue hypoxia. Oxygen desaturation with exercise also may require home oxygen. Home oxygen therapy, 18 h/d, may increase the life span of a patient with COPD by 6 to 7 years.

○ **What percentage of cigarette smokers develop chronic bronchitis?**

10% to 15%. Chronic bronchitis generally develops after 10 to 12 years of smoking.

○ **Other than smoking, what are the risk factors for COPD?**

Environmental pollutants, recurrent upper respiratory infections (especially in infancy), eosinophilia or increased serum immunoglobulin (Ig)E, bronchial hyperresponsiveness, a family history of COPD, and protease deficiencies

○ **Is there any hope for patients with COPD who quit smoking?**

Yes. Symptomatically speaking, coughing stops in up to 80% of these patients. Fifty-four percent of patients with COPD find relief from coughing within a month of quitting.

○ **If a patient with chronic bronchitis has an acute exacerbation of his illness, such as dyspnea, cough, or purulent sputum, what type of oxygen therapy should be initiated?**

We have always been warned against overriding the COPD patient's drive to breathe by overoxygenating him or her. Patients with COPD are no longer prompted to breathe by hypercarbia but by hypoxia alone. However, in the case of acute exacerbation of bronchitis, oxygen therapy should be guided according to pO_2 levels. Adequate oxygen must be maintained at a pO_2 higher than 60 mm Hg, which should be accomplished with the minimal amount of oxygen necessary. The pO_2 must be kept higher than 60 mm Hg, even if the patient loses the drive to breathe.

○ **Which pulmonary function test shows an increase in COPD?**

Residual volume. All other tests (FEV_1, FEV_1/FVC, and forced expiratory volume [FEV] 25%–75%) indicate decreases and diffusion capacity.

○ **Which part of the lung is affected by emphysema? By chronic bronchitis?**

- Emphysema: Terminal bronchi
- Chronic bronchitis: Large airways

○ **What is the risk of placing a patient with COPD on a high fraction of inspired oxygen (FIO_2)?**

Suppression of the hypoxic ventilatory drive, also known as carbon dioxide retention leading to suppression of respiration

○ **What is the definition of chronic bronchitis?**

A productive cough for 3 months of each year for 2 years straight

○ **What is a "blue bloater?"**

An overweight patient with COPD, bronchitis, and central cyanosis. These individuals have normal lung capacity and are hypoxic.

○ **What is a "pink puffer?"**

A patient with COPD and emphysema. These patients are generally thin and noncyanotic. They have an increased total lung capacity and a decreased FEV_1.

O **In treating a patient with a common cold, you prescribe an oral decongestant. Is it necessary to also suggest an antitussant?**

No. Most coughs arising from a common cold are caused by the irritation of the tracheobronchial receptors in the posterior pharynx as a result of postnasal drip. Postnasal drip can be relieved with decongestant therapy, thus eliminating the need for cough suppressant therapy.

O **Should over-the-counter cough medications be used in children?**

Over-the-counter cough medications were removed from the market in the United States in 2008 for children younger than 2 years because of the risk-masking cough, suppressing pulmonary toilet, and hiding symptoms of respiratory distress.

O **What are the most common causes of a chronic cough?**

Postnasal drip (40%), asthma (25%), and gastroesophageal reflux (20%). Other causes include bronchitis, bronchiectasis, bronchogenic carcinoma, esophageal diverticula, sarcoidosis, viruses, and drugs.

O **What drugs can induce a chronic cough?**

ACE inhibitors cause chronic cough as a result of the accumulation of prostaglandins, kinins, or substances that excite the cough receptors. β-Blockers evoke bronchoconstriction, and, thus, coughing by blocking β-2 receptors. Avoid administering β-blockers in patients with asthma or other patients with an airway disease. With careful titration, you can consider selective $β_2$-blockers in patients with coronary artery disease or CHF if they tolerate a low dose.

O **Hoarseness can herald far greater problems than viral laryngitis. At what point is a more thorough workup indicated?**

If hoarseness persists for more than 6 to 8 weeks or is accompanied by a mass, chest pain, weight loss, aspiration dyspnea, or any other signs of malignancy. You should be suspicious of chronic cough or hoarseness in smokers if there is a change in either.

O **Your vitamin-crazed father insists that his daily vitamin C regimen has helped him avoid colds for the past 53 years. Is there any validity to this statement?**

No. Study results have failed to show a prophylactic effect of vitamin C. However, it has been shown that consuming 1 g of vitamin C per day decreases the severity and duration of symptoms associated with the common cold by 23%.

O **What condition must be ruled out when childhood nasal polyps are found?**

Cystic fibrosis

O **What age group has the most colds per year?**

Kindergartners, with an average of 12 colds per year. Second place goes to preschoolers, with 6 to 10 per year. Schoolchildren contract an average of 7 colds per year. Adolescents and adults average only 2 to 4 colds per year.

O **What is the duration of a common cold?**

3 to 10 days (self-limited)

○ **A 2-year-old presents with wheezing; rhonchi; inspiratory stridor; and a sudden, harsh cough that worsens at night. What is the diagnosis?**

Croup, also known as "laryngotracheitis." This condition usually is preceded by an upper respiratory infection and frequently is caused by a parainfluenza virus.

○ **What age group usually contracts croup?**

Children aged 6 months to 3 years. Croup is characterized by cold symptoms; a sudden, barking cough; inspiratory and expiratory stridor; and a slight fever.

○ **A newborn presents with poor weight gain, steatorrhea, and a GI obstruction arising from thick meconium ileus. What test should be performed?**

The sweat test, which detects electrolyte concentrations in the sweat. The infant may have cystic fibrosis, an autosomal recessive defect that affects the exocrine glands, producing higher electrolyte concentrations in the sweat glands.

○ **What result from the sweat test is considered positive for cystic fibrosis?**

A sweat chloride concentration greater than 60 mEq/L.

○ **What is the classic triad of cystic fibrosis?**

1. COPD
2. Pancreatic enzyme deficiency
3. Abnormally high concentration of sweat electrolytes

○ **What is the most common lethal, inheritable disease in the white population?**

Cystic fibrosis, an autosomal recessive disease that occurs in 1 in 2000 births

○ **Empyema is most often caused by what organism?**

Staphylococcus aureus. Gram-negative organisms and anaerobic bacteria also may cause empyema.

○ **What percentage of effusions are associated with malignancy?**

25%

○ **What is the difference between the cough associated with croup and the cough associated with epiglottitis?**

Croup is accompanied by a seal-like barking cough, and epiglottitis is accompanied by a minimal cough. Children with croup have a hoarse voice, and those with epiglottitis have a muffled voice.

○ **What is the tripod sign?**

A small child leans forward to open the airway, often drooling, and refuses to open his or her mouth for examination. This is classic presentation of epiglottitis.

O **What should you do if a child presents with drooling, tripod sign, decreased oral intake, hoarseness, or refusing to eat or talk?**

Do not examine the pharynx unless you have the ability to perform fiber-optic nasal intubation because the epiglottis can swell to obstruct airway within seconds to minutes. Instead, arrange for the child to be examined in a setting such as the emergency department or pediatric intensive care unit where fiber-optic nasal intubation may be possible.

O **What are the pathogens most commonly associated with epiglottitis?**

Haemophilus influenzae type b and group A *Streptococcus*

O **What is the "thumbprint" sign?**

Soft-tissue inflammation of the epiglottis seen on a lateral radiograph of the neck. The epiglottis, normally long and thin, appears swollen and flat at the base of the hypopharynx in patients with epiglottitis.

O **What is the "steeple" sign?**

Subglottic edema, which creates a symmetrically tapered configuration in the subglottic portion of the trachea when imaged at frontal soft-tissue radiography of the neck. This is consistent with croup.

O ***Hantavirus* occurs most commonly in what geographic location?**

Southwestern United States, especially in areas with deer mice

O **What is the definition of massive hemoptysis?**

Coughing of more than 600 mL of blood in 24 hours

O **What are the most common causes of hemoptysis in nonhospitalized patients?**

Bronchitis, bronchogenic carcinoma, TB, pneumonia, abscess, trauma, and idiopathic causes. It also can occur because of bleeding from the nose into the respiratory tract.

O **What systemic illnesses cause hemoptysis?**

Lung cancer, amyloidosis, CHF, mitral stenosis, sarcoidosis, systemic lupus erythematosus, vasculitis, coagulation disorders, pulmonary-renal syndromes, and TB

O **Life-threatening hemoptysis should be suspected when there is:**
- A large volume of blood
- Appearance of a fungus ball in a pulmonary cavity at chest radiography
- Hypoxemia

O **What percentage of people in the Ohio and Mississippi valleys are infected with histoplasmosis?**

100% in endemic areas. However, only 1% of these individuals develop the active disease. The spores of *Histoplasma capsulatum* can remain active for 10 years. For unknown reasons, bird and bat feces promote the growth of the fungus. The disease is transmitted when the spores are released and inhaled.

○ **What is Pancoast syndrome?**

Tumor of the apex of the lung that gives rise to Horner syndrome and shoulder pain. The tumor invades the bronchial plexus.

○ **What is Horner syndrome?**

Miosis, ptosis, and anhydrosis

○ **What are Kerley B lines?**

Short, horizontal white lines found on chest radiographs in patients with pulmonary edema. Fluid in the lung causes waterlogged interlobular septa that then become fibrotic.

○ **What antibiotic is the most effective for treating uncomplicated lung abscesses?**

Clindamycin

○ **True/False: Flora of lung abscesses are usually polymicrobial.**

True

○ **What is the most common cancer in the United States?**

Lung cancer

○ **What are the most common causes of lung cancer?**

- Smoking
- Radon
- Metastatic causes
- Idiopathic causes

○ **What cancers generally metastasize to the lungs?**

Breast, colon, prostate, and cervical cancers

○ **What routine program is recommended for screening for lung cancer in the adult population?**

None. Screening programs for lung cancer have not been demonstrated to produce a decrease in morbidity or mortality. Practitioners must be aware of the signs and symptoms associated with lung cancer, including chronic, nonproductive cough; increased sputum production; hemoptysis; dyspnea; recurrent pneumonia; hoarseness; pleurisy; weight loss; shoulder pain; superior vena cava syndrome; exercise fatigue; and anemia. Incidental findings at chest radiography also should be investigated.

○ **Where do the following cancers most commonly develop within the lung: adenocarcinoma and large cell? Squamous cell and small cell?**

Adenocarcinoma and large cell carcinomas usually are located peripherally; squamous and small cell carcinomas are located centrally.

○   **Which form of lung cancer is the most common?**

Squamous cell carcinoma (40%–50%), followed by adenocarcinoma (35%) and small cell (oat cell) carcinoma (25%)

○   **Name 5 HIV-related pulmonary infections.**

1. *Pneumocystis jiroveci* pneumonia (PCP)
2. TB
3. Histoplasmosis
4. *Cryptococcus*
5. Cytomegalovirus

○   **Describe the chest radiograph of a patient with PCP.**

A reticular pattern ranging from fine to coarse, ill-defined patchy areas, and segmental and subsegmental consolidation

○   **What diagnostic test is helpful for the identification of a subclinical PCP infection?**

Exertional pulse oximetry is indicative of PCP if after 3 minutes of exercise the oxygen saturation decreases by 3% or the alveolar-arterial (A-a) gradient increases by 10 mm Hg from rest.

○   **What laboratory tests aid in the diagnosis of PCP?**

An increasing level of lactate dehydrogenase (LDH) or LDH greater than 450 U/L and an erythrocyte sedimentation rate greater than 50 mm/h. A low albumin level implies a poor prognosis.

○   **The initial therapy for PCP includes which antibiotics?**

Trimethoprim-sulfamethoxazole or pentamidine

○   **What other medication should be prescribed for a patient with PCP?**

Corticosteroids when the pO_2 is less than 70 mm Hg or an A-a gradient is greater than 35 mm Hg.

○   **What 2 drugs are used as prophylactic treatment to prevent PCP in patients with HIV?**

Aerosolized pentamidine or trimethoprim-sulfamethoxazole

○   **Where does pain from pleurisy radiate?**

The shoulder, as a result of referred pain of diaphragmatic irritation

○   **Pneumatoceles (thin-walled, air-filled cysts) on an infant's radiograph are a sign of which type of pneumonia?**

Staphylococcal

○   **What are the most common causes of staphylococcal pneumonias?**

Drug use and endocarditis. This pneumonia produces high fever, chills, and a purulent productive cough.

○ **What are the extrapulmonary manifestations of *Mycoplasma* infection?**

Erythema multiforme, pericarditis, and central nervous system disease

○ **What intracellular atypical pneumonia is associated with atypical pneumonia, acute renal failure, and rash?**

Mycobacterium avium

○ **What is the most frequent cause of nosocomial pneumonia?**

Pseudomonas aeruginosa. There is a high mortality associated with pneumonia caused by *Pseudomonas*. It most frequently occurs in immunocompromised patients or patients receiving mechanical ventilation.

○ **A 67-year-old alcoholic man was found in an alley, covered in his own vomit and beer. At examination, he is shaking, has a fever of 103.5°F, and is coughing up currant jelly sputum. What is the diagnosis?**

Pneumonia induced by *Klebsiella pneumoniae*. This is the most probable cause in alcoholic patients, the elderly, the very young, and immunocompromised patients. Other gram-negative bacteria, such as *Escherichia coli* and other Enterobacteriaceae, may also be contributory causes of the aspiration pneumonia in an alcoholic patient.

○ **Match the pneumonia with the treatment.**

1. *K pneumoniae*	**a.** Erythromycin, tetracycline, or doxycycline
2. *Streptococcus pneumoniae*	**b.** Penicillin G
3. *Legionella pneumophila*	**c.** Cefuroxime and clarithromycin
4. *H influenzae*	**d.** Erythromycin and rifampin
5. *Mycoplasma pneumoniae*	

Answers: (1) c, (2) b, (3) d, (4) c, and (5) a

○ **What are features of patients that could warrant inpatient treatment of community-acquired pneumonia?**

Age older than 50 years; resident of a nursing home; coexisting illnesses, such as active cancer, renal disease, liver disease, stroke, or clinical findings consistent with respiratory distress such as the following: altered mental status; tachypnea greater than 30 breaths per minute; tachycardia of 125 beats per minute or more; hypotension with systolic blood pressure less than 90 mm Hg; high fever or hypothermia; pleural effusion; arterial blood gas with pH less than 7.35 or partial pressure of alveolar oxygen (PAO_2) less than 60 mm Hg (hypoxemia); laboratory test result abnormalities, such as hyponatremia, hyperglycemia, or anemia, with hematocrit less than 30%

○ **What is the recommended treatment regimen for community-acquired pneumonia?**

Whenever possible, sputum culture with Gram stain should be performed, and treatment should be guided by the results. Empiric treatment should be started while sputum culture results are pending. Adults should be treated with a macrolide and possibly a β-lactam antibiotic, since macrolide resistance is increasing. Fluoroquinolone monotherapy has a high rate of resistance and should be reserved for patients at high risk of drug resistant *S pneumoniae* infection.

○ **What groups or patients with pneumonia are at high risk of infection with drug-resistant S *pneumoniae*?**

Persons older than 65 years; persons who have undergone treatment with antibiotic therapy in the last 3 to 6 months; persons with alcoholism; persons with preexisting medical conditions, such as diabetes, end-stage renal disease, cirrhosis, or cancer; persons receiving immunosuppressive therapy; caregivers for small children

○ **Describe the classic chest radiographic findings in a patient with *M pneumoniae*.**

Patchy diffuse areas of opacity involving the entire lung. Pneumatoceles, cavities, abscesses, and pleural effusions can occur but are uncommon. Treat the patient with erythromycin or other macrolide antibiotic.

○ **Describe the classic chest radiographic finding associated with *Legionella* pneumonia.**

Dense consolidation and bulging fissures. Expect elevated liver enzymes and hypophosphatemia. The patient with *Legionella* pneumonia classically presents with relative bradycardia.

○ **A 43-year-old man presents with pleurisy, sudden onset of fever and chills, and rust-colored sputum. What is the probable diagnosis?**

Pneumococcal pneumonia caused by *S pneumoniae*, the most common community-acquired pneumonia. It is a consolidating lobar pneumonia and can be treated with a β-lactam antibiotic and a macrolide such as penicillin G plus erythromycin or with amoxicillin 1 g 3 times daily plus azithromycin.

○ **How long should you continue antibiotics for community-acquired pneumonia?**

Until 48 hours after the last fever. Treatment for 7 to 14 days is common. Results from most studies show adequate treatment with 7 days of antibiotics. Newer regimens for macrolides may allow treatment in 3 days or fewer.

○ **When should chest radiography be repeated to show resolution of pneumonia?**

Chest radiographs will continue to show areas of opacity until 6 to 8 weeks after treatment of pneumonia. In older patients or those with recurrent pneumonia, confirming resolution of the pneumonia with radiographs 2 months after clinical resolution is recommended to confirm that the pneumonia was not masking an underlying malignancy.

○ **A 20-year-old college student is home for winter break and presents complaining of a 10-day history of a nonproductive, dry, hacking cough; malaise; a mild fever; and no chills. What is a possible diagnosis?**

M pneumoniae, also known as "walking pneumonia." Although this is the most common pneumonia that develops in teenagers and young adults, it is an atypical pneumonia and most frequently occurs in close-contact populations (ie, schools and military barracks).

○ **A 56-year-old smoker with COPD presents with chills, fever, green sputum, and extreme shortness of breath. Radiography shows right lower lobe pneumonia. What is expected from the sputum culture?**

H influenzae. This organism generally is found in pneumonia and bronchitis in patients with underlying COPD. The next most common organism detected in this patient population is *Moraxella catarrhalis*. Amoxicillin clavulanate is the drug of choice, but patients at high risk should receive yearly influenza vaccinations.

○ **Describe the different presentations of bacterial pneumonia and viral pneumonia.**

Bacterial pneumonia is typified by a sudden onset of symptoms, including pleurisy, fever, chills, productive cough, tachypnea, and tachycardia. The most common bacterial pneumonia is pneumococcal pneumonia.

Viral pneumonia is characterized by gradual onset of symptoms, no pleurisy, chills or high fever, general malaise, and a nonproductive cough.

○ **What is the most common cause of pneumonia in children?**

Viral etiologies. Infecting viruses typically include influenza and parainfluenza strains.

○ **If a patient has patchy infiltrate at chest radiography and bullous myringitis, what antibiotic should be prescribed?**

Erythromycin for *Mycoplasma*

○ **What secondary bacterial infection often occurs after a viral pneumonia?**

Staphylococcal pneumonia

○ **What 3 findings should be present to consider a sputum sample adequate?**

1. Greater than 25 polymorphonucleocytes (white blood cells)
2. Fewer than 10 squamous epithelial cells per low-powered field
3. A predominant bacterial organism

○ **What degree of leukocytosis is considered a risk factor for poor outcome among patients with bacterial pneumonia?**

Greater than 30,000 cells per mm^3

○ **What bacteria are associated with pneumonia after influenza?**

S pneumoniae, *S aureus*, and *H influenzae*

○ **What is the leading identifiable cause of acute community-acquired pneumonia in adults?**

S pneumoniae

○ **What 2 underlying medical conditions are associated with *H influenzae* pneumonia?**

COPD and HIV infection

○ **At what age should the pneumococcal vaccine be administered among healthy adults with no comorbid conditions?**

65 years or older

○ **What is the most common cause of atypical pneumonia?**

M pneumoniae

○ **What is considered the second most common cause of atypical pneumonia?**

Chlamydia pneumoniae

○ **Of the following organisms, which is commonly spread by person-to-person contact: *L pneumophila* or *M pneumoniae*?**

M pneumoniae

○ **What is the most common cause of community-acquired bacterial pneumonia among patients infected with HIV?**

S pneumoniae

○ **What 3 radiographic findings are associated with a poor outcome in patients with pneumonia?**

1. Multilobe involvement
2. Pleural effusion
3. Cavitation

○ **What are the 2 most important risk factors for the development of anaerobic lung abscess?**

Poor oral hygiene and a predisposition toward aspiration

○ **Which lung segments are most often the site of lung abscess formation?**

The posterior segments of the upper lobe and the superior segments of the lower lobes

○ **What anaerobic respiratory infection is associated with slowly enlarging pulmonary infiltrates, pleural effusions, rib destruction, and fistula formation?**

Actinomycosis

○ **What percentage of patients with pneumonia develop pleural effusions?**

40%

○ **What pathologic process is suggested by an air-fluid level in the pleural space?**

Bronchopleural fistula

○ **What is the definition of nosocomial pneumonia?**

Pneumonia occurring in patients who have been hospitalized for at least 72 hours

○ **What are the 2 most important routes of transmission of nosocomial bacterial pneumonia?**

1. Person-to-person transmission via health care workers
2. Contaminated ventilator tubing

○ **In what season does *Legionella* pneumonia most commonly occur?**

Summer. *L pneumophila* thrive in environments such as the water cooling towers that are used in large buildings and hotels. Staphylococcal pneumonias also occur more frequently in summer.

○ **An older patient with GI symptoms, hyponatremia, and relative bradycardia probably has which type of pneumonia?**

Legionella

○   **What are the most common clinical symptoms of influenza?**
- Sudden onset of high fever [38.6°C (101.5°F) or higher]
- Diffuse body aches (myalgias)
- Headache
- Cough
- Mild to moderate sore throat

○   **What is the window for treatment of influenza with antiviral agents?**

Antiviral agents are not curative, but they lessen symptom severity and duration when started within 48 hours—at most, 72 hours—after onset of flu symptoms. Choice of antiviral agent should be guided by the Centers for Disease Control surveillance data.

○   **What is the swine flu?**

In 2009, a subtype of influenza A identified as H1N1 started in North America and spread to pandemic proportions. Although the symptoms were usually mild, mortality rates were surprisingly high in the teen and young adult populations.

○   **A mother calls your office distraught after hearing about the swine flu on the news. She wants to know if there is any risk of getting the illness by eating pork. What do you tell her?**

You correctly reassure her that there is no risk of transmission with eating cooked pork meat. Influenza A (H1N1) was thought to incubate naturally in pigs and then be transmissible to humans. Since many influenza viruses are zoonotic and able to infect birds and swine, often the infection is mild or clinically undetectable for the animals. The animals can spread the infection via respiratory droplets or feces to other birds, swine, and human animal caretakers.

○   **What is the avian flu?**

In 2003, there was a similar outbreak of a subvariant of influenza virus that was spread to humans in contact with infected birds. Again, eating well-cooked poultry did not spread the disease; the virus was spread from live infected birds to humans.

○   **What is antigenic drift?**

Antigenic drift is a phenomenon that happens every year with viruses such as the seasonal influenza virus. Since viruses grow so much faster than humans do, mutations occur regularly that allow the proteins in the outer viral coat to change as the virus spreads in populations. Antigenic drifts, usually in the hemagglutinin or neuraminidase proteins in the viral outer coat, require a new flu vaccine to be formulated every year as the virus mutates as it spreads across global populations. Antigenic drifts can make the virus more virulent or less virulent. Infections with viruses that undergo antigenic drift cause local outbreaks and usually are less severe or widespread than when antigenic shifts occur.

○   **What is antigenic shift?**

Antigenic shifts usually result in more widespread and severe infections. Antigenic shifts can occur only with type A influenza viruses. Antigenic shifts occur when the genomes of 2 viruses combine to make a novel type of virus. Antigenic shifts usually are involved in worldwide pandemics.

○ **What methods are available to protect against flu?**

- Vaccination yearly
- Hand washing
- Covering your cough
- Masks

○ **Who can use the nasal flu vaccine?**

Healthy persons who do not want to get the flu

○ **Who cannot use the nasal flu vaccine?**

- Persons with asthma
- Persons with diabetes
- Immunosuppressed persons
- Children younger than 2 years
- Adults older than 50 years
- Persons allergic to eggs
- Persons with a history of Guillain-Barré syndrome

○ **What are the clinical symptoms of inhalation anthrax?**

Initially, symptoms are flulike, with fevers, body aches, and headache. But patients with inhalation anthrax quickly and rapidly decline to have hypoxemia and severe respiratory distress, and 50% develop hemorrhagic meningitis. Most will have chest radiographs showing mediastinal widening and pleural effusion. Patients may or may not also have cutaneous lesions of anthrax. Suspicion of bioterrorism should warrant quick isolation and testing as directed by the Centers for Disease Control or local health department.

○ **What percentage of upper respiratory infectious agents are nonbacterial?**

Nonbacterial agents account for more than 90% of cases of pharyngitis, laryngitis, tracheal bronchitis, and bronchitis.

○ **Name 2 antiviral medications that are used for viral pneumonia.**

1. Amantadine for influenza A
2. Aerosolized ribavirin for RSV

○ **What is 1 of the most limiting adverse effects of ribavirin?**

It cannot be used in persons with asthma because of the high risk of bronchospasm.

○ **What is the indication for a chest tube in a patient with pneumothorax?**

More than 15% pneumothorax or a clinical indication, such as respiratory distress or enlarging pneumothorax

○ **What therapy may increase the body's absorption of pneumothorax or pneumomediastinum?**

A high FIO_2

○   **What is the profile of a classic patient with a spontaneous pneumothorax?**

Male, athletic, tall, slim, and aged 15 to 35 years

○   **What is the recurrence rate of spontaneous pneumothoraces?**

30% to 50%

○   **Which types of pneumonia are commonly associated with pneumothorax?**

Staphylococcal, TB, *Klebsiella*, and PCP

○   **What are the most common symptoms of a pulmonary embolism?**

Chest pain (88%) and dyspnea (84%)

○   **What are the most common signs of a pulmonary embolism?**

Tachypnea (92%) and rales (58%)

○   **What is the most common radiographic finding of a pulmonary embolism?**

An elevated hemidiaphragm (41%)

○   **What is the most common electrocardiographic finding of a pulmonary embolism?**

T-wave inversion (42%). The $S_1Q_3T_3$ pattern also is seen.

○   **What percentage of patients with a pulmonary embolism have a normal electrocardiogram?**

13%

○   **What is the anticoagulant treatment schedule for a pulmonary embolism?**

Intravenous (IV) heparin until partial thromboplastin time is 2 to 2.5 times normal. After a day, warfarin is added until the international normalized ratio (INR) is greater than 2.0. If clots recur, consider a Greenfield filter in the inferior vena cava. Pulmonary embolectomy is necessary only in cases of massive embolisms. Enoxaparin may be used instead of heparin.

○   **What 3 syndromes are associated with the various degrees of pulmonary embolism?**

1. Acute cor pulmonale: Occurs with massive embolism that obstructs more than 60% of the pulmonary circulation
2. Pulmonary infarction: Occurs with embolization to the distal branches of the pulmonary circulation
3. Acute dyspnea: Milder obstruction, not enough to warrant infarction

○   **What is pulmonary artery hypertension?**

Pulmonary artery pressure greater than 25 to 30 mm Hg with exercise. Measured ideally during cardiac catheterization.

○   **List the causes of pulmonary artery hypertension.**

Use the VITAMIN C mnemonic again.

Vascular: CHF, mitral stenosis

Infections: HIV

Trauma: Pulmonary embolism

Autoimmune: Collagen vascular disease

Metabolic: Cocaine, methamphetamines, obstructive sleep apnea (often related to morbid obesity), portal hypertension

Inflammatory: COPD

Neoplasms: Obstructing left ventricular outflow

Congenital: Cardiac shunts

○   **How is pulmonary hypertension treated?**

If a cause can be found, treatment should be directed at treating the underlying cause (e.g., treatment and prevention of future pulmonary embolisms or mitral valve replacement for mitral stenosis).

All patients should be encouraged to have regular exercise as tolerated and may need formal pulmonary rehabilitation. Patients with pleural effusions or edema should receive diuretics. Any patient with hypoxemia should receive supplemental oxygen. Some patients may benefit from long-term anticoagulation or digoxin. Patients with New York Heart Association class II, III, or IV may benefit from calcium-channel blockers. More advanced cases of disease may benefit from prostanoids or daily oral sildenafil. Patients not responsive to medical treatment may benefit from surgical therapies, such as atrial septostomy or lung transplantation.

○   **What is the equation for the A-a gradient?**

A-a $= (713 \text{ mm Hg} \times FIO_2)\text{-}PCO_2\text{-}pO_2/0.8)$

The normal A-a gradient is 5 to 15 mm Hg, though it increases with age. The A-a gradient also increases with pulmonary embolism and diffusion defects (ie, pulmonary edema and right to left cardiac shunts).

○   **Most pulmonary embolisms arise from what veins?**

Iliac and femoral veins

○   **Primary pulmonary hypertension is most common in what population?**

Young women. Primary pulmonary hypertension is rapidly fatal within a few years.

○   **What heart sounds accompany pulmonary hypertension?**

A narrowed second heart sound split and a louder P_2

○   **What is the major cause of pulmonary hypertension?**

Chronic hypoxia, most commonly from COPD

○ **True/False: Pulse oximetry is a reliable method for estimating oxyhemoglobin saturation in a patient with carbon monoxide poisoning.**

False. Carboxyhemoglobin has light absorbance that can lead to a falsely high pulse oximeter transduced saturation level. The calculated value from a standard arterial blood gas test also may be falsely high. The oxygen saturation should be determined by using a co-oximeter that measures the amounts of unsaturated oxyhemoglobin, carboxyhemoglobin, and methemoglobin.

○ **What are clinical symptoms of carbon monoxide poisoning?**

- Cherry red skin color
- Fatigue
- Headache
- Hypersomnolence

○ **A newborn is breathing rapidly and grunting. Intercostal retractions, nasal flaring, and cyanosis are noted. Auscultation indicates decreased breath sounds and crackles. What is the diagnosis?**

Neonatal respiratory distress syndrome, also known as "hyaline membrane disease." Radiography shows diffuse atelectasis. Treatment involves artificial surfactant and oxygen administration through continuous positive airway pressure.

○ **Other than avoiding prematurity, what can be done to prevent neonatal respiratory distress syndrome?**

If the fetus is older than 32 weeks, administer betamethasone 48 to 72 hours before delivery to augment surfactant production.

○ **Sarcoidosis is most common in what race and age group?**

African Americans aged between 20 and 40 years

○ **What will the chest radiograph in a patient with sarcoidosis classically reveal?**

Bilateral hilar and paratracheal adenopathy with diffuse nodular-appearing infiltrate. Sarcoidosis can be staged by using chest radiography:

- Stage 0: Normal
- Stage 1: Hilar adenopathy
- Stage 2: Hilar adenopathy and parenchymal infiltrates
- Stage 3: Parenchymal infiltrates only
- Stage 4: Pulmonary fibrosis

○ **What other systems can be affected by sarcoidosis?**

Cardiovascular, GI, immunological, integumental, lymphatic, and ocular systems

○ **Upper lobe nodules and eggshell hilar node calcification are displayed on radiographs of an individual with what disease?**

Silicosis

○ **What is the average exposure time necessary for the development of silicosis after silicon dioxide inhalation?**

20 to 30 years. Employees in mining, pottery, soap production, and granite quarrying are at risk. These populations also have a higher chance of acquiring TB.

○ **What is the indication for long-term tracheostomy?**

Intubation expected to exceed 3 weeks or avoidance of aspiration of oral secretions in patients who are neurologically compromised

○ **Differentiate between "transudate" and "exudate."**

Transudate

- Pleural: Serum protein level lower than 0.5
- Pleural: Serum LDH level lower than 0.6
- Most common with CHF, renal disease, and liver disease

Exudate

- Pleural: Serum protein level higher than 0.5
- Pleural: Serum LDH level higher than 0.6
- Most common with infections, malignancy, and trauma

○ **A patient presents with cough, lethargy, dyspnea, conjunctivitis, glomerulonephritis, fever, and purulent sinusitis. What is the probable diagnosis?**

Wegener granulomatosis. This is a necrotizing vasculitis and pulmonary granulomatosis that attacks the small arteries and veins. Treat the patient with corticosteroids and cyclophosphamide.

○ **What serological test is diagnostic for Wegener granulomatosis?**

Classical antineutrophil cytoplasmic antibody in association with appropriate clinical evidence. A renal, lung, or sinus biopsy also may be helpful in making the diagnosis.

○ **What is the mechanism of alveolar hypoventilation (manifested as high PCO_2) in myxedema?**

Depression of the hypoxic and hypercapnic respiratory drive. Respiratory muscle myopathy and phrenic neuropathy are uncommon.

○ **Should all individuals with chronic unexplained alveolar hypoventilation be tested for hypothyroidism?**

Yes

○ **Is obstructive sleep apnea common in hypothyroidism?**

Yes. Contributing factors include enlarged tongue and myopathy. Hypothyroidism should be excluded in most patients with sleep apnea.

○ **What other endocrine disorder is associated with an increased frequency of sleep apnea?**

Acromegaly. Sleep apnea may be central or obstructive in origin.

○ **What is the most common cause of sleep apnea in adults?**

An upper airway obstruction, generally by the tongue or enlarged tonsils. A medulla that is not responsive to carbon dioxide buildup is the most common cause in children. Obstruction by the tongue or enlarged tonsils also induces sleep apnea in children.

○ **What are the long-term sequelae in untreated obstructive sleep apnea?**

- CHF and pulmonary artery hypertension
- Car accidents due to falling asleep at the wheel

○ **Can β-adrenergic agonists result in tolerance?**

Yes. Repeated administration of β-agonist bronchodilators can result in hyposensitization of the receptors, but this should not preclude their use. Glucocorticoids can restore the depressed receptor responsiveness.

Overuse of β-agonists causes downregulation of receptors, resulting in an increased chance of status asthmaticus no longer responsive to albuterol. This is one of the leading factors suspected in sudden asthma-related death.

○ **Prior steroid administration can precipitate adrenal insufficiency under conditions of stress. How long can this effect last?**

Up to 1 year

○ **What is the common mechanism of hyponatremia in pulmonary tumors and infections?**

Syndrome of inappropriate secretion of antidiuretic hormone

○ **What type of lung cancer commonly is associated with hypercalcemia?**

Squamous cell carcinoma. The production of parathormone-related peptide can produce hypercalcemia even without bony metastases.

○ **Which nonneoplastic pulmonary disease often is associated with hypercalcemia and hypercalciuria?**

Sarcoidosis

○ **What type of lung tumors can cause excessive adrenocorticotropic hormone production and Cushing syndrome?**

Small cell carcinoma and carcinoid tumors

○ **What are the pulmonary manifestations in Paget disease?**

High-output cardiac failure with pulmonary edema, impaired respiratory control from bony involvement at the base of the skull, and vertebral fractures leading to kyphosis and restrictive lung disease

○ **What is acute chest syndrome in sickle cell disease?**

The syndrome includes fever, chest pain, leukocytosis, and pulmonary infiltrate. The major dilemma is in distinguishing infarction from pneumonia. Acute chest syndrome also can be caused by fat embolism and pulmonary edema.

○ **What is sickle cell chronic lung disease?**

It is thought to be the result of years of uncontrolled and often asymptomatic sickling and is characterized by pulmonary hypertension, cor pulmonale, and ventilatory defects.

○ **A 9-year-old African American boy is admitted with chest pain and shortness of breath. His chest radiograph shows bilateral, diffuse hazy infiltrates in a "white-out" pattern. What are the most likely diagnoses?**

- Acute chest syndrome related to sickle cell crisis: Check the complete blood cell count, with peripheral smear to confirm sickling, and follow up with hemoglobin electrophoresis. Administer fluid hydration, pain medication, and oxygen.
- Bilateral acute respiratory distress syndrome (ARDS) related to severe pneumonia. Empiric IV antibiotics also would be appropriate until the diagnosis can be confirmed.

○ **What is the most common cause of pneumonia in sickle cell disease?**

S pneumoniae

○ **What are the most commonly used preventive measures in sickle cell disease?**

Pneumococcal vaccine, *H influenzae* b vaccine, and yearly influenza vaccine in patients with chronic pulmonary symptoms

○ **Which type of pneumonia is often associated with cold agglutinins?**

M pneumoniae

○ **Name some of the hypercoagulable states predisposing individuals to thrombosis and pulmonary embolism.**

Deficiencies of protein C, protein S, and antithrombin III; factor V mutation; antiphospholipid syndrome; malignancy, particularly adenocarcinoma; nephrotic syndrome; protein-losing enteropathy; extensive burns; paroxysmal nocturnal hemoglobinuria; and oral contraceptives; Peripartum; prolonged immobility

○ **What are acceptable methods for preventing pulmonary embolism in hospitalized patients?**

- Thromboembolic disorder hose: For patients who will continue to be mobile
- Sequential compression devices: For patients who will be bed bound
- Subcutaneous heparin: For patients who will be bed bound and unable to tolerate sequential compression devices
- Warfarin: With INR goals between 1.5 and 2.2 for postoperative orthopedic patients

○ **What are the pulmonary manifestations of polycythemia?**

Pulmonary embolism related to hyperviscosity and pulmonary hemorrhage related to an increased bleeding tendency

○ **What is pseudohypoxemia?**

Hypoxemia from consumption of oxygen by cells in blood during transport, as can occur in hyperleukocytosis

○ **Which interstitial lung disease may be associated with diabetes insipidus?**

Eosinophilic granuloma or histiocytosis X

○ **What is the typical time period during which acute radiation pneumonitis develops?**
Within the first 8 weeks after irradiation

○ **What are the factors that increase bleeding complications after transbronchial lung biopsy?**
Renal failure, hemorrhagic diathesis, and lymphoma

○ **An acute chest pain syndrome can occur with which chemotherapeutic agents?**
Methotrexate and bleomycin

○ **What is the earliest radiographic abnormality in bleomycin lung toxicity?**
Bibasilar reticular infiltrates

○ **An unusual manifestation of bleomycin lung toxicity is nodular lesions mimicking pulmonary metastases. What is found pathologically?**
Bronchiolitis obliterans organizing pneumonia

○ **What are 4 distinct manifestations of bleomycin lung toxicity?**
1. Chronic pulmonary fibrosis
2. Hypersensitivity lung reaction
3. Acute pneumonitis
4. Acute chest pain syndrome

○ **What are the risk factors for methotrexate pulmonary toxicity?**
Primary biliary cirrhosis, frequency of administration, adrenalectomy, tapering of corticosteroid therapy, and use in multidrug regimens

○ **What drug will produce hilar and mediastinal adenopathy as a toxic reaction?**
Methotrexate

○ **What is the nature of the lung toxicity associated with the cytokine interleukin-2?**
Massive fluid retention and pulmonary edema

○ **What is the incidence of captopril-induced cough?**
1% to 2%

○ **What is the incidence of enalapril-induced cough?**
24.7%

○ **True/False: Generally, the cough related to ACE inhibitors resolves within a few days after withdrawal of the drug.**

False. Cough resolution may be slow, taking several weeks.

○ **What are 4 syndromes of penicillamine-induced lung toxicity?**
1. Chronic pneumonitis
2. Hypersensitivity lung disease
3. Bronchiolitis obliterans
4. Pulmonary-renal syndrome

○ **What is the incidence of aspirin-induced bronchospasm in patients with nasal polyps?**

As high as 75%

○ **True/False: In aspirin-induced bronchospasm, there can be cross-reactivity with nonsteroidal anti-inflammatory drugs.**

True

○ **What laboratory finding distinguishes primary systemic lupus erythematosus from drug-induced lupus?**

Drug-induced lupus has a positive antinuclear anibody test result but a negative double-stranded DNA test result.

○ **True/False: β-Adrenergic antagonists in massive overdose may cause severe bronchospasm in healthy individuals.**

False

○ **True/False: Cardioselective β-blockers avoid precipitation of bronchospasm in individuals with asthma.**

False

○ **What is the therapeutic drug of choice for β-blocker–induced bronchospasm?**

Inhaled ipratropium bromide. If the bronchospasm is severe, parenteral glucagon can reverse the effects.

○ **Name 4 antibiotics known to have in vitro activity against anaerobic bacteria in virtually all cases.**
1. Metronidazole
2. Chloramphenicol
3. Imipenem
4. β-Lactam/β-lactamase inhibitors

○ **Which gram-negative aerobes are known to cause lung abscess?**

Pseudomonas and *Klebsiella*

○ **What are the 2 major risk factors for the development of anaerobic lung infection?**

1. Periodontal disease

2. Predisposition to aspiration

○ **What is the drug of choice for pneumonias caused by anaerobic bacteria acquired in the outpatient setting?**

Clindamycin

○ **What factor determines the magnitude of injury in gastric acid aspiration?**

Gastric pH. A pH less than 3 produces the most severe injury.

○ **Empyema in the absence of parenchymal lung infiltrate suggests what underlying process?**

Subphrenic or other intraabdominal abscess

○ **What is the incidence of *Bacteroides fragilis* in anaerobic lung infections?**

5% to 7%

○ **What is the recommended duration of antibiotic therapy for necrotizing anaerobic pneumonia, lung abscess, or empyema?**

4 to 8 weeks

○ **Under what circumstances is aspiration of vomitus, oral secretions, or foreign material likely?**

Any situation producing an altered level of consciousness (eg, ethanol, overdose, general anesthesia, stroke), impaired swallowing or abnormal GI motility, or disruption of the esophageal sphincters predisposes a patient to aspiration.

○ **What are the signs of a large obstructing foreign body in the larynx or trachea?**

Respiratory distress, stridor, inability to speak, cyanosis, loss of consciousness, and death

○ **What are the symptoms of a smaller (distally lodged) foreign body?**

Cough, dyspnea, wheezing, chest pain and fever

○ **What is the procedure of choice for foreign body removal?**

Rigid bronchoscopy. Fiber-optic bronchoscopy is an alternate procedure in adults, not in children. If bronchoscopy fails, thoracotomy may be required.

○ **What are the common radiographic findings in foreign body aspiration?**

Normal radiograph, atelectasis, pneumonia, contralateral mediastinal shift (more marked during expiration), and visualization of the foreign body

○ **What are the common directly toxic (noninfected) respiratory tract aspirates?**

Gastric contents, ethanol, hydrocarbons, mineral oil, animal and vegetable fats. All of these produce an inflammatory response and pneumonia. Gastric contents are the most common.

○ **What are the consequences of aspirating acid?**

The response is rapid, with nearly immediate bronchitis, bronchiolitis, atelectasis, shunting, and hypoxemia. Pulmonary edema may occur within 4 hours. The clinical manifestations are dyspnea, wheezing, cough, cyanosis, fever, and shock.

○ **Under what circumstances are antibiotics used in aspiration?**

Aspiration of infected material, intestinal obstruction, immunocompromised host, and evidence of bacterial superinfection after aspiration of a noninfected aspirate (new fever, infiltrates, or purulence after the initial 2 to 3 days)

○ **What are the radiographic manifestations of acid aspiration?**

Varied, may be bilateral diffuse infiltrates, irregular patchy infiltrates, or lobar infiltrates

○ **What outcomes occur in patients who do not rapidly resolve gastric acid aspiration pneumonitis?**

ARDS, progressive respiratory failure and death, bacterial superinfection

○ **What is the most common site of aspiration pneumonitis?**

Right lower lobe

○ **What is the annual US mortality from drowning?**

9000. There are 500 near-drownings for each drowning.

○ **What are the indications for intubation and ventilation after near-drowning?**

Apnea, pulselessness, altered mental status, severe hypoxemia, and respiratory acidosis

○ **What is the frequency of ARDS after near-drowning?**

40%

○ **What are the invasive therapies for massive hemoptysis?**

Thoracotomy, embolization, balloon tamponade (via bronchoscopy), double-lumen tube for lung separation and independent ventilation, and laser bronchoscopy

○ **What is the most feared complication of bronchial artery embolization?**

Anterior spinal artery embolization

○ **What percentage of patients with endobronchial neoplasm and normal chest radiographs present with hemoptysis?**

15%

○ **What is the most common cause of hemoptysis in patients with leukemia?**

Fungal infections, often *Aspergillus*

○ **Which bacterial pneumonias frequently cause frank hemoptysis?**

P aeruginosa, *K pneumoniae*, and *S aureus*

○ **What are the major cardiovascular causes of hemoptysis?**

Mitral stenosis, pulmonary hypertension, and Eisenmenger complex

○ **What is the age-related decrease in PaO_2?**

PaO_2 decreases by 2.5 mm Hg per decade. Given that a PaO_2 of 95 to 100 mm Hg is normal for a 20-year-old person, a PaO_2 of 75 to 80 would be normal for an 80-year-old person.

○ **What are the 4 principal mechanisms that lead to hypoxemia?**

1. Hypoventilation
2. Diffusion limitation
3. Shunt
4. Ventilation-perfusion inequality

A fifth mechanism, low inspired oxygen concentration, is important only at altitudes higher than 8000 feet.

○ **Which of the 4 above mechanisms is the most common?**

Ventilation-perfusion inequality

○ **What are the 3 major mechanisms of hypoventilation and what clinical conditions are associated with each?**

1. Failure of the central nervous system ventilatory centers: Drugs (narcotics, barbiturates) and stroke
2. Failure of the chest bellows: Chest wall diseases (kyphoscoliosis), neuromuscular diseases (amyotrophic lateral sclerosis), and diaphragm weakness
3. Obstruction of the airways: Asthma and COPD

○ **How can hypoxemia secondary to hypoventilation alone be distinguished from the other causes of hypoxemia?**

If the hypoxemia is from hypoventilation alone, the A-a gradient for oxygen is normal. It is elevated in all other causes.

○ **What are the most common clinical conditions in which shunt is the primary mechanism for hypoxemia?**

Alveolar filling with fluid (pulmonary edema) and pus (pneumonia) are the most commonly seen clinically. Any condition that fills or closes the alveoli preventing gas exchange can lead to shunt.

○ **How can shunt be distinguished from the other causes of hypoxemia?**

If administered 100% oxygen, the hypoxemic patient with shunt will not have a significant increase in PaO_2. PaO_2 will increase significantly when 100% oxygen is administered in patients with hypoventilation or ventilation-perfusion inequality.

○ **A leftward shift in the oxyhemoglobin dissociation curve indicates an increased or decreased hemoglobin affinity for oxygen?**

Increased

○ **Changes in temperature, $PaCO_2$ or pH, or the level of 2,3-diphosphoglycerate (2,3-DPG) cause a shift in the oxyhemoglobin dissociation curve. To cause a rightward shift, what are the changes that must occur?**

Increased temperature, increased $PaCO_2$, decreased pH, and increased 2,3-DPG level. An easy way to remember this is that these conditions are often associated with decreased tissue oxygen levels. By shifting the curve right, more oxygen is released from the hemoglobin to the tissues.

○ **What is the Bohr effect?**

The rightward shift of the oxyhemoglobin desaturation curve secondary to decreased pH

○ **Which types of hemoglobin are associated with a leftward shift of the oxyhemoglobin dissociation curve?**

Hemoglobin F (fetal hemoglobin), carboxyhemoglobin, and methemoglobin

○ **Which drugs cause methemoglobinemia?**

Oxidant drugs, such as antimalarial agents, dapsone, nitrites/nitrates (nitroprusside), and local anesthetics (lidocaine). Methemoglobinemia occurs when the iron moiety of hemoglobin is oxidated from the ferrous to the ferric state.

○ **Which common enzyme deficiency predisposes a patient to the development of methemoglobinemia in the presence of the above drugs?**

G-6-PD deficiency

○ **What is the treatment of methemoglobinemia?**

Methylene blue

○ **What are the determinants of the oxygen content of blood?**

Hemoglobin concentration, PaO_2, and SaO_2. The equation to determine the oxygen content of blood is: arterial oxygen concentration $(CaO_2) = (1.34 \times [\text{hemoglobin}] \times SaO_2) + (PaO_2 \times 0.003)$. The first term is the hemoglobin-bound oxygen, and the second is the dissolved oxygen. Dissolved oxygen content is a minor portion of total oxygen content unless PaO_2 is high.

○ **How does the shape of the oxyhemoglobin dissociation curve affect the oxygen content of blood?**

Since SaO_2 does not increase significantly if PaO_2 is greater than 60 mm Hg, the oxygen content of blood will increase significantly above this level only by increasing the hemoglobin concentration.

○ **What are the determinants of oxygen delivery to the peripheral tissues?**

CaO_2 and cardiac output. An increase in either will increase oxygen delivery to the tissues.

○ **What is orthodeoxia?**

A decrease in PaO_2, occurring when the patient moves from the supine to the upright position

○ **What is the difference between anatomic and physiologic dead space?**

"Dead space" refers to areas of lung that are ventilated but not perfused. Anatomic dead space refers to the conducting airways (trachea, bronchi, and bronchioles) where there is no gas exchange because there are no alveoli. Physiologic dead space includes the anatomic dead space and any diseased lung in which there is ventilation but no perfusion.

○ **What is the normal dead space in an average 70-kg subject?**

150 mL

○ **Which pulmonary diseases are most associated with an increased physiologic dead space?**

Asthma and COPD

○ **How is the minute ventilation (V_E) related to alveolar and dead space ventilation (V_D)?**

V_E is the product of tidal volume (V_T) multiplied by breathing frequency ($V_E = V_T \times f$). Alveolar ventilation (V_A) is that portion of the V_E that contributes to gas exchange, whereas V_D is the portion that does not contribute to gas exchange. Thus, $V_E = V_A + V_D$.

○ **What is the effect of increased V_A on $PaCO_2$?**

$PaCO_2$ will decrease as V_A increases.

○ **What is the relationship between V_A, V_E, and the dead space ratio (V_D/V_T)?**

V_A is proportional to both V_E and the term ($1-V_D/V_T$). Any process that decreases V_E or increases the dead space will decrease V_A.

○ **Why do persons with asthma eventually have increased $PaCO_2$ if untreated?**

As an asthma attack continues untreated, the work of breathing will continue to increase. Eventually, the diaphragm fatigues, and the patient hypoventilates. The hypoventilation, in association with the increased dead space and increased carbon dioxide production, increases the $PaCO_2$.

○ **What is the normal $PaCO_2$, and does it vary with age?**

Normal $PaCO_2$ is 35 to 45 mm Hg and does not vary with age.

○ **What is the Haldane effect?**

A decrease in carbon dioxide content with increases in hemoglobin oxygen saturation

○   **What is the normal expected change in pH if there is an acute change in the $PaCO_2$?**

The pH will increase or decrease 0.8 units for every 10 mm Hg decrease or increase in $PaCO_2$.

○   **What is the expected change in serum bicarbonate in chronic respiratory acidosis or alkalosis?**

Bicarbonate increases by approximately 3 mEq/L for each 10 mm Hg increase in $PaCO_2$ in chronic respiratory acidosis. Bicarbonate decreases by 4 to 5 mEq/L for each decrease of 10 mm Hg in $PaCO_2$ in chronic respiratory alkalosis.

○   **What is respiratory alkalosis?**

A pH above 7.45 and a PCO_2 less than 35. Alkalosis shifts the oxygen dissociation curve to the left. It also causes cerebrovascular constriction. The kidneys compensate for respiratory alkalosis by excreting bicarbonate.

○   **What are some common causes of respiratory alkalosis?**

Common causes of respiratory alkalosis include any process that may induce hyperventilation: shock, sepsis, trauma, asthma, pulmonary embolism, anemia, hepatic failure, heatstroke, exhaustion, emotion, salicylate poisoning, hypoxemia, pregnancy, and inadequate mechanical ventilation.

○   **What are the consequences of hypercapnia?**

Acute hypercapnia has physiologic consequences due to the increased $PaCO_2$ itself and the decreased pH. Physiologic effects of the $PaCO_2$ increase include:

- Increases in cerebral blood flow
- Confusion, headache ($PaCO_2 > 60$ mm Hg), obtundation, and seizures ($PaCO_2 > 70$ mm Hg)
- Depression of diaphragmatic contractility

The primary consequences of the decreased pH are on the cardiovascular system, with decreased cardiac contractility, decreased fibrillation threshold, and changes in vascular tone (predominantly vasodilatation).

○   **What are the consequences of hypocapnia?**

Acute hypocapnia has physiologic consequences due to the decreased $PaCO_2$ itself and the increased pH. Physiologic effects of the $PaCO_2$ decrease include:

- Decreases in cerebral blood flow. This reflex is used in the management of neurologic disorders with high intracranial pressures as a short-term measure to decrease the increased intracranial pressure.
- Confusion, myoclonus, asterixis, loss of consciousness, and seizures

The primary consequences of the increased pH are, again, primarily on the cardiovascular system, with increased cardiac contractility and vasodilatation.

○   **A 25-year-old man presents to the emergency department obtunded. Examination results indicate a respiratory rate of 8 breaths per minute and pinpoint pupils. An arterial blood gas test reveals a pH of 7.28, a $PaCO_2$ of 55, and a PaO_2 of 60. What is a likely cause of the hypoxemia and hypercapnia?**

Acute narcotic overdose leading to hypoventilation. Administer naloxone hydrochloride.

○ **Chest radiography reveals no pulmonary parenchymal lesions but shows prominent hila and an enlarged right ventricle. What diagnostic test should be performed?**

The patient has no pulmonary parenchymal lesions to cause a shunt; therefore, the patient most likely has an intracardiac right-to-left shunt (probably a previously undiagnosed atrial septal defect). Echocardiography should be performed.

○ **A 45-year-old obese man presents with dyspnea, peripheral edema, snoring, and excessive daytime sleepiness. A room air arterial blood gas test is performed, and the pH is 7.34, the $PaCO_2$ is 60 mm Hg, the PaO_2 is 58 mm Hg, and the calculated bicarbonate level is 28 mEq/L. What is the acid-base disturbance?**

Chronic, compensated respiratory acidosis. If this were acute respiratory acidosis, the pH would be 7.24, with a normal bicarbonate level.

○ **What is the cause of the hypoxemia?**

Hypoventilation is one cause. However, since the A-a gradient for oxygen is elevated, there is another cause in addition to the hypoventilation. In an obese patient, both ventilation-perfusion inequality and shunt (secondary to atelectasis) can contribute to the development of hypoxemia.

○ **A 50-year-old woman presents with pneumonia in the right lower and middle lobes. While receiving 50% oxygen by face mask, her PaO_2 is 75 mm Hg. Should the patient be positioned right side down or up?**

Up. Blood flow is gravity dependent. If the patient is positioned right side down, blood flow will preferentially go to the right side. However, because of the pneumonia, this will increase the amount of shunt, lowering the PaO_2 further.

○ **True/False: If a patient presents with a $PaCO_2$ of 75 mm Hg, he or she should undergo immediate intubation.**

False. There is no $PaCO_2$ level at which a patient must undergo intubation. Intubation is based on the total clinical condition of a patient, not just a blood gas test result.

○ **A 45-year-old man presents to the emergency department after being rescued from a fire. He is dyspneic and cyanotic. Sao_2 while receiving 50% oxygen by face mask is 84%. The blood gas results, however, reveal a PaO_2 of 125 mm Hg. Why is there a discrepancy?**

A fire survivor is likely to have carbon monoxide poisoning. The carbon monoxide has converted the hemoglobin to carboxyhemoglobin, which decreases the binding of oxygen to hemoglobin and prevents an accurate pulse oximetry reading. However, carbon monoxide does not affect dissolved oxygen, which is what is measured in the arterial blood gas.

○ **What is the treatment for carbon monoxide poisoning?**

100% oxygen, which increases carbon monoxide clearance by competing for binding to hemoglobin. If there is no significant response to 100% oxygen, oxygen provided at higher than atmospheric pressure (hyperbaric oxygen) is an alternative therapy.

○ **A 25-year-old woman with a history of mitral valve prolapse presents with nervousness, chest tightness, hand numbness, and mild confusion. Arterial blood gas results are as follows: pH, 7.52; $PaCO_2$, 25 mm Hg; and PaO_2, 108 mm Hg. What is the diagnosis?**

Acute anxiety attack. She is hyperventilating.

○ **Why is the PaO$_2$ elevated?**

Because the lower PaCO$_2$ means a higher PAO$_2$ (see alveolar gas equation above)

○ **What is the treatment?**

The acute hyperventilation can be terminated by having the patient breathe in and out of a bag. Anxiolytic agents can also be provided.

○ **True/False: Oxygen should never be administered in a hypoxemic patient with COPD who has chronic carbon dioxide retention.**

False. Oxygen should always be administered in a patient who is hypoxemic.

○ **What is the major adverse effect associated with the inhalation of N-acetylcysteine?**

Cough and bronchospasm, most likely due to irritation from the low pH (2.2) of the aerosol solution

○ **What is the effect of macrolide antibiotics (erythromycin, clarithromycin) on mucus hypersecretion?**

Some macrolide antibiotics have the ability to downregulate mucus secretion by means of an unknown mechanism. This is thought to be due to anti-inflammatory activity.

○ **Exposure to what mineral, used as insulation, greatly enhances the carcinogenic potential of exposure to cigarette smoke?**

Asbestos

○ **What other exposures are also factors contributing to the development of bronchogenic carcinoma?**

Radon, uranium, nickel, arsenic, bis(chloromethyl) ether, ionizing radiation, vinyl chloride, mustard gas, polycyclic aromatic hydrocarbons, and chromium

○ **Secondhand cigarette smoke exposure is a risk factor for the development of what 2 major lung diseases?**

1. Lung cancer
2. COPD

○ **Which primary lung cancer is most frequently associated with paraneoplastic syndromes?**

Small cell undifferentiated carcinoma

○ **The incidence of lung cancer is increasing in the United States among members of which sex?**

Women

○ **What accounts for this increase?**

Increased prevalence of cigarette smoking

○ **Which vitamin has been associated with a protective effect against the development of lung cancer?**

Vitamin A

○ **Bilateral periostitis, typically affecting the long bones and associated with lung cancer, is known as what other disease?**

Hypertrophic osteoarthropathy

○ **This finding is most frequently associated with which type of lung cancer?**

Adenocarcinoma

○ **What myopathic syndrome is associated with lung cancer?**

Eaton-Lambert syndrome

○ **What finding at physical examination can be used to differentiate Eaton-Lambert syndrome from myasthenia gravis?**

Muscle function improves with repeated activity in Eaton-Lambert syndrome but degrades in myasthenia gravis.

○ **Tumor involvement in which lymph node location most clearly contraindicates a surgical approach to the therapy of non-small cell lung cancer: hilar, contralateral mediastinal, infrapulmonary, or subcarinal?**

Contralateral mediastinal

○ **Of the following, which pattern of calcification of a solitary pulmonary nodule is most likely to be associated with a malignant lesion: lamellar (onion skin), popcorn, eccentric, or central?**

Eccentric

○ **For a new solitary pulmonary nodule, how often should follow-up chest radiography or computed tomography be performed to evaluate for possible growth?**

Every 3 to 6 months until radiographic stability can be established

○ **Radiographic stability for what period is assumed to indicate benign origin of a solitary pulmonary nodule?**

2 years

○ **What is the initial diagnostic test in a clinically stable patient suspected of having lung cancer?**

Sputum cytologic examination

○ **What finding indicates emergent radiation therapy for superior vena cava syndrome?**

Cerebral edema

○ **What is the major indication for laser bronchoscopy in the treatment of bronchogenic carcinoma?**

Tumor obstruction of large airways

○ **Which of the following is the preferred method for predicting postoperative FEV₁ in patients whose preoperative FEV₁ is less than 2 liters: quantitative perfusion lung scanning, quantitative ventilation lung scanning, split-lung function with use of a Carlens tube, or the lateral position test?**

Quantitative perfusion lung scanning

○ **What is the 5-year survival of all patients with a diagnosis of primary lung cancer?**

Less than 15%

○ **Which primary lung cancer is most likely to cavitate?**

Squamous cell carcinoma

○ **The best 5-year survival for non-small cell carcinoma of the lung is achieved by use of what therapy?**

Surgical resection

○ **The increase in death rate from lung cancer among smokers, as opposed to nonsmokers, is how high?**

8- to 20-fold

○ **Do low-tar cigarettes decrease the risk of lung cancer?**

No

○ **The risk of lung cancer after smoking cessation approaches that of lifelong nonsmokers after how many years?**

15 years

○ **The incidence of lung cancer among urban residents is how many times higher than that among rural residents?**

About 1.5 times higher among urban residents

○ **The most common malignancy associated with asbestos exposure is which of the following: esophageal carcinoma, primary lung cancer, mesothelioma, or gastric carcinoma?**

Primary lung cancer

○ **A solitary pulmonary nodule in an HIV-infected patient may represent which of the following: PCP, histoplasmosis, cryptococcosis, or bronchogenic carcinoma?**

All of the above

○ **What happens to V_E at submaximal work rates in interstitial lung disease?**

V_E increases due to increased V_D. Respiratory rate increases, and V_T decreases.

○ **What is the incidence of postoperative respiratory complications in patients with COPD?**

50% or more

○ **Is cessation of smoking 24 hours preoperatively beneficial?**

Yes. It reduces pulse, blood pressure, and carboxyhemoglobin level.

○ **What medications are available to assist patients with smoking cessation?**

Nicotine replacement, such as patches, gums, and lozenges, are available without a prescription.

Nicotine replacement with an inhaler is available by prescription for patients who struggle more with the oral fixation.

Bupropion is an antidepressant effective in decreasing the severity of cravings during smoking cessation.

Varenicline is a medication that blocks the nicotine receptors in the brain, thus blocking the release of dopamine associated with pleasure from smoking and working at the neurologic receptors related to addiction.

○ **Which neuromuscular and spinal diseases can lead to ventilatory insufficiency?**

Muscular dystrophy, polymyositis, myotonic dystrophy, polyneuritis, Eaton-Lambert syndrome, myasthenia gravis, amyotrophic lateral sclerosis, injury, Guillain-Barré syndrome, multiple sclerosis, Parkinson disease, and stroke

○ **Adequacy of alveolar ventilation is reflected by which component of arterial blood gas analysis?**

$PaCO_2$

○ **Patients receiving mechanical ventilation can develop hypoventilation on the basis of what factors?**

Increased dead space (including length of ventilator circuit proximal to the Y piece separating the inspiratory and expiratory limbs), decreased V_T, overdistension of lung, air leaks, and massive pulmonary embolism

○ **What is the principal mechanism of increased $PaCO_2$ with increased FIO_2?**

Worsening ventilation-perfusion mismatch and the Haldane effect

○ **How does malnutrition contribute to respiratory failure?**

Increase in the oxygen cost of breathing and respiratory muscle weakness

○ **What conditions or commonly used medications result in an increase in serum theophylline concentration?**

Cimetidine, macrolides, quinolones, verapamil, fever, CHF, and liver failure

○ **How can the work of breathing with mechanical ventilation associated with intrinsic positive end-expiratory pressure (PEEP) be reduced?**

Add continuous positive airway pressure, reduce V_T, reduce inspiratory time, and increase expiratory time

○ **Through what mechanism does PEEP decrease cardiac output?**

Reduced preload

○ **Through what mechanism does positive pressure ventilation increase cardiac output?**

Decreased afterload

○ **How can compliance of the lung/chest wall be approximated from airway pressure measurements during mechanical ventilation?**

Compliance = V_T/(inspiratory plateau pressure − end-expiratory pressure)

○ **What evidence of barotrauma can be observed at chest radiography?**

Pneumomediastinum, pneumothorax, pneumopericardium, subcutaneous emphysema, and pulmonary interstitial emphysema

○ **What are the primary determinants of the work of breathing?**

V_E, lung/chest wall compliance, and intrinsic PEEP

○ **How is oxygen delivery calculated?**

Cardiac output × arterial blood oxygen content

○ **What is the primary determinant of the oxygen content of arterial blood?**

The product of hemoglobin concentration and the percentage of hemoglobin oxygen saturation of arterial blood. The amount of oxygen dissolved in the plasma (a function of the PaO_2) is negligible at 1 atm of pressure

○ **What is the maximum acceptable endotracheal tube cuff pressure?**

Approximately 26 cm of water at the end of expiration

○ **What is the potential harm of excess endotracheal tube cuff pressure?**

Excess pressure can induce ischemia and necrosis of the underlying tissue, resulting in tracheomalacia and tracheal stenosis

○ **What is bronchiectasis?**

Bronchiectasis is an abnormal dilatation of the proximal medium-sized bronchi greater than 2 mm in diameter. It is due to the destruction of the muscular and elastic components of their walls, usually associated with chronic bacterial infection and foul-smelling sputum.

○ **Which lung segments are most frequently involved in bronchiectasis?**

Posterior basal segments of the left or right lower lobes

○ **What are the most common causes of upper lobe bronchiectasis?**

TB endobronchitis and ABPA

○ **What physiologic and anatomic alterations have been described in patients with bronchiectasis?**

Impaired tracheobronchial clearance, enlargement of the bronchial arteries and extensive anastomosis between these vessels and the pulmonary arteries, diminished total pulmonary arterial blood flow, functional decrease in the cross-sectional area of the pulmonary vasculature with hypoxia, left-to-right intrapulmonary shunting, and decreased ventilation of bronchographically abnormal areas

○ **What are the symptoms of bronchiectasis?**

Chronic cough, purulent sputum, fever, weakness, weight loss, dyspnea in some patients, and hemoptysis. Hemoptysis is generally mild, originates from bronchial arteries, and is not a common cause of death (<10% of deaths attributed to hemoptysis).

○ **What are the most common complications of bronchiectasis?**

Recurrent attacks of pneumonia, empyema, pneumothorax, and lung abscess

○ **What are the radiographic findings in bronchiectasis?**

• Cylindrical bronchiectasis: Tram tracking thin parallel linear radiolucencies radiating from the hila
• Varicose bronchiectasis: Thick parallel shadows
• Cystic bronchiectasis: Isolated or clustered cystic spaces with air-fluid levels

○ **What laboratory investigations aid in the evaluation of idiopathic bronchiectasis?**

• Serum protein electrophoresis to rule out α1-antitrypsin deficiency
• Ig levels with IgG subclass
• Pilocarpine iontophoresis sweat test
• Serum precipitins for *Aspergillus*
• Electron microscopic examination of sperm or respiratory epithelium for primary ciliary dyskinesia

○ **What is the mainstay of treatment for bronchiectasis?**

Antibiotics

○ **What adjunctive treatment measures may be beneficial in patients with bronchiectasis?**

Chest physiotherapy, nutritional support, inhaled indomethacin bronchodilators (shown to decrease bronchial hypersecretion by inhibiting neutrophil recruitment), supplemental oxygen, Ig administration for Ig deficiency, replacement treatment for patients with α1-antitrypsin deficiency, and recombinant DNAase to reduce sputum viscosity in patients with cystic fibrosis

○ **What is Kartagener syndrome?**

Triad of the following: (1) situs inversus, (2) bronchiectasis, and (3) nasal polyps or recurrent sinusitis

○ **What are the possible manifestations of α1-antitrypsin deficiency?**

Panlobular emphysema, bronchiectasis, and hepatic cirrhosis

○ **Cystic fibrosis is confined predominantly to what part of the lung?**

The conducting airways

○ **Why are patients with advanced cystic fibrosis at an increased risk for pneumothorax?**

Subpleural cysts often occur on the mediastinal surfaces of the upper lobes and are thought to contribute to pneumothorax in patients with advanced disease.

○ **What is the most common site of nonpulmonary disease in cystic fibrosis?**

The GI tract, with striking changes seen in the exocrine pancreas. The islets of Langerhans are spared.

○ **What are the reproductive abnormalities in cystic fibrosis?**

In men, the vas deferens, the tail and body of the epididymis, and the seminal vesicles are either absent or rudimentary. In women, the uterine cervical glands are distended, and the mucous and cervical canals are plugged with tenacious mucus secretions. Endocervicitis also is seen.

○ **What are the most frequent respiratory pathogens in patients with cystic fibrosis?**

S aureus and *P aeruginosa*

○ **What are the immunologic defects in cystic fibrosis?**

Patients with cystic fibrosis have low levels of serum IgG in the first decade of life, but these levels increase dramatically once chronic infection is established. T-lymphocyte numbers are adequate. With advancing severity of pulmonary disease, lymphocytes in patients with cystic fibrosis proliferate less briskly in response to *P aeruginosa* and other gram-negative organisms. Deficient opsonic activity of alveolar macrophages is seen in patients with established *P aeruginosa* infection. The major Ig subclass in serum and lungs in patients with cystic fibrosis is IgG.

○ **At radiography, where are the earliest and most severe changes seen?**

Right upper lobe

○ **What are the various radiographic manifestations of cystic fibrosis?**

Hyperinflation, peribronchial cuffing, mucous impaction in airways seen as branching fingerlike shadows, bronchiectasis, subpleural blebs (most prominent along the mediastinal border), and prominent pulmonary artery segments with advanced disease.

○ **What is the immediate mortality with massive hemoptysis?**

Approximately 10%

○ **What are the diagnostic criteria for cystic fibrosis?**

Primary criteria
- Characteristic pulmonary manifestations and/or
- Characteristic GI manifestations and/or
- A family history of cystic fibrosis

Plus
- Sweat chloride concentration greater than 60 mEq/L (repeat measurement if 50–60 mEq/L)

Secondary criteria
- Documentation of dual cystic fibrosis transmembrane conductance regulator mutations and
- Evidence of 1 or more characteristic manifestations

○ **What are the conditions associated with an elevated level of sweat chloride?**

Cystic fibrosis, hypothyroidism, pseudohypoaldosteronism, hypoparathyroidism, nephrogenic diabetes insipidus, type I glycogen storage disease, mucopolysaccharidosis, malnutrition, prostaglandin E administration, hypogammaglobulinemia, and pancreatitis

○ **What test is recognized by the Cystic Fibrosis Foundation as the definitive diagnostic test for cystic fibrosis?**

Collection of sweat (at least 50 mg in 45 minutes) by means of pilocarpine iontophoresis, coupled with chemical determination of the chloride concentration (>60 mEq/L in children, >80 mEq/L in adults).

○ **What is the effect of nutritional supplementation on cystic fibrosis?**

Patients with adequate nutrition experience a slower rate of decline of lung function

○ **How do you manage the pulmonary complications of cystic fibrosis?**

Pulmonary Complication	Management
Right-sided heart failure	Improve oxygenation through intensive pulmonary therapy
Respiratory failure	Vigorous medical therapy of the underlying lung disease and infection
Atelectasis	Aggressive antibiotic therapy and frequent chest physiotherapy
Pneumothorax	Conservative if less than 10% and patient is asymptomatic; pleurodesis to avoid recurrence
Small-volume hemoptysis	Aggressive treatment of lung infection
Persistent massive hemoptysis	Bronchial artery embolization, along with aggressive treatment of the lung infection

○ **What is the life expectancy of a patient with cystic fibrosis?**

Fifty percent of patients survive to age 28 to 30 years.

○ **Stridor is observed in what phase of respiration?**

Inspiratory

○ **What is stridor caused by?**

With extrathoracic airway obstruction, the pressure inside the extrathoracic part of the airway is negative relative to atmospheric pressure. This results in further narrowing of the larynx during inspiration and, therefore, stridor.

○ **Grunting is observed during what phase of respiration?**

Expiratory—exhalation against a closed glottis.

○ **What is the most common organism isolated from patients with bacterial tracheitis?**

S aureus

○ **How do retropharyngeal abscesses arise?**

Lymphatic spread of infections in the nasopharynx, oropharynx, or external auditory canal

○ **What is the most common type of tracheoesophageal fistula?**

Blind esophageal pouch with a fistulous connection of the trachea to the distal esophagus

○ **What is the narrowest part of the adult airway?**

The glottic opening

○ **A 24-year-old woman has a high fever, hoarseness, and increased stridor of 3 hours' duration. She also has a sore throat. Examination results show an ill-appearing woman with a temperature of 40°C, inspiratory stridor, drooling, and mild intercostal retractions. She prefers to sit up. The most likely diagnosis is:**

Epiglottitis

○ **In the diagnosis of a radiolucent foreign body lodged in the right mainstem bronchus, producing incomplete obstruction, inspiratory and expiratory radiographs show air trapping and increased lucency of the lung on the involved side. This phenomenon is due to:**

Ball-valve air trapping. Air enters around the foreign body during inspiration but is trapped as the airway closes around the foreign body during expiration, preventing emptying of that side.

○ **What are some clinical disorders associated with increased capillary permeability causing exudative pleural effusion?**

Pleuropulmonary infections, circulating toxins, systemic lupus erythematosus, rheumatoid arthritis, sarcoidosis, tumor, pulmonary infarction, and viral hepatitis

○ **What are the clinical features associated with pleural effusion?**

A pleural rub (may be the only finding in the early stages), pleuritic chest pain due to involvement and inflammation of parietal pleura, cough (distortion of lung), dyspnea (mechanical inefficiency of respiratory muscles stretched by outward movement of the chest wall and downward movement of the diaphragm), diminished chest wall movements, dull percussion, decreased tactile and vocal fremitus, decreased breath sounds, and whispered pectoriloquy. With large amounts of pleural effusion, there may be contralateral shift of the mediastinum.

○ **What is the minimum amount of pleural liquid that can be detected radiographically?**

Approximately 400 mL in upright views of the chest. A lateral decubitus radiograph obtained with the patient lying on the affected side can depict as little as 50 mL of liquid.

○ **What is the most common cause of exudative effusion?**

Parapneumonic effusion is the most common cause of exudative effusion.

○ **What are the indications for chest tube placement in parapneumonic effusion?**

A complicated parapneumonic effusion, as evidenced by fever, loculations, gross appearance of purulent fluid (pus), increased white blood cell count and low glucose level (usually <40 mg/dL), decreased pH (<7.0, or 0.15 less than the arterial pH), and elevated LDH (>1000 U/L), are usually considered indications for placement of a chest tube for drainage.

○ **What is the most common cause of transudative pleural effusions?**

CHF

○ **What are the common features of pleural effusions associated with CHF?**

Bilateral effusion, more commonly right sided, associated with cardiomegaly. Fluid is serous transudate, there are fewer than 1000 mononuclear cells, pH is greater than 7.4, and pleural fluid glucose levels are the same as those for serum.

○ **What are the radiographic features of pleural effusion associated with cirrhosis?**

They are small to massive right-sided effusion in 70%, left-sided effusion in 15%, and bilateral effusion in 15%, with normal heart size.

○ **What mechanism of atelectasis is associated with pleural effusion?**

Atelectasis leads to decreased perimicrovascular pressure, resulting in a pressure gradient. Fluid moves from the parietal pleural interstitium into the pleural space because of decreased perimicrovascular pressure.

○ **What is the incidence of pleural effusion associated with nephrotic syndrome?**

Approximately 20%

○ **What is the primary mechanism of pleural effusion in nephrotic syndrome?**

Decreased plasma oncotic pressure due to hypoalbuminemia

○ **What is the incidence of pleural effusion associated with malignancy?**

Malignant pleural effusions are the second most common exudative effusions after parapneumonic effusions. The most common malignancies are lung and breast cancers.

○ **What are the conditions associated with malignant transudative effusions?**

Lymphatic obstruction, endobronchial obstruction, and hypoalbuminemia due to the primary malignancy

○ **What types of effusions are suggestive of malignancy?**

Massive effusions, large effusions without contralateral mediastinal shift, or bilateral effusions with normal heart size suggest malignancy.

○ **What type of pleural effusion is associated with malignant mesothelioma?**

Large unilateral effusions. Contralateral pleural plaques are present in 20% of cases. Loculated pleural masses may be evident after thoracentesis.

○ **What factors play a role in the pathogenesis of pleural effusions associated with pulmonary embolism?**

Effusions are present in 40% to 50% of cases of pulmonary embolism. Increased capillary permeability due to ischemia and leak of protein-rich fluid into the pleural space are the main factors. Atelectasis may contribute to transudate, and lung necrosis can lead to hemorrhage.

○ **What are the characteristics of a pleural effusion associated with chronic pancreatitis?**

Pleural effusions associated with chronic pancreatitis are usually large or massive unilateral effusions that develop rapidly after thoracentesis. The pleural fluid can have high amylase content (>200,000 U/L). Direct fistulous communications from the pancreatic bed are responsible. Failure of conservative treatment is an indication for surgical intervention, such as drainage, in as many as 50% of cases.

○ **What is the incidence of pleural involvement in systemic lupus erythematosus?**

Fifty percent to 75% of patients with systemic lupus erythematosus develop pleural effusion or pleuritic pain during the course of the disease.

○ **What are the clinical features of lupus pleuritis?**

Pleuritic chest pain is the most common manifestation. Other features are cough, dyspnea, pleural rub, and fever. An episode of pleuritis usually indicates exacerbation of lupus.

○ **What are the radiographic features of lupus pleuritis?**

Small to moderate bilateral effusions are most common. Unilateral and massive effusions can occur. Other radiographic abnormalities such as alveolar infiltrates, atelectasis, and increasing cardiac silhouette can occur.

○ **What are the characteristic features of pleural fluid in patients with lupus?**

Lupus erythematosus cells in the pleural fluid. A ratio of pleural fluid to serum antinuclear anibody that is greater than 1.0 is suggestive of lupus.

○ **What kind of pleural effusion is associated with lymphangiomyomatosis?**

Chylothorax

○ **What are some drugs reported to be associated with pleural effusion?**

Procainamide, nitrofurantoin, dantrolene, methysergide, procarbazine, methotrexate, amiodarone, mitomycin, and bleomycin

○ **When may end-tidal carbon dioxide detectors be inaccurate?**

In patients with low blood flow to the lungs, or in those with a large dead space (ie, after a pulmonary embolism)

○ **What is the most common complication of endotracheal intubation?**

Intubation of a bronchus. Other complications include lacerations of the lip, tongue, or pharyngeal or tracheal mucosa, resulting in bleeding, hematoma, or abscess. Tracheal rupture, avulsion of an arytenoid cartilage, vocal cord injury, pharyngeal-esophageal perforation, intubation of the pyriform sinus, aspiration of vomitus, hypertension, tachycardia, or arrhythmias can also occur.

○ **What oxygen concentration will be supplied by a nasal cannula with a flow rate of 1 L/min?**

24%. For each 1 L/min increase in flow, a 4% increase in oxygen concentration will occur; 6 L/min produces a 44% oxygen concentration.

○ **What oxygen flow rate is recommended for face mask ventilation?**

At least 5 L/min. Recommended flow is 8 to 10 L/min, which will produce oxygen concentrations as high as 40% to 60%.

○ **What oxygen concentration can be supplied with a face mask and oxygen reservoir?**

6 L/min provides approximately 60% oxygen concentration, and each liter increases the concentration by 10%; 10 L/min is almost 100%.

○ **You are at a restaurant and the person at the table next to you begins coughing loudly. She stands up and begins wheezing between coughs, but she is still able to say "Help! I'm choking!" How should you help?**

Encourage her to cough deeper and keep breathing. Do not interrupt her spontaneous attempts at expulsion if she still has good air exchange, as evidenced by her state of consciousness and the degree of coughing and wheezing. If she displays severe respiratory difficulty with a weakening cough and the inability to talk, perform the Heimlich maneuver.

○ **What should be done if the above patient is markedly obese and in severe respiratory distress?**

The normal Heimlich maneuver will not be as effective. Instead of positioning your fists above the patient's navel, place your cupped fist on the patient's chest and deliver swift thrusts. This is also the method of choice for pregnant women.

○ **What is Virchow triad?**

1. Injury to the endothelium of the vessels
2. Hypercoagulable state
3. Stasis

These represent risk factors for pulmonary embolus.

○ **What does normal ventilation with decreased lung perfusion suggest?**

Pulmonary embolus

○ **What are the most common signs and symptoms of pulmonary embolism?**

Tachypnea (92%), chest pain (88%), dyspnea (84%), anxiety (59%), tachycardia (44%), fever (43%), deep vein thrombosis (32%), hypotension (25%), and syncope (13%)

○ **Can a patient with a pulmonary embolism have a pO₂ greater than 90 mm Hg?**

Yes, but rarely (5%)

○ **What is the most common chest radiographic finding in pulmonary embolism?**

Elevated dome of 1 hemidiaphragm. This elevation is caused by decreased lung volume, which occurs in 50% of patients with pulmonary embolism. Other common findings include a lack of lung markings in the area perfused by the occluded artery, pleural effusions, atelectasis, and pulmonary infiltrates.

○ **What are 2 relatively specific chest radiographic findings in pulmonary embolism?**

1. Hampton hump: Area of lung consolidation with a rounded border facing the hilus
2. Westermark sign: Dilated pulmonary outflow tract proximal to the emboli, with decreased perfusion distal to the lesion

○ **What test is considered the reference standard for the diagnosis of deep vein thrombosis? For the diagnosis of pulmonary embolism?**

- Deep vein thrombosis: Venography
- Pulmonary embolism: Pulmonary angiography

○ **When treating deep vein thrombosis or pulmonary embolism, when should warfarin therapy be initiated?**

On the first or second day after initiation of heparin therapy. Although heparin should be administered immediately, it can be discontinued when the partial thromboplastin time is 1.5 to 1.8 times normal for at least 3 days.

○ **How long should long-term warfarin therapy be administered as prophylaxis for deep vein thrombosis?**

Warfarin should be administered for at least 3 to 6 months after deep vein thrombosis develops to maintain an INR at 2 to 3 times the normal.

○ **What historical findings suggest embolus, as opposed to thrombosis, in a lower extremity?**

- Embolus: Associated with a history of arrhythmia, valvular disease, myocardial infarction, no skin changes from chronic arterial insufficiency, and no symptoms in the opposite extremity
- Thrombosis: Opposite extremity shows evidence of chronic arterial occlusive disease with history of rest pain and claudication.

○ **How is a thrombus distinguished from an embolus on an arteriogram?**

A thrombus appears as a tapering lumen. An embolus has a sharp cutoff.

○ **What is the risk factor for pulmonary embolism in a patient with an axillary or subclavian vein thrombus?**

About 15%

○ **At what percentage of an airway obstruction will inspiratory stridor become evident?**

70% occlusion

○ **What is the initial treatment for tension pneumothorax?**

Large-bore IV catheter placed in the anterior second intercostal space (not a chest tube)

○ **What is the most important cause of hypoxia in a patient with flail chest?**

Underlying lung contusion

○ **How much fluid must collect in the chest to be detected on a decubitus or upright chest radiograph?**

200 to 300 mL. If the patient is supine, more than 1 L may be necessary to be seen on an anteroposterior chest radiograph.

○ **A foreign body is suspected in the lower airways. What will plain radiographs show?**

Air trapping on the affected side. Inspiration and expiration views demonstrate mediastinal shift away from the affected side.

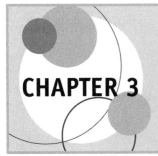

CHAPTER 3   Gastrointestinal

Joe Guidi, DO

○ **A patient states that food sticks in the middle of his chest and then is regurgitated as a putrid, undigested mess. Results from a barium study show a dilated esophagus with a distal "beak." What is the diagnosis?**

Achalasia

○ **What is achalasia?**

Disorder of esophageal motility and incomplete relaxation of the lower esophagus

○ **What is the reference standard for diagnosing achalasia?**

Esophageal manometry

○ **What are the possible findings of an upper gastrointestinal (GI) series in a woman with telangiectasias, tight knuckles, and acid indigestion?**

Aperistalsis, which is characteristic of scleroderma

○ **What is the typical profile of a patient with anorexia nervosa?**

Female, adolescent, upper class, perfectionist

○ **Name some common conditions that mimic acute appendicitis.**

Mesenteric lymphadenitis, pelvic inflammatory disease, mittelschmerz, gastroenteritis, Crohn disease, Meckel diverticulum, and cecal diverticulitis

○ **What are the most frequent symptoms of acute appendicitis in adults?**

Anorexia and abdominal pain. The classic manifestation of anorexia and periumbilical pain with progression to constant right lower quadrant (RLQ) pain is present in only 50% of cases. In children younger than 13 years, pain and vomiting are the 2 most common presenting symptoms.

○ **What percentage of patients with acute appendicitis have an elevated white blood cell (WBC) count?**

An elevated leukocyte count (>10,000 cells/μL) and an elevated absolute neutrophil count are present in 90% of patients; however, up to 60% of patients presenting with abdominal pain and leukocytosis have a noninflamed appendix at pathology examination. In addition, approximately 65% of patients with a perforated appendix do not present with leukocytosis. In children, either the WBC or neutrophil levels are elevated in 96% of patients with appendicitis, though leukocytosis is a nonspecific finding in children with abdominal pain.

○ **Until discounted as a cause, what intraabdominal disease should be assumed for a pregnant woman with right upper quadrant (RUQ) pain?**

Acute appendicitis

○ **Rovsing, psoas, and obturator signs can all indicate an inflamed posterior appendix. Describe these signs.**

- Rovsing sign: RLQ pain with palpation over the left lower quadrant
- Psoas sign: RLQ pain with right thigh extension
- Obturator sign: RLQ pain with internal rotation of the flexed right thigh

○ **How is the diagnosis of Barrett's esophagitis made?**

1. Endoscopic documentation identifying both the squamocolumnar and gastroesophageal junctions of columnar epithelium lining the distal esophagus

2. Histologic confirmation that the columnar epithelium demonstrates specialized intestinal metaplasia

○ **What are frequent complications of Barrett esophagitis?**

Esophageal stricture, ulceration, and hemorrhage

○ **Barrett esophagitis is associated with which type of cancer?**

Esophageal adenocarcinoma. Squamous cell carcinoma is the predominant cancer of the upper esophagus.

○ **Which method is more sensitive for locating the source of GI bleeding: radioactive technetium-labeled red blood cell scanning or angiography?**

Scanning can depict a site bleeding at a rate as low as 0.12 mL/min, whereas angiography requires rapid bleeding (ie, greater than 0.5 mL/min).

○ **A patient with an "acid stomach" develops melena and vomits copious amounts of bright red blood. Is esophagitis a feasible cause?**

No. Capillary bleeding rarely causes impressive acute blood loss. Arterial bleeding from a complicated ulcer, foreign body, Mallory-Weiss tear, or variceal bleeding are much more probable.

○ **Repeated violent bouts of vomiting can result in both Mallory-Weiss tears and Boerhaave syndrome. Differentiate between them.**

Mallory-Weiss tears involve the submucosa and mucosa, typically in the right posterolateral wall of the gastroesophageal junction. Boerhaave syndrome is a full-thickness tear, usually in the unsupported left posterolateral wall of the abdominal esophagus.

○ **Recurrent pneumonias, especially in the right middle lobe or the superior segments of the bilateral upper lobes, are indicative of what syndrome?**

Aspiration associated with motor diseases and gastroesophageal reflux

○ **If medical management fails to relieve symptoms of gastroesophageal reflux after a 1-year trial, what surgical methods might be attempted?**

The Hill gastropexy, the Nissen fundoplication, the Angelchik antireflux prosthesis placement, or the Belsey Mark IV operation. Surgical correction provides a 90% cure rate.

○ **A 6-month-old infant is constipated, flaccid, and only stares straight ahead. His mother states that he does not have a fever; however, she is especially worried because he will not take his bottle, even with honey on the tip. What is the diagnosis?**

Infantile botulism. Infants ingest spores that are in the environment, most commonly in honey. The spores then grow and produce toxins within the host.

○ **How does infantile botulism differ from food-borne botulism?**

Infantile botulism is caused by the spores of *Clostridium botulinum*, whereas adult food-borne botulism arises from the ingestion of *C botulinum* neurotoxins.

○ **What is the antidote for botulism poisoning?**

There are 2 botulism antitoxin therapies available in the United States. Equine serum trivalent botulism antitoxin (types A, B, and E) is used to treat children older than 1 year and adults. Human-derived botulinum immune globulin (called "BIG-IV" or "BabyBIG") is available for intravenous (IV) use in infants younger than 1 year who have a diagnosis of infant botulism. It should be administered as early as possible in the illness.

○ **What is the Murphy sign?**

Pain at palpation of the gallbladder and inspiratory arrest in a patient with acute cholecystitis. Palpation is performed just below the liver edge in the RUQ, the patient is asked to take a deep breath in, and this causes the inflamed gallbladder to descend toward the examining fingers.

○ **What is the most frequent complication of choledocholithiasis?**

Cholangitis (60%). Other complications are bile duct obstruction, pancreatitis, biliary enteric fistula, and hemobilia.

○ **Gallbladder stones are generally formed of what material?**

Cholesterol. The diagnostic test of choice is ultrasonography. This technique may show stones, sludge, bile plugging, or dilated bile ducts.

○ **Acalculous cholecystitis commonly occurs in what type of patients?**

Postoperative, posttraumatic, and burn patients secondary to dehydration and in patients with hemolysis secondary to blood transfusions

○ **A patient with a history of gallstones presents with acute, postprandial RUQ pain. What is the radiograph of the kidneys, ureter, and bladder likely to show?**

Nothing specific. Only about 10% of gallstones are radiopaque. Complications of cholelithiasis, such as emphysematous cholecystitis, perforation, and pneumobilia, are uncommon but useful findings.

○ **A patient presents with acute, postprandial RUQ pain. Abdominal ultrasonography fails to demonstrate the presence of stones. What diagnostic study would be appropriate to evaluate the pain at this point?**

Hepatobiliary iminodiacetic acid (HIDA) scanning can depict gallbladder disease, including acalculous cholecystitis, biliary and/or cystic duct obstruction, and stones not depicted at ultrasonography.

○ **A child with sickle cell disease presents with fever, RUQ abdominal pain, and jaundice. What is the diagnosis?**

The Charcot triad suggests ascending cholangitis. The precipitating cause in this case is probably pigment stones resulting from chronic hemolysis.

○ **A postoperative patient develops RUQ pain, nausea, and low-grade fever. According to his surgeon, the patient's gallbladder did not contain stones. What is the probable diagnosis?**

Acalculous cholecystitis

○ **Eight years after cholecystectomy, a woman develops RUQ pain and jaundice. What is the chance of recurrent biliary tract stones developing?**

At least 10%—because of either retained stones or stones formed in situ by biliary epithelium

○ **List the ultrasonographic findings that are suggestive of acute cholecystitis.**

Formation of gallstones or sludge in acalculous cholecystitis, thickening of the gallbladder wall by more than 5 mm, and presence of pericholecystic fluid. A dilated common bile duct (ie, >10 mm) suggests common duct obstruction.

○ **Name 2 findings in acute cholecystitis that mandate emergency laparotomy.**

1. Emphysematous cholecystitis, which often heralds the development of gangrene and perforation

2. Intractable pain, which typically is caused by perforation

Otherwise, timing of surgery depends somewhat on the institution and the surgeon.

○ **Can acalculous cholecystitis cause perforation?**

Yes. Up to 40% of gallbladder perforations are associated with acalculous cholecystitis.

○ **A 24-year-old man complains that he has had 2 days of rice-water stools, muscle cramps, and extreme fatigue. He looks pale, dehydrated, and ill. The patient states that he has just returned from India. What is the diagnosis?**

Cholera. The incidence of cholera in the United States is 1 in 10,000,000. This disease usually develops in people who have traveled to endemic areas, such as India, Africa, Southeast Asia, southern Europe, Central and South America, and the Middle East. Infection occurs by consuming unpurified water, raw fruits and vegetables, and undercooked seafood.

○ **A patient presents with palmar erythema, spider angiomas, testicular atrophy, and asterixis. What other signs and symptoms may be exhibited?**

Hematemesis, encephalopathy, hepatomegaly, splenomegaly, jaundice, caput medusae, ascites, and gynecomastia may also occur. This patient has cirrhosis.

○   **A patient with cirrhosis vomits bright red blood and has a systolic blood pressure of 90 mm Hg. After aggressive fluid resuscitation with 4 U of packed red blood cells and gastric lavage, his pressure is still 90 mm Hg. What should be done next?**

Assume the patient has coagulopathy. Transfuse fresh frozen plasma, start vasopressin or octreotide, and arrange for emergency endoscopic evaluation and intervention, usually for sclerotherapy or banding.

○   **How does Crohn disease differ from ulcerative colitis?**

Crohn disease is a transmucosal, segmental granulomatous process, whereas ulcerative colitis is a mucosal, juxtapositioned ulcerative process.

○   **At least one-third of patients with Crohn disease develop kidney stones. Why?**

Dietary oxalate is usually bound to calcium and then excreted. When terminal ileal disease leads to decreased bile salt absorption, the resulting fattier intestinal contents bind calcium by means of saponification. Free oxalate is hyperabsorbed in the colon, resulting in hyperoxaluria and calcium oxalate nephrolithiasis.

○   **Complications of Crohn disease include perirectal abscesses, anal fissures, rectovaginal fistulas, and rectal prolapse. What percentage of patients with Crohn disease have perirectal involvement?**

Approximately 90%

○   **What are the signs and symptoms of Crohn disease?**

Fever, diarrhea, RLQ pain with possible mass, fistulas, rectal prolapse, perianal fissures, and abscesses. Arthritis, uveitis, and liver disease are also associated with this condition.

○   **What systemic diseases are associated with Crohn disease?**

Pyoderma gangrenosum, uveitis, episclerosis, scleritis, arthritis, erythema nodosum, and nephrolithiasis

○   **What are the principal signs and symptoms of ulcerative colitis?**

Fever, weight loss, tachycardia, panniculitis, and 6 bloody bowel movements per day

○   **Ulcerative colitis has 2 peaks of incidence. When do they occur?**

In the second and sixth decades

○   **How is ulcerative colitis diagnosed?**

Characteristic history (rectal bleeding and mucus, abdominal pain, tenesmus, and weight loss) coupled with typical endoscopic appearance of mucosa and confirmatory histologic findings obtained by means of biopsy.

○   **Does toxic megacolon commonly occur with ulcerative colitis or with Crohn disease?**

Ulcerative colitis

○   **Which medications may be used for Crohn disease but not for ulcerative colitis?**

Antidiarrheal agents

○   **Does cancer more often develop with ulcerative colitis or Crohn disease?**

Ulcerative colitis. Think of toxic megacolon and cancer. Always avoid antidiarrheal agents in the treatment regimen.

○   **What are the indications for colectomy in a patient with ulcerative colitis?**

Development of toxic megacolon (colonic dilatation of 6 cm or greater) in a patient who appears "toxic" and has not responded to steroid therapy within 72 hours.

○   **What hereditary diseases evident in infancy may cause cirrhosis?**

Glycogen storage disease, cystic fibrosis, galactosemia, fructose intolerance, tyrosinemia, and acid cholesteryl ester hydrolase deficiency

○   **A patient with cirrhosis presents with weakness and edema. What electrolyte imbalances might be present?**

Hyponatremia (dilutional or diuretic induced), hypokalemia (from GI losses, secondary hyperaldosteronism, or diuretics), and hypomagnesemia

○   **What diuretic is the optimal choice for treating most cirrhotic patients with ascites?**

Potassium-sparing agents. Treat the hyperaldosteronism specifically.

○   **A confused patient with cirrhosis enters the hospital. She is afebrile and has asterixis. What should your examination include to determine the precipitant of hepatic encephalopathy?**

Assess her mental status and examine her for localizing neurologic signs suggestive of an occult head injury. Look for dry mucous membranes and low jugular venous pressure, which are indicative of hypovolemia and azotemia. In addition, use a stool guaiac test to assess for GI bleeding. Focused laboratory testing can pinpoint other causes, including diuretic overuse and hypokalemia, hypoglycemia, anemia, hypoxia, and infection. Administer thiamine and folate.

○   **Aside from correcting the problems described above, what therapy is useful for hepatic encephalopathy?**

Lactulose. This synthetic disaccharide produces an acidic diarrhea that traps nitrogenous wastes in the gut.

○   **The portal vein receives blood from what 2 tributaries?**

The splenic vein and the superior mesenteric vein

○   **What is the most common neoplasm of the GI tract?**

Colon cancer. It is also the second most common cause of cancer death in the United States.

○ **What are the current recommendations from the United States Preventive Services Task Force (USPSTF) for routine colon cancer screening?**

For patients aged 50 to 75 years, the USPSTF recommends one of the following screening protocols:
* Annual screening with high-sensitivity fecal occult blood testing
* Sigmoidoscopy every 5 years, with high-sensitivity fecal occult blood testing every 3 years
* Screening colonoscopy every 10 years

The USPSTF recommends against routine screening for colorectal cancer in adults aged 76 to 85 years, although there may be considerations that support colorectal cancer screening in an individual patient.

The USPSTF recommends against screening for colorectal cancer in adults older than 85 years.

○ **Which is the most common type of colon cancer?**

Adenocarcinoma (95%)

○ **Which is the most common type of rectal cancer?**

Adenocarcinoma (95%)

○ **To where on the body does colon cancer most commonly spread?**

The regional lymph nodes. Hematogenous spread occurs most often to the liver or lungs.

○ **Where is the most common site of colorectal cancer?**

For adenocarcinoma, 60% to 65% of cases occur in the distal colon or the rectum, and 35% to 40% occur in the proximal colon. The typical sites for carcinoid tumor, squamous cell cancer, and melanoma are the appendix or rectum, the anal area, and the area adjacent to the dentate line, respectively.

○ **Clinically, differentiate between right-sided and left-sided adenocarcinoma of the colon.**

Right-sided adenocarcinoma: Pain and/or mass in RLQ, occult blood in stool, dyspepsia, fatigue secondary to anemia; stool appearance rarely changes

Left-sided adenocarcinoma: Change in bowel habits, red blood in stool, reduced caliber of stool, and pencil-thin stools

○ **True/False: Serum carcinoembryonic antigen level is a proficient screening tool for colorectal cancer.**

False. Although 70% of patients with colorectal cancer have an elevated level of carcinoembryonic antigen, it is not specific for colorectal cancer. It is, however, a good measure of recurrent colon cancer.

○ **What is the preferred staging system for colorectal cancer?**

The most recent version (2002) of the tumor, node, metastasis (TNM) staging system of the American Joint Committee on Cancer has replaced the older Dukes classification system as the preferred staging system for colorectal cancer.

- Primary tumor (T)
  - Tis: Carcinoma in situ; intraepithelial (within glandular basement membrane) or invasion of lamina propria
  - T1: Tumor invades submucosa
  - T2: Tumor invades muscularis propria
  - T3: Tumor invades through the muscularis propria into the subserosa or into nonperitonealized pericolic or perirectal tissues
  - T4: Tumor directly invades other organs or structures and/or perforates visceral peritoneum
- Regional lymph node (N)
  - NX: Regional nodes cannot be assessed
  - N0: No regional nodal metastases
  - N1: Metastasis in 1 to 3 regional lymph nodes
  - N2: Metastasis in 4 or more regional lymph nodes
- Distant metastasis (M)
  - MX: Distant metastasis cannot be assessed
  - M0: No distant metastasis
  - M1: Distant metastasis
- Stage groupings
  - Stage 0: Tis N0 M0
  - Stage I: T1-2 N0 M0
  - Stage IIA: T3 N0 M0
  - Stage IIB: T4 N0 M0
  - Stage IIIA: T1-2 N1 M0
  - Stage IIIB: T3-4 N1 M0
  - Stage IIIC: Any T N2 M0
  - Stage IV: Any T Any N M1

○ **What is the typical 5-year survival rate for a stage I colon cancer?**

Five-year survival rates according to the most recent staging system are as follows:

- Stage I (T1-2 N0): 93%
- Stage IIA (T3 N0): 85%
- Stage IIB (T4 N0): 72%
- Stage IIIA (T1-2 N1): 83%
- Stage IIIB (T3-4 N1): 64%
- Stage IIIC (Any T N2): 44%
- Stage IV: 8%

Survival rates in patients with stage II and stage III disease are variable and depend on the number of lymph nodes analyzed.

○ **What stool studies are crucial for evaluating acute diarrhea?**

None. Most cases require no testing, just oral rehydration. In patients at risk for complications (ie, at the extremes of age, recently hospitalized, or immunocompromised), enteroinvasive infection should be ruled out with stool guaiac and fecal leukocyte testing. Also consider checking for ova and parasites.

○ **Which diarrheal illnesses cause fecal leukocytes?**

The usual causes are *Shigella*, *Campylobacter*, and enteroinvasive *Escherichia coli*. Others include *Salmonella*, *Yersinia*, *Vibrio parahaemolyticus*, and *Clostridium difficile*. Fecal WBCs are absent in toxigenic and enteropathogenic infection, even with an organism as virulent as *Vibrio cholerae*. Viral and parasitic infections rarely produce fecal WBCs.

○ **Which is the most common form of acute diarrhea?**

Viral diarrhea. It is generally self-limited, lasting only 1 to 3 days.

○ **What are the most common bacterial pathogens causing acute diarrhea in the United States?**

Campylobacter (2.3%), *Salmonella* (1.8%), *Shigella* (1.1%), *E coli* O157:H7 (0.4%)

However, viral infections are the most common cause of acute diarrhea.

○ **Diarrhea that develops within 12 hours after a meal is probably caused by what?**

An ingested preformed toxin

○ **When does travelers' diarrhea typically occur?**

From 4 to 14 days after arrival in or return from a foreign country

○ **What is the treatment for travelers' diarrhea?**

Travelers' diarrhea is usually caused by *E coli*; the preferable treatment is with ciprofloxacin.

○ **What is the definition of chronic diarrhea?**

According to the American Gastroenterological Association, chronic diarrhea should be defined as a decrease in fecal consistency lasting for 4 or more weeks.

○ **A 73-year-old woman with no significant past medical history presents with fever, chills, vomiting, nausea, and an acute onset of pain in the left lower quadrant. Her pain becomes worse after she eats and is mildly relieved after a bowel movement. At physical examination, she has guarding; rebound tenderness; and a firm, nonmobile mass in the left lower quadrant. What is the likely diagnosis?**

Diverticulitis

○ **Where in the colon are diverticula most commonly found?**

The sigmoid colon, which accounts for 95% of diverticular disease

○ **What percentage of patients with diverticula have symptoms?**

20%

○ **What percentage of 45-year-olds have diverticula?**

33%. Sixty-six percent will have diverticula by the age of 85 years.

○ **What are the signs and symptoms of diverticulitis?**

Abdominal pain, generally in the left lower quadrant, a low-grade fever, change in bowel habits, nausea, and vomiting. If there is perforation of the colon, patients may have peritoneal signs and appear "toxic."

○ **What pain medications are theoretically contraindicated for the treatment of pain arising from acute diverticulitis?**

Codeine and morphine. Their use may increase intraluminal colonic pressure.

○ **If bleeding is associated with diverticulitis, where is the bleeding most likely to occur?**

The right side of the colon. Fifty percent of cases of bleeding originate in this area, even though diverticulitis is more common on the left side.

○ **True/False: A barium enema is not a good diagnostic test if diverticulitis is suspected.**

True. If a patient is having an acute attack of diverticulitis, the risk of perforation is too great. Computed tomography (CT) is the preferred diagnostic test for diverticulitis.

○ **What is the treatment for diverticulitis?**

Bowel rest and antibiotics. Outpatient treatment can be performed, unless there are signs of systemic infection or perforation.

○ **Diverticular disease is most common in which part of the colon?**

The sigmoid colon, which accounts for 95% of diverticular disease.

○ **Prescribe an outpatient antibiotic regimen for uncomplicated diverticulitis.**

Ciprofloxacin plus metronidazole

○ **Is diverticulitis the probable diagnosis in a patient with low abdominal pain and bright red blood from the rectum?**

No. Typically, diverticulosis bleeds, whereas diverticulitis does not. Diverticular bleeding is usually painless.

○ **What barium enema findings can be used to distinguish colonic obstruction caused by acute diverticulitis from that caused by colon cancer?**

Diverticulitis is extraluminal. Thus, the mucosa appears intact, and the bowel segments involved are longer. Adenocarcinoma distorts the mucosa, involves a short segment of bowel, and has overhanging edges.

○ **What is the probable cause of colovesicular fistula?**

Sigmoid diverticulitis. Other causes are radiation enteritis, colon carcinoma, and bladder carcinoma. Colovesicular fistula are diagnosed by means of cystoscopy.

○ **What symptoms are usually associated with neuromuscular dysphagia?**

Nasopharyngeal regurgitation and hoarseness

○ **A 40-year-old smoker describes acute crescendo, substernal chest tightness penetrating to his back. The pain is not relieved by antacids. Echocardiography shows ST changes, and his pain resolves 7 to 10 minutes after administration of a nitroglycerin tablet. Is this angina?**

Maybe, although the delayed response to nitrates characterizes esophageal colic, which is caused by segmental esophageal spasm and is often triggered by reflux. Admitting the patient to the hospital to rule out myocardial infarction is still your best plan.

○ **An elderly woman has trouble swallowing solids and later develops difficulty with liquids. She presents with sudden drooling after dinner. What is the concern?**

A peptic stricture or esophageal cancer complicated by bolus obstruction

○ **Name the most common symptom of esophageal disease.**

Pyrosis (heartburn)

○ **What is the first line of treatment for mild gastroesophageal reflux disease?**

Lifestyle modification (elevating the head of the bed, dietary modifications including avoidance of trigger foods, and weight loss) and over-the-counter antacids

○ **What classical features distinguish chest pain of esophageal origin from that of cardiac ischemia?**

None. Exertional pain and palliation with rest or nitroglycerin occur in both groups. Pain relief from nitroglycerin in the GI group usually takes 7 to 10 minutes, whereas ischemic pain usually responds in 2 to 3 minutes.

○ **What is the most common benign esophageal neoplasm?**

Leiomyoma. Papilloma and fibrovascular polyps also occur, but benign esophageal neoplasms are rare.

○ **What percentage of patients with esophageal cancer also have distant metastasis?**

80%. The 5-year survival rate is 5%. If the cancer is squamous and there is no lymph node involvement, the survival rate is 15% to 20%.

○ **What is the most common location of esophageal cancer?**

The lower third (50%), followed by the upper third (30%) and the middle third (20%)

○ **What age and ethnic group is at greatest risk for esophageal cancer?**

Elderly African Americans. Their risk is 4 times higher than that of elderly white Americans. Other ethnic groups at higher risk include those who are Chinese, Iranian, or South African.

○ **A child swallows a coin, and it becomes lodged in the esophagus. How will the coin appear on an anteroposterior chest radiograph?**

Coins in the esophagus lie in the frontal plane, so they will be seen as a round object. Coins in the trachea lie in the sagittal plane, so they will be seen as a narrow line (edge view).

○ **What is the appropriate management for an ingested button battery that is in the stomach?**

In asymptomatic patients, repeat radiographs. Endoscopic retrieval is required if symptoms occur or if the battery does not pass the pylorus after 48 hours.

○ **Foreign bodies tend to lodge at what esophageal level in the pediatric patient?**

Foreign bodies most commonly lodge at the level of the cricopharyngeus muscles. The level of the thoracic inlet, aortic arch, tracheal bifurcation, and lower esophageal sphincter are also possible lodging sites.

○ **In children, what physical findings suggest that a foreign body has been swallowed?**

Distress, a red or scratched oropharynx, dysphagia, a high fever, or peritoneal signs may be evident. In addition, subcutaneous air suggests perforation.

○ **Most objects, even sharp ones, pass thorough the GI tract without incident. When should such objects be removed?**

Remove them if they obstruct or perforate, if they are longer than 5 x 2 cm, and if they are toxic (such as batteries). Sharp or pointed objects, including sewing needles and razor blades, should be removed if they have not yet passed the pylorus.

○ **What is the best way to remove a meat bolus that is causing esophageal obstruction?**

Endoscopy. IV glucagon, 1-mg IV push after a small test dose, then repeated as a 2-mg dose at 20 minutes. Glucagon relaxes esophageal smooth muscle. Meat tenderizer should be avoided because perforation has occurred.

○ **Where are the 3 most common sites of foreign body perforation of the esophagus?**

  1. Cricopharyngeus muscle
  2. Left mainstem bronchus
  3. Gastroesophageal junction

○ **What test must be performed after a food bolus is cleared?**

Either a barium study or endoscopy. These tests can be used to confirm the passage or removal of the foreign body and check for underlying disease, which is present in most adults with obstructing food boluses.

○ **People who live in what countries are at greatest risk for gastric carcinoma?**

Japan, Chile, and Costa Rica. Risk factors include a diet high in additives, achlorhydria, intestinal metaplasia, polyps or dysplasia, *Helicobacter pylori* infection (disputed), familial polyposis, and pernicious anemia.

○ **What is the most common type of gastric carcinoma? What percentages of these are ulcerative, polypoid, or linitis plastica?**

Adenocarcinomas account for 90% of gastric carcinomas. Of these, 75% are ulcerative, 10% are polypoid, and 15% are diffuse infiltrative scirrhous (linitis plastica).

○ **What is a Krukenberg tumor?**

A gastric carcinoma that has metastasized to the ovary

○ **GI cancers are associated with the enlargement of lymph nodes in what distant location?**

Supraclavicular nodes. These are called Virchow nodes.

○ **Which type of hepatitis is characterized by an alanine aminotransferase level greater than the aspartate aminotransferase level?**

Hepatitis A. The alanine aminotransferase level is usually greater than 1000 U/L.

○ **What is the incubation period for hepatitis A?**

30 days. The disease is caused by a retrovirus.

○ **Is hepatitis A associated with jaundice?**

Typically not. More than 50% of the population have serologic evidence of hepatitis and do not recall having symptoms.

○ **Which type of hepatitis is usually contracted through blood transfusions?**

Hepatitis C accounts for 85% of hepatitis infections via this route.

○ **A poor prognosis is associated with which 2 liver function test abnormalities in acute viral hepatitis?**

1. Total bilirubin level greater than 20 mg/dL

2. Prolongation of prothrombin time by more than 3 seconds

The extent of transaminase elevation is not a useful marker.

○ **Match the following hepatitis serologic findings with the correct clinical description.**

1. Hepatitis B surface antigen (HBsAg) (−) and HBsAg antibody (anti-HBs) (+)

2. Immunoglobulin (Ig)M hepatitis B core antigen (HBcAg) (+) and anti-HBs (−)

3. IgG HBcAg (+) and anti-HBs (−)

4. Hepatitis B e antigen (HBeAg) (+)

a. Ongoing viral replication, highly infectious

b. Remote infection, not infectious

c. (−) c. Recent or ongoing infection (a high titer means high infectivity, but a low titer suggests chronic, active infection)

d. Prior infection or vaccination, not infectious

Answers: (1) d, (2) c, (3) b, and (4) a

○ **You stick yourself with a needle withdrawn from a chronic hepatitis B carrier. You have been vaccinated but have never had your antibody status checked. What is the appropriate postexposure prophylaxis?**

Measure your anti-HB titer. If it is adequate (>10 mIU/mL), treatment is not required. If it is inadequate, you need a single dose of hepatitis B immune globulin as soon as possible and a vaccine booster.

○ **What does an elevated level of IgM HBsAg antibody (anti-HBs) indicate?**

Exposure to hepatitis B with antibody to the core antigen. High titers indicate contagious disease; low titers suggest chronic hepatitis B.

○ **Which type of hepatitis is caused by a DNA virus?**

Hepatitis B. The incubation period is 90 days.

○ **What does anti-HBs indicate?**

Prior infection and immunity

○ **List 3 types of internal hernias.**

1. Diaphragmatic hernia
2. Lesser sac hernia (ie, through the foramen of Winslow)
3. Omental or mesenteric hernia

○ **Are small or large hernias more dangerous?**

Small, because incarceration is more likely

○ **What are the borders of the Hesselbach triangle?**

The inguinal ligament, the inferior epigastric vessels, and the lateral border of the rectus abdominis

○ **Which type of hernia passes through the Hesselbach triangle?**

Direct hernias

○ **Among women, which is more common, inguinal or femoral hernia?**

Inguinal. Femoral hernias occur more commonly among women than men, but inguinal hernias are the most common type of hernias in women.

○ **Distinguish between a groin hernia, a hydrocele, and a lymph node.**

Hydroceles are visible at transillumination and are not tender. Lymph nodes are freely moving and firm. Hernias are not visible at transillumination and may produce bowel sounds.

○ **A patient's groin bulged 2 days ago. He then developed severe pain with progressive nausea and vomiting. He has a tender mass in his groin. What should you not do?**

Do not try to reduce a long-standing, tender incarcerated hernia. The abdomen is no place for dead bowel. This situation requires immediate surgical referral because the hernia is either incarcerated or strangulated.

○ **What simple test can help distinguish between conjugated and unconjugated hyperbilirubinemia?**

A dipstick test for urobilinogen, which reflects conjugated (water soluble) hyperbilirubinemia

○ **In addition to conjugated hyperbilirubinemia, what liver function abnormalities suggest biliary tract disease?**

Elevated alkaline phosphatase levels that are out of proportion to transaminase levels

○ **Portal hypertension produces internal hemorrhoids through which veins?**

The superior rectal and inferior mesenteric veins. Internal hemorrhoids are proximal to the dentate line in the 2-, 5-, and 9-o'clock positions in the prone patient and are typically not palpable at rectal examination.

○ **How does transjugular intrahepatic portosystemic shunt aid in alleviating major consequences of portal hypertension?**

Transjugular intrahepatic portosystemic shunt creates a low-resistance channel (via an expandable metal shunt) between the hepatic vein and the intrahepatic portion of the portal vein, which allows blood to return to the systemic circulation.

○ **Currant jelly stool in a child indicates what?**

Intussusception

○ **What is the most common cause of bowel obstruction in children aged between 6 and 36 months?**

Intussusception. Usually the terminal ileum slides into the right colon. The cause remains unknown, but hypertrophied lymph nodes at the junction of the ileum and colon are suspected.

○ **What is the treatment for intussusception?**

Barium enema is both a diagnostic tool and often a cure (ie, it can reduce the intussusception). If the barium enema is unsuccessful, surgical reduction may be required.

○ **List 4 contraindications to the introduction of a nasogastric tube.**

1. Suspected esophageal laceration or perforation

2. Near obstruction due to stricture

3. Esophageal foreign body

4. Severe head trauma with rhinorrhea

○ **How is an ileus treated?**

An ileus of any cause initially is treated conservatively. The patient is maintained with nothing by mouth, a nasogastric tube may or should be placed if the patient is having severe nausea or vomiting, any opioids should be withheld, and the abdomen should be checked frequently, all while a secondary cause is sought.

○ **When is CT of the abdomen warranted in a patient with ileus?**

When the history, physical examination, and other radiologic studies (radiography of the kidneys, ureter, and bladder) cannot help to distinguish between ileus and obstruction of the small bowel.

○ **An elderly patient presents with sudden onset of severe abdominal pain followed by a forceful bowel movement. What is the probable diagnosis?**

Acute mesenteric ischemia. Results of abdominal series may be normal early in acute mesenteric ischemia. Possible late radiographic findings include absent bowel gas, ileus, gas in the intestinal wall, and thumbprinting of the intestinal mucosa. In most cases, radiographic results are normal or not specifically suggestive. Expect heme-positive stools. Patients especially prone to mesenteric ischemia include those with congestive heart failure and chronic heart disease.

○ **What test should be performed when an elderly patient has abdominal pain that is out of proportion to physical examination results?**

Angiography. This test is the reference standard for diagnosing mesenteric ischemia.

○ **Which artery is most likely to be occluded in mesenteric ischemia?**

The superior mesenteric artery (through embolus)

○ **What are some risk factors for mesenteric ischemia?**

Advanced age, atherosclerosis, cardiac arrhythmias, cardiac valvular disease, recent myocardial infarction, and intraabdominal malignancy

○ **What is the defining characteristic for obesity?**

Body mass index of 30 or greater; body mass index between 25 and 30 is categorized as overweight

○ **In order of prevalence, what are the 3 most common causes of colonic obstruction?**

1. Cancer
2. Diverticulitis
3. Volvulus

○ **Describe a patient with sigmoid volvulus.**

Sigmoid volvulus usually affects psychiatric and elderly patients with severe chronic constipation. Symptoms include intermittent cramping, lower abdominal pain, and progressive abdominal distension.

○ **What is the most common cause of sigmoid volvulus in the elderly?**

Constipation

○ **What are the most common causes of hematochezia in adults?**

Diverticulitis (33%), cancer or polyp (19%), colitis or ulcers (18%), and angiodysplasia (8%). Approximately 16% of cases have an unknown cause.

○ **An elderly man is constipated but does not have tenesmus, abdominal pain, nausea, or vomiting. Rectal examination results indicate that he has hard stool in the vault. A radiograph of the kidneys, ureter, and bladder shows a colon full of stool. Is an enema all he needs?**

No. Fecal impaction with obstipation is both common and benign; however, it is usually associated with tenesmus. The patient must also be evaluated for colorectal tumor.

○ **Pseudo-obstruction is typically caused by medications. Name 3 classes of drugs that give rise to pseudo-obstruction.**

1. Anticholinergic agents
2. Antiparkinsonian drugs
3. Tricyclic antidepressants

○ **What is the most frequent cause of small bowel obstruction?**

Adhesions, followed by incarcerated hernias, are the most common causes of extraluminal obstruction. Gallstones and bezoars are the most common causes of intraluminal obstruction.

○ **An elderly woman has a recurrent obstruction of the small bowel with unilateral pain in 1 thigh. What occult process may be present?**

An obturator hernia incarceration. This condition often manifests with pain down the medial part of the thigh to the knee.

○ **What disease is indicated by epigastric pain that radiates to the back and is relieved, to some extent, by sitting up?**

Pancreatitis

○ **What are the major causes of acute pancreatitis?**

Ethanol and biliary stone disease

○ **Is a nasogastric tube always required for acute pancreatitis?**

No, only if nausea and vomiting are severe. Results of 1 study showed that nasogastric tubes contributed to more complications, including aspiration.

○ **When are antibiotics useful in acute pancreatitis?**

Because pancreatitis is a chemical disease, antibiotics are useful only for treating complications, such as abscess or sepsis, and for cases that are associated with choledocholithiasis.

○ **How are patients with severe pancreatitis best supported nutritionally?**

Patients with mild pancreatitis can typically be cared for with IV hydration alone, since recovery time is usually short, but patients with severe pancreatitis require nutritional support. Parenteral nutrition previously has been the standard practice, theoretically to relieve the ileus and abdominal pain and to minimize the stimulation of the pancreas that would occur with enteral feedings; however, most recent data demonstrate that continuous enteral feedings in the distal jejunum are preferable and safe and may actually reduce complications from pancreatitis. (Guidelines from the American College of Gastroenterology and the American Gastroenterological Association)

○ **Where is the most common site of pancreatic cancer?**

The pancreatic duct system (90% to 95%). If results from ultrasonography and CT are negative, endoscopic retrograde cholangiopancreatography (ERCP) may still be used to verify the presence of cancer.

○ **With regard to pancreatic cancer, distinguish between periampullary lesions and lesions of the body and tail.**

Periampullary lesions most commonly develop at the head of the pancreas. These lesions are usually adenocarcinomas and are associated with jaundice, weight loss, and abdominal pain.

Lesions of the body and tail tend to be much larger at presentation because of their retroperitoneal location and their distance from the common bile duct. Weight loss and pain are typical.

○ **What is the most common cause of lower GI perforation?**

Diverticulitis, followed by tumor, colitis, foreign bodies, and instruments

○ **Which types of patients are at risk for gallbladder perforation?**

The elderly, patients with diabetes, and those with recurrent cholecystitis

○ **What do burning epigastric pain shooting to the back, hypovolemic shock, and a high amylase level suggest?**

Posterior perforation of a duodenal ulcer

○ **Enteric-coated potassium tablets, typhoid, tuberculosis, tumors, and a strangulated hernia can all cause what rare process?**

Nontraumatic small bowel perforation

○ **What percentage of patients with a perforated viscus also have radiographic evidence of pneumoperitoneum?**

60% to 70%. Therefore, one-third of patients will not have this sign. Maintain the patient in either the upright or the left lateral decubitus position for at least 10 minutes before radiography.

○ **After a high-speed motor vehicle accident, a driver who had not worn a seat belt develops abdominal and chest pain radiating to the neck. Upper chest radiography shows left-sided pleural fluid. What gastroesophageal event might have occurred?**

Impact against a steering wheel can result in Boerhaave syndrome with esophageal perforation and mediastinitis

○ **What test should be performed if a perforated esophagus is suspected?**

A water-soluble contrast study. In the meantime, start broad-spectrum antibiotics and consult a surgeon immediately.

○ **A former IV drug user with sickle cell disease and a history of splenectomy presents with unremitting fever, crampy abdominal pain, and meningismus. He has no diarrhea but has recently purchased a pet turtle. What bacteria may be the cause?**

Salmonella typhi, the causative agent of typhoid fever. The infection rate is remarkably high for patients who are positive for human immunodeficiency virus (HIV) or sickle cell disease and those who are asplenic. Rose spots occur in 10% to 20% of cases. Relative bradycardia with a high fever and a low to normal WBC with a pronounced left shift are suggestive findings.

○ **What is the treatment for the above patient?**

IV fluoroquinolone, ceftriaxone, or chloramphenicol. Check blood cultures for bacteremia. Avoid antimotility agents.

○ **Is peptic ulcer disease (PUD) more common in men or women?**

Although previously thought to preferentially affect men (3:1), recent data now indicate that PUD is as common in women as it is in men.

○ **Are patients with duodenal PUD usually younger or older?**

Younger. Duodenal PUD is more often associated with *H pylori*. Older people tend to develop gastric ulcers as a result of nonsteroidal anti-inflammatory drug use.

○ **What is the recommended treatment for *H pylori*?**

The regimen most commonly used to treat *H pylori* is triple therapy with a proton pump inhibitor (eg, omeprazole 20 mg twice a day, pantoprazole 40 mg twice a day, lansoprazole 30 mg twice a day, rabeprazole 20 mg twice a day, or esomeprazole 40 mg daily) and dual antibiotic treatment (eg, amoxicillin 1000 mg twice a day and clarithromycin 500 mg twice a day) for 10 to 14 days.

○ **What are some indications for surgery in a bleeding ulcer?**

Failure of endoscopic attempts to achieve hemostasis and/or need for rigorous transfusion (>3 U packed red blood cells)

○ **Do gastric or duodenal ulcers heal faster?**

Duodenal

○ **Are stress ulcers a surgical problem?**

Typically not. The diffuse gastric bleeding that results from central nervous system tumors, head trauma, burns, sepsis, shock, steroids, aspirin, or ethanol is usually mucosal and can be life threatening. However, this condition can usually be managed medically. Endoscopic diagnosis is key.

○ **Are gastric and duodenal perforations more commonly associated with malignant ulcers or with benign ulcers?**

Benign ulcers

○ **What medical conditions are related to an increased incidence of PUD?**

Chronic obstructive pulmonary disease, cirrhosis, and chronic renal failure

○ **Where is the most common location of a perforated peptic ulcer?**

The anterior surface of the duodenum or pylorus and the lesser curvature of the stomach

○ **After fluid and blood resuscitation of a bleeding ulcer, what is the most useful diagnostic test?**

Endoscopy, which can also be therapeutic, with cryo- or electrocautery of a bleeding artery.

○ **What clinical finding essentially eliminates gastric outlet obstruction in a patient with early satiety and ulcer symptoms?**

Bilious vomitus

○ **Name 2 endocrine problems that can cause PUD.**

1. Zollinger-Ellison syndrome
2. Hyperparathyroidism (hypercalcemia)

○ **True/False: Antibiotics are not required after an uncomplicated perirectal abscess is incised and drained.**

True, assuming the patient has no underlying cause of immunoincompetence, such as HIV, diabetes, or malignancy. Primary aftercare includes sitz baths beginning the next day.

○ **Do pilonidal abscesses communicate with the anal canal?**

No. They are virtually always midline and overlie the lower sacrum. Posterior-opening, horseshoe-type anorectal fistulas can find their way to the lower sacrum but are rarely in the midline.

○ **Should pilonidal cysts be excised in the office?**

No. Incision and drainage are acceptable, followed by placement of a bulky dressing, analgesics, and hot sitz baths, which should be initiated the next day. Antibiotics typically are not necessary. Excision should be completed in the operating room once the acute infection clears.

○ **In adults, pruritus ani develops because of dietary factors contributing to liquid stool, such as caffeine and mineral oil, sexually transmitted infections, fecal contamination, overzealous hygiene, and vitamin deficiencies. What is the most common cause in children?**

Enterobius vermicularis, or pinworm. Test for pinworms by applying a piece of transparent adhesive tape, sticky side down, to the perineal area and then use a cotton swab to smooth the tape onto a glass slide. Examine the slide for eggs with a low-power microscope. Treat the pediatric patient with mebendazole, 100 mg in a single dose, and repeat in 2 weeks if necessary.

○ **A patient with a new case of diarrhea and abdominal pain has been receiving antibiotics for sinusitis for 2 weeks. What might sigmoidoscopic examination reveal?**

Yellowish superficial plaques. This finding is indicative of pseudomembranous colitis. Results of stool studies will implicate the *C difficile* toxin.

○ **How is C difficile detected? What is the reference standard for detection?**

Most laboratories use direct stool toxin assays, instead of organism detection assays, because the turnover time for detection of the toxin is much quicker. Of the direct toxin assays, the cytotoxicity assay remains the reference standard for *C difficile* diagnosis (sensitivity, 94%–100%; specificity, 99%); however, most laboratories do not perform this assay because it is considerably more expensive than other assay methods and has a 48-hour turnover time. Enzyme immunoassay has become the preferred diagnostic assay because of its simplicity, ability to detect both toxins A and B, and provide results within 24 hours. Enzyme immunoassay has a relatively high false-negative rate (sensitivity, 60%–95%), and negative results may be confirmed with tissue-culture assay if necessary.

○ **What is the treatment for pseudomembranous colitis?**

Oral vancomycin 125 mg 4 times a day or oral metronidazole 500 mg 4 times a day. Either regimen should be administered for 7 to 10 days. Cholestyramine, which binds the toxin, can help relieve the diarrhea. Perform follow-up stool studies to confirm clearance of the toxin.

○ **Rectal procidentia in adults mandates what intervention?**

Proctosigmoidoscopy and surgical repair. In children, rectal prolapse can be reduced manually with good results.

○ **What is the most common presenting symptom of rectal cancer?**

Persistent hematochezia. Other symptoms include tenesmus and the feeling of incomplete voiding after a bowel movement.

○ **A patient with ascites has a fever but no localizing signs or symptoms of infection. He also has a normal WBC count. Because you know that spontaneous bacterial peritonitis (SBP) can be occult, you perform abdominal paracentesis. What WBC count in the ascitic fluid suggests SBP?**

WBC count greater than 250 cells/mm^3. Also examine the fluid with Gram stain and obtain at least 10 mL of blood in culture bottles. Test the blood for aerobic and anaerobic organisms.

○ **What organism is usually responsible for causing SBP?**

In order of frequency: *E coli*, *Klebsiella*, and *Streptococcus pneumoniae*

○ **What is the best therapy for SBP?**

Third-generation cephalosporins (cefotaxime)

○ **What 2 therapies can reduce the risk of recurrence of SBP?**

1. Diuretics, which decrease ascitic fluid
2. Nonabsorbable oral antibiotics, which decrease the gut bacterial load, thereby limiting bacterial translocation

○ **A patient with chronic and occasionally bloody diarrhea develops severe diarrhea and abdominal pain with marked distension. What diagnosis is confirmed by these signs?**

Toxic megacolon. This condition is a life-threatening complication of ulcerative colitis.

○ **Watery diarrhea with profuse rectal discharge and weakness might suggest which type of uncommon tumor?**

Villous adenoma

○ **A double bubble at radiography or a "bird's beak" and dilated colon at barium enema study indicate what?**

Volvulus

○ **A patient presents with tremor, ataxia, dementia, cirrhosis, and grey-green rings around the edges of his corneas. What is the diagnosis?**

Wilson disease. Kaiser-Fleischer rings (ie, golden brown or grey-green pigmentation around the cornea), central nervous system disturbances, chronic hepatitis, and cirrhosis are all caused by copper retention as a result of impaired copper excretion.

○ **In Wilson disease, what are the levels of copper in the urine and serum?**

Serum copper levels are low because there is a deficiency in ceruloplasmin, the copper-binding protein. However, the level of copper in the urine is high. Treatment for this disease is penicillamine, which chelates copper.

○ **What are the most common cancers of the small bowel?**

Adenocarcinoma, followed by carcinoid tumor, lymphoma, and leiomyosarcoma. The small bowel is not a common site for malignancy and accounts for only 2% of all GI malignancies.

○ **What carcinoid tumors have the highest rate of metastasis?**

Ileal carcinoid tumors. Malignancy is highly dependent on the size of the tumor: only 2% of tumors smaller than 1 cm in diameter are malignant, whereas 80% to 90% of tumors larger than 2 cm are malignant.

○ **Kultschitzsky cells are the precursors to what tumor?**

Carcinoid tumor. A carcinoid tumor can develop anywhere in the GI tract, but its most frequent site of involvement is the appendix.

○ **A patient complains of severe pain when defecating. He is constipated and has blood-streaked stools and a bloody discharge after bowel movements. What is the diagnosis?**

Anal fissure. Ninety percent of anal fissures are located in the posterior midline. If fissures are found elsewhere in the anal canal, then anal intercourse, tuberculosis, carcinoma, Crohn disease, and syphilis should be considered.

○ **What is the initial, conservative treatment for anal fissures?**

Anal fissures are tears in the lining of the anal canal, typically caused by trauma in this area. Once the tear occurs, a cycle of repeated injury is initiated: tear causing pain, pain causing spasm of the internal sphincter muscle beneath the tear, spasm leading to further tearing. The goal of medical therapy is to break the cycle: increase in dietary fiber, stool softeners, warm sitz baths after defecation, and topical anesthetics are used initially. Surgery is reserved for refractory cases.

○ **Differentiate between mucosal rectal prolapse, complete rectal prolapse, and occult rectal prolapse.**

Mucosal rectal prolapse involves only a small portion of the rectum protruding through the anus and has the appearance of radial folds.

Complete rectal prolapse involves all of the layers of the rectum protruding through the anus. Clinically, this condition appears as concentric folds.

Occult rectal prolapse does not involve protrusion through the anus but rather intussusception.

○ **Which are more painful, internal or external hemorrhoids?**

External. The nerves above the pectinate line or dentate line are supplied by the autonomic nervous system and have no sensory fibers. The nerves below the pectinate line are supplied by the inferior rectal nerve and have sensory fibers.

○ **Differentiate between first-, second-, third-, and fourth-degree hemorrhoids.**

- First degree: Appear in the rectal lumen, but do not protrude past the anus
- Second degree: Protrude into the anal canal if the patient strains
- Third degree: Protrude into the anal canal but can be manually reduced
- Fourth degree: Protrude into the canal and cannot be manually reduced

Treatment for first- and second-degree hemorrhoids is a high-fiber diet, sitz baths, and good hygiene. The treatment of choice for third- or fourth-degree hemorrhoids is rubber band ligation. Other treatments are photocoagulation, electrocauterization, and cryosurgery.

○ **Describe the conservative treatment of internal hemorrhoids.**

Conservative measures are successful for most patients with symptomatic (ie, bleeding, irritation and pruritus, and thrombosis) internal hemorrhoids. Increasing dietary fiber (goal of 20–30 g/d) may aid bleeding and help to prevent recurrence, so patients should be encouraged to maintain this as a lifelong regimen. Irritation and pruritus may be managed with analgesic and steroid creams and warm sitz baths (2–3 times each day). Treatment with creams should not be used for longer than 1 week to avoid the potential for contact dermatitis (analgesics) and mucosal atrophy (steroids). Thrombosed hemorrhoids typically undergo clot organization and resorption within several days with these conservative measures.

○ **What are some extraintestinal manifestations of ulcerative colitis?**

Ankylosing spondylitis, sclerosing cholangitis, arthralgias, ocular complications, erythema nodosum, aphthous ulcers in the mouth, thromboembolic disease, pyoderma gangrenosum, nephrolithiasis, and cirrhosis of the liver

○ **If blood is recovered from the stomach after a nasogastric tube is inserted, where is the most likely location of bleeding?**

Above the ligament of Treitz

○ **Where do the majority of Mallory-Weiss tears occur?**

In the stomach (75%), gastroesophageal junction (20%), and distal esophagus (5%)

○ **Where is angiodysplasia most frequently found?**

In the cecum; the proximal ascending colon, sigmoid colon, and rectum are the next most common locations. Lesions are generally singular; bleeding is intermittent and seldom massive.

○ **Are tumors located in the jejunum and ileum more likely malignant or benign?**

Benign. Tumors of the jejunum and ileum constitute only 5% of all GI tumors. The majority are asymptomatic.

○ **What is the most common remnant of the omphalomesenteric duct?**

Meckel diverticulum

○ **What is the Meckel diverticulum rule of 2s?**

Two percent of the population has it; it is 2 inches long and 2 feet from the ileocecal valve; it occurs most commonly in children younger than 2 years: and it causes symptoms in 2% of patients.

○ **What is the most likely cause of rectal bleeding in a patient with Meckel diverticulum?**

Ulceration of the ileal mucosa adjacent to the diverticulum lined with gastric mucosa

○ **What is the difference in the prognosis between familial polyposis and Gardner disease?**

Although both are inheritable conditions of colonic polyps, Gardner disease rarely results in malignancy, whereas familial polyposis virtually always results in malignancy.

○   **How much blood must be lost in the GI tract to cause melena?**

50 mL. Healthy patients normally lose 2.5 mL/d.

○   **What are the most common causes of upper GI bleeding?**

PUD (45%), esophageal varices (20%), gastritis (20%), and Mallory-Weiss syndrome (10%)

○   **What percentage of patients with upper GI bleeding will stop bleeding within hours after hospitalization?**

85%. About 25% of these patients will bleed again within the first 2 days of hospitalization. If no rebleeding occurs in 5 days, the chance of rebleeding is only 2%.

○   **What percentage of patients with PUD bleed from their ulcers?**

20%

○   **How soon after an episode of bleeding has occurred can an ulcer patient be fed?**

12 to 24 hours after the bleeding has stopped

○   **What type of ulcer is more likely to rebleed?**

Gastric ulcers are 3 times more likely to rebleed than are duodenal ulcers

○   **Where is the most common site of duodenal ulcers?**

The duodenal bulb (95%). Surgery is indicated only if perforation, gastric outlet obstruction, intractable disease, or uncontrollable hemorrhage occur.

○   **What is the most common site for gastric ulcers?**

The lesser curvature of the stomach. Surgery is considered earlier in gastric ulcers because of the higher recurrence rate after medical treatment and because of the higher potential for malignancy.

○   **What is the most common cause of portal hypertension?**

Intrahepatic obstruction (90%), which is most often due to cirrhosis. Other causes of portal hypertension are increased hepatic flow without obstruction (ie, fistulas) and extrahepatic outflow obstruction.

○   **What organism causes amebic liver abscesses?**

Entamoeba histolytica. Amebic liver abscesses are found primarily in middle-aged men living in, or who have traveled to, tropical areas. Ninety percent occur in the right lobe of the liver. Treatment is with oral metronidazole.

○   **What are the most commonly isolated organisms in pyogenic hepatic abscesses?**

Streptococcal species, *Pseudomonas,* or mixed gram-negative flora. The source of such bacteria is most likely an infection in the biliary system.

○ **Which has a higher mortality rate: amebic or pyogenic liver abscesses?**

Pyogenic. The mortality rate for a singular pyogenic abscess is 25% and for multiple abscesses is as high as 70%. Amebic abscesses have mortality rates of only 7% if uncomplicated by superinfection. Amebic abscesses are more likely to be singular, whereas pyogenic abscesses can be singular or multiple.

○ **What clinical sign can assist in the diagnosis of cholecystitis?**

Murphy sign: pain at inspiration with palpation of the RUQ. As the patient breathes in, the gallbladder is lowered in the abdomen and comes in contact with the peritoneum just below the examiner's hand. This will aggravate an inflamed gallbladder, causing the patient to discontinue breathing deeply.

○ **What are the main characteristics of cholelithiasis, cholangitis, cholecystitis, and choledocholithiasis?**

- Cholelithiasis: Gallstones in the gallbladder
- Cholangitis: Inflammation of the common bile duct, often secondary to bacterial infection or choledocholithiasis
- Cholecystitis: Inflammation of the gallbladder secondary to gallstones
- Choledocholithiasis: Gallstones that have migrated from the gallbladder to the common bile duct

○ **What percentage of people with asymptomatic gallstones will develop symptoms?**

Only 50%

○ **Which ethnic group has the largest proportion of people with symptomatic gallstones?**

Native Americans. By the age of 60 years, 80% of Native Americans with previously asymptomatic gallstones will develop symptoms, as compared with only 30% of white Americans and 20% of African Americans.

○ **What percentage of patients with cholangitis are also septic?**

50%. Chills, fever, and shock can occur.

○ **What percentage of gallstones can be seen at ultrasonography?**

95%. Ultrasonography is the diagnostic procedure of choice in patients with suspected cholecystitis.

○ **What is the Charcot triad?**

1. Fever
2. Jaundice
3. Abdominal pain

This is the hallmark of acute cholangitis.

○ **What is the Reynolds pentad?**

The Charcot triad plus shock and mental status changes. This is the hallmark of acute toxic ascending cholangitis.

○   **What is the diagnostic test of choice for acute cholecystitis?**

Hepatobiliary iminodiacetic acid (HIDA) scanning (ie, technetium-99-labeled N-substituted iminodiacetic acid scanning). HIDA scanning uses an isotope that emits gamma rays and is selectively extracted by the liver into bile. The labeled bile can then be used to determine if there is cystic duct obstruction or extrahepatic bile duct obstruction, depending on whether the bile fills the gallbladder or enters the intestine. For practical reasons, the diagnosis is frequently made by using clinical impressions, complete blood cell count, and ultrasonography.

○   **Technetium-99m–labeled studies of the gallbladder are viewed every 10 minutes for 1 hour. If the gallbladder is not visible at the 1-hour interval, what does this signify?**

Either complete obstruction of the cystic duct because of inflammation and stones (acute cholecystitis) or partial obstruction with a slow filling rate because of scarring (chronic cholecystitis). Images delayed as long as 4 hours are obtained to rule out the latter possibility.

○   **How effective is oral dissolution therapy with bile acids for those with symptomatic gallstones?**

Oral therapy with bile acids can dissolve up to 90% of stones. However, therapy works only on stones smaller than 5 mm, made of cholesterol, and floating in a functioning gallbladder. Patients are then treated for 6 to 12 months, and 50% have recurrence of gallstones within 5 years.

○   **What are the contraindications to lithotripsy?**

Stones larger than 2.5 cm, more than 3 stones, calcified stones, stones in the bile duct, and poor overall condition of the patient

○   **What electrolyte disturbances are associated with acute pancreatitis?**

Hypocalcemia and hypomagnesemia

○   **The level of serum amylase is frequently elevated in acute pancreatitis. What other conditions can cause a similar increase in amylase level?**

Bowel infarction, cholecystitis, mumps, perforated ulcer, and renal failure. Lipase is more specific. A 2-hour urine amylase test is a more accurate test for pancreatitis.

○   **What are the most common causes of acute pancreatitis?**

Alcoholism (40%) and gallstone disease (40%). The remaining cases of acute pancreatitis are due to familial pancreatitis, hypoparathyroidism, hyperlipidemia, iatrogenic pancreatitis, and protein deficiency.

○   **What are some abdominal radiographic findings associated with acute pancreatitis?**

A sentinel loop of the jejunum, transverse colon, or duodenum; a colon cutoff sign (an abrupt cessation of gas in the middle of the colon or left transverse colon because of inflammation of the adjacent pancreas); or calcification of the pancreas. About two-thirds of patients with acute pancreatitis will have radiographically visible abnormalities.

○   **What is the treatment for pancreatic pseudocysts?**

Initial therapy is to wait for regression (4 to 6 weeks). If no improvement occurs, or if superinfection occurs, surgical drainage or excision is required.

○ **What are the Ranson criteria?**

One of the earliest scoring systems for severity in acute pancreatitis. 0 to 3 criteria = 0% to 3% mortality

At initial presentation	Developing within 24 hours
Older than 55 years	Hematocrit level decrease greater than 10%
WBC count greater than 16,000/μL	Increase in serum urea nitrogen level greater than
Aspartate aminotransferase level higher than	5 mg/dL
250 U/L	Serum Ca^c level less than 8 mg/dL
Serum glucose level higher than 200 mg/dL	Partial pressure of arterial oxygen lower than 60 mm Hg
Lactate dehydrogenase cholesterol level	Base deficit greater than 4 mEq/L
greater than 350 U/L	Fluid sequestration greater than 6 L

0 to 3 criteria = 0% to 3% mortality
3 to 4 criteria = 15% mortality
5 to 6 criteria = 40% mortality
7 to 8 criteria = 100% mortality

Although the system continues to be widely used, results of a meta-analysis of 110 studies indicated that the Ranson score is a poor predictor of severity.

○ **What is the most common cause of pancreatic pseudocysts in adults?**

Chronic pancreatitis. Pseudocysts generally are filled with pancreatic enzymes and are sterile. They manifest about 1 week after the patient has a bout of acute pancreatitis displayed as upper abdominal pain with anorexia and weight loss. Forty percent of cases will regress spontaneously.

○ **What are some other causes of pancreatitis?**

Surgery, trauma, ERCP, viral and *Mycoplasma* infections, hypertriglyceridemia, vasculitis, drugs, penetrating peptic ulcer, anatomic abnormalities around the ampulla of Vater, hyperparathyroidism, end-stage renal disease, and organ transplantation

○ **What are some of the drugs known to cause pancreatitis?**

Sulfonamides, estrogens, tetracyclines, pentamidine, azathioprine, thiazides, furosemide, and valproic acid

○ **What are some of the infectious causes of pancreatitis?**

Mumps, viral hepatitis, *Coxsackie B virus*, and *Mycoplasma*

○ **What are the common symptoms of acute pancreatitis?**

Epigastric or diffuse abdominal pain radiating to the back, nausea, and vomiting

○ **What are the common signs of acute pancreatitis?**

Fever, tachycardia, hypotension, distended abdomen, and guarding with diminished or absent bowel sounds. Rarely seen signs include tender subcutaneous nodules from fat necrosis and hypocalcemic tetany.

○   **What is the mechanism of hypotension in severe cases of acute pancreatitis?**

Fluid sequestration in the intestine and retroperitoneum, systemic vascular effects of kinins, vomiting, and bleeding

○   **What is the Cullen sign?**

Periumbilical ecchymosis indicative of pancreatitis, severe upper bowel bleeding, or ruptured ectopic pregnancy

○   **Does acute pancreatitis commonly progress to chronic pancreatitis?**

No, only rarely.

○   **What are the pathologic spectra in acute pancreatitis?**

Edematous pancreatitis (mild cases) and necrotizing pancreatitis (severe cases). Hemorrhagic pancreatitis may evolve from either of them.

○   **What is the mechanism of necrosis and vascular damage in acute pancreatitis?**

Autodigestion of the pancreas by various proteolytic and lipolytic enzymes

○   **What are the laboratory test abnormalities seen with pancreatitis?**

Leukocytosis, hemoconcentration followed by anemia, hyperglycemia, prerenal azotemia, hypoxemia, hyperamylasemia, and liver function test abnormalities

○   **What are some other causes of hyperamylasemia besides pancreatitis?**

Pancreatic pseudocyst, pancreatic trauma, pancreatic carcinoma, ERCP, perforated duodenal ulcer, mesenteric infarction, renal failure, intestinal obstruction, salivary gland origin, ovarian disorders, prostate tumors, diabetic ketoacidosis, and macroamylasemia.

○   **Does the level of amylase elevation correlate with severity?**

No. Higher levels are seen with biliary pancreatitis.

○   **What is the role of determining serum lipase level?**

Serum lipase is slightly less sensitive than amylase is but much more specific. It is also elevated in renal failure and nonpancreatic acute abdominal conditions. Lipase levels are elevated longer than amylase levels are.

○   **Name a noninvasive technique for evaluating the intrahepatic and extrahepatic bile ducts and the pancreatic duct.**

Magnetic resonance cholangiopancreatography (MRCP) provides accurate depiction and measurements of the bile and pancreatic ducts; associated anatomic variants, such as pancreas divisum and choledochal cysts, can also be seen. The technique is useful for documenting communication between pancreatic cysts and ducts and for evaluating the nature of pancreatic cysts. Unlike with ERCP, it is not necessary to administer contrast material into the ductal system with MRCP, thereby avoiding any potential risks with the procedure or the contrast material. However, MRCP does not allow for any interventional possibilities (eg, stone extraction, biopsy, or stent placement).

○ **Your patient presents with severe RUQ abdominal pain and elevated liver function test results, and MRCP demonstrated cholecystitis with a dilated common bile duct. What is the next step?**

After a noninvasive modality (MRCP) has objectively demonstrated biliary obstruction, then ERCP should be used. ERCP is a relatively complex, invasive, primarily therapeutic, endoscopic procedure, requiring specialized training and equipment, for the management of pancreaticobiliary disorders. Its usefulness in this patient would include sludge or stone removal.

○ **When is surgery indicated in pancreatitis?**

When a patient has infected pancreatic necrosis or abscess that cannot be adequately drained and treated

○ **Should surgery be performed immediately for gallstone pancreatitis?**

No. It should be performed after the pancreatitis has subsided.

○ **What is the Hamman sign?**

Air in the mediastinum after esophageal perforation. This condition produces a crunching sound over the heart during systole.

○ **What are the signs and symptoms of Boerhaave syndrome?**

Substernal and left-sided chest pain with a history of forceful vomiting, leading to spontaneous esophageal rupture

○ **How does a patient present with Boerhaave syndrome?**

Boerhaave syndrome is spontaneous esophageal perforation. It usually occurs after forceful vomiting. The patient has an acute collapse, with chest and abdominal pain. Left pleural effusion is seen at chest radiography in 90% of patients; most have mediastinal emphysema.

○ **What is the most common site of rupture in Boerhaave syndrome?**

The posterior distal esophagus. Boerhaave syndrome is rupture of the esophagus that occurs after binge drinking and vomiting. Patients experience sudden, sharp pain in the lower chest and epigastric area. The abdomen becomes rigid, and shock may follow.

○ **What test should be performed to confirm the diagnosis of Boerhaave syndrome?**

An esophagram. A water-soluble contrast medium should be used in place of barium to confirm the diagnosis.

○ **Which cancer cell types of the esophagus are the most common in African Americans and white Americans?**

Squamous cell carcinoma occurs most frequently in African Americans, and adenocarcinoma is the most common type in white Americans.

○ **What is the major cause of death in patients with Hirschsprung disease?**

Enterocolitis

○ **Is Hirschsprung disease more common in male or in female subjects?**

Male (5:1)

○ **A 41-year-old patient complains of severe but short rectal spasms but has not noticed any bleeding. He is known to be stressed and overtaxed at work. What is your diagnosis?**

Proctalgia fugax. These short rectal spasms last less than 1 minute and occur infrequently. They are associated with people who are anxious or overworked or who have a history of irritable bowel syndrome. No cause is known. Treatment is analgesic suppositories, heating pads, and relaxation techniques.

○ **A patient presents with Mallory-Weiss syndrome. A Sengstaken-Blakemore tube is considered to control the hemorrhage. What prior problem could the patient have had that would prevent its use?**

Hiatal hernia. Neither proper placement of the balloon nor proper traction can be attained in such individuals.

○ **Antacids containing magnesium may cause:**

Diarrhea

○ **Antacids containing aluminum may cause:**

Constipation

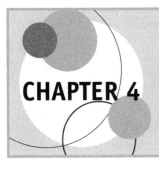

CHAPTER 4 Metabolic and Endocrine

Cynthia M. Waickus, MD, PhD

○ **What are the sodium concentrations of the most common commercially available intravenous (IV) fluids?**

- 0.9 normal saline = 154 mEq/L
- 0.45 normal saline = 77 mEq/L
- 0.3 normal saline = 54 mEq/L
- 0.2 normal saline = 33 mEq/L

○ **What are the signs and symptoms of hyponatremia?**

Weakness, nausea, anorexia, vomiting, confusion, lethargy, seizures, and coma

○ **How does hyperglycemia lead to hyponatremia?**

Glucose stays in the extracellular fluid; hyperglycemia osmotically draws water out of the cell into the extracellular fluid, thus diluting the sodium. Each increase of 100 mg/dL in plasma glucose decreases the serum sodium level by 1.6 to 1.8 mEq/L.

○ **What are the main causes of hypervolemic hyponatremia?**

They are congestive heart failure, liver cirrhosis, and renal diseases such as renal failure and nephrotic syndrome.

○ **How is the sodium deficit calculated?**

Sodium deficit = TBW × (desired sodium − actual sodium)

○ **What 3 conditions may cause sodium concentration to appear falsely low?**

Pseudohyponatremia may be caused by (1) hyperglycemia, (2) hyperlipidemia, or (3) hyperproteinemia.

○ **What is central pontine myelinolysis (osmotic demyelination syndrome)?**

The complication of brain dehydration after the rapid correction of severe hyponatremia. Correct hyponatremia slowly (ie, <12 mEq/h) for chronic hyponatremia.

○ **What are the signs and symptoms of hypernatremia?**

Confusion, muscle irritability, seizures, respiratory paralysis, and coma

○ **What are the most common causes of hypotonic fluid loss leading to hypernatremia?**

Diarrhea, vomiting, hyperpyrexia, and excessive sweating

○ **Hypovolemia is a major concern when treating a patient with hypernatremia. What is the calculation for determining water deficit?**

Water deficit $= (0.6 \times$ weight in kg$) \times$ [(serum sodium/140) $- 1$]

○ **What is syndrome of inappropriate secretion of antidiuretic hormone (SIADH)?**

SIADH is characterized by hyponatremia in the presence of urine that is less than maximally dilute.

○ **A patient presents with a low sodium level and you suspect SIADH. What laboratory test findings would help to confirm the diagnosis?**

Serum osmolality should be low; urine sodium level (ie, >30 mEq/L) and osmolality should be high. Treatment of severe symptomatic hyponatremia includes a loop diuretic, such as furosemide, and the simultaneous infusion of small boluses of 3% saline over 4 hours or normal saline. If hyponatremia is corrected too rapidly, neurologic sequelae may result.

○ **What is the most common cause of euvolemic hyponatremia in children?**

SIADH. Other causes include central nervous system disorders, medications, tumors, and pulmonary disorders.

○ **What specific disease process should be considered in a child who presents with dehydration, hypernatremia, decreased urine osmolarity, and a high level of circulating antidiuretic hormone (ADH)?**

Nephrogenic diabetes insipidus

○ **If nephrogenic diabetes insipidus is assumed, what further pharmacologic treatment may be helpful?**

Thiazide diuretics have a paradoxical effect and may help to decrease fluid losses.

○ **What is the danger of rigorously hydrating a patient who has hypernatremia due to diabetes insipidus?**

Cerebral edema, seizures, and death

○ **What are the most common causes of central diabetes insipidus?**

Most cases of central diabetes insipidus are related to neurosurgery or trauma, primary or secondary tumors, or infiltrative diseases, although 30% to 50% are idiopathic. It is characterized by dilute urine in the absence of renal disease and is caused by insufficient ADH secretion.

○ **A patient with polyuria, low urine osmolality, and high serum osmolality is administered vasopressin, but no change in osmolality is noted. Which type of diabetes insipidus does she have?**

Nephrogenic. Vasopressin will not help because the distal renal tubules are refractory to ADH. In central diabetes insipidus, the disease involves a problem with the production of ADH in the posterior pituitary gland. An increase in urine osmolality of at least 50% will occur with vasopressin administration if the problem is central diabetes insipidus.

○ **What are the echocardiographic findings in a patient with hypokalemia?**

Flattened T waves, depressed ST segments, prominent P and U waves, and prolonged QT and PR intervals

○ **What are the echocardiographic findings in a patient with hyperkalemia?**

Findings include peaked T waves, prolonged QT and PR intervals, diminished P waves, depressed T waves, and QRS complex widening (ie, a classic sine wave), and potassium levels near 10 mEq/L.

○ **What are the causes of hyperkalemia?**

Acidosis, tissue necrosis, hemolysis, blood transfusions, gastrointestinal bleeding, renal failure, Addison disease, primary hypoaldosteronism, excess oral potassium intake, renal tubular acidosis IV, and medications such as succinylcholine, β-blockers, captopril, spironolactone, triamterene, amiloride, and high-dose penicillin

○ **What medications are likely to lead to acute hyperkalemia in a diabetic patient?**

Nonsteroidal anti-inflammatory drugs, angiotensin-converting enzyme inhibitors, β-blockers, potassium-sparing diuretics, and salt substitutes (usually potassium salts)

○ **A young, competitive figure skater complains of generalized weakness after practice. What might be the cause?**

Hypokalemic periodic paralysis is a likely cause of the acute weakness.

○ **How do pH changes affect potassium concentration?**

For a pH increase of 0.1, expect the potassium to decrease by 0.5 mEq/L.

○ **What is the treatment for hyperkalemia?**

- Diuresis with a loop diuretic (ie, furosemide or ethacrynic acid)
- Sodium polystyrene sulfonate cation-exchange resin enema (associated sodium load can cause failure). It may take hours to be effective.
- 1 ampule 50% dextrose (D50) and insulin, 5 to 10 U IV for redistribution, followed by 50 g glucose and 20 U insulin over 1 hour. It takes about 30 minutes to be effective.
- Sodium bicarbonate 50 to 100 mEq IV over 10 to 20 minutes. It takes 5 to 10 minutes to be effective.
- Calcium. Calcium chloride has more calcium per ampule (13.4 mEq) than gluconate (4.6 mEq) does and acts faster. Administer 1 ampule (10 mL) of 10% solution over 10 to 20 minutes. Be careful if prescribing to a patient receiving digitalis; it will potentiate toxicity, and the onset is rapid.
- 3% sodium chloride IV (may serve as a temporary antagonist)
- Peritoneal dialysis or hemodialysis
- Digoxin-specific antibody (Fab) if the cause is secondary to digitalis overdose

○ **What pH decrease is expected with an increase in partial pressure of carbon dioxide (PCO_2) of 10 mm Hg?**

0.08

○ **What pH increase is expected with a decrease in PCO_2 of 10 mm Hg?**

0.13

○ **What pH increase is expected with an increase in bicarbonate of 5.0 mEq/L?**

0.08

○ **What decrease in pH is expected with a decrease in bicarbonate of 5.0 mEq/L?**

0.10

○ **How is the anion gap calculated from electrolyte values?**

Anion gap = sodium − (chlorine − bicarbonate)

The normal anion gap is 12 ± 4 mEq/L.

○ **Name the causes of high anion gap metabolic acidosis.**

The differential diagnosis includes aspirin poisoning, carbon monoxide, diabetic ketoacidosis (DKA), alcoholic ketoacidosis (AKA), iron, isoniazid, lactic acidosis, renal failure or uremia (acute and chronic), starvation, salicylate toxicity, ethylene glycol toxicity, methanol poisoning, and paraldehyde and toluene toxicity.

○ **What are some causes of lactic acidosis?**

Lactic acidosis may be the result of shock, seizures, acute hypoxemia, isoniazid, cyanide, ritodrine, inhaled acetylene and carbon monoxide, and ethanol.

○ **What are the causes of normal anion gap metabolic acidosis?**

Diarrhea, ammonium chloride, renal tubular acidosis, renal interstitial disease, hypoadrenalism, ureterosigmoidostomy, and acetazolamide

○ **Describe the presentation of AKA.**

Nausea, vomiting, and abdominal pain occurring 24 to 72 hours after the cessation of drinking. No specific physical findings are evident, although abdominal pain is a common complaint. AKA is thought to be secondary to increased mobilization of free fatty acids with lipolysis to acetoacetate and β-hydroxybutyrate.

○ **In whom does AKA commonly occur? When?**

It usually occurs in chronic alcoholic patients after an interval of binge drinking followed by 1 to 3 days of protracted vomiting, abstinence, and decreased food intake.

○ **What is the appropriate treatment for a patient with AKA?**

Normal saline and glucose. As acidosis is corrected, potassium level may decrease. Sodium bicarbonate should not be administered unless the pH decreases below 7.1.

○ **What are the potential complications of excess sodium bicarbonate?**

Cerebral acidosis, hypokalemia, hyperosmolality, sodium overload, and an increased binding of hemoglobin to oxygen or impaired oxygen dissociation.

○ **How can the magnitude of the anion gap be useful in narrowing the differential diagnosis of anion gap acidosis?**

An anion gap greater than 35 mEq/L is usually caused by ethylene glycol, methanol, or lactic acidosis. An anion gap of 23 to 30 mEq/L may be due to an increase in organic acids, and an anion gap of 16 to 22 mEq/L may be a result of advanced uremia.

○ **What clinical findings can be used to narrow the differential diagnosis of anion gap acidosis?**

- Methanol: Visual disturbances and headache are common. May produce wide anion gaps because each 2.6 mg/dL of methanol contributes 1 mOsm/L to anion gap. Compare this with ethanol: each 4.3 mg/dL adds 1 mOsm/L to anion gap.
- Uremia: Must be advanced before it causes an anion gap
- Diabetic ketoacidosis: Both hyperglycemia and glucosuria typically occur. AKA is often associated with low blood sugar level and mild or absent glucosuria.
- Salicylates: High levels contribute to anion gap.
- Lactic acidosis: Check serum level. This condition also has a broad differential diagnosis, as cited above.
- Ethylene glycol: Causes calcium oxalate (ie, "hippurate crystals") in urine. Each 5.0 mg/dL contributes 1 mOsm/L to anion gap.

○ **Distinguish between lactic acidosis types A and B.**

Type A is associated with inadequate tissue perfusion, the resultant anoxia, and subsequent lactate and hydrogen ion accumulation. This condition usually occurs because of shock and is often seen in the emergency department. Type B includes all forms of acidosis in which there is no evidence of tissue anoxia.

○ **Diffuse abdominal pain with bloody stools and a high serum lactate level in a diabetic patient might suggest what gastrointestinal disease?**

One should strongly consider ischemic or necrotic bowel.

○ **How is the osmolar gap determined?**

Osmolality is a measure of the concentration of particles in a solution with units of osmoles per kilogram of water. Osmolarity is a measure of osmoles per liter of solution. For dilute solutions, like body fluids, these 2 measures are roughly equivalent. An osmolar gap is the difference between the measured osmolality and the calculated osmolarity, normally 275 to 285 mOsm/L.

The formula for calculating serum osmolality is as follows:

$2Na(mEq/L) + Glu(mg/dL)/18 + BUN (mg/dL)/2.8 = mOsm/kg H_2O$

○ **Name the 2 primary causes of metabolic alkalosis.**

1. Loss of hydrogen and chloride from the stomach
2. Overzealous diuresis with loss of hydrogen, potassium, and chloride

○ **What condition should be suspected in a patient with a serum glucose level of 942 mg/dL, mild ketonuria, depressed sensorium, and positive Babinski sign?**

Hyperosmolar hyperglycemic state

○ **What focal signs may be present in a patient with hyperosmolar hyperglycemic state?**

Hemisensory deficits or perhaps hemiparesis. Ten percent to 15% of these patients will have a seizure.

○ **The term "hyperosmolar hyperglycemic state" has replaced the older term "nonketotic hyperglycemic hyperosmolar coma." What are the criteria for the diagnosis of hyperosmolar hyperglycemic state?**

- Plasma glucose level greater than 600 mg/dL
- Arterial pH greater than 7.30
- Serum bicarbonate level greater than 15 mEq/L
- Variable serum osmolality, but typically greater than 350 mOsm/kg
- Normal anion gap greater than 12 mEq/L
- No more than small serum or urine ketones
- Stuporous or comatose state

○ **What is the treatment for hyperosmolar hyperglycemic state?**

Fluids. Patients can be as much as 12 L deficient. Administer normal saline until adequate blood pressure and urinary output are established. Follow with half normal saline. When the blood glucose level decreases to 250 to 300 mg/dL, the solution should be changed to saline and glucose to avoid cerebral edema.

These patients require little insulin. Administer as little as 5 to 10 U of insulin IV. However, they are commonly deficient in potassium and will need 10 to 15 mEq/hr once urine flow has been established.

○ **What is the overall mortality rate for hyperosmolar hyperglycemic state?**

This disorder has a poor prognosis, with a mortality rate as high as 50% for severe cases.

○ **What are the key factors leading to hypernatremia in a patient with hyperosmolar hyperglycemic state?**

Profound dehydration with greater losses of water than salt, as well as impaired thirst

○ **Differentiate between hyperosmolar hyperglycemic state and DKA.**

Hyperosmolar hyperglycemic state: Glucose level is high (often >600 mg/dL); serum osmolality is high (average about 380 mOsm/kg); and pH is usually maintained at greater than 7.2, since sodium bicarbonate level is normal and nitroprusside test result is negative

DKA: Glucose level is often in the range of 600 mg/dL; serum osmolality is approximately 350 mOsm/kg; and sodium bicarbonate is depleted in DKA and nitroprusside test result is positive

○ **What is the most important initial step in treating DKA?**

Volume replacement, with the first liter administered over about 60 minutes

○ **What laboratory test findings are expected with DKA?**

Elevated β-hydroxybutyrate, acetoacetate, acetone, and glucose levels. Ketonuria and glucosuria are present. Serum bicarbonate levels, PCO_2, and pH are decreased. Potassium levels may be elevated but will decrease when the acidosis is corrected.

○ **Outline the basic treatment for DKA.**

Administer fluids. Start with normal saline (the total fluid deficit may be 5 to 10 L), followed by potassium 100 to 200 mEq in the first 12 to 24 hours. Prescribe insulin 5 to 10 IU/hr. Add glucose to the IV fluid when the glucose level decreases below 250 mg/dL, and administer a phosphate supplement when the levels decrease below 1.0 mg/dL.

For pediatric patients, administer normal saline 20 mL/kg per hour for 1 to 2 hours and insulin 0.1 U/kg per hour IV infusion.

○ **What major insults are likely to lead to DKA in otherwise controlled diabetes?**

Always look for infection (even a minor one), cardiac ischemia, medications, lack of compliance with insulin, and diet.

○ **What are some complications of hypophosphatemia seen in treated DKA?**

Rhabdomyolysis, cardiac dysfunction, arrhythmias, hemolysis, and poor neutrophil function

○ **What do profound polyuria and dehydration in DKA reflect?**

Severe osmotic diuresis caused by glycosuria

○ **What is the most common cause of hypoglycemia seen in the emergency department?**

An insulin reaction in a diabetic patient

○ **In the first 2 years of life, what is the most common cause of drug-induced hypoglycemia?**

Salicylates. Between ages 2 and 8 years, ethanol is the most likely cause, and between ages 11 and 30 years, insulin and sulfonylureas are the primary causes.

○ **What principal hormone protects the human body from hypoglycemia?**

Glucagon

○ **Which is the most common type of hypoglycemia in children?**

Ketotic hypoglycemia. This condition usually develops in boys between ages 18 months and 5 years. Attacks typically arise from caloric deprivation. These attacks may be episodic and are more frequent in the morning and during periods of illness.

○ **What are the neurologic signs and symptoms associated with hypoglycemia?**

Hypoglycemia may produce mental and neurologic dysfunction. Neurologic manifestations can include paresthesias, cranial nerve palsies, transient hemiplegia, diplopia, decerebrate posturing, and clonus.

○ **What are the key predisposing factors to hypoglycemia in diabetic patients receiving insulin?**

Exercise, poor oral intake, worsening renal function, and medications are the key predisposing factors to consider.

○ **What are some common causes of abdominal pain, nausea, and vomiting in a diabetic patient?**

Diabetic gastroparesis, gallbladder disease, pancreatitis, and ischemia bowel

○ **What are some agents used to treat severe diabetic gastroparesis?**

Metachlorpropamide is currently the primary agent. Erythromycin has also been tried in severe cases.

○ **What are the major adverse effects of IV contrast material when administered in diabetic patients?**

Acute tubular necrosis is well known. One should also watch for worsening of congestive heart failure, precipitation of angina pectoris, and hemodynamic compromise.

○ **What causes secondary diabetes mellitus?**

Exocrine pancreatic diseases like cystic fibrosis, pancreatic cancer, and Cushing disease

○ **What is the significance of hemoglobin A_{1c}?**

It represents the fraction of hemoglobin that has been nonenzymatically glycosylated. It provides an accurate estimation of the relative blood glucose level for the preceding 6 to 8 weeks.

○ **What laboratory studies should be performed in elderly patients before prescribing metformin for treatment of diabetes?**

In patients with reduced muscle mass, such as the elderly (especially those older than 80 years), use of serum creatinine concentration to estimate the glomerular filtration rate may be misleading, and creatinine clearance should be determined. If creatinine clearance is less than 70 mL/min, metformin should not be prescribed.

○ **Name some of the many advantages of metformin as a first-line oral antidiabetic agent.**

One of the main advantages of metformin (a biguanide) over some other oral agents is that metformin does not cause hypoglycemia. Lactic acidosis, although rare, can occur in patients with renal impairment who also take metformin. In contrast to most other agents for the control of elevated glucose levels, which often cause weight gain, metformin reduces insulin levels and more frequently has a weight-maintaining or even a weight-loss effect. Gastrointestinal distress is a common adverse effect of metformin, particularly early in therapy.

○ **A 78-year-old man with adequate control of his type 2 diabetes mellitus is scheduled for abdominal computed tomography with oral and IV iodinated contrast material. Which antidiabetic medication should be withheld 48 hours before and after the procedure?**

Metformin should be withheld before and after radiologic procedures with contrast material because of its interaction with iodinated contrast materials. This interaction may cause impaired renal function or lactic acidosis.

○ **Define "impaired fasting glucose" and "impaired glucose tolerance" in the prediabetes state.**

According to the clinical practice guidelines of the American Diabetes Association, impaired fasting glucose is a fasting plasma glucose level of 100 to 125 mg/dL, and impaired glucose tolerance is a 2-hour plasma glucose level of 140 to 199 mg/dL.

These 2 categories have been officially termed "prediabetes" and are considered risk factors for future diabetes and cardiovascular disease.

○ **What are appropriate treatment modalities for prediabetes states?**

Lifestyle modification focusing on weight loss and physical exercise is regarded as first-line therapy for preventing or delaying diabetes in patients with prediabetes. Lifestyle modification (5%–10% weight loss and moderate physical activity of 30 min/d) is associated with a 58% reduction of risk for developing diabetes. Metformin is most effective (reduction in risk of 31%) in prediabetic patients younger than 60 years with a body mass index of at least 35 kg/m².

○ **What are the antihypertensive agents of choice for patients with diabetic nephropathy?**

Nondihydropyridine calcium-channel blockers (diltiazem or verapamil) can reduce overt proteinuria in patients with diabetic nephropathy; however, dihydropyridine calcium-channel blockers (amlodipine or nifedipine) can worsen proteinuria and accelerate the progression of disease in such patients. Diabetic patients treated with dihydropyridine calcium-channel blockers have more severe proteinuria and a more rapid decline in renal function than do patients treated with other antihypertensive agents.

○ **What heralds the onset of renal disease in patients with diabetes?**

Microalbuminuria is the earliest indicator of renal disease in type 2 diabetes. Microalbuminuria is also a strong risk factor for cardiovascular death and coronary heart disease.

○ **Your patient is a 55-year-old man with newly diagnosed type 2 diabetes mellitus. According to the 2008 American Diabetes Association nutrition guidelines, what dietary recommendations should you make regarding dietary fat intake for this patient?**

The primary goal with regard to fat intake in patients with diabetes is to limit saturated fat, trans-fatty acids, and cholesterol. The 2008 American Diabetes Association nutrition guidelines recommend that less than 7% of total calorie intake should be derived from dietary fat and that dietary cholesterol should not exceed 200 mg/d. Intake of trans-unsaturated fatty acids should be minimized, since they increase the low-density lipoprotein cholesterol (LDL-C) and lower the high-density lipoprotein cholesterol (HDL-C). Omega-3 (n-3) fatty acids have a cardioprotective effect; 2 or more servings of fish per week can be recommended to provide an appropriate level of dietary omega-3 fatty acids. A gram of fat contains more than twice the calories of a gram of carbohydrate.

○ **What are the current criteria for diagnosing diabetes mellitus?**

- Fasting plasma glucose level of 126 mg/dL or higher

OR

- 2-hour postload glucose level of 200 mg/dL or higher at oral glucose tolerance testing
- Symptoms of diabetes plus a casual plasma glucose level of 200 mg/dL or higher

○ **What are the current recommendations for screening for type 2 diabetes mellitus?**

Screening is recommended in asymptomatic adults beginning at age 45 years, particularly for those with a body mass index of 25 or greater, and should be repeated at least once every 3 years. Screening should be considered at an earlier age in patients classified at high risk for diabetes; such patients include women with a history of gestational diabetes or of delivering an infant weighing more than 9 lb, persons with a strong family history of type 2 diabetes, certain racial or ethnic groups (eg, Native Americans, African Americans, Hispanics, Asians, and South Pacific Islanders), or persons with conditions associated with insulin resistance (eg, acanthosis nigricans or polycystic ovary syndrome [PCOS]).

Assessing glycosylated hemoglobin level is not recommended as a screening test.

○ **What are the diagnostic criteria for metabolic syndrome?**

Metabolic syndrome is a group of cardiovascular risk factors related to hypertension, abdominal obesity, dyslipidemia, and insulin resistance. Diagnostic criteria for metabolic syndrome include the presence of 3 or more of the following:

- Obesity, with a waist circumference exceeding 102 cm (40 in) in men or 88 cm (35 in) in women
- Blood pressure of 130 mm Hg systolic and/or 85 mm diastolic or higher
- Fasting glucose level of 110 mg/dL or higher
- Serum triglyceride levels of 150 mg/dL or higher
- HDL-C of 40 mg/dL or lower in men or 50 mg/dL or lower in women

○ **What preexisting medical conditions increase the likelihood of insulin resistance syndrome?**

Cardiovascular disease, hypertension, PCOS, acanthosis nigricans, and nonalcoholic fatty liver disease

○ **What are the most effective monotherapy agents for treating hyperglycemia?**

The most effective monotherapy agents for treating hyperglycemia and the typical reduction in hemoglobin A_{1c} are as follows: metformin (0.9%–2.5%), sulfonylureas (1.1%–3.0%), and thiazolidinediones (1.5%–1.6%). Dipeptidyl peptidase-4 inhibitors and α-glucosidase inhibitors are less effective agents, typically reducing hemoglobin A_{1c} by 0.6% to 1.3% and by 0.8%, respectively.

○ **What is used to test lower extremity sensation in patients with diabetes?**

A 10-g monofilament. The failure of the patient to perceive a pressure sensation produced by the Semmes-Weinstein monofilament indicates a loss of protective sensation in the diabetic foot and is highly predictive of foot ulceration.

○ **Which type of hypoglycemic agents are contraindicated in patients with class III or IV heart failure?**

Because of their propensity to expand plasma volume, the use of thiazolidinediones is contraindicated in patients with class III or IV heart failure.

○ **Which oral hypoglycemic agent is most likely to result in weight reduction?**

Metformin. Weight gain is commonly seen in patients treated with sulfonylureas, meglitinides, and thiazolidinediones, and α-glucosidase inhibitors do not typically cause weight loss.

○ **What percentage of weight reduction in patients with impaired glucose tolerance is thought to be sufficient to lower the risk of diabetes?**

Weight reduction as small as 5% to 10% lowers the risk of developing diabetes, often by as much as 58%.

○ **Why is it not advised to combine regular and NPH insulin?**

Although the combination of NPH and regular insulin has been used in an attempt to mimic normal insulin secretion, their erratic absorption and overlapping duration of action not only makes proper dosing a challenge but also increases the risk of hypoglycemia. Hypoglycemic episodes can occur approximately 4 hours after dosing because of the overlap of insulin action seen with regimens combining NPH and regular insulin.

○ **The new insulin analogues more closely mimic physiologic insulin excretion, simplifying insulin dosing and adjustment and providing greater flexibility. Describe the properties of the new insulin analogues: glargine, detemir, lispro, aspart, and glulisine.**

Insulin glargine and insulin detemir are long-acting insulin analogues (genetically modified insulin), with an onset of action of 3 to 4 hours. Glargine is acidic and is only soluble at a pH of 4.0; this reduced solubility at the physiologic pH after subcutaneous injection produces a slow absorption rate. Detemir remains soluble both before and after injection. Both glargine and detemir offer a flat, more prolonged duration of action than NPH does, with less variability in absorption. Glargine's peak action occurs between 8 and 16 hours, and detemir's peak action occurs between 6 and 8 hours.

These basal agents have been shown to cause less hypoglycemia than NPH does. Glargine should not be mixed with other forms of insulin because of the low pH of its diluent.

Insulin lispro, insulin aspart, and insulin glulisine are all rapid-acting insulins with a shorter duration of action than regular insulins; instead of having to be administered 30 minutes before a meal (as required with regular insulin), they may be administered immediately before the meal (onset of action, 15–30 minutes), giving the patient greater flexibility. Compared with regular insulin, lispro, aspart, and glulisine are associated with a lower risk for hypoglycemia when used as a prandial (or bolus) insulin.

○ **Which hormones are responsible for as much as 70% of postprandial insulin secretion?**

Incretin hormones, which include glucagonlike peptide 1 and glucose-dependent insulinotropic polypeptide, are released from the gastrointestinal tract after a meal and are responsible for as much as 70% of postprandial insulin secretion. Exenatide is a synthetic glucagonlike peptide 1 that is administered subcutaneously twice a day and potentiates glucose-mediated insulin secretion. It is thought to lower blood glucose levels by suppressing glucagon secretion and slowing gastric motility.

○ **What are the appropriate parameters for initiating insulin therapy in patients with type 2 diabetes mellitus?**

Insulin therapy should be initiated in patients with fasting blood glucose levels consistently higher than 250 mg/dL. A long-acting insulin should be used initially at a dose of 10 U/d (0.17–0.5 U/kg per day). The dosage should be titrated by 2 U every 3 days to fasting glucose levels lower than 120 mg/dL.

○ **What are the current recommendations for screening for diabetes in children and adolescents?**

The American Diabetes Association recommends screening children with a body mass index at or above the 85th percentile and 2 additional risk factors for diabetes every other year.

○ **What is the predominant energy source used by a healthy subject during starvation?**

Lipids

○ **How long does the body's reserve of carbohydrates last during starvation?**

Glycogen stores are consumed within 24 hours.

○ **What is the equation for nitrogen balance?**

Nitrogen balance = nitrogen intake − nitrogen loss)

$$= [\text{protein (g)}/6.25] - [(\text{urine urea nitrogen}/0.8) + 3]$$

○ **How much protein is required for balance in a healthy stable adult?**

Approximately 0.6 g/kg ideal body weight per day

○ **What is the optimal calorie:nitrogen ratio for critically ill patients?**

100:1 to 200:1

○ **What is the target LDL-C for patients with type 2 diabetes mellitus?**

According to the Third Report of the Expert Panel on Detection, Evaluation, and Treatment of High Blood Cholesterol in Adults (Adult Treatment Panel III, or ATP III) from the National Cholesterol Education Program, a target LDL-C level of 100 mg/dL is optimal for patients with diabetes but without overt cardiovascular disease. However, in patients with overt cardiovascular disease, a lower goal (<70 mg/dL) is preferred.

○ **What effects do bile acid sequestrants such as cholestyramine have on lipid levels?**

Bile acid sequestrants reduce LDL-C by 15% to 30%, increase HDL-C by 3% to 5%, and either produce no change or cause an increase in serum triglyceride levels.

O   **What is the most effective agent for increasing the level of HDL-C?**

Niacin will produce an increase of 15% to 35% in HDL-C level. Fibrates will increase HDL-C level by 10% to 20%, statins by 5% to 15%, and bile acid sequestrants by 3% to 5%. Ezetimibe increases HDL-C levels by 1% to 4%.

O   **What other effects does niacin have on lipid levels, and what is a major adverse effect of niacin?**

Niacin reduces triglyceride levels by 20% to 50% and LDL-C level by 5% to 25%. Hyperglycemia is an adverse effect of niacin therapy, though a dosage of 750 to 2000 mg/day is associated with only moderate increases in blood glucose level and is generally considered a treatment option in patients with diabetes, particularly those with low HDL-C levels.

O   **Patients with what disorder should avoid using the artificial sweetener aspartame?**

Phenylketonuria. Aspartame is completely hydrolyzed in the gut to methanol, aspartic acid, and phenylalanine and is, therefore, contraindicated in patients with phenylketonuria.

O   **What is thyrotoxicosis? What causes it?**

A hypermetabolic state occurring secondary to excess circulating thyroid hormone. Thyrotoxicosis is caused by thyroid hormone overdose, thyroid hyperfunction, or thyroid inflammation.

O   **What are the hallmark clinical features of myxedema coma?**

Hypothermia (75%) and coma

O   **What is the most common precipitant of thyroid storm?**

Pulmonary infections

O   **What signs and symptoms are helpful for diagnosing thyroid storm?**

Eye signs of Graves disease, history of hyperthyroidism, widened pulse pressure, hypertension, palpable goiter, tachycardia, fever, diaphoresis, increased central nervous system activity, emotional lability, heart failure, and coma

O   **Which types of nodules are more likely to be malignant at thyroid scanning: hot or cold?**

Cold. This procedure should not be considered confirmatory. Cysts and benign adenomas can also appear as cold. Some types of thyroid cancers will appear as warm and thus be dismissed. Use caution when interpreting results.

O   **What test should be performed to distinguish a benign cystic nodule from a malignant nodule?**

Fine-needle aspiration biopsy and cytologic evaluation

O   **What is a solitary thyroid nodule most likely to be?**

A nodular goiter (50%). Other possibilities to consider include cancer (20%), adenoma (20%), cyst (5%), or thyroiditis (5%).

O   **What happens to a patient with hyperthyroidism when exogenous thyrotropin-releasing hormone is administered?**

The thyrotropin-releasing hormone receptors are blocked, thus preventing an increase in thyrotropin levels. In a patient with a normal thyroid gland, a concomitant increase in thyrotropin levels would occur.

○ **What are the causes of elevated thyroxine-binding globulin levels?**

Pregnancy, newborn state, estrogens, and heroin

○ **What is the most common cause of acquired hypothyroidism?**

Lymphocytic thyroiditis

○ **What are the clinical manifestations of acquired hypothyroidism?**

Myxedema of the skin, cold intolerance, constipation, low-pitched voice, menorrhagia, mental and physical slowing, dry skin, coarse brittle hair, and decreased energy level with increased need for sleep

○ **What is the most common clinical manifestation of lymphocytic thyroiditis?**

The appearance of a goiter

○ **Patients with lymphocytic thyroiditis are usually: hypothyroid, euthyroid, or hyperthyroid?**

The majority will be euthyroid. However, many will eventually become hypothyroid, but only a few will manifest the symptoms of hyperthyroidism.

○ **What is De Quervain disease?**

A subacute, nonsuppurative thyroiditis. Clinical manifestations involve a tender thyroid gland, fever, and chills, usually remitting within several months.

○ **What is the cause of De Quervain thyroiditis?**

Most likely a viral infection, such as mumps or *Coxsackie virus.*

○ **Which medications commonly cause sporadic goiters?**

Lithium, amiodarone, and iodide-containing asthma inhalers

○ **What is a thyrotropin receptor–stimulating antibody?**

An antibody commonly found in Graves disease, which binds to the thyrotropin receptor leading to thyroid stimulation and goiter production.

○ **Which HLA is associated with Graves disease?**

HLA-DR3. This HLA type is associated with a sevenfold relative risk for Graves disease.

○ **Is Graves disease more common in men or women?**

Women are affected 5 times more than men are.

○ **What are the classical signs and symptoms of Graves disease?**

Emotional lability, autonomic hyperactivity, exophthalmos, tremor, increased appetite with no weight gain or weight loss, diarrhea, and a goiter in nearly all affected individuals

○   **How is Graves disease confirmed with laboratory testing?**

Increased bound and free <u>thyroxine</u> (T_4) and <u>triiodothyronine</u> (T_3) with decreased thyrotropin levels. Frequently, thyroid peroxidase and thyrotropin receptor-stimulating antibodies are present.

○   **What treatment options exist for patients with Graves disease? What treatment is recommended?**

Patients can be treated medically with propylthiouracil or methimazole, surgically with a subtotal thyroidectomy, or with radioiodine therapy. Medical treatment is the treatment of choice.

○   **What are the 3 largest concerns with surgical management of Graves disease?**

1. Hyperthyroidism or hypothyroidism, depending on the amount of tissue removed
2. Vocal cord paralysis
3. Hypoparathyroidism

○   **If fine-needle aspiration biopsy results for a thyroid nodule reveal parafollicular cells, what type of carcinoma should be suspected?**

Medullary carcinoma of the thyroid

○   **How do you manage acute thyrotoxicosis?**

Propranolol 10 mg/kg IV over 10 to 15 minutes for hypertension and increased metabolic rate. Lugol iodine 5 drops orally every 8 hours or sodium iodide 125 to 250 mg/dL IV over 24 hours will stop T_4 production.

○   **What measures can be taken to further reduce peripheral conversion of T_4 to T_3?**

Oral dexamethasone 0.2 mg/kg or oral hydrocortisone 5 mg/kg

○   **What biochemical markers typically are associated with the euthyroid sick syndrome, also known as nonthyroidal illness syndrome (NTI)?**

Low T_3 with normal T_4 levels and low T_3 with low T_4 levels are the most common variants of this syndrome. Thyrotropin level is usually normal but may be high or low.

○   **A small child with failure to thrive has a bone age that is markedly delayed relative to height age and chronologic age. The most likely cause is:**

Hypothyroidism, which is associated with markedly delayed bone age relative to height age and chronologic age

○   **What clinical criteria would increase suspicion for possible thyroid cancer in the evaluation of a patient with a solitary thyroid nodule?**

Male sex; age younger than 20 years or older than 65 years; rapid growth of the nodule; symptoms of local invasion, such as dysphagia, neck pain, and hoarseness; history of head or neck irradiation; family history of thyroid cancer; hard, fixed nodule larger than 4 cm; and cervical lymphadenopathy

○   **Excess thyroid hormone replacement over a number of years in postmenopausal women can lead to:**

Osteoporosis. Even small amounts of thyroid hormone replacement over many years can cause bone mineral resorption, increase serum calcium levels, and lead to osteoporosis.

○ **You have hospitalized a 78-year-old woman for pneumonia. She is mildly dehydrated and slightly lethargic and appears acutely ill. Physical examination results reveal normal height and weight, and chest radiographic findings and physical examination results are consistent with lobar pneumonia. Her laboratory test results reveal an elevated white blood cell count and elevated level of thyrotropin (10.2 mIU/L; normal, 1.0–5.0 mIU/L). What is the next step in the workup of her thyroid abnormality?**

This patient most likely has euthyroid sick syndrome, and the elevated thyrotropin level is due to her illness rather than any underlying thyroid disorder. Subsequent testing (free T_4, T_3) should be performed only if the thyrotropin level remains elevated after resolution of the illness.

○ **What are the causes of thyrotoxicosis characterized by decreased radioactive iodine uptake?**

Subacute thyroiditis, sporadic silent thyroiditis, postpartum lymphocytic thyroiditis, radiation-induced thyroiditis, iodine-induced thyroiditis, thyrotoxicosis factitia, metastatic follicular thyroid cancer, and struma ovarii

○ **What are the causes of thyrotoxicosis characterized by increased radioactive iodine uptake?**

Graves disease, toxic multinodular goiter, solitary hot nodule, thyrotropin-secreting pituitary tumor, molar pregnancy, and choriocarcinoma

○ **What is the treatment of choice for recurrent Graves disease during pregnancy?**

Propylthiouracil has been used extensively during pregnancy and has never been shown to have any teratogenic effect. Methimazole crosses the placenta and is associated with aplasia cutis. Propranolol would control the patient's heart rate but would do nothing about the underlying hyperthyroidism. Radioactive iodine therapy is contraindicated during pregnancy.

○ **An elderly patient presents with an altered mental status, a history of insulin-dependent diabetes mellitus, and hypoglycemia. Core temperature is 32°C. What endocrinologic condition is likely?**

Myxedema coma. Other clues to look for are history of thyroid surgery, hypothyroidism, and use of antithyroid medications.

○ **A patient presents with arms extended and fingers spread apart. Her extremities are flexing and extending in a static-kinetic tremor. This tremor can be associated with what disease?**

Hyperthyroidism

○ **What is another name for "life-threatening hypothyroidism?"**

Myxedema coma. This condition occurs in elderly women during the winter months and is stimulated by infection and stress.

○ **What is the second most common cause of hypothyroidism?**

Autoimmune Hashimoto thyroiditis

○ **How can primary hypothyroidism be distinguished from secondary hypothyroidism?**

- Primary hypothyroidism: Thyrotropin levels are high, patients often have a history of thyroid surgery, and they may have a goiter.
- Secondary hypothyroidism: Thyrotropin levels are low or normal, there is no history of surgery, and no goiter is evident.

○ **What drugs may worsen myxedema?**

Propranolol and phenothiazine

○ **What are the signs and symptoms of hyperthyroidism?**

- Signs: Fever, tachycardia, wide pulse pressure, congestive heart failure, shock, thyromegaly, tremor, liver tenderness, jaundice, stare, hyperkinesis, and pretibial myxedema. Mental status changes include somnolence, obtundation, coma, or psychosis.
- Symptoms: Weight loss, palpitations, dyspnea, edema, chest pain, nervousness, weakness, tremor, psychosis, diarrhea, hyperdefecation, abdominal pain, myalgias, and disorientation

○ **What is the most common cause of hyperthyroidism?**

Graves disease (toxic diffuse goiter)

○ **Is the pituitary gland responsible for parathyroid regulation?**

No. Unlike the thyroid gland, the parathyroid glands are not regulated by the pituitary gland but rather by circulating calcium levels.

○ **What is the difference between primary and secondary hyperparathyroidism?**

In primary hyperparathyroidism, the defect is in the parathyroid gland (ie, an adenoma or hyperplasia), whereas in secondary hyperparathyroidism, the elevated parathyroid hormone (PTH) level is a physiologic response to a low calcium level, usually a result of renal disease.

○ **What are the diagnostic laboratory findings seen in primary hyperparathyroidism?**

Elevated serum calcium and PTH levels, with concomitant decreased phosphorous levels

○ **What is von Recklinghausen disease?**

Hyperparathyroidism leading to cystic changes in bone because of osteoclastic resorption with fibrous replacement, forming nonneoplastic brown tumors.

○ **What is pseudohypoparathyroidism?**

An autosomal recessive disorder characterized by kidney unresponsiveness to PTH, shortened fourth and fifth metacarpals and metatarsals, and short stature, all occurring without evidence of parathyroid dysfunction.

○ **What is the most common cause of hyperparathyroidism?**

Surgery that causes devascularization, removal, or trauma of the parathyroid glands.

○ **What are the indications for parathyroid surgery in patients with repeatedly elevated calcium levels associated with elevated PTH levels?**

Indications for parathyroid surgery include kidney stones, being younger than 50 years, a serum calcium level greater than 1 mg/dL above the upper limit of normal, and reduced bone density.

○ **Which diuretics may exacerbate hypercalcemia associated with primary hyperparathyroidism?**

Thiazide diuretics decrease renal clearance of calcium by increasing distal tubular calcium reabsorption, and although they do not cause hypercalcemia by themselves, they can exacerbate the hypercalcemia associated with primary hyperparathyroidism. Furosemide tends to lower serum calcium levels and is used in the treatment of hypercalcemia.

○ **What is the Trousseau sign, and when is it exhibited?**

A carpal spasm induced when a blood pressure cuff on the upper arm maintains a pressure higher than systolic pressure for approximately 3 minutes. Fingers become spastically extended at the interphalangeal joints and flexed at the metacarpophalangeal joints. The Trousseau sign is a more reliable indicator of hypocalcemia than is the Chvostek sign. Trousseau sign also indicates hypomagnesemia, severe alkalosis, and strychnine poisoning.

○ **What are the causes of hypocalcemia?**

Hypoparathyroidism, shock, sepsis, multiple blood transfusions, vitamin D deficiency, pancreatitis, hypomagnesemia, alkalosis, fat embolism syndrome, phosphate overload, chronic renal failure, loop diuretics, hypoalbuminemia, and tumor lysis syndrome. Medications, such as phenytoin, phenobarbital, heparin, theophylline, cimetidine, and gentamicin, also can cause hypocalcemia.

○ **What are the common causes of hypercalcemia?**

PTH, Addison disease, multiple myeloma, Paget disease, sarcoidosis, cancer, hyperthyroidism, milk-alkali syndrome, immobilization, vitamin D excess, and thiazides.

○ **What are the signs and symptoms of hypercalcemia?**

The most common gastrointestinal symptoms are anorexia and constipation.

- Stones: Renal calculi
- Bones: Osteolysis
- Abdominal groans: Peptic ulcer disease and pancreatitis
- Psychic overtones: Psychiatric disorders

○ **What is the initial treatment for hypercalcemia?**

Restoration of the extracellular fluid with 5 to 10 L of normal saline within 24 hours. After the patient is rehydrated, administer furosemide in doses of 1 to 3 mg/kg. Patients with hypercalcemia are dehydrated because high calcium levels interfere with ADH and the ability of the kidney to concentrate urine.

○ **What are the initial symptoms of a patient with hypocalcemia?**

Paresthesias around the mouth and fingertips, irritability, hyperactive deep tendon reflexes, and seizures

○ **What echocardiographic change is associated with hypocalcemia?**

Prolonged T waves

○ **What metabolic disorder is associated with hypercalcemia?**

Hypokalemia

○ **What is a positive Chvostek sign?**

A twitch in the corner of the mouth that occurs when the facial nerve in front of the ear is tapped. It is present in approximately 10% to 30% of healthy persons. Eyelid muscle contraction resulting from the Chvostek maneuver generally indicates hypocalcemia.

○ **What other mineral must be considered in the patient who appears hypocalcemic?**

Magnesium. Calcium alone will not correct the problem; however, administration of magnesium will correct both the calcium level and the magnesium level.

○ **A patient with a history of ethanol abuse presents after a recent tonic-clonic seizure. What particular electrolyte abnormality should be considered and treated during evaluation?**

Hypomagnesemia. Treat the patient with magnesium sulfate 2 g IV over 1 hour. Total deficit is often 5 to 10 g.

○ **What are the most common causes of hyperphosphatemia?**

Acute and chronic renal failure

○ **What vital sign might be affected with hypermagnesemia?**

Hypermagnesemia causes hypotension because it relaxes vascular smooth muscle. Deep tendon reflexes may disappear.

○ **What is the most common cause of hypermagnesemia in a patient with renal failure?**

Patient use of compounds high in magnesium, such as antacids. This can result in neuromuscular paralysis.

Consider IV calcium. Saline- and furosemide-assisted diuresis may not help a patient with renal failure, so consider dialysis as well.

○ **What hormones are produced by the adrenal cortex?**

Mineralocorticoids, glucocorticoids, and androgenic steroids (remember: salt, sugar, sex)

○ **What is the major mineralocorticoid?**

Aldosterone. Regulated by the renin-angiotensin system, it increases sodium reabsorption and hydronium and potassium excretion.

○ **What is the major glucocorticoid?**

Cortisol

○ **What hormones are produced by the medulla of the adrenal gland?**

Epinephrine and norepinephrine

○ **Name 4 conditions that can be attributed to hyperadrenocortical stimulation.**

1. Cushing syndrome
2. Hyperaldosteronism
3. Adrenogenital syndrome
4. Feminization

○ **What is Cushing disease?**

Pituitary adenomas leading to increased corticotropin secretion with resultant bilateral adrenal hyperplasia and elevated cortisol levels.

○ **What is the differentiation between Cushing disease and Cushing syndrome?**

The term "Cushing syndrome" is used to describe a condition resulting from long-term exposure to excessive glucocorticoids, most commonly from exogenous administration; "Cushing disease" refers to excessive secretion of endogenous corticotropin by a pituitary tumor as the cause of the syndrome.

○ **What are the clinical manifestations of Cushing syndrome?**

Patients with Cushing disease usually present with 1 or more signs and symptoms secondary to the presence of excess cortisol or corticotropin: hypertension, sudden weight gain and central obesity, buffalo hump, facial plethora (moon facies), acne, hypertrichosis, hirsutism, violet striae, glucose intolerance or diabetes mellitus, decreased libido, menstrual disorders, proximal muscle weakness, and depression are most common.

○ **What tests are used to diagnose Cushing syndrome?**

The diagnosis is confirmed when at least 2 of these 3 tests have positive results:

1. Late night salivary cortisol
2. Urinary cortisol
3. Low-dose dexamethasone suppression test

○ **What is the primary clinical manifestation of acute adrenal crisis?**

Adrenal crisis most commonly manifests as hypotension and shock; however, diffuse abdominal pain, anorexia, nausea, vomiting, weakness, fatigue, lethargy, fever, and confusion or coma are also common.

○ **What are the causes of acute adrenal crisis?**

Major stress, such as surgery, severe injury, myocardial infarction, or any other acute illness, in a patient with primary or secondary adrenal insufficiency, although the most common cause is abrupt withdrawal of steroids

○ **Define Waterhouse-Friderichsen syndrome.**

Adrenal insufficiency due to adrenal hemorrhage. It is typically caused by septicemia secondary to meningococcemia with associated bilateral adrenal gland hemorrhage. The patient will have a petechial rash, purpura, shaking, chills, and a severe headache.

○ **What is the characteristic hemodynamic pattern of adrenal insufficiency?**

Predominantly, decreased systemic vascular resistance; to a lesser degree, decreased cardiac contractility, depending on the volume status

○ **What symptoms should increase the suspicion of adrenal insufficiency in the critically ill?**

Unexplained circulatory instability, high fever without cause, unresponsiveness to antibiotics, hypoglycemia, hyponatremia, hyperkalemia, neutropenia, eosinophilia, unexplained mental status changes, disparate anticipated severity of disease, and the actual state of the patient

○   **What are the current dosing recommendations for stress doses of hydrocortisone in patients suspected of having adrenal insufficiency?**

- Minor stress: 25 mg/24 h
- Moderate stress: 50 to 75 mg/24 h
- Major stress: 100 to 150 mg/24 h

○   **What is the emergent steroid replacement in adrenal insufficiency?**

Hydrocortisone 50 to 100 mg IV every 8 hours initially

○   **What is the daily replacement of hydrocortisone once the patient is stabilized?**

Hydrocortisone 15 mg in the morning and 10 mg at night. The dose should be the smallest possible to alleviate clinical symptoms yet prevent weight gain and osteoporosis. Measurements of urinary cortisol levels may help determine the appropriate dosing.

○   **Which patients should receive fludrocortisone?**

Patients with primary adrenal insufficiency should receive 50 to 200 μg/dL of fludrocortisone as a substitute for aldosterone, with the dosage determined according to measurements of blood pressure, potassium level and plasma renin activity.

○   **How long after routine surgery do the serum corticotropin and cortisol concentrations return to normal?**

24 to 28 hours

○   **What is the amount of increased cortisol production that accompanies surgery?**

It depends on the surgery: 85% above baseline for as long as 2 days after laparotomy and 35% above baseline for more minor procedures involving joints, breasts, or neck.

○   **Which drugs can increase the metabolism of cortisol?**

Phenytoin, phenobarbital, and rifampin

○   **Is there any evidence to support the use of corticosteroids for septic shock?**

No beneficial effects of corticosteroids have been shown in sepsis or septic shock. In fact, they may be harmful, according to results from several studies.

○   **Results from randomized prospective trials have shown benefit from corticosteroids for which disease states?**

Bacterial meningitis, acute spinal injury, typhoid fever, *Pneumocystis jirovecii* pneumonia, and possibly the fibroproliferative phase of acute respiratory distress syndrome.

○   **Which study is probably the best predictor of adrenal adequacy in patients previously receiving steroids who are scheduled for surgery?**

Although the insulin-induced hypoglycemia test and metyrapone tests can be useful, the best indicator of maximal serum cortisol concentration during surgery is the peak cortisol level after administration of corticotropin.

○ **What is the normal daily production of cortisol?**

It was previously thought to be 12 to 15 μg/dL, but current estimates are 5 μg/dL. This correlates to about 10 to 12 mg of oral hydrocortisone replacement per square meter because of decreased bioavailability secondary to first-pass hepatic metabolism.

○ **What are the adverse effects of excessive cortisol dosing for stress?**

Catabolic effects on muscle, impaired wound healing, antagonizing insulin, effects on glucose metabolism, and anti-inflammatory effect on active infection

○ **What are the main causes of death during an acute adrenal crisis?**

Circulatory collapse and cardiac arrhythmias induced by hyperkalemia

○ **In a critical care setting, adrenal insufficiency is likely in patients with conditions refractory to which types of medications?**

Catecholamines and vasopressors

○ **What are the common clinical features of chronic adrenal insufficiency?**

Fatigue worsened by exertion and improved with rest, lethargy, anorexia, weight loss, hyperpigmentation, hyponatremia, and hyperkalemia are common. Depression, dizziness, orthostatic hypotension, nausea and vomiting, diarrhea, lymphocytosis, increased level of eosinophils, and normocytic-normochromic anemia are also significant manifestations. Hypoglycemia is not common.

○ **What are the 3 types of adrenal insufficiency?**

1. Primary: Disease at the adrenal level, involving destruction of the steroid-secreting cortex
2. Secondary: Any process that involves the pituitary gland and interferes with corticotropin secretion from the pituitary gland
3. Tertiary: Interference with corticotropin-releasing hormone secretion by the hypothalamus gland

○ **What are the major differences in clinical manifestation between primary adrenal insufficiency and secondary or tertiary adrenal insufficiency?**

Primary adrenal insufficiency is manifested by both glucocorticoid and mineralocorticoid deficiency and, in women, androgen deficiency. Since mineralocorticoid activity remains intact in secondary and tertiary adrenal insufficiency, hyperpigmentation (corticotropin is not increased), hyperkalemia (aldosterone is still present), and dehydration are not present; hypotension is less prominent and gastrointestinal symptoms are less common, though hypoglycemia is more common.

○ **What is the cause of primary adrenal insufficiency?**

Failure of the adrenal cortex (also known as Addison disease)

○ **What are the causes of acute abrupt primary adrenal insufficiency?**

Adrenal hemorrhage, necrosis, thrombosis in meningococcal disease, sepsis, anticoagulation therapy, or antiphospholipid syndrome

○   **What are the causes of primary adrenal insufficiency (Addison disease)?**

Autoimmune disease (autoimmune adrenalitis) is responsible for 70% to 90%, with the remainder being caused by infectious diseases (tuberculosis or fungal infection, such as histoplasmosis, blastomycosis, or cryptococcosis), AIDS (cytomegalovirus or Kaposi sarcoma), replacement by metastatic cancer (lung, breast, or kidney) or lymphoma, adrenal hemorrhage or infarction, or drugs.

○   **What are the signs and symptoms of Addison disease?**

Hyperpigmentation, hyperkalemia, alopecia, and ascending paralysis secondary to hyperkalemia. Hyperpigmentation of the skin and mucosal membranes due to high corticotropin levels as a consequence of cortisol feedback and salt craving are the most specific signs of primary adrenal insufficiency.

○   **What characteristic laboratory test findings are associated with primary adrenal insufficiency?**

Hyponatremia due to mineralocorticoid deficiency and increased vasopressin secretion caused by cortisol deficiency, hyperkalemia due to mineralocorticoid deficiency, azotemia (if volume depleted), and mild metabolic acidosis. Hypercalcemia may occur, but is rare, and hypoglycemia is rare in adults in the absence of infection, fever, or ethanol ingestion, or prolonged fasting.

○   **Are imaging studies of the adrenal glands necessary in the diagnosis of primary adrenal insufficiency?**

Yes. In cases other than autoimmune or adrenal myeloneuropathy, computed tomography of the adrenal glands should be performed to aid in the differential diagnosis. Enlarged glands with or without calcifications in patients with tuberculosis are a sign of active disease and warrant anti-infective therapy. Enlargement also occurs with other fungal infections, lymphoma, cancer, and AIDS. Biopsy performed with computed tomographic guidance may also be helpful.

○   **The use of which sedating agent has been shown to increase mortality in critically ill patients by inducing primary adrenal insufficiency?**

Etomidate. This sedating agent is a selective inhibitor of adrenal 11-hydroxylase, the enzyme that converts deoxycortisol to cortisol. Mortality reportedly increased in a trauma unit that began using etomidate as continuous infusion for sedation, so etomidate is not used for continuous sedation in the critically ill.

○   **What effect does Addison disease have on cortisol and aldosterone levels?**

It lowers them. Low cortisol levels induce nausea, vomiting, anorexia, lethargy, hypoglycemia, water intoxication, and the inability to withstand even minor stress without shock. Low aldosterone levels cause sodium depletion, dehydration, hypotension, and syncope.

○   **What are the causes of secondary adrenal insufficiency?**

Any process that involves the pituitary and interferes with corticotropin secretion can cause secondary adrenal insufficiency: pituitary infarction (Sheehan syndrome), pituitary tumor, infectious disease or hemorrhage, and head trauma.

○   **Secretion of which adrenal hormone is not impaired by secondary adrenal insufficiency?**

Aldosterone. Aldosterone secretion depends more on angiotensin II than on corticotropin, and aldosterone deficiency is not a problem in hypopituitarism. Selective aldosterone hypersecretion can manifest as a result of increased renin and angiotensin II formation.

○ **What are the 3 tests used to evaluate secondary adrenal insufficiency?**

1. Insulin-induced hypoglycemia
2. Short-term metyrapone tests
3. Corticotropin-releasing hormone test

○ **What is the basis of the insulin-induced hypoglycemia test for secondary adrenal insufficiency?**

Hypoglycemia induced by 0.1 U of insulin per kilogram of body weight stimulates the entire hypothalamic-pituitary-adrenal, sympathetic nervous system, and plasma cortisol levels should exceed 20 μg/dL. This test is contraindicated in patients with cardiac disease and a history of seizures, as well as in patients with low basal cortisol levels.

○ **What is the short-term metyrapone test?**

Metyrapone (30 mg/kg administered with a snack at midnight) inhibits adrenal 11-hydroxylase. Normally, the cortisol precursor 11-deoxycortisol level increases to at least 7 μg/dL in response to the decreased production of cortisol and loss of negative feedback of cortisol to the hypothalamic-pituitary-adrenal axis; hence, corticotropin production is stimulated. This indicates secondary adrenal insufficiency only in the setting of a previously measured cortisol level of 8 μg/dL or lower.

○ **How can the corticotropin-stimulation test result be normal for secondary adrenal insufficiency of recent origin?**

The results of a corticotropin-stimulation test can show a normal cortisol production response because the gland has not yet atrophied and retains the ability to be stimulated. The 250-μg dose of corticotropin is also far in excess of the 5 or 10 μg that maximally stimulates a normal adrenal cortex. A stimulation test with a low dose of 1 μg corticotropin may allow for assessment of mild insufficiency.

○ **What is the most common cause of tertiary adrenal insufficiency?**

Abrupt cessation of high-dose glucocorticoid therapy or correction of Cushing syndrome

○ **Does a normal cortisol level in a critically ill patient rule out adrenal insufficiency?**

No. With critical illness, one should expect a cortisol level greater than normal, and a normal level could be considered relatively insufficient. An absolute level of 25 μg/dL probably rules out adrenal insufficiency, although the lower cutoff is unknown.

○ **How is a corticotropin-stimulation test performed to rule out adrenal insufficiency?**

After a baseline cortisol level is measured, 250 μg of cosyntropin is administered IV (or intramuscularly), and cortisol levels are measured at 30 and 60 minutes after injection. Adrenal function is thought to be normal if the cortisol level measured at 30 or 60 minutes is 20 μg/dL or higher.

○ **What added precautions should be taken by all patients with adrenal insufficiency?**

They should wear a medic alert bracelet, carry a card detailing their medications and the recommendations for treatment in emergencies, and double or triple their dose of hydrocortisone when they sustain injury or illness. They should secure ampules of glucocorticoids for self-injection or suppositories when vomiting or unable to take oral steroids.

○   **What accounts for the almost immediate effect of cortisol on blood pressure in patients with adrenal insufficiency?**

Cortisol exerts a permissive effect on catecholamine vascular responsivity and plays a vital role in the maintenance of vascular tone, vascular permeability, and distribution of body water within the vascular compartment.

○   **If autoimmune adrenal disease is the underlying disorder, which zone of the adrenal gland is spared?**

Medulla

○   **What is the function of aldosterone?**

Aldosterone causes sodium conservation and potassium excretion. As a result, it causes increased resorption of sodium and fluid.

○   **What is Conn syndrome?**

Primary hyperproduction of adrenal mineralocorticoids, usually caused by an aldosterone-producing adenoma

○   **What are the clinical features of primary hyperaldosteronism?**

Hypertension and hypokalemia are the 2 major clinical findings in primary aldosteronism. The clinical features are determined by the actions of the aldosterone. There is an increase in the number of open sodium channels in the cortical collecting tubules, causing increased sodium and water reabsorption (mild hypernatremia), leading to volume expansion and hypertension and to renal excretion of potassium (hypokalemia) and hydrogen ions (metabolic alkalosis). Mild urinary magnesium wasting may also occur (hypomagnesemia).

○   **Define the medical therapeutic approach to primary hyperaldosteronism due to bilateral adrenal hyperplasia.**

The goals of therapy include correction of hypokalemia, restoration of normal blood pressure, and reversal of the effects of hyperaldosteronism on the heart. Spironolactone, a mineralocorticoid receptor antagonist, is the drug of choice and is titrated to a normal serum potassium level without the aid of potassium supplements. A thiazide diuretic or an angiotensin-converting enzyme inhibitor can be added if hypertension persists.

○   **What is a pheochromocytoma?**

A rare catecholamine-secreting tumor of the adrenal medulla (tumoral hypersecretion of norepinephrine, epinephrine, and dopamine); when the catecholamine-secreting tumor arises from the sympathetic ganglia, it is referred to as an "extra-adrenal catecholamine-secreting paraganglioma," although the clinical manifestations are the same.

○   **Define the classic triad of symptoms in patients with pheochromocytoma.**

1. Headache
2. Sweating
3. Tachycardia

About half of patients have paroxysmal hypertension, though most have what appears to be essential hypertension.

○   **What autosomal dominant diseases are associated with a higher prevalence of pheochromocytoma?**

von Hippel-Lindau syndrome, multiple endocrine neoplasia type II, and neurofibromatosis type 1

○ **What laboratory tests are used to confirm the diagnosis of pheochromocytoma?**

The diagnosis is typically confirmed with measurements of 24-hour urinary metanephrines and catecholamines (epinephrine, norepinephrine, metanephrine, and vanillylmandelic acid); measurement of fractionated plasma free metanephrines lacks specificity and is reserved only for cases for which the index of suspicion is high. The clonidine-suppression test is a confirmatory test intended to distinguish between pheochromocytoma and false-positive increases in plasma catecholamines and fractionated plasma metanephrines.

○ **Which medications interfere with the diagnostic tests for pheochromocytoma?**

Tricyclic antidepressants interfere most frequently with the interpretation of 24-hour urinary catecholamine and metabolite tests. Although it is preferable that patients not receive any medication during the diagnostic evaluation, treatment with most medications may be continued.

○ **What is the typical size of an adrenal carcinoma when diagnosed?**

Ninety percent are larger than 6 cm in diameter.

○ **Pheochromocytomas produce what compounds?**

Catecholamines. This group of chemicals results in increased blood pressure, perspiration, heart palpitations, anxiety, and weight loss.

○ **If vanillylmandelic acid, normetanephrine, and metanephrine are detected in the urine, what is the likely cause?**

Pheochromocytoma

○ **Where are most pheochromocytomas located?**

Ninety percent are found in the adrenal medulla. The remainder are located in other tissues originating from neural crest cells.

○ **What is the pheochromocytoma rule of 10s?**

Ten percent are malignant, 10% are multiple or bilateral, 10% are extraadrenal, 10% occur in children, 10% recur after surgical removal, 10% are familial.

○ **Which class of antihypertensive medications is used preoperatively to control blood pressure (including preventing a hypertensive crisis during surgery) and volume expansion in patients with pheochromocytoma?**

α-Adrenergic blocking agents like phenoxybenzamine should be started 7 to 10 days preoperatively to normalize blood pressure and expand the contracted blood volume.

○ **How do you manage a hypertensive crisis in a patient with pheochromocytoma?**

1 mg IV phentolamine or 0.5 to 0.8 mg/kg per minute of sodium nitroprusside

○ **What are the hormones produced in the anterior pituitary gland?**

Six well-characterized hormones are secreted by the anterior pituitary gland: (1) corticotropin, (2) thyrotropin, (3) luteinizing hormone (LH), (4) follicle-stimulating hormone (FSH), (5) growth hormone, and (6) prolactin.

○   **What is the most common cause of hypopituitarism?**

The most common cause of hypopituitarism is the presence of a pituitary tumor. Although they are true neoplasms, most pituitary adenomas are benign. Hypothalamic tumors are responsible for about 13% of cases of hypopituitarism. Pituitary infarction (Sheehan syndrome) accounts for only 0.5% of cases. Treatment involves replacement of the deficient hormone.

○   **What are the most common causes of hyperprolactinemia?**

Hyperprolactinemia results almost exclusively from diseases that cause hypersecretion of prolactin by the lactotroph cells. The most common causes are categorized as physiologic (pregnancy, nipple stimulation, and stress) and pathologic (prolactinomas, decreased inhibition of prolactin secretion, and decreased prolactin clearance). Many drugs, including antipsychotic drugs, phenothiazines, haloperidol, butyrophenones, metoclopramide, domperidone, antihypertensive drugs, methyldopa, and verapamil (though other calcium-channel blockers do not), can cause hyperprolactinemia.

○   **What are the clinical manifestations of hyperprolactinemia?**

Hyperprolactinemia in premenopausal women causes hypogonadism, manifested as infertility, oligomenorrhea, or amenorrhea and, less often, as galactorrhea. Since postmenopausal women are already hypogonadal and hypoestrogenemic, galactorrhea is rare, and hyperprolactinemia is recognized only when a lactotroph adenoma becomes so large that it causes headaches or vision disturbances. In men, hyperprolactinemia causes hypogonadotropic hypogonadism manifested as decreased libido, impotence, infertility, gynecomastia, and (rarely) galactorrhea.

○   **What options exist for the treatment of prolactinomas?**

Medical therapy with dopamine agonists (bromocriptine, cabergoline, or pergolide) to decrease prolactin levels or surgery by means of a transsphenoidal approach

○   **What is the best radiologic modality to evaluate a sellar mass?**

Magnetic resonance imaging (MRI) is the single best imaging procedure for most sellar masses.

○   **What are the clinical manifestations of acromegaly?**

Acromegaly is the clinical syndrome that results from excessive secretion of growth hormone. Common clinical manifestations include macrognathia, enlarged hands and feet, coarse facial features, macroglossia, deepening of the voice, skin thickening, and excessive hair growth.

○   **What pituitary tumor is the most common?**

Prolactinoma

○   **What are the common presenting signs of prolactinoma?**

Headache, amenorrhea, and galactorrhea

○ **After an endocrinologic diagnosis has been established with hormonal studies, what would be the radiologic study of choice to assess for pituitary or hypothalamic tumor?**

Magnetic resonance imaging (MRI) with analysis of the sagittal and coronal sections. Computed tomography can be helpful if bony invasion is suspected.

○ **What clinical findings will there be in a 7-year-old with an ovarian granulosa cell tumor?**

Pseudoprecocious puberty. She may have vaginal bleeding, axillary hair, and early breast budding.

○ **How is primary hypogonadism defined in a male patient?**

Hypogonadism in a male patient refers to a decrease in 1 or both of the 2 major functions of the testes—sperm production or testosterone production—resulting from disease of the testes.

○ **What are the clinical manifestations of primary hypogonadism?**

Failure of development of the secondary sexual characteristics, with abnormally small penis and testes

○ **How is primary hypogonadism diagnosed?**

The levels of FSH and LH are abnormally elevated for the corresponding age. Testosterone levels remain low and show little response to the administration of human chorionic gonadotropin.

○ **What is the deficient hormone in secondary hypogonadism?**

FSH or LH. The defect is in the pituitary gland rather than in the testes or ovaries.

○ **How is primary hypogonadism differentiated clinically from secondary hypogonadism?**

By measurement of the serum LH and FSH levels. The patient has primary hypogonadism if the serum testosterone concentration and/or the sperm count are lower than normal and the serum LH and/or FSH concentrations are higher than normal. The patient has secondary hypogonadism (disease of the pituitary or hypothalamus gland) if the serum testosterone concentration and/or the sperm count are subnormal and the serum LH and/or FSH concentrations are normal or reduced.

○ **What is hypogonadotropic hypogonadism?**

A delayed onset of puberty caused by decreased levels of FSH and LH, with functioning ovaries or testes

○ **What is Kallmann syndrome?**

Hypogonadotropic hypogonadism associated with anosmia

○ **What is the most common disorder of sexual differentiation?**

Klinefelter syndrome is the most common congenital abnormality causing primary hypogonadism and occurs in approximately 1 in 1000 live male births. The primary abnormality is the presence of 2 or more X chromosomes; most commonly the genotype is 47,XXY.

○ **Describe the cause of PCOS.**

Insulin resistance with compensatory hyperinsulinemia is thought to play a major role in the cause of this syndrome, which is characterized by anovulation and hyperandrogenism. PCOS affects an estimated 6% of women of reproductive age.

○ **What are the clinical manifestations of PCOS?**

Obesity, hirsutism, secondary amenorrhea, and bilaterally enlarged polycystic ovaries

○ **What agents reduce insulin resistance in patients with PCOS?**

Metformin and troglitazone are oral hypoglycemic agents that reduce insulin resistance and have been shown to increase the frequency of ovulation in patients with PCOS. Other thiazolidinediones have not been shown to have a similar effect.

○ **What treatments are used for PCOS?**

Oral contraceptive pills for menstrual regulation and ovarian suppression

○ **What laboratory findings are seen in PCOS?**

Most patients have an increased ratio of LH to FSH and an increased amount of LH because of an exaggerated response to gonadotropin-releasing hormone.

○ **What joint is most commonly affected with gout?**

The hallux metacarpophalangeal joint

○ **What joint is most commonly affected with pseudogout?**

The knee. The causative agent is calcium pyrophosphate crystals.

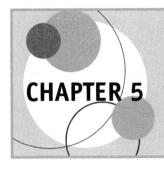

CHAPTER 5 Neurology

Raj C. Shah, MD

○ **What is the significance of bilateral nystagmus with cold caloric testing?**

It signifies that an intact cortex, midbrain, and brain stem are present.

○ **Differentiate between decerebrate and decorticate posturing.**

Decerebrate posturing: Elbows and legs are extended (indicative of a midbrain lesion).

Decorticate posturing: Elbows are flexed and legs extended (suggestive of a thalamic lesion).

(Remember: de**COR**ticate = hands by the heart)

○ **What area of the brain is dysfunctional when a patient has Cheyne-Stokes respiration?**

The cortex. The nervous system is relying on diencephalic control.

○ **What are common electrocardiographic changes seen in brain injuries?**

Sinus tachycardia, QT-interval prolongation, and pan precordial T-wave inversion. More severe findings include QRS widening and ventricular tachycardia.

○ **What is the single most important modifiable risk factor for stroke?**

Hypertension

○ **What is the risk of cerebral infarction in the first 5 years after posterior circulation transient ischemic attacks?**

35%

○ **What are major risk factors for carotid artery stenosis?**

Older age, male sex, hypertension, smoking, high cholesterol level, and heart disease

○ **Carotid endarterectomy is indicated for patients who have symptoms and what degree of stenosis?**

70% or greater

○ **Heterozygotes for homocystinuria can manifest what problem in adulthood?**

Adults who are heterozygous for homocystinuria can present with a history of stroke at a younger age than would otherwise be expected. Deficiency of cystathionine β-synthase is the most common cause of homocystinuria. Homozygous persons present early in life with ectopia lentis, intellectual disability, and early strokes.

○ **What artery is most commonly involved in stroke?**

The middle cerebral artery

○ **A patient with aphasia most likely had a stroke involving which hemisphere?**

The dominant hemisphere. Patients who have a stroke in the nondominant hemisphere have apraxia and sensory neglect.

○ **What is the difference between dysarthria and aphasia?**

Dysarthria is a disorder of speech, a motor function. Aphasia is a disorder of language, a higher cortical function.

○ **A patient has an irritative lesion in the left hemisphere. Which way do the eyes deviate?**

To the right

○ **What visual deficit is typically associated with lesions at the optic chiasm?**

Bitemporal hemianopsia

○ **Which is the most common cause of cerebral artery occlusion: embolic or thrombotic?**

Thrombotic

○ **What signs occur with an anterior cerebral artery infarct?**

Leg weakness greater than arm weakness on the contralateral side and incontinence. No aphasia will be evident.

○ **What signs are displayed in a middle cerebral artery stroke?**

Contralateral hemiplegia or hemiparesthesia, homonymous hemianopsia, speech disturbance, and arm and face weakness greater than leg weakness

○ **What motor function is spared in locked-in syndrome?**

Upward gaze

○ **Unilateral occlusion of the vertebrobasilar arterial distribution results in what kind of symptoms?**

Ipsilateral cranial nerve abnormalities and contralateral motor and sensory deficits

○ **If a lesion is in the brain stem, which way will the eyes deviate?**

Away from side of the lesion in the brain stem

○ **What is the risk of symptomatic intracranial hemorrhage in patients who receive tissue plasminogen activator?**

6%. The risk of fatal intracranial hemorrhage is 3%.

○ **What treatment decreases morbidity or mortality in patients with acute ischemic stroke?**

Aspirin in a daily dose of 160 to 300 mg initiated within 48 hours after symptom onset resulted in a decrease in 6-month morbidity and mortality caused by acute ischemic stroke.

○ **What are the antiplatelet mechanisms of action of aspirin and ticlopidine?**

Aspirin interferes with platelet function by inhibiting the enzyme cyclooxygenase. Ticlodipine inhibits adenosine diphosphate–induced platelet aggregation.

○ **What potential adverse effect requires monitoring in patients treated with ticlopidine?**

Neutropenia

○ **What is the usual localization of the pure sensory stroke?**

Thalamus

○ **A patient presents with facial droop on the left and weakness of the right leg. Where is the most likely site of the lesion?**

The brain stem, specifically the left pons

○ **What are the signs and symptoms of posterior inferior cerebellar artery syndrome?**

Cerebellar dysfunction, such as vertigo, ataxia, and dizziness

○ **Describe the key features of vertebrobasilar insufficiency.**

Vertigo (nearly always positional accompanied by nystagmus). Other signs of arteriosclerosis may be found. Vertebrobasilar insufficiency is typically prevalent in older persons and may occur with other symptoms of brain-stem ischemia.

○ **For the following clinical presentations, identify which are associated with peripheral vertigo and which are associated with central vertigo.**

1. Intense spinning, nausea, hearing loss, diaphoresis
2. Swaying or impulsion, worse with movement, tinnitus, acute onset
3. Unidirectional nystagmus inhibited by ocular fixation, fatigable
4. Mild vertigo, diplopia, and ataxia
5. Multidirectional nystagmus not inhibited by ocular fixation, nonfatigable

Answers: Peripheral vertigo: (1), (2), and (3); central vertigo: (4) and (5)

○   **Which of the following signs is not part of the classic Wallenberg syndrome: nystagmus, Horner syndrome, contralateral hemiparesis, ipsilateral ataxia, or contralateral loss of pain and temperature sense?**

Hemiparesis

○   **A 36-year-old presents with altered mental status and history of a fall with severe headache. What is the diagnosis after viewing only the computed tomographic (CT) scan?**

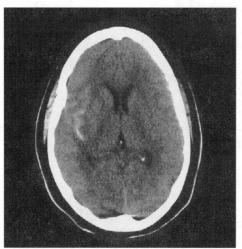 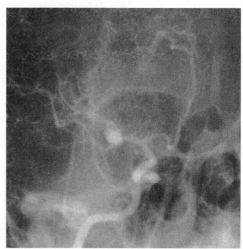

Fig. A   Fig. B

Acute right-sided subarachnoid hemorrhage confined mostly to the sylvian fissure. (Fig. A) The differential diagnosis is between trauma and ruptured intracerebral aneurysm. In this patient, a large, right, middle cerebral artery trifurcation aneurysm is confirmed by means of contrast material–enhanced angiography. (Fig. B)

○   **What are the causes of cerebral hemorrhage?**

Trauma, hypertension, ruptured aneurysms, cerebral amyloid angiopathy, vascular malformations, hemorrhage into a tumor (eg, melanoma, choriocarcinoma, renal cell carcinoma), anticoagulant use, hemophilia, thrombocytopenia, stimulant drugs (amphetamines, cocaine, phenylpropanolamine), and vasculitis (eg, Wegener granulomatosis)

○   **Lesions containing what substances are of high attenuation on CT scans obtained without the use of contrast material?**

Blood, calcium, or melanin. High attenuation with blood results from the protein fraction of hemoglobin (92%–93%) rather than from that of iron, which contributes only 7% to 8% to the brightness.

○   **Carotid bifurcation aneurysms may cause intracerebral hemorrhage into what areas of the brain?**

Frontal lobe, temporal lobe, and basal ganglia

○   **Where is the most common intraparenchymal site of intracranial bleeding?**

The putamen

○   **Where are congenital berry aneurysms located?**

In the circle of Willis

○ **What are the complications that occur after subarachnoid hemorrhage?**

Vasospasm, recurrent hemorrhage, hydrocephalus, seizures, cardiac arrhythmias, hypertension, neurogenic pulmonary edema, stress ulcers, and syndrome of inappropriate secretion of antidiuretic hormone

○ **How is a subarachnoid hemorrhage diagnosed?**

CT may show blood in the suprasellar cistern, interhemispheric fissure, sylvian fissure, or surface of the brain. If CT findings are normal, a spinal tap may show xanthochromia or blood.

○ **What is the most common cause of subarachnoid hemorrhage?**

Saccular aneurysm

○ **What are other common causes of subarachnoid hemorrhage?**

Rupture of cerebral artery aneurysm and arteriovenous malformation. Patients present with an abrupt, severe headache that can progress to syncope, nausea, vomiting, nuchal rigidity, and nonfocal neurological changes.

○ **What drug will reduce the risk of vasospasm after subarachnoid hemorrhage?**

Nimodipine

○ **When is maximum cerebrospinal fluid (CSF) xanthochromia observed after subarachnoid hemorrhage?**

48 hours

○ **What is the Cushing reflex?**

The elevation in blood pressure and reduction in pulse that follow an increase in intracranial pressure. It is a brain-stem–mediated reflex.

○ **Below what value of cerebral perfusion pressure is autoregulation of cerebral blood flow impaired?**

Below 40 to 50 mm Hg: CPP = MAP − ICP, where CPP is cerebral perfusion pressure, MAP is mean arterial pressure, and ICP is intracranial pressure

○ **When should steroids be used in the treatment of increased intracranial pressure?**

Steroids are beneficial in the treatment of vasogenic edema, so they should be used to treat increased intracranial pressure associated with tumors, abscesses, and brain trauma.

○ **At lumbar puncture, opening pressure is markedly elevated. What should be done?**

Close the 3-way stopcock, remove only a small amount of fluid from the manometer, abort the lumbar puncture, and initiate measures to decrease the intracranial pressure.

○ **What are the earliest clinical features of uncal herniation?**

Uncal herniation begins with a unilateral enlarged pupil and a sluggish pupillary light reaction

○ **Rank the following vascular malformations in order of risk of hemorrhage: arteriovenous malformation, capillary telangiectasia, cavernous malformation, and venous angioma.**

    1. Arteriovenous malformation

    2. Cavernous malformation

    3. Capillary telangiectasia

    4. Venous angioma

○ **What stroke type is increased most in the postpartum period?**

Cerebral venous thrombosis

○ **What disorder manifests with ischemic and hemorrhagic stroke associated with progressive occlusion of the arteries at the circle of Willis?**

Moyamoya disease

○ **Bilateral cortical hemorrhagic infarcts associated with increased intracranial pressure are observed in what stroke syndrome?**

Superior sagittal sinus syndrome

○ **What disorder manifests with chemosis, proptosis, and an ocular bruit?**

Carotid cavernous fistula

○ **What diagnosis must be investigated in the patient presenting with pulsating exophthalmos?**

Carotid cavernous fistula. Patients without a history of trauma, usually women, older than 40 years, often present with orbito-fronto-temporal headache, dilated conjunctival veins, and possibly a sixth-nerve palsy.

○ **What are the most common clinical problems at the initial manifestation of an intracranial arteriovenous malformation?**

Seizures and hemorrhage

○ **What is the management of an incidental venous angioma of the brain?**

No treatment is necessary.

○ **Damage to the middle meningeal artery results in what kind of hematoma?**

Epidural

○ **A 29-year-old drunken man presents after having his head pounded on the concrete. The patient had a brief syncopal episode but was then ambulatory and alert. Now he appears drowsy and just vomited. What is the probable diagnosis?**

Epidural hematoma

○ **Which is more common: subdural or epidural hemorrhaging?**

Subdural. Subdural hemorrhaging can result from the tearing of the bridging veins. Bleeding occurs less rapidly because the veins, not the arteries, are damaged.

○ **What is the most common anatomic source of a subdural hematoma?**

Bridging veins

○ **A 71-year-old man presents with a unilateral burning headache that is worse around his temples and his eye. He also complains of visual disturbances and pain in his jaw after heavy use. At examination, you palpate a prominent temporal artery that is tender. What tests should be performed to make a diagnosis?**

Biopsy of the temporal artery. This patient most likely has temporal arteritis or giant cell arteritis. A sedimentation rate higher than 50 mm/h suggests this diagnosis.

○ **Why is the above case a medical emergency?**

Giant cell arteritis affects the large blood vessels. It usually involves the arteries branching off of the carotids. Therefore, involvement of the temporal artery may also indicate involvement of the central retinal artery. Twenty-five percent of patients with temporal arteritis have thromboses in the central retinal artery, which leads to blindness. An immediate course of high-dose prednisone should be started to decrease the inflammation in all patients.

○ **What conditions are included in the autism spectrum disorders?**

Autistic disorder, Asperger syndrome, and pervasive developmental disorder not otherwise specified

○ **What are the impairments in autism?**

Autism is characterized by qualitative impairments in communication and social interaction and by restricted, repetitive, and stereotyped patterns of behaviors and interests. Abnormal development is present before age 3 years. One-third of patients develop epilepsy, and three-fourths have intellectual disability.

○ **How many adults with autism live independent lives?**

15%. Another 15% to 20% live alone with community support. The remainder require full-time care.

○ **What are the clinical findings of Kleine-Levin syndrome?**

This syndrome occurs in adolescent boys and manifests as episodes of hypersomnia, hyperphagia, and frontal lobe–type personality changes.

○ **Differentiate between dementia and delirium.**

Dementia is irreversible, impaired functioning secondary to changes and deficits in memory, spatial concepts, personality, cognition, language, motor and sensory skills, judgment, or behavior. There is no change in consciousness.

Delirium is a reversible, organic mental syndrome reflecting deficits in attention, organized thinking, orientation, speech, memory, and perception. Patients are frequently confused, anxious, and excited and have hallucinations. A change in consciousness may be evident.

○ **What is the most common pathophysiologic cause of delirium?**

Acetylcholine deficiency

○ **What are the typical features of transient global amnesia?**

Abrupt onset of amnesia that spares personal identity, resolves within 24 hours, has no other neurologic deficits, and occurs typically between ages 50 and 70 years.

○ **The postconcussive syndrome includes what symptoms?**

Headaches, dizziness, impaired memory and concentration, irritability, and depression

○ **A 25-year-old man was knocked unconscious for 10 seconds while playing touch football 1 week ago. Since then, he has had intermittent vertigo, nausea, vomiting, blurred vision, headache, and malaise. His neurologic examination and CT results are normal. What is the diagnosis?**

Postconcussive syndrome. Most individuals recover fully over 2 to 6 weeks. A small percentage of patients with postconcussive syndrome will have persistent deficits.

○ **What is the most common nontraumatic cause of dementia?**

Alzheimer disease. At the age of 65 years, 10% of the population has Alzheimer disease; by 85 years, 50% does. Multi-infarct dementia is the second most common cause of nontraumatic dementia.

○ **What are the 2 pathologic findings used to confirm the diagnosis of Alzheimer disease?**

The quantity of neurofibrillary tangles and senile plaques. Other findings include neuronal loss and amyloid degeneration.

○ **What types of memory are impaired earliest in Alzheimer disease?**

Episodic, explicit, declarative, and short-term memory

○ **What is the first symptom of Alzheimer disease?**

Progressive memory loss, followed by disorientation, personality changes, language difficulty, and other symptoms of dementia

○ **Apart from the Mini-Mental State Examination, what are brief screening instruments for dementia that take 3 to 5 minutes to administer in a primary care setting?**

The General Practitioner Assessment of Cognition (GPCOG), the Memory Impairment Screen (MIS), and the Mini-Cog Assessment Instrument (Mini-Cog) have accuracy similar to or better than that of the Mini-Mental State Examination and have been validated in the primary care setting. The GPCOG has 6 items for the patient being evaluated, with an optional set of 6 questions for someone who knows the patient well. The MIS involves immediate and delayed recall (with prompting if necessary) of 4 words, with a delay filled by counting from 1 to 20 forward and backward. The Mini-Cog involves immediate and delayed recall of 3 words with a clock-drawing test used between the word recall tests. The GPCOG was 82% sensitive and 70% specific, the MIS was 86% sensitive and 91% specific, and the Mini-Cog was 99% sensitive and 93% specific. As an initial screening for dementia, the higher the sensitivity to rule out cases, the better the screening test. A positive screen result would lead to further detailed dementia testing.

○ **How do donepezil, rivastigmine, and galantamine treat Alzheimer disease?**

All are acetylcholinesterase inhibitors and help compensate for the cholinergic deficits in Alzheimer disease.

○ **What is the prognosis for patients with Alzheimer disease?**

Alzheimer disease is irreversible. Death occurs about 10 years after presumptive diagnosis but can range anywhere from 3 to 20 years.

○ **What are the major risk factors for Alzheimer disease?**

Age, Down syndrome (trisomy 21), and family history

○ **Patients with which type of apolipoprotein are more likely to acquire Alzheimer disease?**

Apolipoprotein E type 4

○ **What percentage of patients with primary Alzheimer disease will present with secondary depression?**

30% to 35%

○ **What is sundown syndrome?**

Hallucinations and delusions that occur at nighttime because of decreased sensory stimulation

○ **What functions are preserved in frontotemporal dementias (eg, Pick disease) as compared with Alzheimer disease?**

Memory, calculations, and visuospatial abilities. Both are associated with language disturbances, and personality alterations are prominent in frontotemporal dementias.

○ **What is the characteristic triad of normal pressure hydrocephalus?**

Dementia, incontinence, and gait ataxia (often described as a "magnetic" gait because of difficulty picking up the feet)

○ **What is meant by the term "communicating" (or "nonobstructive") hydrocephalus?**

All of the ventricles are dilated, including the cerebral aqueduct and basal cisterns. Obstructive hydrocephalus is secondary to either aqueductal stenosis or CSF outflow blocked by a mass.

○ **What is the Wernicke-Korsakoff syndrome?**

Chronic, severe impairment in anterograde amnesia (Korsakoff syndrome) with acute confusion, ataxia, ophthalmoplegia, and nystagmus (Wernicke encephalopathy). This syndrome results from lesions of the dorsomedial nuclei of the thalamus and mamillary bodies.

○ **How should Wernicke encephalopathy be treated?**

Immediate intravenous (IV) thiamine replacement

○ **Differentiate between Korsakoff psychosis and Wernicke encephalopathy.**

Korsakoff psychosis is the inability to process new information (ie, to form new memories). This is a reversible condition resulting from brain damage induced by a thiamine deficiency that is generally secondary to chronic alcoholism.

Wernicke encephalopathy is also due to an ethanol-induced thiamine deficiency. This is an irreversible disease in which the brain tissues break down, become inflamed, and bleed. Patients experience decreased muscle coordination, ophthalmoplegia, and confusion.

○ **What type of physical activity can improve cognitive function in older adults?**

Aerobic physical activity in persons older than 55 years is associated with improved cognitive speed and auditory and visual attention but not other cognitive functions. Because aerobic physical activity has been the most studied, it is not clear if other forms of exercise are as beneficial.

○ **A 9-month-old boy is having frequent convulsions and cannot control his muscles enough to hold up his head. You noted a developmental roadblock at the age of 6 months, and now it seems the child is regressing in both motor and cognitive skills. At examination, the patient has a cherry red macula. What is the patient's prognosis?**

This patient probably has Tay-Sachs disease. As the disease progresses, the child will lose his sight, have dementia, and become paralyzed. Death will occur before age 4 years.

○ **What is the probable ethnic background of the patient described in the above case?**

Eastern European, Jewish, or French Canadian

○ **What causes cerebral palsy?**

Seventy percent of cases are idiopathic. Other causes include in utero infection, chromosomal abnormality, or stroke. Cerebral palsy is a defect of the central nervous system (CNS) that occurs prenatally, perinatally, or before age 3 years.

○ **Which subtypes of cerebral palsy are associated with intellectual disability?**

Spastic and sometimes athetotic. Intellectual disability occurs in 25% of patients with cerebral palsy.

○ **Describe the common findings of benign essential tremors?**

Tremulousness of speech and nodding of the head. This is an action tremor that is usually familial and is often treated with atenolol, propranolol, diazepam, and ethanol.

○ **What body parts are most commonly affected in an essential tremor?**

Head and upper extremities. Essential tremors are sporadic and slowly progressive. These tremors are rare at rest but become worse when the limbs are used.

○ **If a patient with a tremor drinks ethanol and the tremor temporarily subsides a bit, what kind of tremor is it?**

An essential tremor or a familial tremor. Botulinum toxin injections, β-blockers, and primidone are the conventional treatments.

○ **A resting tremor is usually related to what disease?**

Parkinson disease. Parkinson tremors are generally asymmetrical and have the characteristic "pill-rolling" appearance.

○ **A patient with a stooped posture, festinating gait (small shuffling steps) masklike facies, poor balance, slow starting speech, decreased movement, muscular rigidity, and a "pill-rolling" tremor should be treated with what?**

Dopaminergic agonists such as amantadine, bromocriptine, and levodopa and cholinergic antagonists such as benztropine. Parkinsonism syndrome is caused by a loss of dopaminergic cells in the substantia nigra. Most people lose these neurons at a rate of 0.5% a year. Individuals with Parkinson disease lose them at a rate of 1% per year.

○ **What is the most common presenting symptom in Parkinson disease?**

Tremor. The brain lesion is located in the substantia nigra.

○ **List, by order of initiation, drugs used for the treatment of Parkinson disease.**

Start with amantadine and trihexyphenidyl; if this fails, use a combination of levodopa and carbidopa. Pergolide and bromocriptine can be used to treat episodes of immobility.

○ **Parkinson-like adverse effects are common with which class of drugs?**

Neuroleptic agents. Parkinson-like adverse effects can develop with perphenazine, chlorpromazine, reserpine, haloperidol, metoclopramide, and the illicit meperidine analog 1-methyl-4-phenyl-1,2,3,6-tetrahydropyridine.

○ **Describe the signs and symptoms of neuroleptic malignant syndrome.**

Patients present with muscle rigidity, autonomic disturbances, acute organic brain syndrome, and a fever as high as 42°C (108°F). Blood pressure and pulse fluctuate wildly. Muscle necrosis may occur with resultant myoglobinuria.

○ **What is the most common medication associated with neuroleptic malignant syndrome?**

Haloperidol. Other drugs, especially antipsychotic medications, are also causative.

○ **What is the hallmark motor finding in neuroleptic malignant syndrome?**

Lead-pipe rigidity

○ **What is the treatment for neuroleptic malignant syndrome?**

Rapid cooling methods and immediate withdrawal of the neuroleptic drugs. Carbidopa/levodopa, bromocriptine, or dantrolene may be used as needed.

○ **What is Shy-Drager syndrome?**

A rare, gradually progressive nerve disorder characterized by low blood pressure, lack of coordination, muscle wasting, stiffness, and lack of bladder and/or bowel control. This syndrome occurs most often in young people.

○ **A man developed Huntington chorea at the age of 44 years. What are the chances of his daughter developing the same disease?**

50%. Huntington chorea is an autosomal dominant disorder that first manifests itself between ages 30 and 50 years. Symptoms include dementia, amnesia, delusions, emotional instability, depression, paranoia, antisocial behavior, and irritability. If the daughter inherits the disease, she will also develop chorea, bradykinesia, hypertonia, hyperkinesia, clonus, schizophrenia, intellectual impairment, and bowel incontinence. She will eventually die a premature death about 15 years after the onset of her symptoms.

○ **What chromosome carries the genetic defect for Huntington chorea?**

The short arm of chromosome 4

○ **Which neurons are spared in Huntington disease?**

Cholinergic interneurons whose axons terminate in the striatum and interneurons expressing somatostatin and neuropeptide Y

○ **What percentage of adults experience restless leg syndrome?**

10%

○ **What are the diagnostic criteria for restless leg syndrome?**

Urge to move legs that is usually accompanied or caused by uncomfortable or unpleasant sensations in the legs. The urge to move or unpleasant sensation begins or worsens during periods of rest or inactivity, is partially or totally relieved by movement as long as activity continues, and is worse in the evening or at night than during the day.

○ **What is the first-line therapy for moderate to severe symptomatic, daily restless leg syndrome?**

Dopamine agonists. Pramipexole and ropinirole are indicated by the United States Food and Drug Administration (FDA) for the treatment of moderate to severe restless leg syndrome.

○ **What is Tourette syndrome?**

A tic disorder with motor and vocal tics developing before age 18 years. Vocal tics may be unformed or formed (words). Coprolalia (cursing) and echolalia may occur. Tourette syndrome may be accompanied by attention-deficit disorder and obsessive compulsive disorder.

○ **What are tics?**

Tics are involuntary or semivoluntary, sudden, brief, intermittent repetitive movements (motor) or sounds (phonic). Simple motor tics involve a single muscle or group of muscles. Simple phonic tics are often meaningless utterances or noises. Complex motor tics result in more coordinated movement mimicking normal motor function. Complex phonic tics are words or phrases, echoing what others say (echolalia), and repeating one's own utterances (paliphrasia).

○ **By age 18 years, what percentage of individuals with Tourette syndrome have complete resolution of tics?**

50%

○ **What other psychiatric comorbidities are associated with Tourette syndrome?**

Fifty percent of children may experience a psychiatric comorbidity. The most common are attention-deficit/hyperactivity disorder or obsessive compulsive disorder. Depression, anxiety, and behavioral problems may also be present.

○ **What are the goals of treatment for children with Tourette syndrome?**

Improve social functioning, self-esteem, and quality of life

○ **What are the agents approved by the FDA for the treatment of tics and Tourette syndrome?**

Haloperidol and pimozide (dopamine-receptor blocking agents). Haloperidol is often avoided because of its less favorable adverse-effect profile. Although its use for Tourette syndrome is off label, clonidine (an α_2-adrenergic agonist) is commonly used as a first-line treatment when symptoms are mild.

○ **What are symptoms of attention-deficit disorder?**

Impulsivity, distractibility, and often hyperactivity

○ **What is the most commonly diagnosed neurodevelopmental disorder in children and adolescents?**

Attention-deficit/hyperactivity disorder, with an estimated 2% to 16% of school-aged children having this diagnosis.

○ **What are the 3 common subtypes of attention-deficit/hyperactivity disorder?**

The predominantly hyperactive-impulsive type is characterized by excessive fidgeting and restlessness, with the possibility of not setting physical boundaries or exhibiting destructive behavior. The predominately inattentive type is characterized by easy distractibility, forgetfulness, and difficulty completing tasks. The combined hyperactive-impulsive and inattentive type has features of both.

○ **What is the first-line medication for attention-deficit/hyperactivity disorder?**

Use of stimulants such as methylphenidate, dexmethylphenidate, or dextroamphetamine. Common adverse effects of stimulant use include appetite suppression, weight loss, abdominal pain, headache, irritability, insomnia, and tics. The FDA has added warnings to psychostimulants as being associated with increased risk of sudden death and cardiovascular problems including heart attacks.

○ **What are common causes of excessive daytime sleepiness?**

The most common causes are secondary hypersomnias. Sleep deprivation, medication effects, illicit substance use, obstructive sleep apnea, depression, and medical conditions (including head trauma, stroke, cancer, inflammatory conditions, encephalitis, and neurodegenerative conditions). Primary hypersomnias (including narcolepsy and hypersomnia) are rare.

○ **What is the most common manifestation of obstructive sleep apnea?**

Excessive daytime sleepiness, which has been reported to be present in approximately 23% of women and 16% of men

○   **What are the criteria for chronic insomnia?**

Chronic insomnia involves difficulty with maintaining or initiating sleep or experiencing nonrestorative sleep. It should last for at least 1 month and cause significant daytime impairment.

○   **What modality should be used as the initial treatment for chronic insomnia?**

Cognitive behavioral therapy. Results from 1 meta-analysis of 59 trials with 2102 patients with chronic insomnia showed that 5 hours of therapy time resulted in a decrease in sleep latency (time to fall to sleep) by 43% compared with a decrease of 30% with pharmacotherapy alone and that clinical improvements were maintained after an average of 6 months of follow-up. Cognitive behavioral therapy can consist of cognitive therapy (to identify dysfunctional beliefs about sleep, challenge their validity, and replace them with more adaptive substitutes), sleep hygiene education (good sleep habits), stimulus control (eliminating distractions and associating the bedroom with only sleep and sex), sleep restriction (limiting the time in bed to maximize sleep efficiency), paradoxical intention (remove fear of not being able to fall asleep by advising patient to remain awake), and relaxation therapy.

○   **When does the onset of epilepsy usually occur?**

Before age 20 years

○   **How long must a generalized tonic-clonic seizure last without a period of consciousness to be considered status epilepticus?**

30 minutes. Status epilepticus may result from grand mal seizures or anticonvulsant therapy withdrawal.

○   **What electrocardiographic finding makes phenytoin relatively contraindicated?**

Second- or third-degree heart block. If the patient is in status epilepticus, there may be no other choice. Phenytoin is relatively ineffective for seizures due to cyclic antidepressant overdose.

○   **What is the classic electroencephalographic finding associated with petit mal seizures?**

A 3-second spike-and-wave pattern

○   **What is the drug treatment for convulsive status epilepticus?**

Lorazepam (0.1 mg/kg) administered at 2 mg/min, followed by IV fosphenytoin (18 mg of phenytoin equivalent per kilogram)

○   **Which antiepileptic drugs seem to have a higher risk for interfering with the effectiveness of oral contraceptives?**

Cytochrome P450 enzyme–inducing drugs increase the breakdown of estrogen and progesterone into inactive metabolites and potentially reduce the contraceptive effectiveness of these compounds. Cytochrome P450 enzyme–inducing antiepileptic drugs include carbamazepine, felbamate, oxcarbazepine, phenobarbital, phenytoin, and topiramate. Although no direct studies exist to show that these agents decrease the effectiveness of oral contraceptives, guidelines by many organizations suggest increasing the dose of the estrogen in the oral contraceptives.

○   **What are febrile seizures?**

Events in infancy or childhood (usually occurring between 3 months and 5 years of age) that are associated with fever without evidence of intracranial infection or a defined cause of seizure. Simple febrile seizures are generalized in onset, last less than 15 minutes, and do not occur more than once in 24 hours. Complex seizures last longer, have focal symptoms, and can recur within 24 hours.

○ **What percentage of children in the United States and Western Europe will experience at least 1 febrile seizure by 5 years of age?**

2% to 5%

○ **Is treatment for a simple febrile seizure recommended?**

No. No clear information is available if antipyretic drugs help reduce the risk of subsequent seizures. Intermittent use of anticonvulsants are likely to be ineffective or harmful. Long-term use of anticonvulsants requires weighing the benefits and harms in preventing further episodes in a child with a history of simple febrile seizures and must reduce the risk of subsequent epilepsy as much as 12 years later.

○ **Recurrent seizures in patients with a history of a febrile seizure generally occur in what time frame?**

About 85% occur within the first 2 years. The younger the child, the more likely recurrence is. If a patient has a febrile seizure in the first year of life, the recurrence rate is 50%. If it occurs in the second year, the recurrence rate is only 25%.

○ **Why is diazepam avoided in neonatal seizures?**

It may cause hyperbilirubinemia by uncoupling the bilirubin-albumin complex.

○ **What are some disorders of myelination in the CNS?**

Multiple sclerosis (MS) is an autoimmune disorder of central myelin. Pelizaeus-Merzbacher disease is a hereditary CNS demyelinating disorder caused by a mutation in myelin proteolipid protein. Metabolic demyelinating diseases include metachromatic leukodystrophy (deficiency of arylsulfatase A), adrenoleukodystrophy (faulty metabolism of very long-chain fatty acids), and Krabbe globoid cell leukodystrophy. Central pontine myelinolysis, a catastrophic disruption of corticospinal pathways in the brain stem resulting in a locked-in syndrome, occurs with overrapid correction of hypo- or hypernatremia. Progressive multifocal leukoencephalopathy is a viral patchy white matter encephalopathy caused by JC virus but associated with human immunodeficiency virus infection.

○ **A 28-year-old woman complains of a 2-day history of weakness and tingling in her right arm and leg. She reports a previous episode of right eye pain and blurred vision that resolved over 1 month but that occurred 2 years ago. She also recalls a 2-week episode of intermittent blurred vision the previous year. What is the diagnosis?**

Presumptive MS. Confirm with magnetic resonance (MR) imaging and CSF testing (look for oligoclonal bands).

○ **What is the most common presenting symptom with MS?**

Optic neuritis (about 25%)

○ **A patient with MS presents with a fever. The nurse asks, "Should I give the patient acetaminophen?" What is your response?**

Yes. Reducing a fever is important for MS patients. Existing signs and symptoms can worsen with small increases in temperature.

○ **Are there any psychiatric symptoms seen in MS?**

In about 50% of cases, depression, irritability, low mood, anxiety, and poor concentration occur. Less common is confusion and psychosis.

○   **Does MS affect cognition?**

Yes, in 50% of cases, manifesting mostly as deficits in short-term memory, attention, and speed of processing, with frank dementia in fewer than 5% of cases

○   **What percentage of MS patients will never experience a relapse?**

15%

○   **What exogenous factors may exacerbate MS?**

Interferon gamma and tumor necrosis factor-α produced by the immune cells during viral infections

○   **What is the cause of MS?**

Demyelination of CNS (white matter) with relative axonal preservation, although there is evidence of a moderate degree of axonal loss and some plaques encroaching on the cortex with sparing of neuronal cell bodies and axis cylinders.

○   **What are good prognostic indicators for MS?**

Female sex, younger age at onset, relapsing-remitting form, lower rate of relapses early in the course, long first interattack interval, and an initial symptom of sensory or cranial nerve dysfunction

○   **What other conditions can produce MR imaging findings similar to those of MS?**

Ischemia, systemic lupus erythematosus, Behcet disease, other forms of vasculitis, human T-lymphotropic virus 1, and sarcoidosis

○   **What is the preferred therapy for acute MS?**

High-dose IV methylprednisolone (6–15 mg/kg) for 3 to 5 days, with or without a taper of oral prednisone, will induce objective improvement in more than 85% of cases.

○   **What therapies are commonly used for symptoms of MS?**

- Fatigue: Amantadine, pemoline, and fluoxetine
- Pain: Carbamazepine, misoprostol (prostaglandin E analog), tricyclic antidepressants, phenytoin, baclofen, and divalproex
- Spasticity: Baclofen, benzodiazepines, and dantrolene
- Intention tremor: Clonazepam, propranolol, and trihexyphenidyl

○   **A 26-year-old woman complains of a throbbing, dull unilateral headache that lasts for hours then goes away with sleep. She also has been nauseated and has vomited twice. She reports small areas of visual loss plus strange zigzag lines in her vision. What is the most likely diagnosis?**

Classic migraine headache. Classic migraine accounts for only 1% of migraines. It can be differentiated from the common migraine because it involves visual disturbances of scotomata and fortification spectra, in addition to all the other migraine symptoms.

○ **What factors may precipitate migraine headaches?**

Bright lights, cheese, hot dogs and other foods containing tyramine or nitrates, menstruation, monosodium glutamate, and stress

○ **A 30-year-old man with severe orbital and temporal pain on the right side has tearing from the right eye but not the left. The patient's pain tends to occur when he arrives home from work. He also knows he will get a headache if he drinks beer. The headaches last only about an hour. What syndrome can be associated with this man's headache?**

Horner syndrome (anhidrosis, miosis, and ptosis). This man has a cluster headache, which typically occurs in men ranging from ages 20 to 50 years. A cluster headache can recur at the same time and location each day and is exacerbated by ethanol and vasodilators. Relief is achieved with 100% oxygen, ergots, lithium, or prednisone. Intranasal viscous lidocaine can also be effective.

○ **Which type of headache do adults usually have?**

Tension headaches. This is a bilateral, bandlike fronto-occipital headache accompanied by constant pain. Tension headaches are generally muscular in nature, so a patient may also have tense neck and scalp muscles.

○ **Describe the key signs and symptoms of common, classic, ophthalmoplegic, and hemiplegic migraine headaches.**
- Common: This headache is the most common. It is a slowly evolving headache that lasts for hours to days. A positive family history and 2 of the following are prevalent: nausea or vomiting, throbbing quality, photophobia, unilateral pain, and increase with menses. A lack of visual symptoms distinguishes common migraine from classic migraine.
- Classic: The prodrome lasts up to 60 minutes. The most common symptom is visual disturbance (homonymous hemianopsia, scintillating scotoma, fortification spectra, and photophobia). Lip, face, and hand tingling; aphasia; extremity weakness; nausea; and vomiting may occur.
- Ophthalmoplegic: These headaches are most common in young adults. The patient has an outwardly deviated, dilated eye with ptosis. The third, fourth, and sixth nerves are usually involved.
- Hemiplegic: Unilateral motor and sensory symptoms and mild hemiparesis to hemiplegia are exhibited.

○ **How can you tell if a headache is caused by an intracranial tumor?**

Through CT or MR imaging. However, everyone who seeks treatment for a headache cannot undergo CT or MR imaging. Patients complaining of serious headaches should undergo imaging and lumbar puncture. Other signs that may suggest a serious underlying disease are headaches that (1) wake patients from their sleep (although cluster headaches may do this), (2) are worse in the morning, (3) increase in severity with postural changes or Valsalva maneuvers, (4) are associated with nausea and vomiting (though migraines have similar symptoms), (5) are associated with focal defects or mental status changes, and (6) occur with a new onset of seizures.

○ **What is the most common type of primary brain tumor in adults?**

Neuroglial tumors from astrocytes, oligodendrocytes, or ependymal cells account for 80% of primary brain tumors. Glioblastoma multiforme is the most common type of glioma. Meningiomas account for about 20% of primary brain tumors. The third most common type are primary CNS lymphoma tumors.

○   **What is the most common malignant brain tumor in adults?**

Glioblastoma

○   **What is the most common benign brain tumor in adults?**

Meningioma

○   **A 69-year-old presents with confusion of new onset. What is the diagnosis after viewing the CT scan?**

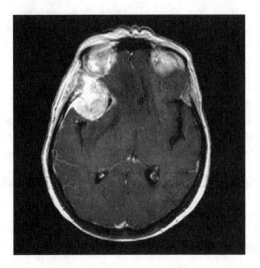

A large dural enhancing mass with a dural tail arises near the greater wing of the sphenoid at the junction of the right frontal and temporal lobes. The mass has characteristics of an extra-axial lesion and is consistent with a meningioma. Note that the finding of a small dural tail of enhancement along the edge of the mass is characteristic of meningioma, along with its broad-based dural attachment based dural attachment.

○   **What is the most common symptom of a glioblastoma multiforme?**

Headache, in three-fourths of patients

○   **In what age group does the incidence of primary brain tumors in adults peak?**

65 to 79 years

○   **What are the most common origins of metastatic brain lesions in adults?**

Breast adenocarcinoma, bronchogenic carcinoma, and malignant melanoma. Twenty percent of adult brain tumors are metastatic.

○   **What is the treatment for cerebral metastatic brain tumors?**

High-dose corticosteroids to reduce the mass effect from cerebral edema and usually radiation therapy. Surgery replaces radiation therapy if biopsy for the diagnosis of a metastatic lesion is required or if a single metastatic lesion is present.

○ **These images were obtained in a 68-year-old with new onset right homonomous hemianopsia. On the basis of these images, what is the diagnosis?**

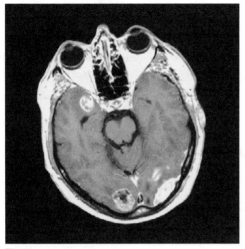
Fig. A

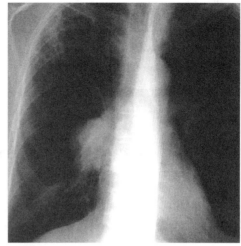
Fig. B

Multiple inhomogeneously enhancing lesions, several of which are shown on the CT scan (Fig. A), are present throughout the brain. The left occipital lesion would explain the patient's visual symptoms. The chest radiograph (Fig. B) demonstrates a large mass in the right hilum in this patient with lung carcinoma and multiple brain metastases.

○ **What are the most common brain tumors in children?**

Cerebellar astrocytomas and medulloblastomas

○ **What is the most common tumor of the sellar and parasellar regions?**

Pituitary adenoma

○ **What is the most common endocrine disorder associated with suprasellar extension of pineal tumors?**

Diabetes insipidus

○ **What are the common presenting symptoms of a glomus jugulare tumor?**

Hearing loss and pulsatile tinnitus

○ **Distinguish between the gait of a patient with a cerebellar lesion and that of a patient with an extrapyramidal lesion.**

A patient with a cerebellar lesion will have truncal ataxia and an unsteady, irregular gait with broad steps. A patient with an extrapyramidal lesion will have a festinating gait, with several small, shuffling steps taken without swinging the arms.

○ **What is encephalitis?**

Inflammation of the brain tissue, which often manifests with altered mental status, fever, and headache

○ **Headache, altered mentation, seizures, and an electroencephalogram showing periodic lateralized epileptiform discharges suggest what diagnosis?**

Herpes simplex encephalitis

○ **What is meningitis?**

Inflammation of the meninges, which often manifests with altered mental status, fever, and headache

○ **At what age is bacterial meningitis most common?**

In infants younger than 1 year

○ **What bacteria is the most common cause of meningitis in infants younger than 1 year?**

Group B streptococci and *Escherichia coli*

○ **What organism is frequently responsible for bacterial meningitis in adults?**

Neisseria meningitidis

○ **How does bacterial meningitis differ from viral meningitis in terms of the corresponding CSF laboratory test values?**

Bacterial meningitis is associated with low glucose and high protein levels, whereas viral meningitis is associated with normal glucose and normal protein levels.

○ **A patient presents with acute meningitis. When should antibiotics be initiated?**

Immediately. Do not wait for results of lumbar puncture. Patients should undergo CT before lumbar puncture only if papilledema or a focal deficit is present.

○ **What is the most worrisome diagnosis of a purpuric, petechial rash in an infant?**

Meningococcemia

○ **Which type of bacteria is most commonly cultured from brain abscesses: aerobic or anaerobic?**

Anaerobic

○ **What are the microorganisms most commonly found in brain abscesses?**

The enteric gram-negative bacilli, anaerobes, *Nocardia*, staphylococci, streptococci, and *Toxoplasma*

○ **What are the causes of subdural empyema?**

Sinusitis, meningitis, head trauma, otitis, and osteomyelitis

○ **What is the recommended duration of antibiotic therapy for brain abscess?**

The recommended duration is 6 to 8 weeks of IV antibiotics.

○ **What are the 2 organisms that most commonly cause meningitis in patients with ventriculoperitoneal shunts?**

1. *Staphylococcus epidermidis*
2. *Staphylococcus aureus*

○ **Which vitamin should be administered routinely during the treatment of tuberculous meningitis?**

Vitamin B6. Isoniazid can induce peripheral neuropathy, which can be prevented by coadministration of vitamin B6 (pyridoxine).

○ **A ring lesion is noted on a CT scan of the brain of an immunocompromised patient. The patient is confused and has lymphadenopathy, fever, and headache. What is the probable diagnosis?**

Toxoplasmosis caused by *Toxoplasma gondii* cyst. The disease is typically treated with pyrimethamine and sulfadiazine.

○ **What cutaneous manifestation is seen in patients with Sturge-Weber disease?**

A port-wine stain, or angiomatous nevus, is seen in the distribution of cranial nerve V. This may be associated with pial angiomas. Seizures are the main clinical manifestation, but hemiparesis may also occur.

○ **What is the CSF volume in a typical adult?**

150 mL

○ **Rapid correction of chronic hyponatremia will cause which neurologic disorder?**

Central pontine myelinolysis may be caused by rapid correction of serum sodium level (>0.5 mEq/L per hour).

○ **What symptoms form the classic tetrad seen in kernicterus?**

1. Choreoathetosis
2. Supranuclear ophthalmoplegia
3. Sensorineural hearing loss
4. Enamel hypoplasia

○ **What are the 2 main forms of neurofibromatosis?**

1. Neurofibromatosis type 1 (NF1), von Recklinghausen disease or peripheral neurofibromatosis: Consists of cafe au lait spots, neurofibromas, plexiform neuromas, iris hamartomas (Lisch nodules), optic gliomas, and osseous lesions. NF1 is caused by a mutation in the gene on chromosome 17 and accounts for 85% of all neurofibromatoses.
2. Neurofibromatosis type 2 (NF2), central neurofibromatosis: involves tumors of cranial nerve VIII, and the gene is linked to chromosome 18.

○ **What is the enzyme defect in Lesch-Nyhan disease?**

Hypoxanthine-guanine phosphoribosyltransferase

○ **What is the most common cause of syncope?**

Vasovagal or simple fainting (50%)

○ **In order for a patient to faint from cardiac causes, to what level must the cardiac output decrease?**

50% of normal capacity. Cardiac syncope can occur because of mechanical causes, such as aortic or pulmonic obstruction and arrhythmias, or because of ischemic causes, such as myocardial infarction or aortic dissection.

○ **What is neuritis?**

Inflammation of the peripheral nerves. Often manifests with radicular pain or weakness, peripheral neuropathy, or cranial nerve palsy.

○ **Describe the symptoms of optic neuritis.**

Variable loss of central visual acuity with central scotoma and change in color perception. The disc margins are blurred from hemorrhage, the blind spot is increased, and the eye is painful.

○ **What is a Marcus Gunn pupil?**

An afferent pupillary defect. Shining a light into the affected eye causes sluggish constriction. Swinging the light from the normal eye to the affected one dilates both pupils because the brain perceives less light via the abnormal eye.

○ **What is an Argyll Robertson pupil?**

A small and irregular pupil that can narrow to focus but not in response to light. This can be a sign of neurosyphilis. Other symptoms include headache, dizziness, diplopia, nuchal rigidity, weakness, paralysis, tabes dorsalis, memory loss, dementia, lethargy, and delusions.

○ **What happens if light is directed into the eyes of a patient who is in a diabetic coma?**

The pupils will constrict.

○ **What is the legal definition of blindness?**

Visual acuity of 20/400 at best, with external correction such as glasses or contact lenses

○ **A child with blurry vision has an abnormal pupillary reflex and a white reflex at funduscopic examination. What is the treatment?**

Surgical removal of the eye. This is a retinoblastoma that can grow to other sites in the brain or body. This condition is inheritable, so the parents should be counseled about the risks.

○ **Are fixed and dilated pupils found only with structural dysfunction?**

No. Metabolic dysfunction (eg, hepatic encephalopathy) or toxins (eg, atropine) can produce enlarged unreactive pupils.

○ **What are pontine pupils?**

Pinpoint, but reactive, pupils secondary to injury of the sympathetic fibers descending through the tegmentum. It results from intrinsic pontine tegmental injury or from cerebellar or other posterior fossa mass effect causing compression of the tegmentum. Narcotic administration causes similar pupillary findings.

○ **What conditions are associated with sudden, unilateral, transient vision loss?**

Nonischemic central retinal vein occlusion, early retinal detachment, embolism to the eye, uveitis, and vasospasm

○ **What conditions are associated with sudden, bilateral, transient vision loss?**

Atherosclerotic (occlusive) disease of the internal carotid artery, migraine headache, and transient ischemic attack of the visual cortex

○ **What are conditions associated with sudden, bilateral, persistent vision loss?**

Bilateral occipital lobe ischemia, giant cell arteritis, lymphoma, and posterior ischemic neuropathy

○ **What are the most common neurologic findings in adult botulism cases?**

Eye and bulbar muscle deficit

○ **Which cranial nerve is the most affected in pseudotumor cerebri?**

Cranial nerve IV can be involved, with clinical signs of diplopia. Other findings include decreased visual acuity and restricted peripheral fields with enlargement of the blind spot.

○ **What deficits can result from ocular motor nerve paralysis?**

Ptosis, which can be caused by levator palpebrae superioris muscle/cranial nerve III injury. Lateral nerve gaze is controlled by cranial nerve VI, and the corneal reflex is controlled by the cranial nerve V. The superior oblique muscle moves the gaze downward and laterally and is controlled by cranial nerve IV.

○ **A 67-year-old woman complains of severe episodes of pain in her nose, cheek, and upper lip. She says it feels like a lightning bolt is hitting her face. What is the diagnosis?**

Tic douloureux or trigeminal neuralgia. This is a nerve condition of unknown cause, possibly microvascular compression causing a neuronal breakdown. It involves the trigeminal nerve and is most common in the ophthalmic and maxillary branches, although it may affect all 3 branches.

○ **How is the above patient treated?**

Perform MR imaging to rule out a brain-stem process, such as a tumor. Carbamazepine is used to treat trigeminal neuralgia.

○ **What symptoms are associated with trigeminal neuralgia?**

Trigeminal neuralgia is defined as sudden, usually unilateral, severe, brief, stabbing, recurrent episodes of pain in 1 or more branches of the trigeminal nerve (the fifth cranial nerve). Classic trigeminal neuralgia requires the absence of any clinically evident neurologic deficit. Symptomatic trigeminal neuralgia requires identifying a structural abnormality other than vascular compression (such as MS plaques, tumors, and abnormalities of the skull base).

○ **What is probably the best test to differentiate classic trigeminal neuralgia from symptomatic neuralgia?**

Abnormal trigeminal reflexes have a high specificity of 94% and a sensitivity of 87%.

○ **What treatment has the best evidence to support it for managing the pain from classic trigeminal neuralgia?**

Carbamazepine (200 to 1200 mg/d). Oxcarbazepine (600 to 1800 mg/d) is probably the next best treatment choice, followed by baclofen, lamotrigine, and pimozide.

○ **How are upper motor neuron lesions of cranial nerve VII (facial nerve) distinguished from peripheral lesions?**

Upper motor neuron: A unilateral weakness of the lower half of the face. Peripheral: Involves the entire half of the face, as seen in Bell palsy

○ **What is the most common cranial neuropathy seen in borreliosis (Lyme disease)?**

Unilateral or bilateral facial palsy. Less frequently, cranial nerve VIII is affected.

○   **The Weber test is performed in a patient complaining of hearing loss. The patient hears sounds more loudly in his right ear. Which types of hearing loss may this patient have?**

Conductive hearing loss on the right or sensory hearing loss on the left

○   **Describe the Rinne test and explain the normal findings.**

The Rinne test is performed by placing the tip of a tuning fork on the mastoid process until the patient can no longer hear the tone. The fork is then relocated to just in front of the pinna until the patient can no longer hear the tone. In healthy patients, the ratio is 1:2 for the duration of time the patient can hear the tuning fork.

○   **A 50-year-old woman with hearing loss over the last 6 months presents at 2 AM with vertigo that has progressively become worse over the last 2 months. At examination, she is mildly ataxic. What is the diagnosis?**

Eighth nerve lesion, possibly an acoustic schwannoma or meningioma

○   **What is a vestibular schwannoma?**

An acoustic neuroma or a tumor of the eighth cranial nerve. In addition to hearing loss and vertigo, patients also present with tinnitus. Surgical removal is the treatment of choice because this tumor may spread to the cerebellum and the brain stem.

○   **Describe the signs and symptoms of acoustic neuroma.**

Unilateral high-tone sensorineural hearing loss, tinnitus, and unsteadiness. Decreased corneal sensitivity, diplopia, headache, facial weakness, and positive radiographic findings are also possible. Vertigo usually appears late, is more often exhibited as a progressive feeling of imbalance, and can be provoked by changes in head movement. Nystagmus is frequently present and is usually spontaneous. The CSF may have elevated protein levels.

○   **A 35-year-old woman with a history of flulike symptoms (upper respiratory infection) 1 week ago presents with vertigo, nausea, and vomiting. No auditory impairment or focal deficits are noted. What is the likely diagnosis?**

Labyrinthitis or vestibular neuronitis

○   **What are the key features of viral labyrinthitis or vestibular neuronitis?**

Severe vertigo (usually lasting 3 to 5 days), with nausea and vomiting. Symptoms generally regress over 3 to 6 weeks. Nystagmus may be spontaneous during the severe stage.

○   **A 50-year-old woman with acute vertigo, nausea, and vomiting reports similar episodes over the last 20 years that are sometimes associated with hearing change, hearing loss, and tinnitus. She has permanent right > left sensorineural hearing loss. What is the diagnosis?**

Ménière disease.

○   **Describe the key features of Ménière disease.**

Vertigo, hearing loss, and tinnitus. Ménière disease typically manifests with the rapid onset of vertigo, nausea, and vomiting that lasts for hours to 1 day. Nystagmus may be spontaneous during the critical stage. Tinnitus may be present and is louder during attacks, and sensorineural hearing loss may occur. There also may be an aura with a sensation of fullness in the ear during an attack. Symptoms are unilateral in more than 90% of patients, and recurring attacks are typical.

○　**What are the distinguishing characteristics of benign positional vertigo?**

Benign positional vertigo is usually provoked by certain head positions or movements. Nystagmus is always positional, of brief duration, and with fatigability.

○　**What is myelitis?**

Inflammation of the spinal cord that often manifests with paralysis or diffuse neuropathic pain

○　**A 62-year-old patient presents with right shoulder pain. What is the diagnosis after viewing the CT scans?**

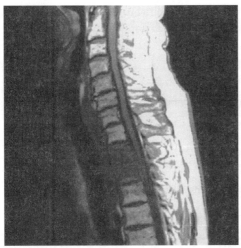

Fig. A

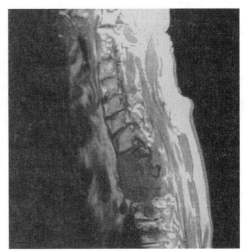

Fig. B

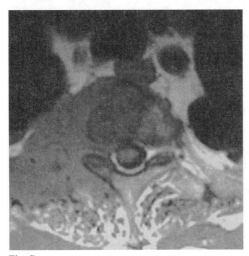

Fig. C

Sagittal (Figs. A and B) and transverse T1-weighted (Fig. C) noncontrast material–enhanced sections through the upper thoracic spine demonstrate a mass involving both vertebral bodies and the nearby lung pleura, with some extension into the epidural space on the right. Subsequent biopsy results showed a Pancoast tumor.

○ **Injury to what cervical area results in Horner syndrome (ptosis, miosis, and anhidrosis)?**

Disruption of the cervical sympathetic chain at C7 to T2

○ **You see a patient with an obvious traumatic spinal cord lesion. At physical examination, he has motor paralysis, loss of gross proprioception, loss of vibratory sensation on 1 side, and loss of pain and temperature sensation on the opposite side. What is the diagnosis?**

Brown-Séquard syndrome

○ **Describe the presentation of a patient with anterior cord syndrome.**

Complete motor paralysis and loss of pain and temperature sensations distal to the lesion. Posterior column sparing results in intact proprioception and vibration sense. The cause is occlusion of the anterior spinal artery or the protrusion of fracture fragments into the anterior canal.

○ **What are the signs of an upper motor neuron lesion?**

Upper motor neuron lesions involve the corticospinal tract. The lesions usually induce paralysis with:

- Initial loss of muscle tone and then increased tone, resulting in spasticity
- Babinski sign
- The loss of superficial reflexes
- Increased deep tendon reflexes

A lower motor neuron lesion is associated with the anterior horn cell axons. These lesions cause paralysis with decreased muscle tone and prompt atrophy.

○ **What is the first-line treatment for neurogenic bladder?**

Clean, intermittent self-catheterization

○ **What symptoms related to lumbar disk herniation are indications for emergency surgery?**

Urinary retention, perineal numbness, and motor weakness of more than a single nerve root. These are findings suggestive of cauda equina compression.

○ **What are common findings associated with cauda equina syndrome?**

Cauda equina syndrome is a neurologic emergency. It is associated with compression of the nerve fibers from the base of the spinal cord. Findings include fecal incontinence, urinary retention, and saddle anesthesia.

○ **What is the most common cause of sciatica?**

Sciatica is defined as pain originating in the lower back and radiating down the posterior or lateral thigh. After important syndromes associated with cord compression, infection, fracture, and neoplasm are ruled out, the most common cause is lumbar disk herniation.

○ **How often is radiologically detectable lumbar disk herniation found in patients with acute lumbar pain with sciatica?**

4% of the time

○ **What reflexes, motor finding, and sensory loss finding are associated with L4 nerve root (L3-L4 disk) sciatica?**

Patellar reflex loss, ankle dorsiflexion motor loss, and medial malleolus sensory loss

○ **What reflexes, motor finding, and sensory loss finding are associated with L5 nerve root (L4-L5 disk) sciatica?**

No reflex loss, hallux dorsiflexion motor loss, and dorsal third metatarsophalangeal joint sensory loss

○ **What reflexes, motor finding, and sensory loss finding are associated with S1 nerve root (L5-S1 disk) sciatica?**

Achilles reflex loss, ankle plantar flexion motor loss, and lateral heel sensory loss

○ **What is the first treatment option for acute sciatica without "red-flag" symptoms?**

Conservative management for 6 weeks before imaging or considering surgical approaches and continued physical activity rather than bed rest to avoid muscle deconditioning. Nonsteroidal anti-inflammatory drugs, acetaminophen, and muscle relaxants have been studied extensively in lumbar disk herniation pain but may be effective in nonspecific low back pain. Systemic steroids are no better than placebo in the treatment of lumbar disk herniation pain. Physical therapy has been used in conservative management of lumbar disk herniation, but the best evidence suggests little to support its use in improving pain or functional status.

○ **How many people achieve resolution of acute sciatica symptoms after 6 weeks of conservative therapy?**

90%

○ **What is the drug treatment for acute traumatic spinal cord injury?**

The treatment for acute (<8 hours) spinal cord injury is methylprednisolone 30 mg/kg bolus followed by 5.4 mg/kg per hour for the next 23 hours.

○ **What are the clinical features of spinal cord compression from metastatic cancer?**

Localized spinal tenderness, radicular pain, sensory level, paraparesis or quadriparesis, bowel and bladder incontinence, brisk deep tendon reflexes, upgoing plantar reflexes, and spasticity

○ **What is the treatment for acute spinal cord compression from metastatic cancer?**

Usually high-dose corticosteroids and radiation therapy. Surgical therapy is used instead of radiation therapy if the primary cancer type is unknown, the tumor is radioresistant, spinal instability makes surgery necessary, or the patient has received the maximum radiation dose.

○ **What are the clinical features of epidural abscess?**

Spinal tenderness, fever, radicular pain, myelopathy, elevated CSF protein level, and CSF pleocytosis

○ **What is the treatment of epidural abscess?**

Immediate laminectomy, drainage of the abscess, and antibiotic therapy. A delay may result in permanent myelopathy.

○ **What is the prognosis for a patient with recently diagnosed amyotrophic lateral sclerosis?**

Death 3 to 10 years after the onset of symptoms. Amyotrophic lateral sclerosis, also known as Lou Gehrig disease, involves a progressive loss of the anterior horn cell function of the motor neurons. No sensory abnormalities are involved, just gradual weakness and atrophy of the muscles.

○ **Do individuals infected with the rabies virus really foam at the mouth?**

Yes, hypersalivation is 1 of the symptoms of furious rabies, along with hyperactivity, fear of water, hyperventilation, aerophobia, and autonomic instability. Patients with paralytic rabies develop either ascending paralysis or paralysis that affects 1 or more limbs individually. Rabies is 100% fatal once symptoms are exhibited.

○ **What are the features of botulism infection?**

A history of recent ingestion of home canned or prepared foods, followed by sudden onset of diplopia; dysphagia; muscle weakness; dry mouth; fixed, dilated pupils; and respiratory paralysis. Treatment is with botulism antitoxin.

○ **What is tabes dorsalis?**

Progressive loss of all or part of the body's reflexes. The large joints of affected limbs are destroyed. Patients experience severe, stabbing pains in their legs, sensory deficits, and difficulty walking. Forty percent of patients with neurosyphilis have tabes dorsalis.

○ **Which 3 bacterial illnesses manifest with peripheral neurologic findings?**

1. Botulism

2. Tetanus

3. Diphtheria

○ **Where does botulism toxin exert its effects?**

At the myoneural junction. The toxin prevents the release of acetylcholine.

○ **Describe botulism intoxication.**

Acute food poisoning caused by *Clostridium botulinum*. Neurologic symptoms usually occur within 24 to 48 hours of ingestion of contaminated foods. Botulism poisoning often manifests with ocular bulbar deficits. Rapid, symmetrical descending weakness, usually with no sensory abnormalities, also develops. Other classical symptoms include dysphagia, dry mouth, diplopia, and dysarthria. Deep tendon reflexes may be decreased or absent.

○ **What are some disorders of peripheral nervous system myelin?**

Guillain-Barré Syndrome (GBS, also known as acute inflammatory demyelinating polyradiculoneuropathy) is an autoimmune attack on peripheral myelin, often after a viral or bacterial illness, resulting in sudden, rapidly progressive weakness and areflexia. Electromyographic testing shows slowing of nerve conduction and conduction block. The prognosis is worse if *Campylobacter jejuni* is involved. Treatment options include plasma exchanges or IV immunoglobulin G. Chronic inflammatory demyelinating polyradiculoneuropathy (CIDP) is a chronic or relapsing form of GBS. CIDP responds to steroids; GBS does not. Charcot-Marie-Tooth is an autosomal recessive (usually) or X-linked (rarely) distal peripheral neuropathy; mutations in myelin membrane-binding proteins or connexin gap junction proteins result in progressive demyelination, distal weakness, and atrophy with foot drop and a storklike gait. There is also an axonal form (HSMN2).

○ **Describe GBS.**

A lower motor neuron disease that commonly affects people in their 30s and 40s. Symptoms include ascending weakness in the legs and arms. A sensory component may be present. Bulbar muscles are usually involved late in the course of the disease. Reflexes are affected early. Paralysis can progress rapidly; recovery is usually slow, but it is almost always complete.

○ **What are some predisposing factors to GBS?**

Viral infection, gastrointestinal infection, immunization, or surgery often precede the neurological symptoms by 5 days to 3 weeks.

○ **Does early treatment with IV immunoglobulin or plasmapheresis accelerate recovery from GBS?**

Yes. It also diminishes the incidence of long-term neurologic disability.

○ **How would you differentiate acute anterior poliomyelitis from GBS?**

Acute anterior poliomyelitis shows asymmetry of paralysis, signs of meningeal irritation, fever, and CSF pleocytosis.

○ **When considering GBS as a diagnosis, what other conditions should be part of the differential?**
- Porphyria
- AIDS
- Hypophosphatemia
- Toxic neuropathies (hexane, thallium, arsenic)
- Botulism

○ **A 32-year-old woman who complains of periods of weakness, especially when she chews her food, presents with ptosis, diplopia, and dysarthria. Her muscles weaken with repetitive exercise. What test can be used to confirm the diagnosis of myasthenia gravis?**

Administration of exogenous anticholinesterase. Myasthenia gravis produces autoimmune antibodies against the acetylcholine receptors in the neuromuscular junction. Therefore, administering exogenous anticholinesterase will lead to an increase of acetylcholine and relieve the symptoms.

○ **Describe the initial symptoms and signs of myasthenia gravis.**

Weakness and fatigue, with ptosis, diplopia, and blurred vision. Bulbar muscle weakness is also prevalent, with dysarthria and dysphagia.

○ **What neoplastic process is most commonly associated with myasthenia gravis?**

Thymoma

○ **What is myasthenic crisis?**

A patient with myasthenia gravis with significant impairment in respiratory function. Myasthenic crisis may require emergency intubation and assisted ventilation.

○ **Eaton-Lambert syndrome is associated with which class of diseases?**

Malignancies, particularly oat cell carcinoma. Symptoms include aching muscle pain and weakness; cranial nerves are usually not involved. Muscle strength may increase with repeated use in Eaton-Lambert syndrome, whereas it will decrease with use in myasthenia gravis.

○ **Deep tendon reflexes are usually maintained in which of the following diseases: myasthenia gravis, GBS, or Eaton-Lambert syndrome?**

Myasthenia gravis. Reflexes are usually depressed in Eaton-Lambert syndrome and absent in GBS.

○   **Mononeuropathies are most commonly induced by what?**

Trauma that results in compression or entrapment of the involved nerve

○   **Which is the most common type of muscular dystrophy?**

Duchenne muscular dystrophy

○   **Which forms of muscular dystrophy are autosomal dominant and which forms are X linked?**

Myotonic dystrophy and facioscapulohumeral dystrophy are autosomal dominant. Duchenne dystrophy and Becker type tardive muscular dystrophy are X linked.

○   **Pseudohypertrophy of the calves is characteristic of which type of muscular dystrophy?**

Duchenne muscular dystrophy. Hypertrophy is caused by fatty infiltration of the muscles.

○   **How many minutes of cerebral anoxia will result in irreversible brain injury?**

Oxygen deprivation for more than 4 minutes will typically cause irreversible brain injury.

○   **Match the following conditions and symptoms.**
   1. Neuropraxia   **a. Damage to the axon, no damage to the sheath**
   2. Axonotmesis   **b. Temporary loss of function, no damage to the axon**
   3. Neurotmesis   **c. Damage to the axon and the sheath**
   Answers: (1) b, (2) a, and (3) c

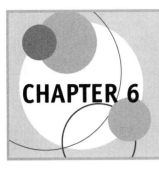

CHAPTER 6

Clinical Pharmacology and Toxicology

Robert L. Barkin, MBA, PharmD, FCP, DAAPM

○ **What is the clinical manifestation of anticholinergic poisoning?**

Mydriasis, tachycardia, hypoactive bowel sounds, urinary retention, dry axillae, hyperthermia, and mental status changes. Remember:

- Dry as a bone
- Red as a beet
- Mad as a hatter
- Hot as Hades
- Blind as a bat

○ **Name 7 primary actions of cyclic antidepressant overdose.**

1. Inhibition of amine reuptake
2. Sodium-channel blockade, which causes negative inotropy
3. Anticholinergic effects, primarily antimuscarinic, cardiac toxicity, quinidine-like events, and QRS duration longer than 100 milliseconds
4. Central nervous system (CNS) depression, agitation, hallucinations
5. α-Adrenergic antagonism, which contributes further to hypotension
6. Seizures
7. QTc interval greater than 440 millisecond prolongation

○ **What is the appropriate treatment for QRS widening in tricyclic antidepressant (TCA) poisoning?**

Sodium bicarbonate is administered intravenously (IV) for patients with QRS widening greater than 100 milliseconds. Initial 50-mEq bolus followed by 0.5 to 2 mEq/kg are initially administered and repeated until the blood pH is between 7.45 and 7.55. A continuous infusion of sodium bicarbonate, 3 ampules in 1 L of dextrose 5% water, may then be initiated and titrated in over 4 to 6 hours to maintain an appropriate pH; if hypotension does not respond, consider vasopressors (norepinephrine), 0.1 to 0.2 mg/kg, and contact and consult the regional poison control center. Potassium levels must be closely monitored because supplementation may be required to prevent hypokalemia. For arrhythmias that are not responsive, consider lidocaine (1 mg/kg IV).

○   **What is the appropriate treatment for TCA-induced seizures?**

Benzodiazepines (lorazepam/diazepam IV) and barbiturates (IV phenobarbital or propofol) are the agents of choice. Phenytoin is not generally effective but may be tried for recurrent seizures or in those unresponsive to treatment. Bicarbonate and alkalosis are the mainstays of treatment because acidosis worsens cardiovascular toxicity.

○   **What 4 mechanisms induce TCA toxicity?**

1. Anticholinergic atropine-like effects secondary to competitive antagonism of acetylcholine
2. Reuptake blockage of norepinephrine
3. Quinidine-like action on the myocardium
4. α-Blocking action

○   **What is the treatment for TCA-induced hypotension?**

Isotonic saline and alkalinization. If the patient is resistant to fluid resuscitation, a directly acting α-agonist, such as norepinephrine, should be started. Dopamine acts in part by releasing norepinephrine, which may already be depleted by the reuptake inhibition of some cyclic antidepressants and by stress.

○   **What period of observation (monitoring vital signs, cardiac rhythm, serial electrocardiogram [ECG], and mental status) is required before medically clearing a TCA overdose?**

6 hours

○   **A 32-year-old woman is prescribed meperidine for acute pain due to an open fracture. The patient is using long-term fluoxetine. What is a potential complication?**

Serotonin syndrome. Meperidine is also a reuptake blocker of norepinephrine and serotonin.

○   **What signs and symptoms are typical of serotonin syndrome's 3 categories (mental status changes, autonomic changes, and neuromuscular changes)?**

Agitation, anxiety, altered mental status, delirium, obtundation, ataxia, diaphoresis, poor coordination, sinus tachycardia, hyperthermia, shivering, tremor, hyperreflexia, myoclonus, muscular rigidity, and diarrhea

○   **What are potential pharmacologic treatments for serotonin syndrome?**

Serotonin antagonists, such as cyproheptadine. Benzodiazepines, barbiturates, and nitroprusside have each been successfully used to control CNS and hypertensive events.

○   **A patient who has ingested a toxic quantity of a monoamine oxidase inhibitor (MAOI) is in a hyperadrenergic state, with blood pressure of 240/160 mm Hg. What is the appropriate pharmacologic treatment?**

Short-acting antihypertensives for hypotension episodes. Norepinephrine, phentolamine, or nitroprusside should be used because the patient may soon develop refractory hypotension; benzodiazepines may be used to treat agitation.

○   **What are the major pharmacologic effects of neuroleptic agents?**

Blockade of dopamine; α-adrenergic, muscarinic, anticholinergic, and antiserotonin effects; and histamine receptors

○   **Describe the signs and symptoms of neuroleptic malignant syndrome.**

Patients present with muscle rigidity, autonomic disturbances or instability, acute organic brain syndrome (altered mental status), respiratory failure, acute renal failure, cardiovascular collapse, and a fever as high as 108°F (42°C). Blood pressure and pulse fluctuate wildly. Rhabdomyolysis may occur with resultant myoglobinuria.

○ **Although lithium levels correlate poorly with toxicity, what signs and symptoms may indicate lithium toxicity?**

If lithium levels are 2.0 mEq or lower, the patient may have diarrhea, emesis, ataxia, drowsiness, muscular weakness, or lack of coordination.

If lithium levels are 3 to 6 mEq, the patient may have giddiness, ataxia, blurry vision, tinnitus, or a large volume of dilute urine.

○ **What are the signs and symptoms of lithium toxicity?**

Neurological signs and symptoms include tremor, cerebellar and cognitive defects, neuroleptic malignant syndrome hyperreflexia, clonus, fasciculations, seizures, and coma. Gastrointestinal (GI) signs and symptoms consist of nausea, vomiting, and diarrhea. Cardiovascular effects include hypotension ST-T wave changes, bradycardia, conduction defects, and arrhythmia.

○ **What is the treatment for lithium toxicity?**

Supportive care, normal saline diuresis, hemodialysis in patients with clinical signs of severe poisoning (ie, seizures and arrhythmias, renal failure, or decreasing urine output). Hypotension should be managed with norepinephrine.

○ **What is the pharmacologic effect of barbiturates and benzodiazepines?**

Both enhance chloride influx through the γ-aminobutyric acid (GABA) receptor–associated chloride channel. Benzodiazepines increase the frequency of channel opening, whereas barbiturates increase the duration of channel opening.

○ **What are the common effects of barbiturate overdose?**

Hypothermia, hyperventilation, venodilation with hypotension, and negative inotropic effect on the myocardium. Clear vesicles and bullae may also develop.

○ **How should barbiturate poisoning be treated?**

Support, charcoal, alkalinization of the urine, charcoal hemoperfusion, or hemodialysis

○ **When is alkalization of the urine beneficial to enhance renal excretion in the management of severe barbiturate toxicity accompanied by life-threatening signs and symptoms?**

With use of long-acting barbiturates, such as phenobarbital; barbiturates are acidic compounds.

○ **What are the end products of methanol, ethylene glycol, and isopropyl ethanol metabolism?**

- Methanol: Formate
- Ethylene glycol: Oxalate and formate
- Isopropyl alcohol: Acetone

○ **Ingestion of which type of ethanol is associated with hypocalcemia?**

Ethylene glycol

○ **Ingestion of which type of ethanol is associated with hemorrhagic pancreatitis?**

Methanol

○   **What alcohol poisoning is suggested by a plasma bicarbonate level of zero?**

Methanol. It also produces a large osmolal gap and a large anion gap. Methanol poisoning is treated with IV ethanol and hemodialysis.

○   **What are the signs and symptoms of isopropanol poisoning?**

Sweet-smelling breath from acetone, isopropanol's metabolite; hypotension; hemorrhagic gastritis; and CNS depression from isopropanol and acetone

○   **At what rate is ethanol metabolized in an acutely intoxicated person?**

About 20 mg/dL per hour

○   **What is a pharmacologic treatment for ethanol withdrawal?**

Benzodiazepines. Propofol may be used for delirium refractory to benzodiazepine use.

○   **Isopropanol is metabolized by what enzyme to what metabolite?**

Isopropanol is slowly metabolized by Class I isoenzymes of hepatic alcohol dehydrogenase to acetone in the liver, and acetone is metabolized to acetate, formate, and carbon dioxide.

○   **An alcoholic patient presents with complaints of abdominal pain and blurred vision. The patient is photophobic, and blood gas levels indicate metabolic acidosis. What is the diagnosis?**

Methanol poisoning. Patients may describe seeing something resembling a snowstorm.

○   **What are the toxic metabolic end products of methanol poisoning?**

Formaldehyde, initially, and then formic acid, which causes metabolic acidosis and retinal toxicity

○   **What cofactor is required to convert formic acid to carbon dioxide and water?**

Folate. Leucovorin (folinic acid) the active form of folate used to enhance formate degradation, is preferentially administered at 1 mg/kg. Folate may be substituted at the same dose if leucovorin is not available.

○   **What is the lethal dose of methanol?**

30 mL. Formate levels from methanol poisoning are greatest in the vitreous humor.

○   **Birefringent calcium oxalate crystals in the urine are pathognomonic for poisoning with what substance?**

Ethylene glycol. The lethal dose of ethylene glycol is 100 mL.

○   **What are the signs and symptoms of ethylene glycol poisoning?**

Hallucinations, nystagmus, ataxia, papilledema, and a large anion gap

○   **What cofactors are administered in a patient with ethylene glycol poisoning?**

Thiamine and pyridoxine. These cofactors will aid in transforming glyoxylic acid to nontoxic metabolites. Both are administered daily as 100-mg IV increments.

○ **Name the 3 clinical phases of ethylene glycol poisoning.**

1. Stage 1: Neurological symptoms (ie, inebriation and euphoria)
2. Stage 2: Metabolic acidosis, cardiovascular instability, and cardiopulmonary instability
3. Stage 3: Renal failure and bone marrow depression

○ **How should ethylene glycol poisoning be treated?**

Gastric lavage, sodium bicarbonate, thiamine and pyridoxine, IV ethanol, and hemodialysis

○ **When should hemodialysis be initiated in a patient with ethylene glycol poisoning?**

When the serum level of ethylene glycol is higher than 50 mg/dL or when renal insufficiency, severe metabolic acidosis, or severe fluid and electrolyte abnormalities occur

○ **What is the toxic dose of naloxone?**

None. Naloxone is a safe drug and may be administered in large quantities. The usual initial adult dosage is up to 2 mg IV; the usual pediatric dose is 0.01 mg/kg. Naloxone may precipitate acute withdrawal and may therefore be titrated to effect.

○ **What medications are appropriate in the treatment of a patient with tachycardia resulting from cocaine abuse?**

Benzodiazepines may sedate the patient and decrease tachycardia. Nitroprusside may be administered to treat hypertension. Caution must be used with β-adrenergic antagonist agents alone because these medications may leave α-adrenergic stimulation unopposed, thereby increasing the patient's risk for intracranial hemorrhage or aortic dissection.

○ **What metabolite of cocaine is measured in clinical urine drug testing?**

Benzoylecgonine

○ **Name the specific antagonist (competitive inhibitor) of alcohol dehydrogenase; this drug may also serve as an alternative to ethanol in the treatment of ethylene glycol poisoning.**

Fomepizole

○ **How does treatment for a cocaine-induced myocardial infarction differ from a typical myocardial infarction?**

Both are treated the same way except that β-blockers are not used for a cocaine-induced myocardial infarction because of potential unopposed α-adrenergic activity and increased vasoconstriction. The tachycardia associated with a cocaine-induced myocardial infarction is first treated with benzodiazepine sedation and nitroglycerin for chest pain.

○ **What metabolite appears at confirmatory urine testing that indicates coingestion of ethanol and cocaine?**

Cocaethylene

○ **What syndrome is associated with smoking jimsonweed?**

Anticholinergic poisoning

○   **What are the signs of salicylate poisoning?**

Hyperventilation, hyperthermia, mental status change, nausea, vomiting, abdominal pain, dehydration, diaphoresis, ketonuria, metabolic acidosis, and respiratory alkalosis

○   **Describe the effects of salicylate poisoning on the CNS.**

Lethargy, confusion, seizures, and respiratory arrest

○   **What are the common signs and symptoms of chronic salicylism?**

Fever, tachypnea, CNS alterations, acid-base abnormalities, electrolyte abnormalities, chronic pain, ketonuria, and noncardiogenic pulmonary edema

○   **What is the mechanism of salicylate toxicity?**

Salicylates uncouple oxidative phosphorylation and thereby halt cellular adenosine triphosphate production.

○   **Which acid-base disturbance is typical for salicylate poisoning?**

Mixed respiratory alkalosis secondary to central respiratory center stimulation and metabolic acidosis secondary to uncoupling of oxidative phosphorylation

○   **A patient has an arterial pH of 7.5 through alkalization, but her urine pH is still low. What electrolyte is probably responsible?**

Potassium. When reabsorbing sodium, the renal tubules will preferentially excrete hydrogen ions rather than potassium ions into the tubular lumen. Thus, the potassium level should be maintained at 4.0 mEq/L.

○   **What order is the kinetics of elimination for acetylsalicylic acid overdose?**

Zero-order elimination, with hepatic enzymatic clearance saturated and renal clearance becoming important

○   **What dose (mg/kg) of nonenteric-coated acetylsalicylic acid must be exceeded in an acute ingestion to cause toxicity?**

150 mg/kg

○   **Metabolic acidosis favors the formation of which form of salicylate: ionized or unionized?**

Unionized. This is crucial in 2 respects:

1.   It is the reason to therapeutically produce alkaline urine. More of the free salicylate is thereby converted to the ionized form, which cannot be reabsorbed by tubules and is excreted instead.

2.   It is the reason for large changes in the amount of free drug that diffuses into the tissue. Small decreases in pH result in decreased protein binding. Therefore, more salicylate in the unionized form diffuses into tissue, increasing its volume of distribution. Always treat the patient and not the level because serum levels can decrease as salicylate moves into tissue.

○   **Is hemodialysis used to treat salicylate toxicity?**

Yes. For severely poisoned patients (ie, those with refractory acidosis, CNS toxicity, renal failure, coma, acute respiratory distress syndrome, cardiac toxicity, serum salicylate levels >80–100 mg/L, acute overdose, and 50–60 mg/L in chronic intoxication) and for patients who are unresponsive to maximal therapy

○ **What is the treatment for salicylate overdose?**

Decontamination, lavage and charcoal, replacement of fluids, supplementation with potassium, alkalizing the urine with bicarbonate, cooling for hyperthermia, administration of glucose for hypoglycemia, administration of oxygen and positive end-expiratory pressure for pulmonary edema, multiple-dose activated charcoal, and dialysis

○ **What is the treatment for prolonged prothrombin time in salicylate poisoning?**

Parenteral vitamin K administration. Salicylates inhibit vitamin K epoxide reductase in poisoning, resulting in an ability for the inactive vitamin K epoxide to be regenerated into the active vitamin K.

○ **Can a patient present with salicylate poisoning and a therapeutic prothrombin level?**

Yes. Patients with chronic salicylate poisoning have a large volume of distribution, so they may present with mental status changes and a therapeutic prothrombin level.

○ **What are the 4 stages of acetaminophen (APAP) poisoning?**

1. Stage I: 30 minutes to 24 hours—nausea and vomiting
2. Stage II: 24 to 48 hours—abdominal pain and elevated liver function test results
3. Stage III: 72 to 96 hours—liver function test results peak, nausea, and vomiting
4. Stage IV: 4 days to 2 weeks—resolution or fulminant hepatic failure

○ **APAP poisoning produces what type of hepatic necrosis?**

Centrilobular necrosis. The toxic metabolite of APAP is generated in the liver by means of the cytochrome P450 system, which is located in the centrilobular region.

○ **What is the toxic metabolite of APAP?**

N-acetyl-para-benzoquinoneimine (NAPQI). When the glucuronidation and sulfation pathways are saturated, APAP is metabolized by the CYP 450 system to the toxic metabolite NAPQI, which is glutathione dependant.

○ **How is APAP usually metabolized in nonoverdose conditions?**

Most APAP is metabolized by glucuronidation. However, some APAP metabolism occurs in conjugation with sulfate, and this percentage increases with decreasing age. Four percent or less of APAP is transformed into an extremely toxic intermediary compound (NAPQI) by CYP 450 mixed function oxidase. Theoretically, this toxic intermediary immediately conjugates with glutathione and is harmlessly excreted in the urine.

○ **How does N-acetylcysteine work in APAP overdose?**

The precise mechanism is still not well understood. However, it is known that N-acetylcysteine enters cells and is metabolized to cysteine, which serves as a glutathione precursor.

○ **Which measure of hepatic function is the best prognostic indicator in acute APAP overdose: liver enzyme levels, bilirubin level, prothrombin time, serum α-glutathione S-transferase level, serum interleukin-6 level, or C-reactive protein level?**

All are of equal prognostic value.

○ **An acutely intoxicated, nonalcoholic, otherwise healthy patient ingests APAP. Is this patient more or less likely than the alcoholic patient to develop hepatotoxicity?**

Less likely. Short-term ingestion of ethanol will engage the CYP 450 system and thereby inhibit NAPQI formation. A patient with chronic alcoholism has an induced CYP 450 system and will have greater APAP hepatotoxicity through increased NAPQI formation.

○ **What is the minimum dose of APAP that can cause hepatotoxicity in a child? In an adult?**

- Child (aged 1–5 years): More than 250 mg/kg
- Adult (or child 6 years or older): 200 mg/kg (or about 7.5–10 g)

○ **What is an antidote for APAP poisoning?**

N-acetylcysteine 140 mg/kg for the first hour, followed by 17 doses of 70 mg/kg every 4 hours for all the doses until completion

○ **According to the Rumack-Matthew nomogram, at what 4-hour APAP level should treatment be initiated for acute poisoning?**

150 mg/mL

○ **What is the appropriate initial treatment for theophylline-induced seizures?**

Benzodiazepines (IV diazepam or lorazepam), barbiturates, and phenobarbital but not phenytoin, which is not effective for theophylline-induced seizures. Theophylline-induced seizures warrant hemodialysis or charcoal hemoperfusion; if the seizure is recurring, consider midazolam infusions.

○ **What is the treatment for theophylline-induced hypotension?**

Fluid administration and β-blockers. Theophylline-induced cardiovascular instability is secondary to β-agonist effects. Therefore, β-blockers can be beneficial in the treatment of arrhythmias and hypotension.

○ **What are absolute indications for hemodialysis or hemoperfusion in theophylline toxicity?**

Seizures or arrhythmias that are unresponsive to conventional therapy and a theophylline level higher than 80 μg/mL in acute poisoning or 40 to 60 μg/mL in chronic poisoning

○ **What abnormal laboratory test results are typical in a patient with acute theophylline poisoning?**

Hypokalemia, hyperglycemia, and leukocytosis. The β-agonist properties of theophylline produce these abnormalities. Monitor creatine kinase level, renal function, and acid-base balance in patients with seizures, compartment syndrome, and severe toxicity.

○ **What factors and substances decrease theophylline metabolism and increase theophylline levels?**

- Factors: Age greater than 50 years, prematurity, hepatic and renal disease, pulmonary edema, congestive heart failure, pneumonia, obesity, and viral illness in children
- Substances: Drugs that increase theophylline levels include cimetidine, erythromycin, allopurinol, troleandomycin, biphasic calcium phosphates, and quinolone antibiotics.

In smokers, the theophylline half-life is decreased, which causes the serum theophylline levels to decrease. Phenobarbital, phenytoin, rifampin, carbamazepine, marijuana smoking, exposure to environmental pollutants, and the consumption of charcoal-broiled foods can also decrease serum theophylline levels.

○ **What electrolyte change is expected with ingestion of a large amount of digoxin?**

Expect hyperkalemia. After administration of digoxin-specific antibody fragments (Fab), the potassium level may decrease quickly, and the patient may become hypokalemic. Monitor the potassium level carefully.

○ **What are the absolute indications for Fab administration in digoxin poisoning?**

Severe acute ventricular arrhythmias, hemodynamically significant progressive bradyarrhythmias, second- or third-degree heart block that is unresponsive to standard therapy (ie, atropine), and potassium level greater than 5.0 mEq/L

○ **Why is calcium chloride administration contraindicated in digoxin poisoning?**

Digoxin inhibits the phosphorylation of sodium, potassium, and adenosine triphosphatase. This mechanism increases the intracellular concentration of sodium. The sodium-calcium exchange pump is then activated, which leads to high intracellular concentrations of calcium. Calcium chloride administration would further increase intracellular calcium, which would cause myocardial irritability.

○ **A patient receiving Fab is bradycardic and hypotensive and exhibits significantly peaked T waves at ECG. What is the initial treatment?**

Administer 10 vials of IV Fab while simultaneously treating the presumed hyperkalemia with insulin and glucose, sodium bicarbonate, and sodium polystyrene sulfonate. After the Fab is administered, hyperkalemia-induced arrhythmias may safely be treated with calcium chloride.

○ **What is the antidote for β-blocker poisoning?**

Glucagon. Glucagon receptors, located on myocardial cells, are G protein-coupled receptors that activate adenylate cyclase, leading to increased levels of intracellular cyclic adenosine monophosphate. Thus, glucagon administration causes the same intracellular effect as does a β-agonist, so it is effectively a β-adrenergic blocker antagonist.

○ **What are potential treatment modalities for calcium-channel blocker poisoning?**

Therapeutic interventions include IV calcium chloride; insulin and dextrose; isoproterenol; glucagon; transvenous pacemaker placement; atropine; and vasopressors, such as norepinephrine, epinephrine, dopamine, amrinone, and phenylephrine.

○ **What is clonidine's mechanism of action?**

Clonidine is a central-acting α-agonist. It leads to decreased sympathetic outflow and lowers catecholamine levels.

○ **What are the mechanism and treatment for clonidine-induced hypotension?**

- Treatment: IV fluid administration, dopamine, and norepinephrine
- Mechanism: Decreased cardiac output secondary to decreased sympathetic outflow from the CNS

○ **What typical eye response is related to clonidine and tizanidine poisoning?**

Pinpoint pupils (miosis)

○ **At what adrenergic receptor are clonidine and tizanidine active?**

Clonidine and tizanidine are both imidazoles and α_2-agonists.

○ **What is the pharmacologic basis of the anticonvulsant effect of phenytoin?**

Sodium-channel blockade. Phenytoin causes an increasing efflux or a decreasing influx of sodium ions across cell membranes in the motor cortex during generation of a nerve impulse.

○ **Why does IV phenytoin administration lead to cardiovascular toxicity?**

The propylene glycol diluent is a myocardial depressant and vasodilator.

○ **What are the 4 stages of iron poisoning?**

1. Stage 1: 0 to 6 hours: Abdominal pain, nausea, vomiting, and diarrhea secondary to the corrosive effects of iron; in more severe cases, hematemesis, hypotension, and altered mental status

2. Stage 2: 6 to 24 hours: Quiescent period during which iron is absorbed; in severe poisoning, latent period may be absent

3. Stage 3: 12 to 24 hours: GI hemorrhage, shock, metabolic acidosis, heart failure, cardiovascular collapse, coma, seizures, coagulopathy, and hepatic and renal failure

4. Stage 4: 4 to 6 weeks after ingestion: Gastric outlet or small bowel obstruction secondary to scarring

○ **What dose of iron is expected to produce clinical toxicity?**

60 mg/kg of elemental iron. Generally, 20 mg/kg or less is not toxic; the estimated lethal dose is 0.3 g/kg body weight.

○ **What iron level is generally considered toxic 4 hours after ingestion?**

300 to 350 μg/dL

○ **What is the antidote for a toxic ingestion of iron?**

Deferoxamine chelates only free iron. It should be administered if the iron level is greater than 350 μg/dL.

○ **What are indications for deferoxamine therapy?**

• Patients exhibiting symptoms that are more than merely transient
• Patients with lethargy, significant abdominal pain, hypotension, mental status changes, hypovolemia, or metabolic acidosis
• Patients with positive results at radiography of the kidneys, ureter, and bladder
• Patients with symptoms who have an iron level greater than 300 μ/dL

○ **What laboratory test can aid in the evaluation of possible toxic iron ingestion?**

Total iron-binding capacity measured 3 to 5 hours after ingestion. If the serum iron level is significantly less than the total iron-binding capacity, toxic iron ingestion is less likely.

○ **What symptom warrants evaluation after hydrocarbon ingestion?**

Coughing. Any patient who coughs after ingesting a hydrocarbon has the potential for developing chemical pneumonitis.

○ **At what point can a patient who has ingested a hydrocarbon be discharged safely?**

After 6 hours. Patients without symptoms with normal chest radiographs and pulse oxygen levels may be discharged to home.

○ **What drug is absolutely contraindicated when treating hydrocarbon poisoning?**

Epinephrine. It sensitizes the myocardium and potentially leads to arrest.

○ **What metabolic complication is encountered in chronic solvent abuse?**

Renal tubular acidosis

○ **Carbon tetrachloride poisoning produces what type of liver damage?**

Centrilobular necrosis

○ **Methylene chloride is metabolized to which toxin?**

Carbon monoxide

○ **What are the most common complaints in a patient with carbon monoxide poisoning?**

A headache is most common, followed by dizziness, weakness, and nausea.

○ **A 2-year-old boy is asymptomatic after ingestion of a button battery. Radiography of the kidneys, ureter, and bladder reveals the foreign body in his stomach. What is the disposition for this patient?**

Discharge to home. If the battery is lodged in the esophagus, endoscopy must be performed immediately. Otherwise, reassure the patient's parents and instruct them to check their son's stools.

○ **A patient presents with miotic pupils, muscle fasciculations, diaphoresis, and diffuse oral and bronchial secretions. The patient has a garlic odor on his breath. What is your diagnosis?**

Organophosphate poisoning

○ **What enzyme is inhibited by organophosphates?**

Acetylcholinesterase

○ **How do organophosphates enter the body?**

They can be inhaled, ingested, or absorbed through the skin.

○ **What are the signs and symptoms of organophosphate poisoning?**

One to two hours after poisoning patients may have GI upset, bronchospasm, miosis, bradycardia, excessive salivation and sweating, tremor, respiratory muscle paralysis, muscle fasciculations, agitation, seizures, coma, and death.

SLUDGE

Salivation

Lacrimation

Urinary incontinence

Diarrhea

Gastric upset

Emesis

○ **What ECG changes may be associated with organophosphate poisoning?**

Prolongation of the QT interval and ST-segment and T-wave abnormalities

○ **What is the key laboratory finding in the diagnosis of organophosphate poisoning?**

Decreased red blood cell cholinesterase activity. The serum cholinesterase level (pseudocholinesterase) is more sensitive but less specific. Red blood cell cholinesterase is regenerated slowly and can take months to approach normal levels.

○ **What is the treatment for organophosphate poisoning?**

Decontamination, charcoal, atropine, and pralidoxime as needed

○ **What antihypertensive agent may induce cyanide poisoning?**

Nitroprusside. One molecule of sodium nitroprusside contains 5 molecules of cyanide. Preventing toxicity with infusions of long duration requires infusing sodium thiosulfate with sodium nitroprusside at a ratio of 10:1. Beware of thiocyanate toxicity.

○ **What are the signs and symptoms of cyanide overdose?**

Dryness and burning in the throat, air hunger, and hyperventilation. If the individual is not removed from the toxic environment, loss of consciousness, seizures, bradycardia, and apnea will occur, followed by asystole.

○ **Cyanide binds to metals and disrupts the function of metal-containing enzymes. Which is the most important of these enzymes?**

Cytochrome A, also known as "cytochrome oxidase," which is necessary for aerobic metabolism

○ **What is the appropriate treatment for cyanide poisoning?**

Amyl nitrite and sodium nitrite IV, followed by sodium thiosulfate IV

○ **Why administer nitrites for cyanide poisoning?**

Nitrites form methemoglobin, which strongly bind to cyanide.

○ **Why prescribe sodium thiosulfate for cyanide poisoning?**

Rhodanese, an intrinsic enzyme, transfers cyanide from its attachment to methemoglobin to sulfur, thereby forming thiocyanate, which is then excreted. Sodium thiosulfate acts as a sulfur donor for this process.

○ **What is the antidote for isoniazid-induced seizures?**

Pyridoxine

○ **What regions of the liver lobules contain the greatest amount of CYP 450–related mixed-function oxidases?**

The centrilobular regions, accounting for primarily centrilobular necrosis

○ **Clonidine is a centrally acting presynaptic α_2-adrenergic agonist that decreases the central sympathetic outflow. Although its primary use is to treat hypertension, clonidine has additional emergency value in blunting withdrawal symptoms from opiates and ethanol. A clonidine overdose closely resembles an overdose with which other class of drugs?**

Opiates

○ **Toxicity from clonidine usually occurs within what time period?**

4 hours

○ **Which agent is a useful antidote for clonidine overdose?**

Naloxone

○ **Name a few substances that have anticholinergic properties.**

Antihistamines, cyclic antidepressants, phenothiazine, atropine, and, jimsonweed

○ **What ECG abnormality is most common in patients who have anticholinergic toxicity?**

Sinus tachycardia. Other dangerous arrhythmias include conduction problems and ventricular tachycardia.

○ **True/False: A patient with acute digitalis toxicity presents with frequent multifocal premature ventricular contractions, peaked T waves, and a potassium level of 6.2 mEq/L. The correct treatment is to first administer calcium chloride because this is the fastest acting agent for reducing hyperkalemia.**

False. Although calcium chloride is the fastest acting agent for decreasing hyperkalemia, you should not administer any excess calcium in a patient with digitalis-induced cardiac toxicity.

○ **What drugs increase the half-life of phenytoin?**

Sulfonamides, isoniazid, dicumarol, and chloramphenicol

○ **What are the cardiac effects of phenytoin?**

It inhibits sodium channels and decreases the effective refractory period and automaticity in the Purkinje fibers. It has little effect on QRS width or action potential duration.

○ **What is the lethal dose of phenytoin?**

20 mg/kg

○ **What symptoms are expected with a phenytoin level of higher than 20, higher than 30, and higher than 40 μg/mL?**

Higher than 20 μg/mL: Lateral gaze nystagmus
Higher than 30 μg/mL: Lateral gaze nystagmus plus increased vertical nystagmus with upward gaze
Higher than 40 μg/mL: Lethargy, confusion, dysarthrias, and psychosis

○ **True/False: Phenytoin is the drug of choice for a patient with nonketotic hyperosmolar coma who experiences a seizure.**

False. Phenytoin is contraindicated in patients with hyperglycemic, hyperosmolar, nonketotic coma. The drugs of choice for this seizure disorder are lorazepam or diazepam. Phenobarbital use is also appropriate.

○ **What are the signs and symptoms of phenytoin toxicity?**

Seizure, heart blocks, bradyarrhythmias, tachyarrhythmias, hypotension, cerebellar dysfunction, and coma. All dangerous cardiovascular complications of phenytoin overdose result from parenteral administration. High levels after oral administration do not cause such signs in a stable patient.

○ **What is the treatment for phenytoin overdose?**

Systemic support, charcoal, atropine, epinephrine, dopamine, bradyarrhythmias, and phenobarbital (20 mg/kg IV) for seizures

○ **Name the 3 main effects β-adrenergic antagonists have on the heart.**

1. Negative chronotropy
2. Negative inotropy
3. Decreased atrioventricular nodal conduction velocity (negative dromotropy)

○ **True/False: β-Adrenergic antagonists can cause mental status changes and seizures.**

True

○ **What is the treatment for opiate overdose?**

Naloxone, 0.4 to 2.0 mg initially in an adult and 0.01 mg/kg in a child. Naloxone's duration of action is about 1 hour. Higher doses and continuous infusion may be required.

○ **Describe the features of the 3 stages of phencyclidine (PCP) intoxication.**

1. Stage I: Agitation or violence and normal vital signs
2. Stage II: Tachycardia, hypertension, and no response to pain
3. Stage III: Unresponsiveness, depressed respirations, seizures, and death

○ **Which types of nystagmus are expected with PCP overdose?**

Vertical, horizontal, and rotary. Vertical nystagmus is not common with other conditions and ingestions. The most common findings with PCP overdose are hypertension, tachycardia, and nystagmus.

○ **How can PCP enter the body?**

Through inhalation, skin, and ingestion

○ **What is the clinical manifestation of PCP intoxication?**

Irritation of skin, eyes, and upper respiratory tract; headache; vomiting; weakness; sweating; hyperthermia; tachycardia; tachypnea; convulsions; coma; pulmonary edema; cardiovascular collapse; and death

○ **What is the most common cause of chronic heavy metal poisoning?**

Lead. Arsenic is the most common cause of acute heavy metal poisoning.

○ **A child presents with bluish discoloration of the gingiva. What is the probable diagnosis?**

Chronic lead poisoning. Expect the erythrocyte protoporphyrin level to be elevated with this condition.

○ **Organophosphates are found in what kinds of compounds?**

Pesticides, flame retardants, and plasticizers

○ **What is the rate-limiting step in the metabolism of ethanol?**

The conversion of ethanol to acetaldehyde by alcohol dehydrogenase

○ **What is the most common arrhythmia induced by long-term, heavy ethanol binging?**

Atrial fibrillation

○ **What blood ethanol level will cause confusion or stupor in a person who does not drink?**

180 to 300 mg/dL. The minimum blood ethanol level that can cause coma in a person who does not drink is 300 mg/dL.

○ **In chronic ethanol use, ethanol withdrawal seizures occur approximately how many hours after cessation of heavy ethanol consumption?**

6 to 48 hours from the time of the last drink

○ **Delirium tremens occurs how long after the cessation of heavy ethanol consumption?**

On average, 3 to 5 days

○ **Is there a role for phenytoin in the prevention or treatment of pure ethanol withdrawal seizures?**

No. Careful titration of benzodiazepines or phenobarbital should be used if necessary.

○ **True/False: Status epilepticus is commonly seen in ethanol withdrawal seizures.**

False. Status epilepticus is rare in ethanol withdrawal seizures and should suggest the need to find other causative disease.

○ **What is the classic triad of Wernicke encephalopathy?**

1. Global confusion
2. Oculomotor disturbances
3. Gait ataxia

○ **What constellation of findings should prompt consideration of ethylene glycol toxicity?**

Ethanol-like intoxication (with no odor), large anion gap acidosis, increased osmolal gap, altered mental status leading to coma, and calcium oxalate crystals in the urine

○ **True/False: Lithium has a narrow therapeutic toxic range.**

True. Therapeutic lithium levels are between 0.5 and 1.5 mEq/L and must be monitored closely.

○ **How is lithium eliminated after metabolism?**

Through renal excretion

○ **Which electrolyte abnormality may enhance lithium toxicity?**

Hyponatremia. Reabsorption of lithium will be enhanced.

○ **What are the typical CNS findings in mild lithium toxicity?**

Rigidity, tremor, and hyperreflexia

○ **What are the typical CNS findings in severe lithium toxicity?**

Seizures, coma, and myoclonic jerking

○ **What are the indications for hemodialysis in lithium toxicity?**

Serum lithium level higher than 4.0 mEq/L, renal failure, and severe clinical symptoms (eg, stupor or seizures)

○ **True/False: Permanent neurologic sequelae (ie, encephalopathy) can develop from lithium toxicity.**

True

○ **A 30-year-old man presents to the emergency department 20 minutes after ingesting 30 tablets of amitriptyline. What is the preferred method of gastric emptying?**

Immediate gastric lavage with a large (34–36 French) orogastric tube. Ipecac should not be used because of the potential for rapid deterioration in mental status and seizures.

○ **What class of antiarrhythmics are contraindicated in cyclic antidepressant overdoses?**

Types 1A and 1C antiarrhythmics. They have quinidine-like effects on the sodium channels and will enhance the cardiotoxicity of the cyclic antidepressants.

○ **The onset of toxicity of MAOIs can occur for how long after ingestion?**

12 to 24 hours

○ **What over-the-counter cold medications should not be used by people taking MAOIs?**

Decongestants, antihistamines, and products containing dextromethorphan

○ **A 45-year-old woman presents with a diagnosis of depression, anxiety, and insomnia and is currently using tramadol, flecainide, and tamoxifen. Can you prescribe a selective serotonin reuptake inhibitor (SSRI) for her?**

No. SSRIs are CYP 450 2D6 inhibitors, and the drugs she is using use CYP 450 2D6 for their metabolism.

○ **Name 5 herbal remedies associated with bleeding.**

1. Ginger
2. Garlic
3. Ginkgo
4. Ginseng
5. Feverfew

○ **What herbal remedies are associated with CNS stimulation?**

Guarana, ma huang, St Johns wort, yohimbe, and ginseng

○ **Can a patient with sulfonamide or acetylsalicylic acid allergy be prescribed a cyclooxygenase 2 inhibitor?**

No. Celecoxib is a sulfonamide.

○ **Which opiate combination is associated with arrhythmias, pulmonary edema, and hepatic failure and is banned in the United Kingdom?**

Propoxyphene N 100 plus APAP

○ **A person working in a plant making chemical deodorizers was exposed to phenol. What is a possible field treatment?**

Clean him or her with olive oil and water.

○ **Ingestion of benzene (an ingredient in pesticides, detergent, and paint remover) causes dermatitis, leukemia, and aplastic anemia. How can it be identified as a causative agent in such illnesses?**

Phenol, the metabolite, can be found in the urine.

○ **What drug blocks the uptake of radioactive iodine?**

Potassium iodide

○ **Isoniazid and *Gyromitra* mushroom poisoning is best treated with what drug?**

Pyridoxine

○ **The psilocybin mushroom is associated with what symptom?**

Hallucinations

○ **How are the effects of pancuronium reversed?**

Atropine and neostigmine

○ **What adverse effect of propranolol may be of concern to a diabetic patient?**

Hypoglycemia

○   **What is the treatment for propranolol overdose?**

Glucagon

○   **What is the most common complication of verapamil, and how should it be treated?**

Hypotension, which should be treated with calcium gluconate IV over several minutes. This can be followed by glucagon.

○   **What are common adverse effects of danazol?**

Hirsutism, amenorrhea, deepening of the voice, acne, weight gain, hot flashes, labile emotions, and decreased vaginal lubrication

○   **What are the adverse effects of phenothiazine therapy?**

Parkinsonism, dystonia, and akathisia (ie, the neuroleptic triad). These adverse effects can be treated with antiparkinsonian medication.

○   **What is the rationale for pretreating a patient with a subpolarizing (defasciculating) dose of a nondepolarizing agent before treatment with succinylcholine?**

Attenuation of fasciculations from succinylcholine-induced depolarization, which may decrease subsequent muscle pain. Increased intragastric and intraocular pressure is associated with the administration of succinylcholine.

○   **Is succinylcholine a depolarizing or a nondepolarizing neuromuscular blocking agent?**

Depolarizing. Succinylcholine is the only commonly used depolarizing agent. It binds to postsynaptic acetylcholine receptors, thereby causing depolarization. The material is enzymatically degraded by pseudocholinesterase (serum cholinesterase). Onset is within 1 minute; paralysis last 7 to 10 minutes.

○   **What dosage of midazolam causes a loss of consciousness and amnesia during rapid sequence induction?**

0.1 mg/kg. Five milligrams is effective for most people.

○   **Loss of consciousness usually occurs within 15 seconds after thiopental is administered. What is the usual duration of action?**

2 to 30 minutes, depending on the source. Less than 5 minutes is commonly referenced.

○   **What drugs should be avoided in glucose-6-phosphate dehydrogenase deficiency?**

Acetylsalicylic acid, phenacetin, primaquine, quinine, quinacrine, nitrofurans, sulfamethoxazole, sulfacetamide, and methylene blue

○   **What are the common anticholinergic compounds?**

Atropine, TCAs, antihistamines, phenothiazine, antiparkinsonian drugs, belladonna alkaloids, and some Solanaceae plants (ie, deadly nightshade and jimsonweed)

○ **Describe the action and adverse effects of diazoxide.**

Action begins within 1 to 2 minutes and lasts as long as 12 hours. Adverse effects may include nausea, vomiting, fluid retention, and hyperglycemia. Diazoxide is a direct arterial vasodilator. It is contraindicated in patients with aortic dissection or angina.

○ **What is the antidote for gold?**

British anti-Lewisite

○ **What is the antidote for nitrites?**

Methylene blue 1%, 0.2 mL/kg IV over 5 minutes. Severe methemoglobinemia requires an exchange transfusion.

○ **What are common entities in the differential diagnosis of pinpoint pupils?**

Narcotic overdose; clonidine overdose; and sedative hypnotic overdose, including ethanol; cerebellopontine angle infarct; and subarachnoid hemorrhage

○ **What are the effects of dopamine at various doses?**

- 1 to 10 mg/kg: Renal, mesenteric, coronary, and cerebral vasodilation
- 10 to 20 mg/kg: Both α- and β-adrenergic effects
- 20 mg/kg: Primarily α-adrenergic effects

○ **List 5 toxic syndromes and the hepatotoxic drugs that cause them.**

1. Acute hepatitis: Halothane, methyldopa, and isoniazid

2. Cholestatic jaundice: Anabolic steroids, oral contraceptives, oral hypoglycemic agents, and erythromycin estolate

3. Massive hepatic necrosis: Carbon tetrachloride, phosphorus, APAP, and *Amanita* mushrooms

4. Chronic active hepatitis and cirrhosis: Vinyl chloride and arsenic

5. Steatosis and hepatocellular necrosis: Ethanol

○ **Which street drug commonly causes both horizontal and vertical nystagmus?**

Phencyclidine (PCP)

○ **Name 5 drugs or conditions that cause hypertension or tachycardia.**

SWAMP

1. Sympathomimetics

2. Withdrawal

3. Anticholinergics

4. MAOIs

5. PCP

○   **Name 6 common drugs that can cause hyperthermia.**

SANDS-PCP

1. **S**alicylates
2. **A**nticholinergics
3. **N**euroleptics
4. **D**initrophenols
5. **S**ympathomimetics
6. **P**CP

○   **What drugs cause an acetone odor on the breath?**

Ethanol, isopropanol, and salicylates. Ketosis is often accompanied by the same odor.

○   **What substances induce an odor of almonds on the breath?**

Cyanide, laetrile, and apricot pits (the latter 2 containing amygdalin)

○   **What drugs induce a garlic odor on the breath?**

Dimethyl sulfoxide, organophosphates, phosphorus, arsenic, arsine gas, and thallium

○   **What drugs are commonly excreted by means of alkaline diuresis?**

Long-acting barbiturates; isoniazid; TCAs; salicylates; and, less commonly, lithium

○   **What is a potential adverse effect of the use of sodium polystyrene sulfonate?**

Sodium polystyrene sulfonate exchanges sodium for potassium. As a result, sodium overload and congestive heart failure may occur.

○   **What is the therapy of choice to neutralize heparin in a patient who has inadvertently received too much?**

Protamine. One milligram of protamine will neutralize about 100 U of heparin. The maximum dose of protamine is 100 mg.

○   **What is the best diluent for treating the ingestion of solid lye?**

Milk

○   **A patient presents with belladonna alkaloid poisoning resulting in anticholinergic effects. Explain the dangers of treating this patient with physostigmine.**

Physostigmine increases acetylcholine levels. In doing so, it can precipitate a cholinergic crisis, resulting in heart block and asystole. As a result, physostigmine should be reserved for life-threatening anticholinergic complications.

○   **What is the treatment for chloral hydrate overdose?**

Hemodialysis and/or charcoal hemoperfusion will clear the active metabolite, as well as trichloroethanol.

○   **What is the ferric chloride test, and what toxic ingestion does it detect?**

Add a few drops of 10% ferric chloride solution to a few drops of urine. A purple color indicates the presence of salicylic acid. Ketones or phenothiazine can lead to false-positive results.

○   **What is the antidote for phosphorus poisoning?**

Copper sulfate, 1% solution. Remove phosphorus within 30 minutes after exposure. Phosphorus can be identified by the formation of an insoluble black precipitate after swabbing with copper sulfate.

○   **What is vitamin K used to treat?**

Warfarin overdose

○   **What is methylene blue used to treat?**

Methemoglobinemia

○   **If a patient is prescribed only morphine for pain, which of the following opioids will not be revealed by confirmatory clinical urine drug testing (ie, gas chromatography-mass spectrometry or liquid chromatography-mass spectrometry): hydromorphone, codeine, oxycodone, or morphine?**

Oxycodone. All the others will be detected at gas chromatography-mass spectrometry. Standard tests for opiates are responsive to morphine and codeine but have a lower sensitivity for semisynthetic and synthetic opioids, such as oxycodone.

○   **Which of the following 4 opioids will not be revealed by clinical urine drug testing (gas chromatography coupled to tandem mass spectrometry or liquid chromatography coupled to tandem mass spectrometry) when the patient is prescribed only codeine for pain: hydrocodone, codeine, hydromorphone, and morphine?**

Hydromorphone. Codeine ingestion will produce all the other metabolites revealed by this test.

○   **True/False: Codeine, a poor analgesic, is metabolized by CYP 450 2D6; the analgesic effects of codeine depend on conversion to morphine.**

True. Codeine's true effectiveness is with its conversion to morphine.

○   **Propoxyphene is banned in the United Kingdom for prescribing. What are the toxic effects of this drug?**

Propoxyphene is a poor analgesic and produces a cardiopulmonary toxic metabolite: norpropoxyphene. Multiple deaths have been caused by cardiac effects (prolonged QT interval) and pulmonary edema after use of the drug.

○   **What are the toxic effects of methadone?**

Methadone has been implicated in contributing to QT prolongation and arrhythmias. Methadone has a long half-life and may accumulate in the body with prolonged use; therefore, starting doses should begin low (ie, 25 mg) for initiating analgesia.

○   **With use of enzyme immunoassay (EIA) for presumptive testing of urine, what is the typical time period during which the following drugs can be detected: codeine, hydrocodone, hydromorphone, morphine, oxycodone, oxymorphone, and tramadol?**

As long as 4 days. Because of limitations of detection at EIA, these drugs will not be detected after 4 days. Other methods (eg, gas chromatography-mass spectrometry) can be used to detect these drugs in the urine for longer periods.

○   **What drug may produce a false-positive finding with EIA cross-reactivity for opioids?**

Levofloxacin. Like that of opioids, the metabolic structure of levofloxacin is not discernible at EIA.

○   **With use of EIA for detection, what drug may produce a false-positive test result for tetrahydrocannabinol (*Cannabis*)?**

Pantoprazole. Tetrahydrocannabinol and pantoprazole are structurally similar at EIA.

○   **How do the processes of pharmacokinetics and pharmacodynamics differ?**

Pharmacokinetics describes what the body does to the drug, and pharmacodynamics describes what the drug does to the body.

○   **Define phase I drug metabolism.**

During phase I (nonsynthetic) metabolic reactions, a compound acquires hydrophilic functional groups through oxidation, reduction, and hydrolysis by mixed function oxidases within the liver. The CYP 450 system typically is involved in these oxidative reactions. The formation of highly polar metabolites in phase I reactions facilitates renal excretion of the drug.

○   **Define phase II drug metabolism.**

During phase II (synthetic) metabolic reactions, which do not require CYP 450 interactions, conjugation occurs between metabolites, parent compounds, and endogenous substrates (glucuronic acid, glutathione, or amino acids) to produce a polar molecule that is water soluble and, therefore, more easily excreted renally.

○   **Why is propoxyphene overdose not treated with naloxone?**

Because when propoxyphene is converted into norpropoxyphene, it is no longer an opioid and, therefore, not reversible by naloxone

○   **What therapeutic outcome can be expected when using 2 drugs that both rely on CYP 450, with 1 drug as an inducer of that enzyme system?**

Induction by definition involves augmentation of metabolism of the other drug, resulting in decreased effectiveness and producing an effect that is less than therapeutic.

○   **What significant adverse effect may occur when tramadol is taken at doses exceeding the maximum daily dose of 400 mg recognized by the U.S. Food and Drug Administration?**

Patients have a greater risk of seizure when tramadol doses exceed 400 mg/d.

○ **Tramadol, trazodone, cyclobenzaprine, an SSRI, and triptans (such as sumatriptan or rizatriptan) all augment and use the serotonin receptor binding pathways. What adverse effects (syndromes) can occur when these agents are coprescribed?**

Hypertensive crisis, serotonin syndrome, neuroleptic malignant syndrome, and extrapyramidal symptoms all can be the result of coprescribing 2 or more of these drugs.

○ **What electrolyte abnormality may occur with the use of the SSRIs (eg, sertraline, paroxetine, and fluoxetine) and selective serotonin reuptake inhibitors (eg, as venlafaxine, duloxetine, and desvenlafaxine)?**

All of the SSRIs and selective serotonin reuptake inhibitors are implicated in producing hyponatremia. Monitor the sodium levels.

○ **What are the Beers criteria?**

The Beers criteria are a list of medications generally considered inappropriate for administration in elderly people. The Beers criteria are now highly recognized and are a commonly used and quoted source of pharmacotherapies to avoid in patients older than 65 years.

○ **According to the Beers criteria, which of the following nonsteroidal anti-inflammatory drugs (NSAIDs) may be used safely in elderly patients: indomethacin, celecoxib, ketorolac, piroxicam, and oxaprozon?**

Celecoxib is the only NSAID listed that would meet the Beers criteria for safe use in patients older than 65 years. The remaining NSAIDs all have long half-lives, low creatinine clearance (<50 mL/min/1.73 m^2), and cyclooxygenase 1–mediated GI adverse effects, and they decrease platelet efficacy.

○ **NSAIDs are associated with a relatively high incidence of renal impairment. NSAIDs should be prescribed with caution in patients with renal function below what level?**

The renal caution for NSAIDS is a creatinine clearance of 50 mL/min/1.73 m^2 or less.

○ **You are having a hard time remembering which anesthetics are amides and which anesthetics are esters. What is a fairly easy way of telling these 2 classifications apart?**

With the exception of the suffix "-caine," only the anesthetics in the amide classification include the letter "i":

Amides
- Lidocaine
- Bupivacaine
- Mepivacaine

Esters
- Procaine
- Cocaine
- Tetracaine
- Benzocaine

○ **Do local anesthetics freely cross the blood-brain barrier?**

Yes. Most systemic toxic reactions to local anesthetics involve the CNS or cardiovascular systems.

○ **Of the following anesthetics, which has the shortest duration of action: lidocaine, procaine, bupivacaine, or mepivacaine?**

Procaine

○ **Activated charcoal is not indicated for which types of overdose?**

Ethanol ingestion, electrolytes, heavy metals, lithium, hydrocarbons, and caustic ingestions

○ **What are some common adverse effects of phenothiazine use?**

Malaise, hyperthermia, tachycardia, anticholinergic effects, and quinidine-like membrane stabilization. The most dangerous adverse effect is neuroleptic malignant syndrome.

○ **How should stable ventricular tachyarrhythmias associated with phenothiazine overdose be treated?**

Lidocaine and phenytoin

○ **Hepatic failure is commonly associated with what anticonvulsant?**

Valproic acid

○ **What is the main excitatory neurotransmitter in brain?**

Glutamate

○ **What is the main inhibitory neurotransmitter in the brain?**

GABA

○ **What drugs act at GABA receptors?**

Benzodiazepines (eg, diazepam), barbiturates (eg, phenobarbital), neurosteroids, and the novel anticonvulsant loreclezole enhance GABA receptors. GABA receptors are inhibited by convulsants, including bicuculline, picrotoxin, penicillin, and Zn^{++}.

○ **What are the major monoamine neurotransmitters in the CNS?**

Acetylcholine, epinephrine, norepinephrine, serotonin, dopamine, and histamine

○ **What drugs act at CNS muscarinic acetylcholine receptors?**

Antimuscarinic agents (eg, atropine and scopolamine) and antimuscarinic adverse effects of other agents (eg, TCAs) cause initial CNS excitation, irritability, hallucinations, or delirium, progressing to coma and respiratory paralysis. Clinical uses include decreasing secretions or GI motility, paralyzing the iris, reversing bradycardia or bronchospasm, preventing motion sickness, and inducing sleep. Anticholinergics are sometimes helpful in treating early Parkinson disease, especially for tremor, but can cause confusion, dry mouth, and urinary retention.

Anticholinesterases (eg, physostigmine and neostigmine) are used to treat hypotonic bladder, glaucoma, and myasthenia gravis. Tacrine and donepezil modestly improve symptoms of Alzheimer disease.

Organophosphate insecticides irreversibly inhibit acetylcholine esterase, resulting in sweating, salivation, lacrimation, urination, defecation (SLUD), bradycardia, hypotension, and death.

○ **What is the role of acetylcholine in CNS disease?**

Loss of cholinergic neurons may be responsible for some of the symptoms of Alzheimer disease and has led to use of acetylcholine esterase inhibitors in treatment. A mutation in the membrane-spanning region of the a4 subunit of nicotinic acetylcholine receptor is likely responsible for autosomal dominant frontal lobe epilepsy; the disease mechanism is unknown.

○ **What diseases are associated with dopamine?**

Parkinson disease results from loss of substantia nigra pars compacta dopaminergic neurons. Schizophrenia is undoubtedly related to dopamine receptor function, but the cause remains elusive. Long-term treatment with neuroleptic agents can result in dopamine receptor upregulation and tardive dyskinesia or dystonia.

○ **What drugs act at CNS dopamine receptors?**

A preparation of levodopa and carbidopa that prevents peripheral metabolism of levodopa and reduces adverse effects, such as nausea. Bromocriptine is a direct dopamine agonist used occasionally in Parkinson disease, used for suppression of pituitary prolactinomas, and formerly used to stop lactation, but it is now restricted because of the incidence of hypertension, seizure, and stroke with its use. Antidopaminergics (neuroleptics) are used to treat psychosis, schizophrenia, and other problems. Clozapine is an antipsychotic D4 receptor antagonist that does not exacerbate Parkinson disease. Deprenyl, a type B MAOI, provides minimal symptom relief in early Parkinson disease; results from the latest analyses of the DATATOP study data no longer support a protective effect on substantia nigra pars compacta neurons.

○ **What drugs act as adrenergic receptors?**

α_2-Agonist agents (eg, clonidine) suppress sympathetic outflow in hypertension. $\beta 1$ receptors are found in the cerebral cortex, and $\beta 2$ receptors are found in the cerebellum. Isoproterenol is a relatively pure β-agonist. Deprenyl and pargyline are antidepressants that inhibit catabolism of epinephrine and norepinephrine by blocking monoamine oxidase. Desipramine and other TCAs block norepinephrine reuptake. Amphetamine blocks reuptake and facilitates increased release of norepinephrine. β-Blockers (eg, propranolol, nadolol, and atenolol) are used for hypertension, to prevent arrhythmias, and in migraine prophylaxis.

○ **What are the major peptide neurotransmitters in the CNS?**

Opioid peptides; substance P; neuropeptide Y; and gut peptides, including somatostatin, cholecystokinin, neurotensin, vasoactive intestinal peptide, calcitonin gene-related peptide, and corticotropin-releasing factor, are present in neurons and may act as neurotransmitters or neuromodulators. Substance P is 1 of several tachykinin peptides present in dorsal root ganglion neurons that project to the substantia gelatinosa of the dorsal spinal cord (involved in pain modulation) and in projection neurons from the striatum back to the substantia nigra.

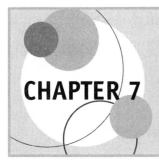

CHAPTER 7 # Infectious Disease

Andrew H. Zalski, MD

○ **Describe the pathophysiologic features of human immunodeficiency virus (HIV).**

HIV attacks the T4 helper cells. The genetic material of HIV consists of single-strand RNA. HIV has been found in semen, vaginal secretions, blood and blood products, saliva, urine, cerebrospinal fluid (CSF), tears, alveolar fluid, synovial fluid, breast milk, transplanted tissue, and amniotic fluid. There has been no documentation of infection from casual contact.

○ **How quickly do patients infected with HIV develop symptoms?**

Five percent to 10% develop symptoms within 3 years of seroconversion if untreated. Predictive characteristics include a low CD4 count and a hematocrit less than 40%. The mean incubation time is about 8.23 years for adults and 1.97 years for children younger than 5 years.

○ **An HIV-positive patient presents with a history of weight loss, diarrhea, fever, anorexia, and malaise. She is also dyspneic. Laboratory study results reveal abnormal liver function test results and anemia. What is the most likely diagnosis?**

Mycobacterium avium intracellularae. Laboratory test results are confirmed by using acid-fast staining of body fluids or by using a blood culture.

○ **How many years does a patient usually live after HIV is diagnosed?**

The prognosis for patients with HIV has greatly improved since the introduction of protease inhibitors and highly active antiretroviral therapy (HAART) in the mid-1990s. A computer simulation published in *Medical Care* in November 2006 estimated the median life span of an adult entering HIV care to be 24.2 years. Results from other studies have suggested life spans of 24 to 35 years after diagnosis. The bottom line is that patients with HIV entering treatment today may expect a nearly normal life span and are more likely to die from causes not related to HIV.

○ **What is the most common cause of focal encephalitis in patients with AIDS?**

Toxoplasmosis. Symptoms include focal neurologic deficits, headache, fever, altered mental status, and seizures. Ring-enhancing lesions are evident at computed tomography (CT).

○ **Which drugs are used to treat central nervous system (CNS) toxoplasmosis in patients with AIDS?**

Pyrimethamine plus sulfadiazine

○   **What does the differential diagnosis of ring-enhancing lesions in patients with AIDS include?**

Lymphoma, cerebral tuberculosis, fungal infection, cytomegalovirus, Kaposi sarcoma, toxoplasmosis, and hemorrhage

○   **What are the signs and symptoms of CNS cryptococcal infection in a patient with AIDS?**

Headache, depression, light-headedness, seizures, and cranial nerve palsies. A diagnosis is confirmed with an India ink preparation or a fungal culture or by testing for the presence of cryptococcal antigens in the CSF.

○   **What is the most common eye finding in patients with AIDS?**

Cotton wool spots. Cotton wool spots may be associated with *Pneumocystis jiroveci* pneumonia (PCP). Cotton wool spots may be difficult to differentiate from the fluffy, white, often perivascular retinal lesions associated with CMV.

○   **What is the most common cause of retinitis in patients with AIDS?**

CMV. Findings include photophobia, redness, scotoma, pain, or a change in visual acuity. At examination, fluffy, white retinal lesions may be evident.

○   **What is the most common opportunistic infection in patients with AIDS with a CD4 count less than 200?**

PCP. Symptoms may include a nonproductive cough and dyspnea. Chest radiography may reveal diffuse interstitial infiltrates, or it may not. Although gallium scanning is more sensitive, false-positive results occur. Initial treatment includes trimethoprim and sulfamethoxazole. Pentamidine is an alternative.

○   **What is HAART?**

HAART is a combination of antiretroviral medications that can nearly completely suppress HIV viral replication. Medications used are nucleoside and nonnucleoside reverse transcriptase inhibitors, protease inhibitors, integrase inhibitors, C-C chemokine receptor type 5 blockers, and fusion inhibitors.

○   **What is PEP, and when can it be used?**

PEP is postexposure prophylaxis. It is a combination of HIV medications used to try to prevent HIV infection in individuals who have been exposed to HIV. It should be used as soon as possible but definitely within 72 hours.

○   **How is candidiasis of the esophagus diagnosed?**

Air-contrast barium swallow study showing ulcerations with plaques. In contrast, herpes esophagitis produces punched-out ulcerations with no plaques. Definitive diagnosis is made by means of upper gastrointestinal (GI) endoscopy and fungal and viral cultures.

○   **What is the most common GI complaint in patients with AIDS?**

Diarrhea. Many of the medications used to treat HIV have GI adverse effects. Hepatomegaly and hepatitis are also typical. Conversely, jaundice is an uncommon finding. *Cryptosporidium* and *Isospora* are common causes of prolonged watery diarrhea.

○   **A patient is infected with *Treponema pallidum*. What is the treatment?**

The type of treatment depends on the stage of the infection. Primary and secondary syphilis are treated with benzathine penicillin G, 2.4 million U intramuscularly (IM)] in 1 dose. Tertiary syphilis is treated with benzathine penicillin G, 2.4 million U IM in 3 doses 3 weeks apart. According to Centers for Disease Control and Prevention recommendations, patients with known penicillin allergies should undergo penicillin allergy skin testing and penicillin desensitization, if necessary.

○ **Describe the lesions associated with lymphogranuloma venereum.**

Lymphogranuloma venereum, caused by *Chlamydia*, manifests as painless skin lesions with lymphadenopathy. Lesions may be papular, nodular, or herpetiform vesicles. Sinus formation, involving the vagina and rectum, are common in women.

○ **What is the cause of chancroid?**

Haemophilus ducreyi. Patients with this condition present with 1 or more painful necrotic lesions. Suppurative inguinal lymphadenopathy may also be present.

○ **What is the cause of granuloma inguinale?**

Calymmatobacterium granulomatis. Onset occurs with small papular, nodular, or vesicular lesions that develop slowly into ulcerative or granulomatous lesions. Lesions are painless and are located on mucous membranes of the genital, inguinal, and anal areas.

○ **What causes tetanus?**

Clostridium tetani. This organism is a gram-positive rod; it is vegetative and forms spores. It produces tetanospasmin, an endotoxin, which induces the disinhibition of the motor and autonomic nervous systems and, thus, the exhibition of the clinical symptoms of tetanus.

○ **What is the incubation period of tetanus?**

Hours to more than 1 month. The shorter the incubation period, the more severe the disease. Most patients who contract tetanus in the United States are older than 50 years.

○ **What is the most common presentation of a patient with tetanus?**

Generalized tetanus, with pain and stiffness in the trunk and jaw muscles. Trismus develops and results in risus sardonicus ("devil's smile).

○ **Outline the treatment for tetanus.**
- Respiratory: Administer succinylcholine for immediate intubation, if required
- Immunotherapy: Human tetanus immune globulin will neutralize circulating tetanospasmin and the toxin in the wound. However, it will not neutralize toxin fixed in the nervous system. Dose tetanus immune globulin 3000 to 5000 U. Prescribe tetanus toxoid, 0.6 mL IM, at 1 week, 6 weeks, and 6 months.
- Antibiotics: Penicillin G, which has been used widely for years, is no longer the drug of choice. Metronidazole (eg, 0.5 g every 6 hours) has comparable or better antimicrobial activity, and penicillin is a known antagonist of γ-aminobutyric acid, as is tetanus toxin.
- Muscle relaxants: Administer diazepam or dantrolene
- Neuromuscular block: Prescribe pancuronium bromide, 2 mg plus sedation
- Autonomic dysfunction: Prescribe labetalol, 0.25 to 1.0 mg/min intravenously (IV), or magnesium sulfate, 70 mg/kg IV load, then 1 to 4 g/h continuous infusion to treat autonomic dysfunction. Administer magnesium sulfate, 5 to 30 mg IV infusion every 2 to 8 hours, and clonidine, 0.1 to 0.3 mg every 8 hours nasogastrically.

Note: Fatal cardiovascular complications have occurred in patients treated with β-adrenergic blocking agents alone. Adrenergic blocking agents used to treat autonomic dysfunction may precipitate myocardial depression.

○ **Which is the most common tapeworm in the United States?**

Hymenolepis nana. Infections occur in institutionalized patients.

○ **Where is the hookworm *Necator americanus* infection acquired?**

In areas where human fertilizer is used and people do not wear shoes. Patients present with chronic anemia, cough, low-grade fever, diarrhea, abdominal pain, weakness, weight loss, eosinophilia, and guaiac-positive stools. The diagnosis is confirmed if ova are present in the stool. Treatment includes mebendazole, albendazole, or pyrantel pamoate.

○ **What are the signs and symptoms of *Trichuris trichiura*?**

This roundworm lives in the cecum. Complaints include anorexia, abdominal pain (especially in the right upper quadrant), insomnia, fever, diarrhea, flatulence, weight loss, pruritus, eosinophilia, and microcytic hypochromic anemia. *T trichiura* is diagnosed by examining the stool for ova. Mebendazole is the treatment of choice.

○ **A patient attended a walrus, bear, and pork roast. He now has nausea, vomiting, diarrhea, fever, urticaria, myalgia, splinter hemorrhages, muscle spasm, headache, and a stiff neck. What physical finding will clinch the diagnosis?**

Periorbital edema is pathognomonic for infection with *Trichinella spiralis*. Patients may have acute myocarditis, nonsuppurative meningitis, catarrhal enteritis, and bronchopneumonia. Laboratory study results may reveal leukocytosis, eosinophilia, electrocardiographic changes, and an elevated creatine kinase level. Diagnosis is confirmed with a latex agglutination, skin, complement fixation, or bentonite flocculation test. Stool examination is not helpful for confirming the diagnosis after the initial GI phase.

○ **List 3 common protozoa that can cause diarrhea.**

1. *Entamoeba histolytica*: Found worldwide. Although half of the infected patients have no symptoms, the usual symptoms consist of nausea, vomiting, diarrhea, fever, anorexia, abdominal pain, and leukocytosis. Determine the presence of this organism by ordering stool tests and performing an ELISA for extraintestinal infections. Treatment is with metronidazole or tinidazole followed by chloroquine phosphate.

2. *Giardia lamblia*: Found worldwide. This organism is 1 of the most common intestinal parasites in the United States. Symptoms include explosive watery diarrhea, flatus, abdominal distension, fatigue, and fever. The diagnosis is confirmed by examining the stool. Treatment is with metronidazole.

3. *Cryptosporidium parvum*: Found worldwide. Symptoms are profuse watery diarrhea, cramps, nausea, vomiting, fever, and weight loss. Treatment is supportive care. Medications may be needed for immunocompromised patients.

○ **Explain the pathophysiology of rabies.**

Infection occurs within the myocytes for the first 48 to 96 hours. It then spreads across the motor end plate and ascends and replicates along the peripheral nervous system and axoplasm and into the dorsal root ganglia, spinal cord, and CNS. From the gray matter, the virus spreads by means of peripheral nerves to tissues and organ systems.

○ **What is the characteristic histologic finding associated with rabies?**

Eosinophilic intracellular lesions within the cerebral neurons called Negri bodies, which are the sites of CNS viral replication. Although these lesions occur in 75% of rabies cases and are pathognomonic for rabies, their absence does not eliminate the possibility of rabies.

○ **What are the signs and symptoms of rabies?**

Incubation period of 12 to 700 days, with an average of 20 to 90 days. Initial signs and systems are fever, headache, malaise, anorexia, sore throat, nausea, cough, and pain or paresthesias at the bite site.

During the CNS stage, agitation, restlessness, altered mental status, painful bulbar and peripheral muscular spasms, bulbar or focal motor paresis, and opisthotonos are exhibited. As in the Landry-Guillain-Barré syndrome, 20% of cases develop ascending, symmetric flaccid and areflexic paralysis. In addition, hypersensitivity to water and sensory stimuli of light, touch, and noise may occur.

The progressive stage includes lucid and confused intervals with hyperpyrexia, lacrimation, salivation, and mydriasis along with brain-stem dysfunction, hyperreflexia, and extensor plantar response.

Final stages include coma, convulsions, and apnea, followed by death between the fourth and seventh day for the untreated patient.

○ **What is the diagnostic procedure of choice in rabies?**

Fluorescent antibody testing

○ **In the United States, what animals are most likely to be infected with the rabies virus?**

Bats, skunks, and raccoons. Dogs are the usual carriers in developing countries.

○ **Can rabies be transmitted via a rat bite?**

No. Rodents do not carry the virus, and bats are not rodents.

○ **Do individuals infected with the rabies virus foam at the mouth?**

Yes. Hypersalivation is 1 of the symptoms of furious rabies, along with hyperactivity, fear of water, hyperventilation, aerophobia, and autonomic instability. Patients with paralytic rabies develop either ascending paralysis or paralysis that affects 1 or more limbs individually. Rabies is 100% fatal once symptoms are exhibited.

○ **How is rabies treated?**

Wound care includes debridement and irrigation. The wound must not be sutured; it should remain open, which will decrease the rabies infection by 90%.

Rabies immune globulin 20 IU/kg, half at the wound site and half in the deltoid muscle, should be administered, along with human diploid cell rabies vaccine, 1-mL doses IM on days 0, 3, 7, 14, and 28, also in the deltoid muscle.

○ **A patient has a 40°C fever and an erythematous, macular, and blanching rash that becomes deep red, dusky, papular, and petechial. The patient is vomiting and has a headache, myalgias, and cough. Where did the rash begin?**

Rocky Mountain spotted fever (RMSF) rash typically begins on the flexor surfaces of the ankles and wrists and spreads centripetally and centrifugally.

○ **Which test confirms the diagnosis of RMSF?**

Immunofluorescent antibody staining of a skin biopsy specimen or serologic fluorescent antibody titer. The Weil-Felix reaction and complement fixation tests are no longer recommended.

O **Which antibiotics are prescribed for the treatment of RMSF?**

Tetracyclines are the drugs of choice, even in children younger than 9 years, despite the risk of staining the teeth. Chloramphenicol is now rarely used. Antibiotic therapy should not be withheld pending serologic confirmation.

O **What is the most deadly form of malaria?**

Plasmodium falciparum

O **What is the vector for malaria?**

The female *Anophelese* mosquito

O **What laboratory test findings are expected for a patient with malaria?**

Normochromic-normocytic anemia, a normal or depressed leukocyte count, thrombocytopenia, an elevated sedimentation rate, abnormal kidney and liver function test results, hyponatremia, hypoglycemia, and a false-positive VDRL test result.

O **How is malaria diagnosed?**

Visualization of parasites on Giemsa-stained blood smears. In early infection, especially with *P falciparum*, parasitized erythrocytes may be sequestered and undetectable.

O **How is *P falciparum* diagnosed at blood smear?**

- Small ring forms with double chromatin knobs within the erythrocyte
- Multiple rings infected within red blood cells
- Rare trophozoites and schizonts on smear
- Pathognomonic crescent-shaped gametocytes
- Parasitemia exceeding 4%

O **What is the drug of choice for treating *Plasmodium vivax, ovale*, and *malariae*?**

Chloroquine

O **How is uncomplicated chloroquine-resistant *P falciparum* treated?**

Quinine plus pyrimethamine-sulfadoxine plus doxycycline or clindamycin or mefloquine

O **What are the adverse effects of chloroquine?**

Nausea, vomiting, diarrhea, fever, pruritus, headache, dizziness, rash, and hypotension

O **Name the most common intestinal parasite in the United States.**

Giardia lamblia. Cysts are obtained from contaminated water or hand-to-mouth transmission. Symptoms include explosive foul-smelling diarrhea, abdominal distension, fever, fatigue, and weight loss. Cysts reside in the duodenum and upper jejunum.

○ **How is Chagas disease transmitted?**

Through the bloodsucking Reduviid "kissing" bug, blood transfusion, or breast feeding. A nodule or chagoma develops at the site. Symptoms include fever, headache, conjunctivitis, anorexia, and myocarditis. Congestive heart failure and ventricular aneurysms can occur. The myenteric plexus is involved, and megacolon may develop. Laboratory test findings include anemia, leukocytosis, elevated sedimentation rate, and electrocardiographic changes, such as PR interval, heart block, T-wave changes, and arrhythmias.

○ **Which 2 diseases are transmitted by the deer tick, *Ixodes scapularis*?**

1. Lyme disease
2. Babesiosis

○ **How do patients with *Babesia* infection present?**

Intermittent fever, splenomegaly, jaundice, and hemolysis. The disease may be fatal in patients without spleens. Treatment is with clindamycin and quinine.

○ **What is the most frequently transmitted tick-borne disease?**

Lyme disease. The causative agent is a spirochete (*Borrelia burgdorferi*), and the vectors are *I scapularis*, *Ixodes pacificus*, *Amblyomma americanum*, and *Dermacentor variabilis*.

○ **What areas of the United States report the highest incidence of Lyme disease?**

The New England, middle Atlantic, and upper Midwestern states

○ **What are the signs and symptoms of Lyme disease?**

• Stage I: In the first month after the tick bite, patients present with fever, fatigue, malaise, myalgia, headache, and a circular macule or papule lesion with a central clearing at the site of the tick bite that gradually enlarges (erythema chronicum migrans).
• Stage II: Occurring weeks to months later, this stage involves neurological abnormalities such as meningoencephalitis, cranial neuropathies, peripheral neuropathies, myocarditis, and conjunctivitis to blindness.
• Stage III: Occurring months to years later, migratory oligoarthritis of the large joints, neurological symptoms such as subtle encephalopathy (mood, memory, and sleep disturbances), polyneuropathy, cognitive dysfunction, and incapacitating fatigue may develop.

○ **How is Lyme disease diagnosed and treated?**

A patient who presents with a typical solitary erythema migrans rash requires no laboratory testing and is presumed to have Lyme disease. Immunofluorescent and immunoabsorbent assays can be used to identify the antibodies to the spirochete; interpretation of these tests is complex. Seroconversion may take several weeks, so results may be seronegative early in the infection Treatment includes doxycycline or tetracycline, amoxicillin, cefuroxime, IV ceftriaxone, IV penicillin, or erythromycin. Cefuroxime is the only drug for Lyme disease approved by the US Food and Drug Administration.

○ **Which type of paralysis does tick paralysis cause?**

Ascending paralysis. The venom that causes the paralysis is probably a neurotoxin. A conduction block is induced at the peripheral motor nerve branches that prevents the release of acetylcholine at the neuromuscular junction; 43 species of ticks have been implicated as causative agents.

○ **What tick-borne disease is also harbored in wild rabbits?**

Tularemia

○ **What are the signs and symptoms of tularemia?**

Indurated skin ulcers at the site of inoculation, regional lymphadenopathy, fever, shaking chills, cough, hemoptysis, shortness of breath, rales or pleural rub, hepatosplenomegaly, and a maculopapular rash

○ **What is the treatment for tularemia?**

Streptomycin is the treatment of choice. Gentamycin, which is more widely available, may also be used. Alternative therapies include doxycycline and ciprofloxacin and would be recommended in a mass casualty situation, such as a terrorist attack. The mortality rate is 5% to 30% without antibiotic treatment.

○ **A patient presents with sudden onset of fever, lethargy, a retro-orbital headache, myalgias, anorexia, nausea, and vomiting. She is extremely photophobic. The patient has been on a camping trip in Wyoming. What tick-borne disease might cause these symptoms?**

Colorado tick fever. This is caused by a virus of the genus *Orbivirus* and the family *Reoviridae*. The vector is the tick *Dermacentor andersoni*. The disease is self-limited; treatment is supportive.

○ **What is the most common cause of cellulitis?**

Streptococcus pyogenes. *Staphylococcus aureus* can also cause cellulitis, though it is generally less severe and more often associated with an open wound.

○ **What is the most common cause of cutaneous abscesses?**

S aureus

○ **What are the most common microorganisms found in brain abscesses?**

The enteric gram-negative bacilli, anaerobes, *Nocardia*, staphylococci, streptococci, and *Toxoplasma*

○ **What organism is commonly found in infected wounds caused by animal bites?**

Pasteurella multocida. The second most common organism is *S aureus*.

○ **What percentage of dog and cat bites become infected?**

About 10% of dog bites and 50% of cat bites become infected. *P multocida* is the causative agent for 30% of dog bites and 50% of cat bites.

○ **A 6-year-old child presents with headache, fever, malaise, and tender regional lymphadenopathy about a week after a cat bite. A tender papule develops at the site. What is the diagnosis?**

Cat scratch disease. This condition usually develops 3 days to 6 weeks after a cat bite or scratch. The papule typically blisters and heals with eschar formation. A transient macular or vesicular rash may also develop.

○ **What is the probable cause of an animal bite infection that develops in less than 24 hours? More than 48 hours?**

- Less than 24 hours: *P multocida* or streptococci
- More than 48 hours: *S aureus*

○ **What is the most common cause of gas gangrene?**

Clostridium perfringens

○ **What is the most common site of a herpes simplex 1 infection?**

The lower lip. These lesions are painful and can frequently recur since the virus remains in the sensory ganglia. Recurrences are generally triggered by stress, sun, and illness.

○ **Is the vasculitis seen in syphilis a large- or a small-vessel disease?**

Both. Large-vessel disease (Huebner arteritis) is caused by adventitial lymphocytic proliferation of large vessels and is commonly seen in the late meningovascular syphilis. Small-vessel vasculitis (Nissl-Alzheimer) is the dominant vasculitic pattern in paretic neurosyphilis.

○ **What is the recommended treatment for neurosyphilis?**

IV penicillin G. Follow-up CSF examinations are mandatory.

○ **What complication may arise from aggressive treatment of neurosyphilis with penicillin?**

Jarisch-Herxheimer reaction. It is due to a release of endotoxin when large numbers of spirochetes are lysed during the penicillin treatment. It consists of mild fever, malaise, headache, and arthralgia and may produce a temporary worsening of the neurological status.

○ **At which stage of Lyme disease does neurological involvement occur?**

The second and third stages. At the second stage, cranial neuropathies, meningitis, and radiculoneuritis may develop. At the third stage, encephalitis and a variety of CNS manifestations, including stroke-like syndromes, and extrapyramidal and cerebellar involvement may develop.

○ **What is Weil disease?**

Weil syndrome is the less common variety of leptospirosis, with icterus, marked hepatic and renal involvement, and bleeding diasthesis being the main features, hence the name "leptospirosis-icterohemorrhagica."

○ **What is the most common neurological feature of leptospirosis?**

Aseptic meningitis, which is present in more than 50% of cases.

○ **What clinical feature of leptospirosis sets it apart from other infections of the nervous system and hints at the diagnosis?**

Hemorrhagic complications. These are common, and intraparenchymal and subarachnoid hemorrhages have been reported.

○ **What are the neurological features of brucellosis?**

Mainly, chronic meningitis and its vascular complications. However, cranial neuropathies, demyelination, and mycotic aneurysms have all been described.

○ **How is brucellosis spread?**

By ingestion of contaminated milk and milk products. It may also be spread by contact with an infected animal (usually cattle). *Brucella melitensis* is the causative agent.

○ **Which infectious disease characteristically causes dementia and supranuclear palsy?**

Whipple disease, which is caused by a gram-positive argyrophilic bacillus

○ **What neurological findings are found almost exclusively in Whipple disease?**

Oculo-facial-skeletal-myoarrythmia. In this condition, there is a convergence of the eyes or a pendular nystagmus that is synchronous with movements of the jaw or other parts of the body.

○ **What is the neuropathological characteristic of Whipple disease?**

Nodular ependymitis, mainly of the third and fourth ventricles and the cerebral aqueduct. There is also a microgranulomatous polioencephalitis that may involve inferior frontal, temporal cortex and cerebellar nuclei. Spinal cord gray matter may be involved.

○ **What are the characteristic features of cerebral amebiasis, and what is the pathogenic organism?**

Cerebral amebiasis is usually a secondary infection, and patients often have intestinal or hepatic amebiasis. The causative organism is *E histolytica*. The clinical features are that of intracerebral abscesses causing focal neurological signs. Frontal lobes and basal nuclei are common sites of abscess formation.

○ **What is the treatment for amebiasis with neurological involvement?**

E histolytica is treated with metronidazole, emetine, and chloroquine. Metronidazole can cross the blood-brain barrier. *Naegleria* is treated with amphotericin and rifampicin.

○ **What pathological findings are seen in the brain biopsy specimen for *Toxoplasma* encephalitis?**

Tachyzoites around the necrotic lesion

○ **What are some important radiological differences between intracranial toxoplasmosis and lymphoma?**

- Intracranial toxoplasmosis usually manifests as multiple lesions, whereas lymphomas usually are solitary, at least in the beginning.
- Enhancement. Both may enhance with gadolinium-based contrast material on magnetic resonance (MR) images; however, *Toxoplasma* lesions are usually round and discrete in comparison to lymphoma lesions.
- Thallium 201 single photon emission CT. Lymphomas usually show increased activity at thallium scanning compared to toxoplasmosis, which has poor uptake.
- Location. Toxoplasmosis is usually in the deeper structures, such as basal ganglia, or the gray-white junction, whereas lymphomas usually manifest in the periventricular areas. However, biopsy is still necessary to make the diagnosis, since imaging study results may be similar for the 2 diseases.

○ **What is the current recommended treatment for intracranial toxoplasmosis with HIV disease?**

Treatment is usually a combination therapy with sulfadiazine, pyrimethamine, and folinic acid.

○ **What is the nature of CNS lymphoma in AIDS?**

Tumors are almost all of B-cell origin. Tumors may be large cell immunoblastic or small noncleaved cell lymphoma.

○ **Which virus is considered responsible for AIDS-associated CNS lymphoma?**

Epstein-Barr virus

○ **What is the typical clinical manifestation of progressive multifocal leukoencephalopathy (PML)?**

PML commonly manifests with focal neurological signs, such as hemisensory or motor signs, and visual field deficits.

○ **Which virus is responsible for causing PML?**

JC virus, which is a Papovavirus that infects oligodendrocytes

○ **PML is seen in which other immune disorders?**

Cell-mediated immunodeficiency. It is seen in HIV disease, chronic myeloid leukemia, and Hodgkin disease; it is seen in patients undergoing chemotherapy; and, rarely, in sarcoidosis.

○ **What are the common radiological features of PML?**

Areas of hypoattenuation in the subcortical white matter at CT. T1-weighted images of the brain at MR imaging show PML lesions as hypointense, and T2-weighted images show PML lesions as hyperintense. PML lesions are not contrast material enhanced and usually start in the parietooccipital region of the subcortical white matter.

○ **Which virus is considered responsible for tropical spastic paraparesis?**

Human T-lymphotropic virus 1

○ **What are the modes of transmission of human T-lymphotropic virus 1?**

- Vertical: Mother to child
- Horizontal: Through sexual contact and blood transfusion

○ **What are 4 other infectious causes of paraparesis?**

1. Syphilis
2. Tuberculosis with Pott disease of the spine
3. Leptospirosis
4. Varicella zoster virus

○ **What is the single most helpful antemortem test to support the diagnosis of Creutzfeldt-Jakob disease?**

Electroencephalogram showing triphasic sharp waves at 1 to 2 cycles per second that are superimposed on a depressed background. The cycles are usually asymmetrical and slow with advancing disease.

O   **How is botulism contracted, and what are the principal clinical features?**

Botulism is contracted by consumption of contaminated foods, by injury from nonsterile objects (wound botulism), and in infants from intestinal colonization by *Clostridium botulinum* (lack of normal intestinal flora permit this colonization). The clinical features are that of a descending paralysis with complete ophthalmoplegia and bulbar and somatic palsy.

O   **Is the motor paralysis induced by botulinum toxin reversible?**

It is an irreversible paralysis, and recovery is from axonal sprouting from old sarcolemmal areas to a new locus.

O   **Which condition resembles Guillain-Barré syndrome, the appropriate treatment of which results in complete improvement, often within a day?**

Tick paralysis, which results in an ascending paralysis within a few days of attack by *D variabilis*, a hard tick. This tick releases a toxin in its saliva, which is responsible for the neuromuscular blockade. Within hours after removal of the tick, resolution of the weakness begins.

O   **What is the cause of Sydenham chorea, and what are the principal clinical features?**

Sydenham chorea is caused by an immunological cross-reaction after group A streptococcal infections. The chorea often occurs several months after the acute infection. It is characterized by the development of involuntary choreiform movements that may be unilateral, and it remits spontaneously after a while. There are also associated behavioral changes that may reach the severity of obsessive-compulsive disorder.

O   **What is epidemic pleurodynia (Bornholm disease)?**

An upper respiratory tract infection followed by pleuritic chest pain and tender muscles. Coxsackie viruses are a group of enteroviruses responsible for the epidemic myalgia (Bornholm disease) in which pleurodynia is also a common feature. Specifically, the disease is thought to be caused by a *Coxsackie B virus*.

O   **What is the CSF characteristic of polio?**

In the acute stages, it is associated with lymphocytic pleocytosis and elevated protein and normal glucose levels. There may be a neutrophilic response early in the disease. In chronic residual polio, CSF is normal.

O   **To which group of viruses does the Poliovirus belong?**

Poliovirus is an enterovirus that belongs to the picornavirus group.

O   **What is the meaning of the term "reverse transcriptase" in the description of HIV?**

Under normal circumstances, the transcription of a protein in a human cell occurs in a forward direction, going from DNA to RNA. With a reverse transcriptase, the transcription proceeds from RNA to DNA. HIV is a reverse transcriptase, or retrovirus, that needs to be incorporated into the human genome by the reverse transcription before replicating.

O   **Is AIDS dementia a cortical or subcortical dementia?**

Cortical. There is no evidence of myelin breakdown in AIDS dementia. The white matter pallor is probably secondary to blood-brain barrier breakdown.

○ **A 31-year-old man stepped on a nail at his job. The nail pierced through his sneaker and into his foot. His tetanus status is up-to-date. What is the main concern?**

Infection with *Pseudomonas* that can lead to osteomyelitis. Pseudomonal infection is most commonly associated with hot, moist environments, such as sneakers.

○ **How do viral meningitis and bacterial meningitis differ with regard to CSF pressure? CSF leukocytes? CSF glucose?**

CSF pressure in bacterial meningitis is increased, whereas it is normal or only slightly increased in viral meningitis. Leukocytosis is greater than 1000 cells/μL (as high as 60,000 cells/μL) in bacterial meningitis but is rarely higher than 1000 cells/μL in viral meningitis. Glucose concentration is decreased in bacterial meningitis but is generally normal in viral meningitis.

○ **What is the essential presenting feature of botulism poisoning?**

Bulbar palsy

○ **What is thought to be the mode of inoculation in cat scratch disease?**

Contact with a cat, usually a kitten, often with a history of being bitten or scratched by a cat. Rubbing the eye after contact with a cat can also be a mode of inoculation.

○ **A patient has a diagnosis of group A streptococcal impetigo. What sequelae should you monitor for?**

Acute poststreptococcal glomerulonephritis. It will not, however, lead to rheumatic fever, for reasons that are not fully understood but possibly because the strains for pharyngitis and impetigo are different.

○ **What are the major Jones criteria used to diagnose rheumatic fever?**

Carditis, Sydenham chorea, erythema marginatum, migratory polyarthritis, and subcutaneous nodules. The diagnosis requires either 2 major or 1 major and 2 minor criteria, with evidence of previous streptococcal infection.

○ **What is the drug of choice for meningococcal disease?**

Aqueous penicillin G (250,000–300,000 U/kg per day IV in 6 doses) is the ideal, though treatment can be started effectively with empiric cefotaxime or ceftriaxone if meningococcal disease is suspected and if patients are allergic to penicillin.

○ **Should people who have had contact with patients with meningococcal meningitis receive prophylactic antibiotics?**

Yes. Rifampin or ceftriaxone are recommended.

○ **What is the most common cause of aseptic meningitis?**

Enteroviruses

○ **What is the recommended initial treatment for gonorrhea?**

Third-generation cephalosporins ceftriaxone or cefixime plus either doxycycline (100 mg twice a day for 7 days) or azithromycin (1 g orally for 1 dose) for presumptive coinfection with chlamydia.

○ **What is the cause of epidemic keratoconjunctivitis?**

Adenovirus

○ **After finishing the prescribed dosage of penicillin for pharyngitis, your patient's repeat culture still grows** *Streptococcus.* **What do you do?**

Nothing. Most people are asymptomatic carriers, and in most cases it is inconsequential.

○ **What are the most common causes of herpangina?**

Coxsackie A and *B viruses* and *Echovirus*

○ **Why does therapy for tuberculosis take several months when other infections usually clear in a matter of days?**

Because the mycobacteria divide slowly and have a long dormant phase when they are not responsive to medications.

○ **What is the most common adverse effect of rifampin?**

Orange discoloration of urine and tears

○ **What are 5 infectious diseases that produce false-positive results for treponemal tests (fluorescent treponemal antibody, microhemagglutination-*Treponema pallidum*, *Treponema pallidum* immobilization) for syphilis?**

1. Yaws
2. Pinta
3. Leptospirosis
4. Rat-bite fever (*Spirillum minus*)
5. Lyme disease

○ **What are 5 diseases that produce false-positive results for nontreponemal tests (VDRL, rapid plasma reagin) for syphilis?**

1. Infectious mononucleosis
2. Connective tissue diseases
3. Tuberculosis
4. Endocarditis
5. IV drug abuse

○ **In what disease is CSF albuminocytologic dissociation seen, and what does it mean?**

Guillain-Barré syndrome. An increase in CSF protein without a corresponding increase in CSF white cells is referred to as "albuminocytologic dissociation."

○ **How is histoplasmosis diagnosed?**

By means of culture or staining of specimens from sputum, bronchoalveolar lavage, or tissue and by means of positive serologic test results

○ **How is coccidioidomycosis diagnosed?**

By means of culture or staining of specimens from sputum, bronchoalveolar lavage, or tissue and by means of positive serologic test results

○ **How is pulmonary zygomycosis diagnosed?**

By means of biopsy

○ **How does one definitively diagnose invasive aspergillosis?**

By means of biopsy

○ **What are 5 infectious agents associated with erythema nodosum?**

Erythema nodosum has been associated with many infectious and some noninfectious processes. Some of its better known associates are group A streptococcus, meningococcus, syphilis, *Mycobacterium tuberculosis*, and *Mycobacterium leprae*, as well as histoplasmosis, coccidioidomycosis, blastomycosis, and herpes simplex virus. Some of the less common associates of erythema nodosum include *Chlamydia trachomatis*, *Chlamydophila psittaci*, *Corynebacterium diphtheriae*, *Campylobacter*, *H ducreyi*, *Yersinia*, *Rochalimaea henselae*, *Trichophyton*, filariasis, sarcoidosis, and various drugs.

○ **What is the risk of transmission of HIV from an HIV-infected person after needle-stick exposure?**

0.3% to 0.5%, on average, though this varies with the needle gauge and depth and with the site of insertion

○ **What 2 common urinary pathogens do not produce positive urine nitrite test results?**

1. *Enterococcus*
2. *Staphylococcus saprophyticus*

Acinetobacter also fails to produce positive urine nitrite test results.

○ **What are the features of typhoid fever?**

BIRDS FLEW

Bradycardia

Insidious onset

Rose spots

Dicrotic pulse

Splenomegaly

Fever

Leukopenia

Epidemic

Widal reaction

○ **In a patient who presents with diarrhea, high fever, headache, lethargy, and confusion and has normal lumbar puncture results, 45% band forms on the differential white blood cell count, and blood culture positive for *Escherichia coli*, what is the most likely cause of the diarrhea?**

Shigella. Blood cultures in *Shigella* diarrhea are almost never positive for *Shigella*. When the results are positive, they are more likely to be positive for *E coli*. Perhaps this is because *Shigella*, although locally invasive at the mucosal level, is poorly invasive at the systemic level. Resident *E coli* in the gut, however, take advantage of the disrupted mucosa and invade the blood stream.

○ **Which hemoglobin provides the greatest innate resistance to falciparum malaria?**

Erythrocytes in patients who are heterozygous for sickle cell hemoglobin (ie, those with sickle cell trait) are resistant to malaria.

○ **What is the most common infectious disease complication of both measles and influenza?**

Pneumococcal pneumonia

○ **On Tuesday, you are driving home from work in rural California and pass 3 dead squirrels. On Wednesday, taking a different route, you pass 2 more dead squirrels. The following morning you see a 26-year-old man with enlarged tender nodes and lymphadenitis and a fever of 105°F. What illness might you suspect?**

Cases of human plague (*Yersinia pestis*) are sometimes heralded by squirrel die-offs. A squirrel die-off occurs when the organism is introduced into a highly susceptible mammalian population, causing a high mortality rate among infected animals. This is referred to as "epizootic plague."

○ **One day after a previously healthy adult has been admitted to the hospital after an accidental overdose of oral iron, she appears to develop sepsis. What organism is most likely causing her sepsis?**

Yersinia enterocolitica. The growth of *Y enterocolitica* appears to be enhanced after exposure to excess iron. This growth, combined with intestinal mucosal damage by the iron, may play a role in pathogenesis.

○ **If the test result of a patient's purified protein derivative (PPD) is read as 3 mm of induration, and then 15 mm of induration after placement of a second PPD 2 weeks later, which study result should be considered more reliable?**

The second, showing induration of 15 mm. With time, the body's memory of tuberculosis infection may wane, and PPD placement may stimulate that memory, which is referred to as the "booster phenomenon." The boosted result is considered the reliable result.

○ **A patient from the Philippines has a hypopigmented patch lacking in sensation. What is the most likely cause of his problem?**

Leprosy (*M leprae*)

○ **Which intestinal parasites cause anemia as their major manifestation?**

Hookworms. Three species of hookworms affect humans: *Ancylostoma duodenale*, *N americanus*, and *Ancylostoma ceylanicum*.

○ **What is the most common symptom of tularemia?**

Skin sores at the site of inoculation and lymphadenopathy (75%). Other symptoms include pneumonia, lesions in the GI system, infection of the eyes, fever, and headache.

○ **How is tularemia most commonly transmitted?**

Ticks and exposure to rabbits. Tularemia is caused by *Francisella tularensis*.

○ **Which has a longer incubation period: staphylococci or salmonellae?**

Salmonellae, which generally are ingested in small doses; they then multiply in the GI tract. Symptoms occur 6 to 48 hours after ingestion. *S aureus* has an incubation period of just 3 hours.

○ **Which antibiotics most commonly produce diarrhea secondary to *Clostridium difficile*?**

Cephalosporins, ampicillin/amoxicillin, and clindamycin. Vancomycin or metronidazole are the antibiotics of choice for treatment.

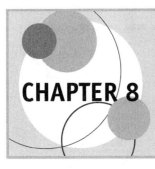

CHAPTER 8 Rheumatology, Immunology, and Allergy

Joel Augustin, MD

○ **Which class of immunoglobulins is responsible for urticaria (hives) and angioedema?**

Immunoglobulin (Ig) E

○ **Which class of immunoglobulins is responsible for food allergies?**

IgE

○ **What are the most common food allergens?**

Dairy products, eggs, and nuts

○ **When do the clinical manifestations of a new drug allergy usually become apparent?**

1 to 2 weeks after starting the drug

○ **Which class of drugs is commonly associated with angioedema?**

Angiotensin-converting enzyme (ACE) inhibitors. A patient who has had angioedema from 1 ACE inhibitor should not be prescribed another. Complications can result from any member of this class of antihypertensive agents. ACE-triggered angioedema can occur at any time during the course of therapy.

○ **What drug is the most common pharmaceutical cause of true allergic reactions?**

Penicillin. It accounts for approximately 90% of true allergic drug reactions and more than 95% of fatal anaphylactic drug reactions. Parenterally administered penicillin is more than twice as likely to cause a fatal anaphylactic reaction as is orally administered penicillin.

○ **How long after exposure to an allergen will anaphylaxis typically occur?**

Seconds to 1 hour

○ **After penicillin, what is the next most common cause of anaphylaxis-related deaths?**

Insect stings. Approximately 100 deaths occur in the United States annually because of anaphylaxis induced by insect stings.

○ **A patient receiving β-blockers who develops anaphylactic cardiovascular collapse may not respond to epinephrine or dopamine infusions. What drug should be used in this setting?**

Glucagon, 5 to 15 mg/min intravenously (IV)

○ **What percentage of patients with Kawasaki disease also develop acute carditis?**

50%, usually myocarditis with mild to moderate congestive heart failure. Pericarditis, conduction abnormalities, and valvular disturbances may occur but are less common.

○ **Are the nodules of erythema nodosum more often symmetrical or asymmetrical in distribution?**

Symmetrical. These nodules are distinctive, bilateral, tender nodules with underlying red or purple shiny patches of skin that develop in a symmetric distribution along the shins, arms, thighs, calves, and buttocks.

○ **Is there an effective treatment for erythema nodosum?**

No. The disease usually lasts several weeks, but the pain associated with the tender lesions can be relieved with nonsteroidal anti-inflammatory drugs (NSAIDs).

○ **A patient presents with fever and acute polyarthritis or migratory arthritis a few weeks after a bout of streptococcal pharyngitis. What disease should be suspected?**

Acute rheumatic fever. Although the early symptoms may be nonspecific, physical examination eventually reveals signs of arthritis (60%–75%), carditis (30%), choreiform movements (10%), erythema marginatum, or subcutaneous nodules.

○ **What treatment should be started when acute rheumatic fever is diagnosed?**

Penicillin or erythromycin. This treatment should be started even if cultures for group A streptococci are negative. High-dose aspirin therapy is used at an initial dose of 75 to 100 mg/kg per day. Carditis or congestive heart failure is treated with prednisone, 1 to 2 mg/kg per day.

○ **What is Lhermitte sign in ankylosing spondylitis?**

A sensation of electric shock that radiates down the back when the neck is flexed. This is a sign that atlantoaxial subluxation and cervical spine instability may be present. Lhermitte sign may also be present in patients with rheumatoid arthritis and multiple sclerosis.

○ **What rheumatic syndrome may lead to corneal irritation, ulceration, and infection?**

Sjögren syndrome. This syndrome involves the lymphocytic infiltration of the lacrimal and salivary glands and may occur as an independent entity or as an accompaniment to other rheumatologic diseases. Patients with Sjögren syndrome present with dry mouth and eyes.

○ **Describe a patient presenting with Sjögren syndrome.**

Sjögren syndrome usually occurs in women older than 50 years. Symptoms often include diminished lacrimal and salivary gland secretions, salivary gland enlargement, and arthritis. Sjögren syndrome predisposes a patient to corneal irritation, ulceration, and superimposed infection. It may complicate many rheumatic diseases or may occur independently. The most probable cause of Sjögren syndrome is lymphatic infiltration of the lacrimal and salivary glands, which results in dry eyes and mouth.

○   **What organisms are typically responsible for septic arthritis and osteomyelitis of the foot in an immunocompetent adult?**

Staphylococcus, Haemophilus influenzae, and *Pseudomonas* in people using IV drugs

○   **With what are rhomboid-shaped crystals obtained by means of joint aspiration associated?**

Pseudogout

○   **With what are needle-shaped crystals associated?**

Gout

○   **What is the cause of pseudogout?**

Release of crystals of calcium pyrophosphate dihydrate into joints

○   **How is gout distinguished from pseudogout by using a microscope with a polarizing filter?**

When the plane of polarization is perpendicular to the crystal, pseudogout (calcium pyrophosphate) crystals appear yellow and rhomboidal, and gout (uric acid) crystals appear blue and needle shaped. The mnemonic "CUB," for "crossed urate blue," is a reminder.

○   **Is the onset of pain more rapid in gout or in pseudogout?**

Gout. The onset of pain in acute gouty arthritis occurs over a few hours, whereas the pain associated with pseudogout usually evolves over a day or more.

○   **What is the acute treatment for gout?**

Colchicine, indomethacin, and other NSAIDs

○   **There are 4 types of hypersensitivity reactions. Name them in order and cite an example.**

Hypersensitivity	Reaction	Mediator	Example
Type I	Immediate	IgE binds allergen, includes mast cells and basophils	Food allergy Asthma in children
Type II	Cytotoxic	IgG and IgM antibody reactions to antigen on cell surface activate complement and killers	Blood transfusion reaction Idiopathic thrombocytopenic purpura, hemolytic anemia The least common reaction
Type III	Immune complex Arthus reaction	Complexes activate complement	Tetanus toxoid in sensitized persons Poststreptococcal glomerulonephritis
Type IV	Cell mediated, delayed	Activated T lymphocytes	Skin tests

○ **What is the common name for granulomatous arteritis of the thoracic aorta and its branches? What are its common symptoms?**

Temporal arteritis. Symptoms include tender scalp, headache, fluctuating vision, reduced brachial pulse, and jaw or tongue pain.

○ **Myocardial infarction can occur with which 2 rheumatic diseases?**

1. Kawasaki disease
2. Polyarteritis nodosa

○ **What is the most common cause of anaphylactoid reactions?**

Radiologic contrast media. Other causes include acetylsalicylic acid, NSAIDs, and codeine.

○ **What is the difference between anaphylactoid and anaphylaxis reactions?**

Anaphylactoid reactions resemble anaphylaxis reactions in symptoms but do not require prior exposure and are not immunologically mediated. Anaphylactoid reactions are caused by a toxic reaction, rather than the immune system mechanism that occurs with true anaphylaxis.

○ **There are a bacterial infection and an allergic phenomenon that can both cause a generalized confluent exfoliation of the skin; what are the 2 diseases? What test should be performed to distinguish between them?**

1. Bacterial infection: Ritter disease. This disorder is caused by *Staphylococcus* and thus is also known as "staphylococcal scalded skin syndrome." Ritter disease causes exfoliation at the superficial granular layer of the epidermis.
2. Allergic phenomenon: Toxic epidermal necrolysis (TEN)

Skin biopsy can be used to distinguish between the 2 conditions because the exfoliative cleavage plane is deeper at the dermal-epidermal junction or lower with TEN.

○ **How is mucocutaneous lymph node syndrome (Kawasaki disease) diagnosed in a young patient with prolonged fever?**

Diagnosis requires 4 of the following findings:

1. Conjunctival inflammation
2. Rash
3. Adenopathy
4. Strawberry tongue and injection of the lips and pharynx
5. Erythema and edema of extremities

Desquamation of the fingers and the toes may be striking, but it is a late finding and is not 1 of the key clinical features of the disease.

○ **What is the treatment of choice for a patient in anaphylactic shock?**

Epinephrine
- Mild anaphylaxis (urticaria, rhinitis, mild bronchospasm): 0.3 to 0.5 mL 1:1,000 subcutaneously
- Moderate (generalized urticaria, angioedema, hypotension): 1 to 5 mL 1:10,000 intramuscularly every 5 to 20 minutes, 3 times
- Severe (laryngeal edema, respiratory failure, shock): 1 to 5 mL IV over 10 minutes; if no improvement, start an epinephrine IV drip

○ **How long should a patient with a generalized anaphylactic reaction be observed?**

24 hours. Recurrence of hemodynamic collapse and airway compromise is common within this period. Treat with antihistamines and steroids for 72 hours.

○ **How does relapsing polychondritis affect the airway?**

Approximately 50% of patients with relapsing polychondritis have airway involvement and may present with pain and tenderness over the cartilaginous structures of the larynx. Dyspnea, stridor, cough, hoarseness, and erythema and edema of the oropharynx and nose may also occur.

○ **How should airway involvement from relapsing polychondritis be managed?**

Admit these patients for high-dose steroids and for close observation. Repeated exacerbations may lead to severe airway compromise and asphyxiation.

○ **In what patient populations is systemic lupus erythematosus (SLE) most commonly found?**

Women, those aged 15 to 45 years, African Americans, and Hispanics

○ **What laboratory result is most associated with SLE?**

98% of patients with SLE have positive antinuclear antibody (ANA) test results.

○ **How common is pleurisy in patients with SLE?**

Approximately half of the patients with SLE will develop symptoms of pleurisy at some time.

○ **What is the diagnostic approach for SLE with a pleural effusion?**

All pleural effusions in patients with rheumatic disease require thoracentesis to distinguish inflammatory effusions from infectious effusions. Pulmonary embolisms are common in patients with SLE; thus, nuclear ventilation-perfusion scanning is also indicated.

○ **What are the cerebral manifestations of SLE?**

Aseptic meningitis, headaches, seizures, organic brain syndrome, psychosis, depression, acute stroke syndromes, transverse myelitis, and movement disorders

○ **What are the most common causes of death with SLE?**

Infection, CNS lupus, cardiovascular disease, and renal failure

○ **What drugs can induce a lupus-like disease and produce positive ANA test results?**

A variety of drugs have been identified as being possible causes for SLE or lupus-like reactions. Those with the highest incidence of inducing SLE are procainamide, hydralazine, and penicillamine. Minocycline, methyldopa, chlorpromazine, diltiazem, isoniazid, quinidine, phenytoin, and rifampin are among others also thought to have a probable association with the disease.

○ **What percentage of patients with Kawasaki disease will develop coronary artery aneurysms if not treated?**

Approximately 20%. One percent to 2% of these patients will die from acute myocardial infarction during the resolution phase of the illness.

○   **What cardiac complication commonly occurs with isoniazid, juvenile rheumatoid arthritis (JRA), and rheumatoid arthritis?**

Pericarditis

○   **What is the normal atlantodental distance on lateral flexion views of the cervical spine? What rheumatologic diseases commonly alter this?**

As much as 3.5 mm in adults and 4 mm in children. Ankylosing spondylitis and rheumatoid arthritis can destroy ligamentous supporting structures and produce atlantoaxial subluxation with widening of this space.

○   **What are the symptoms of atlantoaxial subluxation?**

Changes in bowel or bladder function, limb paresthesias, or new weakness

○   **What vascular disease is accompanied by polymyalgia rheumatica in 10% to 30% of cases?**

Temporal arteritis

○   **In polymyalgia rheumatica, what does SECRET stand for?**

Stiffness and pain
Elderly
Constitutional symptoms, white
Rheumatism (arthritis)
Elevated erythrocyte sedimentation rate
Temporal arthritis

○   **Who is the typical patient with polymyalgia rheumatica?**

Women older than 60 years, whites

○   **How long should patients with polymyalgia rheumatica be treated with prednisone?**

Because of frequent relapses, the ideal treatment time is 1 year, with initial rapid tapering of prednisone to 5 mg/d.

○   **What are the most common initial presentations for giant cell arteritis?**

Headache, polymyalgia rheumatica, fever, visual symptoms, and fatigue

○   **A patient is suspected of having a new onset of acute gouty arthritis. What must be determined?**

The exclusion of septic arthritis must assume top priority because the signs and symptoms of the 2 diseases may be indistinguishable.

○   **What 5 joints are most commonly involved in rheumatoid arthritis?**

1. Metacarpophalangeal joint
2. Wrist
3. Metatarsophalangeal joint
4. Knee
5. Proximal interphalangeal joint

○ **What complication of rheumatoid arthritis requires emergency treatment?**

Vasculitis. This condition should be treated promptly with systemic steroids. If treatment is delayed, irreversible neuropathy may occur.

○ **What is Felty syndrome?**

Rheumatoid arthritis with splenomegaly and neutropenia. It is a late complication of rheumatoid arthritis.

○ **What complication of rheumatoid arthritis may produce signs and symptoms that mimic those of deep vein thrombosis?**

Baker cyst. This cyst can occasionally be distinguished clinically from deep vein thrombosis when deep hemorrhage from the ruptured cyst produces bruising or staining in a purple crescent below the malleoli or when localized swelling at the site of the ruptured popliteal cyst spares the more distal parts of the leg and the foot.

○ **Arthritis of the elbow joint causes limitation of all motion at the joint. In what way does olecranon bursitis differ?**

Pain from olecranon bursitis may limit flexion and extension at the elbow, but it usually does not affect pronation and supination.

○ **How should potentially septic olecranon bursitis be treated?**

Aspirate as much fluid as possible from the bursa via a large-bore needle. Antibiotics should be started immediately.

○ **How does the white blood cell count in fluid aspirated from septic bursitis differ from that detected from septic arthritis?**

The white blood cell count in the fluid from a septic joint is usually 10 times higher than the white blood cell count in the fluid from septic bursitis.

○ **What are the articular symptoms of disseminated, stage 2 Lyme disease?**

Migratory arthritis, bursitis, and tendonitis. The attacks associated with migratory arthritis are usually brief.

○ **What are the articular symptoms of late, stage 3 Lyme disease?**

Chronic arthritis, especially in the knee; periostitis; and tendonitis

○ **How should new monoarthritis be approached in a patient with rheumatoid arthritis?**

Assume it is septic until proved otherwise. The risk for infection is higher in a joint that has been previously injured or affected by arthritis.

○ **A 10-year-old child is limping; he complains of several weeks of groin, hip, and knee pain that worsens with activity. What diseases should be considered?**

Transient tenosynovitis of the hip, slipped capital femoral epiphysis, Legg-Calvé-Perthes syndrome, suppurative arthritis, rheumatic fever, JRA, and tuberculosis of the hip

○ **What is Legg-Calvé-Perthes disease? How does it manifest? Who is affected?**

Legg-Calvé-Perthes disease is avascular necrosis of the femoral head, manifesting in children between 4 and 13 years of age as subacute groin, hip, and knee pain that worsens with activity. The disease is also known as "coxa plana." The cause is unknown, but there appears to be a male predominance.

○ **What is the diagnosis for a preadolescent child with activity-related knee pain and a thickened and tender patellar tendon?**

Osgood-Schlatter disease. This disease is an inflammatory repetitive injury process in which cartilaginous fragments are pulled loose from the tibial tuberosity by the ligamentum patellae of the quadriceps tendon. Treatment involves several months of restriction from excessive physical activity.

○ **What disease is suspected in an adolescent with a tender, purpuric dependent rash on the lower extremities, colicky abdominal pain, migratory polyarthritis, and microscopic hematuria?**

Henoch-Schönlein purpura, a leukocytoclastic vasculitis. Intestinal or pulmonary hemorrhage may occur, and 7% to 9% of the patients will develop chronic renal sequelae. Salicylates are effective for the arthritis. Other treatments are directed at the symptoms. Steroids are not particularly effective.

○ **A child has painful, swollen joints, along with a spiking high fever, shaking chills, signs of pericarditis, and a pale erythematous coalescing rash on the trunk, palms, and soles. Hepatosplenomegaly is found. What is the diagnosis?**

Systemic JRA. Arthrocentesis is necessary to eliminate the possibility of septic arthritis. The rheumatoid factor and ANA test results usually are negative; one-fourth of patients will develop joint destruction. This is the least common of the 3 types of JRA.

○ **What treatment, besides aspirin, prevents the complications of Kawasaki disease?**

IV immunoglobulins can reduce the incidence of coronary artery aneurysms to less than 5%. Corticosteroids are thought to increase the likelihood of development of coronary artery disease.

○ **What are the 3 types of JRA?**

1. Pauciarticular disease type 1: This is the most common type of JRA; 30% to 40% of all patients with JRA have type 1. JRA type 1 begins before the age of 4 years, and 90% of cases have positive ANA test results. The most commonly affected joints are the knees, ankles, and elbows. The hips are spared. Serious disabilities or joint destruction is uncommon, but these patients are prone to eye problems.

2. Pauciarticular disease type 2: Ten percent to 15% of all patients with JRA have type 2. JRA type 2 is found predominantly in those older than 8 years. Rheumatoid factor and ANA test results are usually negative, and 75% of patients are HLA-B27 positive. Large joints, particularly the lower extremities, including the hip and spine, are affected.

3. Systemic onset JRA type 3: JRA type 3 has prominent extraarticular manifestations, particularly high fever and rashes; 10% to 20% of patients with JRA present this way; and sex distribution is approximately equal. Patients seem ill and will often have hepatosplenomegaly and lymphadenopathy. Patients may have pleural thickening and pericarditis. Articular symptoms manifest within months of onset of symptoms. Systemic symptoms are unlikely to recur after puberty.

○ **What are the cardiovascular manifestations of rheumatoid arthritis?**

Pericarditis and aortitis

○ **What are the indications for intraarticular hyaluronic acid injections for arthritis of the knee?**

Inadequate response to pharmocologic therapy, symptoms after debridment (arthroscopic surgery), or inability to tolerate total knee replacement

○ **Which patients are more likely to get recurrences of rheumatic fever?**

Recurrences are most common in children and patients who have had carditis during the initial episode; 20% of these patients will have a second episode within 5 years.

○ **What is relapsing polychondritis?**

A rare disease of unknown cause that is characterized by destructive lesions of cartilaginous structures, principally the ears, nose, trachea, and larynx

○ **A 70-year-old patient has had progressive pain and motion restriction of the shoulder for several months. There is minimal tenderness at palpation, but active and passive range of motion are limited in abduction and rotation. What is the probable diagnosis?**

Adhesive capsulitis. The pain is usually a poorly localized diffuse ache that is often worse at night. The cause is unclear, but the condition commonly follows injury or chronic inflammation, particularly after immobilization.

○ **What is the treatment for adhesive capsulitis?**

An intensive physical therapy program with range-of-motion exercises, intraarticular steroids, and NSAIDs

○ **A 40-year-old patient complains of sudden onset right shoulder pain while at rest. Any shoulder movement reproduces the pain. There is crepitus with motion, and the point of maximum tenderness is over the proximal humerus at the insertion of the rotator cuff. What might a radiograph reveal? What is the diagnosis?**

The radiograph might reveal calcified deposits in the rotator cuff, typical of calcific tendonitis. The cause is unknown, but the calcific deposits are painless until they begin to undergo spontaneous resorption. The symptoms are self-limited.

○ **What disease produces erythematous plaques with dusky centers and red borders resembling bull's-eye targets?**

Erythema multiforme. This disease can also produce nonpruritic urticarial lesions, petechiae, vesicles, and bullae.

○ **What is the appropriate management for TEN?**

Admit the patient for treatment similar to that required for extensive second-degree burns. The mortality rate of patients with TEN can be as high as 50% because of fluid loss and secondary infections.

○ **What drugs are most commonly implicated in TEN?**

Sulfonamides and sulfones, phenylbutazone and related drugs, barbiturates, antiepileptic drugs, and antibiotics

○ **What can cause erythema multiforme?**

Viral or bacterial infections, drugs of nearly all classes, and malignancy

○ **What is the most common cause of allergic contact dermatitis?**

Toxicodendron species, such as poison oak, poison ivy, and poison sumac. These allergens are responsible for more cases than all other allergens combined.

○ **Why does scratching spread poison oak and poison ivy?**

The antigenic resin contaminates hands and fingernails. A single contaminated finger can produce more than 500 reactive groups of lesions.

○ **How is the antigen of poison oak or poison ivy inactivated?**

Careful washing with soap and water destroys the antigen. Special attention must be paid to the fingernails; otherwise, the antigenic resin can be carried for weeks.

○ **What underlying illnesses should be considered in a patient with nontraumatic uveitis?**

Collagen vascular diseases, sarcoidosis, ankylosing spondylitis, Reiter syndrome, tuberculosis, syphilis, toxoplasmosis, JRA, and Lyme disease

○ **What is the difference between episcleritis and scleritis?**

Both are associated with collagen vascular disorders; however, episcleritis is a benign superficial inflammation of the tissues between the sclera and the conjunctiva. Conversely, scleritis is a more severe and more painful inflammation of the deep sclera, and it can result in vision loss.

○ **What bony abnormality can produce Horner syndrome, radicular symptoms without neck pain, vertebrobasilar insufficiency, and painless weakness in an upper extremity myotome?**

Osteophytes encroaching on cervical neural foramina

○ **A patient presents with acute lower back pain. What are the criteria for admission?**

Paralysis, paraparesis, loss of bowel or bladder function, inability to stand or sit, the need to sleep in an upright position, intractable pain, spasticity, or metastatic cancer

○ **In what way does trochanteric bursitis mimic lumbar radiculopathy?**

Both conditions produce pain that involves the hip and radiates along the iliotibial band to the lateral knee.

○ **A patient with sudden, symmetric, multilevel areflexia; lower extremity muscle weakness; and bowel or bladder incontinence may have what neurologic problem?**

A midline herniation of a lumbar disk, with compromise of the distal cauda equina. Emergency decompression may restore function and prevent permanent paraparesis.

○ **A patient has myalgias, arthralgias, headache, and an annular erythematous lesion accompanied by central clearing. What is the diagnosis?**

Stage 1 Lyme disease with the classic lesion of erythema chronicum migrans. The primary lesion occurs at the site of the tick bite.

○ **What rheumatologic ailments produce pulmonary hemorrhage?**

Goodpasture disease, SLE, Wegener granulomatosis, and nonspecific vasculitides

○ **How are antineutrophil cytoplasmic antibodies (ANCAs) helpful in differentiating vasculitides?**

Cytoplasmic ANCA is highly specific for Wegener granulomatosis, and perinuclear ANCA may be found in Churg-Strauss syndrome, and microscopic polyangiitis.

○ **What rheumatologic ailments can produce pulmonary fibrosis?**

Ankylosing spondylitis, scleroderma, and rheumatoid arthritis (less common)

○ **What rheumatologic ailments can produce respiratory muscle failure?**

Dermatomyositis and polymyositis

○ **What rheumatologic ailments can produce acute airway obstruction?**

Relapsing polychondritis and rheumatoid arthritis

○ **What are the most common endocrine diseases that have rheumatologic manifestations?**

Diabetes mellitus, Cushing syndrome, acromegaly, hypoparathyroidism, hypothyroidism, hyperthyroidism, and hyperparathyroidism

○ **What infectious agents can produce chronic smoldering arthritis with sterile aspiration culture results?**

Tuberculosis and fungal infections. Synovial biopsy may be required to confirm the diagnosis.

○ **How is septic bursitis contracted?**

A puncture wound or overlying cellulitis are the typical sources for septic bursitis.

○ **What lymphocyte surface molecule is responsible for activating the alternate T-cell activation pathway?**
CD2

○ **What lymphocyte surface molecule is responsible for HLA class II antigens?**
CD4

○ **Which are the only complement-fixing immunoglobulins?**
IgG and IgM

○ **Which immunoglobulin is the major host defense against parasites?**
IgE

○ **What are the 2 main functions of T cells?**
1. To signal B cells to make antibody
2. To kill virally infected or tumor cells

○ **What are the most reliable and cost-effective tests for assessing T-, B-, and NK-cell function?**

Complete blood cell count and sedimentation rate. If the sedimentation rate is normal, chronic bacterial infection is unlikely. If the absolute lymphocyte count is normal, the patient is not likely to have a severe T-cell defect. If the red blood cells are without Howell-Jolly bodies, congenital splenism is excluded. If the platelet count is normal, then Wiskott-Aldrich syndrome is excluded.

○ **Blood products administered in an individual with selective IgA deficiency must be prepared in what way?**

Washed normal donor erythrocytes or blood products. Forty-four percent of IgA-deficient patients have IgA autoantibody. When present, it may precipitate anaphylaxis and result in death from transfusion of unprepared donor cells.

○ **What complex syndrome exhibits clinical features that include progressive cerebellar ataxia, oculocutaneous telangiectasia, chronic sinopulmonary infections, high incidence of malignancy (lymphoreticular being the most common), and variable cellular and humoral immunodeficiency?**

Ataxia-telangiectasia

○ **Which X-linked recessive syndrome is characterized by atopic dermatitis, thrombocytopenic purpura, small defective platelets, and undue susceptibility to infection?**

Wiskott-Aldrich syndrome

○ **Which rare primary immunodeficiency manifests with recurrent severe staphylococcal abscesses, sinopulmonary tract infections, allergic rhinitis, asthma, keratoconjunctivitis, and markedly elevated levels of serum IgE and IgD?**

Hyper-IgE or Job syndrome

○ **A patient presents with classic amalar rash, fever, fatigue, myalgia, and arthralgia. Kidney biopsy results demonstrated membranoproliferative glomerulonephritis. However, all SLE serologic test results are negative. What disease is most likely?**

Deficiency of the complement component C1q

○ **X-linked agammaglobulinemia (Bruton syndrome) and C3 complement deficiency share what common clinical feature?**

Susceptibility to pyogenic infections

○ **Why do patients with C1 esterase inhibitor deficiency have hereditary angioedema?**

Episodic localized, nonpitting edema results from vasodilatory effects of kinins on the postcapillary venule because of uncontrolled C1 activity, so C4 and C2 break down with kinin release.

○ **What causes fatality in hereditary angioedema?**

Edema of the larynx or pharynx

○ **Patients with SLE and their asymptomatic family members often have a partial deficiency of which complement component?**

Deficiency of complement receptor 1, which increases the risk of developing immune complex disease

○ **Patients with familial Mediterranean fever have a genetic deficiency in a protease the function of which is to inactivate chemotactic factor C5a and interleukin-8. How does the disease manifest clinically?**

Patients with this rare disorder have recurrent episodes of fever, with associated painful inflammation of joints and pleural and peritoneal cavities.

○ **Reactive leukocytosis, which can resemble leukemia, can occur in what clinical scenarios?**

Sepsis, hepatic failure, diabetic acidosis, and azotemia

○ **What is the definition of neutropenia?**

Absolute neutrophil count (ANC) lower than 1500 cells/μL

○ **Aside from chemotherapeutics, which suppress bone marrow, what other agents are most commonly implicated in neutropenia?**

Phenothiazines, semisynthetic penicillin, NSAIDs, aminopyrine derivatives, and antithyroid medications

○ **What is the most common cause of transient neutropenia?**

Viral infections, which most commonly include hepatitis A, hepatitis B, influenza A and B, measles, rubella, and varicella.

○ **How long would the neutropenia be expected to persist?**

It may persist for the first 3 to 6 days of the acute viral syndrome.

○ **What nutritional deficiencies may precipitate neutropenia?**

Vitamin B12, folic acid, and copper

○ **Neutropenia and bacterial infection may herald the onset of what?**

Overwhelming sepsis

○ **Briefly explain the cellular basis for the type I hypersensitivity reaction (wheal and flare). Give a clinical example.**

This immediate type or anaphylactic hypersensitivity is mediated by circulating basophils and mast cells, which become activated by cross-linking of IgE on their membrane surfaces. IgE has a high affinity for its receptor on mast cells and basophils. The prototypic IgE-mediated disease is ragweed hay fever. Other, sometimes fatal, anaphylactic reactions are the classic allergies induced by insect venom or food.

○ **Briefly explain the cellular basis for the type II hypersensitivity reaction (cytotoxic). Give a clinical example.**

These immune interactions involve integral cellular antigen components and IgG and IgM antibody formation to these foreign antigen determinants. The classic example is immune mediated hemolysis, such as that seen in transfusion reaction, or hemolytic disease of the newborn.

○   **Briefly explain the cellular basis for the type III hypersensitivity reaction (Arthus reaction or immune complex). Give a clinical example.**

Tissue injury is caused by immune complex deposition in various tissues (mostly of IgG and possibly of IgM), which are toxic to that tissue, by mechanisms such as complement activation or proteolytic enzyme release. Examples include immune complex pericarditis and arthritis after meningococcal or *Haemophilus influenzae* infection.

○   **In type IV hypersensitivity reaction (cell mediated or delayed type), pathologic changes follow interaction of antigen with what cellular component of the immune system?**

Antigen-specific sensitized T cells

○   **What features should be highlighted during examination of a patient with atopic disease?**

Height, weight, pulsus paradoxus, alae nasi flaring, mouth breathing, allergic shiner, allergic salute (transverse nasal creasing from habitual nose wiping), and Dennie lines (wrinkles beneath lower eyelids)

○   **What other conditions would you see with eosinophilia?**

Neoplasm (eg, Hodgkin lymphoma), immunodeficiency, parasitic infestation, Addison disease, collagen vascular disease, cystic fibrosis, infections (cytomegalovirus, Epstein-Barr virus, leprosy, systemic candidiasis, coccidioidomycosis), Guillain-Barré syndrome, hemosiderosis, interstitial nephritis, and Kawasaki disease

○   **What are some possible adverse effects of long-term steroid use?**

Posterior subcapsular cataract, osteoporosis, hypertension, diabetes mellitus, cushingoid body habitus, infections, pancreatitis, gastritis, and myopathy

○   **What is the basis of antigen desensitization?**

Injection of antigenic extract into patients blunts the anamnestic increase in IgE via production of IgG, which effectively sequesters antigen by binding it. A cell exposed to a relevant agonist becomes hyporesponsive to the same agent.

○   **What are the likely causative agents implicated in perennial allergic rhinitis?**

Components of house dust, feathers, allergens, dander of household pets, and mold spores are the most common inciting agents.

○   **What constitutes triad asthma?**

The syndrome of nasal polyps, asthma, and aspirin intolerance comprises triad asthma (also called "Samter triad").

○   **What is the most effective treatment of allergic rhinitis?**

Topical use of corticosteroids, such as beclomethasone nasal spray

○   **What is extrinsic asthma?**

Asthmatic exacerbation after environmental exposure to allergens, such as dust, pollens, and dander

○ **What is intrinsic asthma?**

Asthmatic exacerbation not associated with an increase in IgE or positive skin test results. It is a nonseasonal, nonallergic form of asthma.

○ **What is atopic dermatitis?**

An inflammatory, chronic, relapsing skin disorder characterized by erythema, edema, pruritus, exudation, crusting, and scaling. Eighty percent of patients have elevated serum IgE levels.

○ **What is the most effective treatment for control of urticaria?**

0.5 mg/kg hydroxyzine is the most effective therapy, but diphenhydramine is also useful. First-generation antihistamines are used in acute or refractory cases. Second-generation antihistamines, such as loratadine, are used for chronic urticaria.

○ **What are typical initial symptoms of an anaphylactic reaction?**

Initially, patients usually report a tingling sensation around the mouth, followed by a warm feeling and tightness in the chest or throat.

○ **Patients with severe allergic reaction to eggs should avoid receipt of which vaccines?**

Influenza and yellow fever vaccines

○ **What is the most serious complication of serum sickness?**

The most serious complications are Guillain-Barré syndrome and peripheral neuritis, most commonly of the brachial plexus.

○ **What is the major cause of serum sickness?**

Drug allergy, particularly penicillin

○ **What may be administered as part of the preparative regimen to lessen the likelihood of rejection in patients with aplastic anemia who have received transfusions?**

Antithymocyte globulin with cyclophosphamide

○ **Of what treatment does immediate postoperative immunosuppression in cardiac transplant patients consist?**

- Cyclosporine 10 mg/kg/24 h
- Azathioprine 2 mg/kg/24 h
- Prednisone 0.6 mg/kg/24 h
- Antilymphocyte preparation within the first 1 to 2 weeks

○ **In what postoperative period is acute rejection the greatest?**

3 months after transplant

○ **What is the most commonly seen adverse effect of cyclosporine therapy?**

Hypertension, as a result of plasma volume expansion and defective renal sodium excretion. It occurs in 50% of patients after renal transplant and in most cardiac transplant patients.

○ **What commonly used immunosuppressive agent would be contraindicated in heart-lung transplant patients?**

Steroids. Their use may affect airway healing. However, in some studies, no increase in morbidity and mortality could be found after lung transplant with preoperative administration of 0.3 mg/kg per day of prednisolone.

○ **What is the most sensitive and specific sign of an infectious disease in an immunocompromised host?**

Fever

○ **At what ANC are neutropenic patients at risk for serious infection, and what 2 types of infectious agents are most responsible?**

At ANC less than 500 cells/μL, the risk for infection is inversely proportional to the cell count, with the most common infectious agents being (1) bacterial or (2) fungal.

○ **At what CD4 cell count is prophylaxis indicated in these patients, and what antimicrobial agent is used?**

Just as with immunodeficiency virus, a CD4 count of less than 200 cells/μL is indication for prophylaxis with trimethoprim and sulfamethoxazole.

○ **What is the most important care for a patient before liver transplant?**

Ensure adequate nutritional status with regard to caloric intake, vitamins, and mineral supplementation.

○ **What viral antibody titers must be tested in both the donor and the recipient before renal transplant?**

Hepatitis A, B, and C; Epstein-Barr; cytomegalovirus; herpes; and varicella

○ **A renal transplant patient, 30 days after transplant, presents with fever, oliguria, hypertension, and an elevated serum creatinine level. What 2 diagnostic tests would you perform next?**

1. Renal ultrasonography
2. Renal scanning to evaluate renal blood flow

○ **What diagnostic study is necessary to differentiate rejection reaction, acute tubular necrosis, cyclosporine toxicity, and recurrence of renal disease?**

Renal biopsy

○ **Sequential immunosuppression after transplant commonly includes which drugs?**

Azathioprine, cyclosporine, and prednisone

○ **What is the major cause of death in renal transplant recipients 1 year after transplant?**

Infection

○ **What is the most common infection seen in renal transplant patients?**

Cytomegalovirus

○ **In transplant patients receiving immunosuppressive therapy, how does one evaluate abdominal pain?**

Long-term steroid use often masks abdominal catastrophes. Therefore, abdominal pain in a transplant patient is a surgical emergency until proved otherwise.

○ **What immunosuppressive agents have the highest risk of reactivating cytomegalovirus infection?**

Azathioprine and OKT3/antilymphocyte globulin

○ **After an acute episode of cytomegalovirus, what are patients with renal or liver transplants at increased risk for?**

Graft rejection. Cytomegalovirus has been shown to upregulate major histocompatibility complex (MHC) class II D/DR in allografts, which may precipitate rejection reaction.

○ **A liver transplant patient presents with increased levels of liver aminotransferase and direct bilirubin without pain or fever. Which diagnostic test would be most useful?**

Doppler flow study to rule out arterial thrombosis

○ **What would you suspect if a liver transplant patient presented with rapidly increasing ascites and liver dysfunction?**

Portal vein thrombosis

○ **What is the immunosuppressive mechanism of IV immunoglobulin or colloidal gold?**

Inhibition of phagocytosis

○ **What is the immunosuppressive mechanism of hydroxychloroquine?**

Alkalinization of proteolytic vesicles

○ **Anti-double-stranded DNA antibodies are most indicative of what disease?**

SLE

○ **The presence of cytoplasmic ANCA with a diffuse staining pattern at serum immunofluorescence is most commonly associated with what disease?**

Wegener granulomatosis. It can also be seen in human immunodeficiency virus and Kawasaki disease.

○ **Patients with antiphospholipid antibodies in either primary or secondary antiphospholipid syndromes are at increased risk for what diseases?**

- Thrombotic events
- Thrombocytopenia
- Hemolytic anemia
- Stroke
- Chorea
- Transverse myelitis
- Vascular heart disease

○ **What are the HLA allele associations for the following types of JRA: pauciarticular types 1 and 2 and polyarticular rheumatoid factor positive?**

- JRA pauciarticular type 1: HLA-DR5, -DR6, and -DR8
- JRA pauciarticular type 2: HLA-B27
- Polyarticular rheumatoid factor positive: HLA-DR4

○ **In which 2 subgroups of JRA is joint destruction more likely?**

Polyarticular rheumatoid factor positive and systemic onset JRA. Fifty percent will develop severe arthritis.

○ **What forms of JRA are ANA negative?**

Pauciarticular type 2 and systemic onset

○ **Regardless of joint disease activity, what should all children with pauciarticular onset disease be screened for and how?**

Children with this form of JRA are at increased risk of chronic ocular inflammation, regardless of systemic activity, so serious sequelae, such as cataracts, glaucoma, ocular globe degeneration, and permanent blindness, can result. Therefore, slit-lamp examinations are mandatory every 3 to 4 years in these children.

○ **In pauciarticular JRA type 1, would one expect positive rheumatoid factor test results?**

No. More than 90% of patients, however, will be ANA positive.

○ **Which type of JRA predominantly affects boys older than 8 years?**

Pauciarticular disease type 2

○ **What are the most common manifestations of JRA?**

High intermittent fever, rheumatoid rash, arthralgia or myalgia during febrile episodes, and persistent arthritis lasting longer than 6 weeks

○ **What is the overall prognosis for JRA patients?**

At least 75% of patients with JRA will have long-term remissions without significant residual deformity or loss of function.

○ **How does ankylosing spondylitis differ from rheumatoid arthritis?**

Involvement of the sacroiliac joints and lumbodorsal spine, predilection for males, occurrence of aortitis, familial incidence, negative rheumatoid factor test results, and lack of rheumatoid nodules or incidence of acute iridocyclitis characterize ankylosing spondylitis.

○ **Reiter disease may occur after infection with which microbial agents?**

Shigella, Yersinia enterocolitica, Campylobacter, and *Chlamydia*

○ **What triad is associated with Reiter syndrome?**

Nongonococcal urethritis, polyarthritis, and conjunctivitis. Conjunctivitis is the least common and occurs in only 30% of patients. Acute attacks respond well to NSAIDs.

○ **What percentage of patients with inflammatory bowel disease have articular manifestations of the disease?**

10%

○ **What are the most frequent early symptoms of SLE?**

The most frequent early symptoms in children are fever, malaise, arthritis or arthralgia, and rash.

○ **What is the most sensitive serum marker in SLE?**

ANA test results are positive in 95% to 100% of patients with SLE, but it is not specific. ANA test results are also positive in rheumatoid arthritis, hepatitis, and interstitial lung disease.

○ **What hematologic conditions are seen in patients with SLE?**

Anemia, thrombocytopenia, and leukopenia occur frequently.

○ **What pharmacologic agents are most commonly associated with drug-induced lupus?**

Anticonvulsants, hydralazine, and isoniazid

○ **What are the major causes of SLE mortality?**
- Nephritis, with resultant renal failure
- Central nervous system complications
- Infection
- Pulmonary lupus
- Myocardial infarction

○ **When is anticoagulation therapy indicated in SLE?**

In patients with the persistent presence of antiphospholipid antibodies (because of the risk of venous or arterial thrombosis), migraine, recurrent fetal loss, transient ischemic attack, stroke, avascular necrosis, transverse myelitis, pulmonary hypertension or embolus, livedo reticularis, leg ulcers, or thrombocytopenia

○ **What are the possible complications of Kawasaki disease during the acute phase of the illness?**
- Arthritis
- Myocarditis
- Pericarditis
- Mitral insufficiency
- Congestive heart failure
- Iridocyclitis
- Meningitis
- Sterile pyuria

○ **What are the diagnostic criteria for Kawasaki disease?**

Illness not explained by any other known disease process, fever lasting at least 5 days, and the presence of 4 of the following 5 conditions:

1. Bilateral nonpurulent conjunctival injection
2. Changes in the mucosa of the oropharynx, including infected pharynx, dry fissured lips, and strawberry tongue
3. Changes in peripheral extremities, such as edema and/or erythema of the hands or feet, and desquamation
4. Primarily truncal rash
5. Cervical lymphadenopathy

○ **A 30-year-old patient presents with progressive destruction and ulcerations of the upper respiratory tract and associated arthritis and acute glomerulitis. The presumptive diagnosis of Wegener granulomatosis is made. What are the therapeutic options?**

Corticosteroids, cyclosporine, or trimethoprim-sulfamethoxazole

○ **Which calcium-channel blockers are effective in treating the symptoms of Raynaud phenomenon?**

Nifedipine and diltiazem are effective; verapamil has no effect.

○ **What will the clinical histologic biopsy results show in a patient with scleroderma?**

Fibrosis with minimal inflammation and occlusive vasculitis affecting the capillaries and small blood vessels

○ **What clinical manifestations differentiate systemic from focal scleroderma?**

In focal scleroderma, one sees cutaneous fibrosis and no systemic involvement, such as diffuse fibrosis or Raynaud phenomenon, both of which are components of systemic scleroderma.

○ **What characteristic features differentiate eosinophilic fasciitis from systemic scleroderma?**

In eosinophilic fasciitis, one sees isolated inflammation of the fascial layers, particularly the limbs, with sparing of the skin, prominent eosinophilia, and absence of Raynaud phenomenon. Joint contractures of the hand are characteristic of both diseases.

○ **An 18-year-old woman presents with complaints of fever and malaise 1 week before the development of 1- to 3-cm painful, red, ovoid nodules on her shins bilaterally. The patient's mother states that the patient also had an episode of severe sore throat the previous week. Hilar lymphadenopathy is demonstrated at chest radiography. What is the diagnosis?**

Erythema nodosum

○ **Behcet syndrome is characterized by recurrent oral and genital ulcers and ocular inflammation. What additional symptoms are associated with a particularly poor prognosis?**

CNS abnormalities, such as cranial nerve palsies and psychosis

○ **The combination of pain, tenderness, and swelling of the costosternal junction is referred to as what syndrome?**

Tietze syndrome or costochondritis

○ **What is the clinical scenario of familial Mediterranean fever, and what is the attributed cause?**

Amyloid deposition is the cause of this condition, which manifests with proteinuria that progresses to nephrotic syndrome and renal failure. Colchicine may greatly lessen the occurrence of amyloid deposition.

○ **What inflammatory conditions might one expect in secondary amyloidosis?**

JRA, cystic fibrosis, inflammatory bowel disease, and chronic infections, such as tuberculosis

○ **What connective tissue disease is characterized by sicca complex and anti-SSA and -SSB autoantibodies?**

Sjögren syndrome

○ **Which vasculitis affects predominantly the extracranial vessels?**

Takayasu arteritis

○ **A patient presents with pain along the radial aspect of the wrist extending into the forearm. What is the diagnostic test of choice?**

Finkelstein test. This test confirms the diagnosis of de Quervain tenosynovitis, an overuse inflammation of the extensor pollicis brevis and the abductor pollicis where they pass along the groove of the radial styloid. The Finkelstein test is performed by instructing the patient to make a fist with the thumb tucked inside the other fingers. The test is positive if pain is reproduced when the examiner gently deviates the fist in the ulnar direction.

○ **In carpal tunnel syndrome, the Tinel sign is produced by tapping the volar wrist over the median nerve. If the test is positive, what does the patient experience?**

Paresthesias extending into the thumb and first two fingers.

○ **Name some diseases and conditions often associated with carpal tunnel syndrome.**
PRAGMATIC
Pregnancy
Rheumatoid arthritis
Acromegaly
Glucose (diabetes mellitus)
Mechanical (overuse)
Amyloid (amyloidosis)
Thyroid (hypothyroidism)
Infection (tubercular, fungal)
Crystals (gout, pseudogout)

○ **What are the 3 most common cervical problems that produce pain radiating to the shoulder?**

1. Degenerative disease of the cervical spine
2. Degenerative disk disease
3. Herniated nucleus pulposus

○   **What herniated cervical disk causes pain that mimics the pain of a rotator cuff injury?**
C5 to C6

○   **What is the most common manifestation of a Charcot joint?**
A swollen ankle and a "bag of bones" appearance at radiography

○   **What is the most common cause of Charcot joints?**
Diabetic peripheral neuropathy

○   **What are the 2 most common organisms to infect a prosthetic joint at the time of surgery?**
1. *Staphylococcus epidermidis*
2. *Staphylococcus aureus*

○   **What does EMS stand for?**
Eosinophilia-myalgia syndrome, which has myalgias, rash, edema, fever, fatigue, cough, and weight loss as the most common clinical features. It was first described in 1989, initially in New Mexico.

○   **What is the shoulder-hand syndrome?**
Vasomotor changes of reflex sympathetic dystrophy that accompany a frozen shoulder.

○   **In hypothyroidism, what does TRAP stand for?**
Tunnel (carpal tunnel syndrome)
Raynaud phenomenon
Aching muscles (as in fibromyalgia)
Proximal muscle weakness

○   **What are the most common areas involved in vascular necrosis?**
Femoral head, humeral head, femoral condyles, and proximal tibia

CHAPTER 9 Genitourinary

Cynthia M. Waickus, MD, PhD

○ **What are the 2 most common causes of acute kidney injury?**

1. Prerenal disease (volume depletion, hypotension, edematous states, and renal ischemia)
2. Acute tubular necrosis (from postischemic states and nephrotoxins)

○ **What is the definition of oliguria? Of anuria?**

- Oliguria: Urine output less than 500 mL/d
- Anuria: Urine output less than 50 mL/d

○ **What is the leading cause of end-stage renal disease?**

Diabetic nephropathy develops in 20% to 40% of patients with diabetes and is the leading cause of chronic and end-stage renal disease.

○ **What type of acute renal failure is seen in a patient with systemic lupus erythematosus (SLE)?**

SLE with diffuse proliferative glomerulonephritis (GN) is likely to cause renal failure, nephrotic syndrome, hematuria, and cylindruria. This acute renal failure may be treated with steroids and intravenous (IV) cyclophosphamide pulse therapy.

○ **What are the indications for emergency dialysis in acute renal failure?**

Refractory fluid overload, hyperkalemia (plasma potassium >6.5 mEq/L) or rapidly increasing potassium levels, signs of uremia (pericarditis, neuropathy, or unexplained mental status changes), and metabolic acidosis (pH <7.1)

○ **What does acute renal failure in a patient with alcoholic cirrhosis and a urine sodium level of less than 10 mEq/L suggest?**

Prerenal azotemia or hepatorenal syndrome

○ **Total and persistent anuria with renal failure should prompt a workup for what?**

These patients are presumed to have obstruction until proved otherwise.

○ **Which hypertensive agent may unmask underlying renal artery stenosis?**

The development of azotemia suggests the presence of underlying renal artery stenosis in a patient taking an angiotensin-converting enzyme (ACE) inhibitor. ACE inhibitor–induced renal insufficiency is potentiated by sodium depletion and preexisting renal dysfunction, and it often provides an indication that critical renovascular disease is present.

○ **What diagnostic test is useful for differentiating prerenal azotemia from acute tubular necrosis?**

Fractional urinary excretion of sodium

○ **What is the earliest sign of end-stage renal disease nephropathy in patients with type 1 diabetes?**

Persistent albuminuria in the range of 30 to 200 mg/24 hr (microalbuminuria) is the earliest sign of nephropathy in patients with type 1 diabetes and is a marker for nephropathy in type 2 diabetes.

○ **What is the role of antihypertensive therapy in diabetic patients?**

Antihypertensive therapy is administered for both renal and cardiovascular protection, since chronic kidney disease and diabetes are independently associated with a marked increase in cardiovascular risk.

○ **What is the target blood pressure goal for patients with diabetic nephropathy?**

The goal in patients with diabetic nephropathy is to reduce the blood pressure to less than 130/80 mm Hg. In patients with protein excretion exceeding 0.5 to 1.0 g/24 hr, even lower systolic pressure may be more effective in slowing progressive renal disease.

○ **What class of antihypertensive agents is recommended in diabetic patients for primary prevention of diabetic nephropathy?**

In addition to their effectiveness in diabetic patients with established diabetic nephropathy, ACE inhibitors or angiotensin II receptor blockers have demonstrated effectiveness in the primary prevention of diabetic nephropathy. The renal protective benefit of ACE inhibitors has been well established in patients with type 1 diabetes; in patients with type 2 diabetes, more data are available on the renoprotective effects of angiotensin II receptor blockers, though a similar benefit is likely present with ACE inhibitors.

○ **How frequently should diabetic patients be screened for microalbuminuria?**

Patients with either type 1 or type 2 diabetes should be screened yearly for the presence of microalbuminuria by using the albumin-to-creatinine ratio in an untimed urine sample. In addition, the serum creatinine concentration and estimation of the glomerular filtration rate (GFR) should also be measured.

○ **At what GFR will patients with chronic renal failure (CRF) due to diabetes need to start dialysis?**

Dialysis is usually begun with GFR of 10 to 15 mL/min.

○ **What are some of the acute complications that occur during hemodialysis?**

Hypotension (25%–55%), muscle cramping (5%–20%), nausea and vomiting (5%–15%), headache (5%), chest pain (2%–5%), back pain (2%–5%), generalized itching (5%), and fever and chills (1%)

○ **Name an abnormal ultrasonographic finding that suggests CRF.**

Kidneys less than 9 cm in length are abnormal. A difference in length of more than 1.5 cm between the 2 kidneys suggests unilateral kidney disease. Kidneys with a small or absent renal cortex are also indicative of CRF.

○ **What is the life expectancy of CRF patients after the disease has progressed to dialysis?**

Patients younger than 60 years have a 4- to 5-year life expectancy. Patients older than 60 years have a 2- to 3-year life expectancy. Patient survival among those with diabetes who are receiving maintenance dialysis is lower than that seen in those without diabetes who have end-stage renal failure due to chronic glomerular disease or hypertension.

○ **What percentage of kidney transplants donated from a relative (usually a parent) are still functional after 3 years?**

75% to 80%

○ **What types of immunosuppressants are administered in renal transplant recipients to prevent acute rejection and loss of the allograft?**

The major immunosuppressive agents that are currently being used in various combination regimens are corticosteroids, cyclosporine, tacrolimus, azathioprine, mycophenolate mofetil, everolimus, mycophenolate sodium, and rapamycin. Dosing of the immunosuppressant regimen must be adequate to decrease the immune response to the allograft, but these levels are slowly decreased over time to help lower the risk of malignancy and infection.

○ **What are the first-line oral phosphate binders used in CRF?**

Calcium carbonate and calcium acetate. Phosphate binders are most effective if taken with meals to bind dietary phosphate. Aluminum-containing agents are best avoided because of the possibility of aluminum toxicity. Likewise, magnesium-containing agents should be avoided because of the risk of hypermagnesemia and the development of diarrhea, and calcium citrate should be avoided because it increases aluminum absorption.

○ **What comorbid factors are likely to increase the risk of contrast material–induced acute tubular necrosis?**

Azotemia, diabetic nephropathy, congestive heart failure, multiple myeloma, and dehydration

○ **Which modalities are effective when administered before contrast material to reduce the risk for contrast material–induced renal failure?**

Current methods for reducing the risk of renal failure induced by contrast material include adequate hydration and the use of N-acetylcysteine.

○ **What are the causes of high levels of parathyroid hormone in CRF?**

Hyperphosphatemia, hypocalcemia due to deficiency of vitamin D, and parathyroid receptor resistance

○ **How can the development of secondary hyperparathyroidism in patients with chronic kidney disease be forestalled?**

By limiting the dietary intake of phosphate to no more than 800 mg/d. This can only be achieved by also limiting protein, which may be difficult for many patients.

○ **At what concentration should serum phosphorous levels be maintained in patients with end-stage renal failure?**

Current guidelines recommend that serum phosphorus levels should be maintained between 3.5 and 5.5 mg/dL for end-stage renal disease (stage 5) and between 2.7 and 4.6 mg/dL for patients with stage 3 or 4 chronic kidney disease.

○ **What is the cause of CRF associated with cerebral berry aneurysms?**

Adult polycystic kidney disease is associated with cerebral berry aneurysms.

○ **CRF with hypertension, small shrunken kidneys, and gout at an early age should suggest what?**

Lead nephropathy should be considered.

○ **What disease is usually seen in patients with CRF, nephrotic syndrome, and AIDS?**

Usually focal segmental glomerulosclerosis is seen at biopsy.

○ **Acute renal failure after use of cocaine may be due to what?**

Rhabdomyolysis leading to acute tubular necrosis

○ **Which radiologic procedure is most appropriate for a patient with a high index of suspicion for renovascular hypertension and diminished renal function but whose GFR is greater than 60 mL/min per 1.73 m^2?**

Magnetic resonance angiography of the kidney

○ **How are the causes of kidney disease classified?**

Both acute and chronic kidney disease are classified by the anatomic portion of the kidney most affected by the disorder. These include prerenal, vascular, glomerular, tubulointerstitial, and obstructive disease.

○ **Describe the signs and symptoms of patients presenting with kidney disease.**

Patients with renal disease may present in a variety of ways, including with asymptomatic elevations in the plasma creatinine concentration; abnormalities at urinalysis; or symptoms of renal failure, systemic symptoms and findings, and/or incidental findings at radiographic testing performed for some other reason.

○ **What is the most important noninvasive test in the diagnostic evaluation of renal failure?**

Microscopic urinalysis because findings of the urine sediment strongly suggest certain diagnoses

○ **What methods are used to assess the degree of renal dysfunction (GFR) in patients with CRF?**

The most commonly used methods to estimate the GFR are the serum creatinine concentration, the creatinine clearance, and estimation equations based on the serum creatinine concentration (Cockcroft-Gault equation and Modification of Diet in Renal Disease study equation).

○ **Why is assessment of the degree of renal dysfunction (GFR) not a reliable indicator of renal dysfunction in patients with acute renal injury?**

Because with acute renal injury, the GFR is reduced out of proportion to serum creatinine levels, as there has not yet been time for the creatinine to accumulate, and the serum creatinine level does not accurately reflect the degree of renal dysfunction.

○ **How is renal tubular acidosis (RTA) classified?**

Into 1 of 3 types:
- Type 1: Distal RTA
- Type 2: Proximal RTA
- Type 4: Mineralocorticoid deficiency (hypoaldosteronism)

There is no type 3.

○ **What are the mechanisms for the different types of RTA?**

In type 1, there is a deficiency in the secretion of the hydrogen ion by the distal tubule and collecting duct. In type 2, there is a decrease in the bicarbonate reabsorption in the proximal tubule. In type 4, there is hyperkalemia due to hypoaldosteronism. The degree of acidosis is generally mild, with plasma bicarbonate concentration higher than 17 mEq/L.

○ **Which isolated form of RTA will be most likely to lead to renal failure?**

Distal (type 1), though most cases of type 1 RTA have an excellent prognosis

○ **What are the characteristic acid-base electrolyte abnormalities associated with RTA types 1 and 2?**

Hypokalemic, hyperchloremic metabolic acidosis

○ **What are the characteristic acid-base and electrolyte abnormalities associated with RTA type 4?**

Hyperkalemic, hyperchloremic metabolic acidosis

○ **What are the characteristic anion gap findings with RTA?**

All forms of RTA have a normal anion gap (hyperchloremic) metabolic acidosis, resulting from either a net retention of hydrogen chloride or its equivalent (such as ammonium chloride) or a net loss of sodium bicarbonate or equivalent base.

○ **What is the major cause of normal anion gap acidosis in patients without renal failure?**

Diarrhea

○ **What diseases are associated with RTA type 4?**

Diseases of the adrenal gland, most commonly Addison disease and congenital adrenal hyperplasia

○ **What 2 common medications can induce nephrogenic diabetes insipidus?**

Lithium and amphotericin B

○ **A patient with nephrogenic diabetes insipidus has a serum sodium level of 117 mEq/L. How do you determine how much sodium chloride to administer to keep the risk of cerebral edema to a minimum?**

Amount of sodium chloride to add in mEq/L = $0.6 \times$ weight (in kg) $\times$ (140 − serum sodium)

○ **Patients born with what disease are more likely to have horseshoe kidneys?**

Turner syndrome

○ **What treatments are used to ameliorate bleeding in a uremic patient?**

Dialysis may lessen bleeding, as may desmopressin, cryoprecipitate, or even platelet transfusions. Estrogens may lessen bleeding from angiodysplasia.

○ **What type of nephrotoxicity is associated with proton pump inhibitor use?**

Acute interstitial nephritis

○   **What are the most common clinical finding with acute GN?**

Red blood cell casts in the urine is the classic finding at urinalysis in a patient with acute GN. Patients also present with hypertension. Children typically present with brown or cola-colored urine, which may be painless or associated with mild flank or abdominal pain.

○   **What are the most common causes for acute GN in children?**

Immunoglobulin A nephropathy (typically directly after an acute upper respiratory tract infection) and acute poststreptococcal GN (PSGN) after a streptococcal throat or skin infection (usually 7–21 days later).

○   **What is the most common cause of postinfectious GN (PSGN)?**

Poststreptococcal group A β-hemolytic. However, other infections may also produce GN-related infections. GN is caused by an immune complex deposition in glomeruli. Most patients recover renal function spontaneously within a few weeks.

○   **What is the classic presentation of PSGN?**

Sudden development of gross hematuria, hypertension, edema, and renal insufficiency after a throat or skin infection with group A β-hemolytic *Streptococcus*. Patients frequently also have generalized complaints of fever, malaise, lethargy, and abdominal pain.

○   **How early in the development of "strep throat" will antibiotic therapy decrease the risk for PSGN?**

Antibiotics do not decrease the risk for PSGN.

○   **What laboratory test result best confirms PSGN as the diagnosis?**

Anti-DNase B antibody titer

○   **What is the most common form of SLE nephritis?**

Diffuse proliferative nephritis (World Health Organization class IV). Unfortunately, this is also the most severe form.

○   **Acute renal failure caused by Wegener granulomatosis may respond best to what treatments?**

This is usually rapidly progressive GN and responds to high-dose steroids and cyclophosphamide.

○   **What are some causes of false-positive hematuria results?**

Food coloring, beets, paprika, rifampin, phenothiazine, phenytoin, myoglobin, or menstruation

○   **What is the preferred imaging study in the workup for hematuria?**

Multi-detector row computed tomographic (CT) urography is preferred over traditional CT.

○   **If a urine dipstick is positive for blood, but a urinalysis is negative for red blood cells, what is the probable disease?**

Rhabdomyolysis. Severe muscle damage can result in free myoglobin in the blood. High levels can lead to acute renal failure.

○ **The laboratory test results from a patient with hematuria show depressed levels of C3. What causes should you suspect?**

Chronic infection, SLE, PSGN, or membranoproliferative GN

○ **What medications may be associated with hemolytic uremic syndrome?**

Mitomycin, estrogens, and cyclosporin

○ **What is the most common cause of proteinuria in children?**

Orthostatic proteinuria accounts for as much as 60% of all cases of asymptomatic proteinuria reported in children, with an even higher incidence in adolescents.

○ **What is the most common cause of nephrotic syndrome in children? In adults?**
- Children: Minimal change disease
- Adults: Idiopathic GN

○ **What is the diagnostic triad of the nephrotic syndrome?**

Edema, hyperlipidemia, and proteinuria with hypoproteinemia

○ **What syndrome is characterized by a rapidly progressive, antiglomerular basement membrane antibody–induced GN that is preceded by pulmonary hemorrhage and hemoptysis?**

Goodpasture syndrome

○ **What is the most common manifestation of Goodpasture disease?**

Hemoptysis. These patients usually develop pulmonary hemorrhage before any signs of renal failure develop.

○ **What factors predispose one to acute papillary necrosis?**

Analgesic abuse, sickle cell disease, diabetes mellitus, and alcoholism are usual predisposing factors.

○ **What is the best study for confirming the diagnosis of a urinary tract stone?**

Unenhanced helical CT scan of the abdomen and pelvis has replaced the former reference standard, IV pyelography (IVP).

○ **What percentage of urinary calculi are radiopaque?**

90%

○ **What is the most common type of kidney stone?**

80% of patients with nephrolithiasis form calcium stones, most of which are composed primarily of calcium oxalate or, less often, calcium phosphate.

○ **What are the principal risk factors for the development of calcium stones?**

High urine calcium and oxalate levels, low urine citrate level, and urine volume; low intake of fluid, calcium, potassium, and phytate; and high intake of sodium, sucrose, vitamin C, and protein. In addition, primary hyperparathyroidism, obesity, gout, diabetes, and medullary sponge kidney may all increase the risk.

○ **What are the admission criteria for patients with renal calculi?**

Infection with concurrent obstruction, a solitary kidney and complete obstruction, uncontrolled pain, intractable emesis, or large stones. Only 10% of stones larger than 6 mm pass spontaneously. Other indications include renal insufficiency and complete obstruction or urinary extravasation, as demonstrated at IVP.

○ **What percentage of patients with urinary calculi do not have hematuria?**

10%

○ **A urinary pH of 7.3 is conducive to the formation of what kind of stones?**

Struvite and phosphate stones. Alkalotic urine inhibits the formation of uric acid and cystine stones. Conversely, struvite and phosphate stones are inhibited by a more acidic urine.

○ **Which type of stone formation is caused by a genetic error?**

Cystine stones. These stones are produced because there is an error in the transport of amino acids that results in cystinuria.

○ **Where is kidney stone formation most likely to occur?**

In the proximal portion of the collecting system

○ **What is the 5-year recurrence rate for kidney stones?**

50%. The 10-year recurrence rate is 70%.

○ **What percentage of patients spontaneously pass kidney stones?**

80%. This depends largely on size. Seventy-five percent of stones smaller than 4 mm pass spontaneously, whereas only 10% of those larger than 6 mm pass spontaneously. Analgesics and increased fluid intake aid in outpatient management of kidney stones.

○ **Which bacterium is associated with magnesium ammonium phosphate ureterolithiasis?**

Proteus, a bacterium that produces urease. These stones are infected and must be removed. Antibiotics will help treat the urinary tract infection (UTI) and will generally stop stone formation and urinary acidification. A urease inhibitor such as acetohydroxamic acid will also prevent stone growth.

○ **What is the most common form of incontinence?**

Detrusor instability

○ **What is the postvoid residual volume that suggests urinary retention?**

A volume greater than 60 mL

○ **Which fluoroquinolones should not be used in the treatment of UTIs?**

Moxifloxacin should not be used in the management of UTIs because it fails to achieve adequate urinary concentrations.

○ **What is the most common clinical presentation for acute pyelonephritis?**

Acute pyelonephritis typically manifests as high fever and costovertebral angle or flank pain and tenderness. Patients may also appear to have sepsis, and white blood cell casts are seen at urinalysis.

○ **What are appropriate antibiotic regimens for pyelonephritis in a pregnant patient?**

Ampicillin is widely used as the agent of first choice, but because of variable drug resistance, some studies suggest adding an aminoglycoside for seriously ill patients. Alternatively, extended-spectrum penicillin or a third-generation cephalosporin may be used.

○ **Outpatient management of pyelonephritis should be reserved for which patients?**

Young, otherwise healthy patients who are not vomiting, are hemodynamically stable, are defervescing with antipyretics, and are able to drink fluids. These patients should be treated with IV fluids, antipyretics, and a dose of IV antibiotics, such as gentamicin, a third-generation cephalosporin, or trimethoprim-sulfamethoxazole (TMP-SMX).

○ **What are the risk factors for subclinical pyelonephritis?**

Multiple prior UTIs, longer duration of symptoms, recent pyelonephritis, diabetes, anatomic abnormalities, being immunocompromised, and being indigents

○ **What is the most common cause of UTIs?**

Escherichia coli (80%). *E coli* is also the most common cause of pyelonephritis and pyelitis because of its ascension from the lower urinary tract. *Staphylococcus saprophyticus* accounts for 5% to 15% of UTIs.

○ **What is the most common anomaly associated with UTIs in children?**

Vesicoureteral reflux occurs in 30% to 50% of children with UTIs.

○ **What diagnostic studies are used to confirm the diagnosis of posterior urethral valves?**

The diagnosis can be confirmed by means of voiding cystourethrography or endoscopy of the urethra.

○ **Describe the clinical guidelines for treating infants and young children aged 2 to 24 months with febrile UTI.**

According to the American Academy of Pediatrics, ultrasonography and either voiding cystourethrography or radionuclide cystography should be performed in all infants and young children to rule out vesicourethral reflux after the first episode of febrile UTI. All children should have urine for culture collected by means of suprapubic aspiration or urethral catheterization, and a 7- to 14-day course of parenteral or oral antibiotics is recommended, with prophylactic oral antibiotics recommended until imaging studies are completed.

○ **What is the most common cause of urethritis in male patients?**

Neisseria gonorrhoeae (gonococcal urethritis) or *Chlamydia trachomatis* (nongonococcal urethritis). Gonorrhea manifests with a purulent discharge from the urethra, whereas chlamydia is generally associated with a thinner, white mucous discharge. Treatment should cover both gonorrhea and chlamydia because there is a high incidence of coinfection. Ceftriaxone for gonorrhea and doxycycline or tetracycline for chlamydia are the drugs of choice.

○ **Describe the clinical symptoms of urethral syndrome.**

Urethral syndrome is characterized by dysuria and pyuria with culture results negative for uropathogens. Frequency and urgency are often absent.

○ **What organisms are typically associated with urethral syndrome?**

The most common organism is *C trachomatis*, although other organisms, such as *Ureaplasma urealyticum* and *Mycoplasma* species, may be involved.

○ **What is the initial treatment for priapism?**

Terbutaline, 0.25 to 0.5 mg subcutaneously

○ **What is the treatment of choice for chronic nonbacterial prostatitis?**

α-Blockers, quinolone antibiotics, nonsteroidal anti-inflammatory drugs, and finasteride are all effective, although the cause of chronic nonbacterial prostatitis is unknown.

○ **What are the causative organisms of prostatitis?**

E coli (80%), *Klebsiella*, *Enterobacter*, *Proteus*, and *Pseudomonas*

○ **What is the outpatient treatment for prostatitis?**

TMP-SMX, double strength orally twice a day for 30 days, or ciprofloxacin, 500 mg orally twice a day for 30 days, or norfloxacin, 400 mg orally twice a day for 30 days

○ **A 75-year-old diabetic man presents with a fever, appearing toxic, complaining of acute onset of pain and swelling in his scrotum. He denies urinary symptoms and has a painful, erythematous, edematous scrotum with crepitus. What is the diagnosis and treatment?**

Fournier gangrene. This usually develops in immunocompromised elderly patients and is due to infection or trauma of the perianal area. *Bacteroides fragilis* and *E coli* are usually the cause. Treatment is supportive and includes broad-spectrum parenteral antibiotics against anaerobes and gram-negative enteric organisms. Urological consult for surgical debridement is necessary.

○ **Which organism is the most common cause of epididymitis in patients younger than 14 years and older than 35 years?**

E coli

○ **What is the most common cause of epididymitis in the following age groups: prepubertal boys, men younger than 35 years, and men older than 35 years?**

- Prepubertal boys: Coliform bacteria
- Men younger than 35 years: *C trachomatis* or *N gonorrhoeae*
- Men older than 35 years: Coliform bacteria

Epididymitis is also frequently caused by urinary reflux, prostatitis, or urethral instrumentation.

○ **What does epididymitis in childhood suggest?**

Obstructive or fistulous urinary defects. Epididymitis is rare in children.

○ **How does the pain associated with epididymitis differ from that produced by prostatitis?**

- Epididymitis: Pain begins in the scrotum or groin and radiates along the spermatic cord. It intensifies rapidly, is associated with dysuria, and is relieved with scrotal elevation (Prehn sign).
- Prostatitis: Patients have frequency, dysuria, urgency, bladder outlet obstruction, and retention. They may have low back pain and perineal pain associated with fever, chills, arthralgias, and myalgias.

○ **What percentage of patients with epididymitis will also have pyuria?**

25%

○ **How is testicular torsion distinguished clinically from epididymitis?**

The rate of the pain onset. Torsional pain typically begins instantaneously at maximum intensity, whereas epididymal pain grows steadily over hours or days. In torsion, there classically is a loss of the cremasteric reflex and a swollen, firm high-riding testicle. Clinically, elevation of the scrotum may relieve pain related to epididymitis but is not effective with torsional pain (Prehn sign). This test is not, however, considered diagnostic.

○ **What is the classic physical finding most consistent with testicular torsion?**

Increased pain with elevation of the testes

○ **How is testicular torsion diagnosed?**

Emergency surgical exploration. A Doppler examination is also sensitive but should not delay treatment.

○ **What is testicular viability after 6, 10, and 24 hours of ischemia?**

- 6% to 80%
- 10% to 20%
- 24% to near 0%

○ **What does a blue dot sign suggest?**

Torsion of the epididymis or appendix testis. With transillumination of the testis, a blue reflection occurs. When detected early, torsion of the appendix testis will cause intense pain near the head of the epididymis or testis, which is frequently associated with a palpable tender nodule. If normal flow to the affected testis can be confirmed by means of testicular ultrasonography, immediate surgery can be avoided. Most appendages will calcify or degenerate within 14 days without harm to the patient.

○ **Testicular torsion is most common in which age group?**

Boys aged 14 years. Two-thirds of cases occur in the second decade of life. The next most common group is newborns.

○ **True/False: Testicular torsion frequently follows a history of strenuous physical activity or occurs during sleep.**

True

○ **True/False: Forty percent of patients with testicular torsion have a history of similar pain in the past that resolved spontaneously.**

True

○ **What is the definitive treatment for testicular torsion?**

Bilateral orchiopexy in which the testes are surgically attached to the scrotum

○ **A 4-year-old boy presents with a painless mass in his scrotum that fluctuates in size with palpation. The mass is visible at transillumination. What is the probable diagnosis?**

Communicating hydrocele. Inguinal scrotal ultrasonography should be used to distinguish hydrocele from bowel, and testicular nuclear scanning should help to rule out testicular torsion.

○ **What test result can be used to confirm sterility after vasectomy?**

A single postvasectomy semen sample at 12 weeks that shows rare, nonmotile sperm or azoospermia is acceptable for confirmation of sterility.

○ **Varicoceles are most common on which side of the scrotum?**

The left. Varicoceles are a collection of veins in the scrotum. Patients with varicoceles have a higher incidence of infertility, presumably because of the increased temperature of the testes surrounded by the warm blood of the varicocele. Incidentally, the left testis is the first to descend and also hangs lower than the right in most men. Hernias are also more common on the left side.

○ **What is the most common systemic cause of impotence?**

Diabetes

○ **What is the US Preventive Services Task Force recommendation on prostate cancer screening?**

There is insufficient evidence to assess the balance of benefits and harms of prostate cancer screening in men younger than 75 years.

○ **When is retrograde urethrography necessary to evaluate a penile fracture?**

Patients with hematuria, blood at the urethral meatus, or the inability to void should undergo this procedure to rule out urethral injury. A penile fracture is a rupture of the corpus cavernosum with tearing of the tunica albuginea. It occurs as a result of a blunt trauma to the erect penis. Urethral injury occurs in approximately 10% of patients with a penile fracture.

○ **Why is surgical correction of cryptorchidism important?**

Surgical correction is required to preserve fertility, but the procedure has no bearing on the future development of testicular cancer. Surgery must be performed before age 5 years to preserve fertility.

○ **What is the most common neoplasm in men younger than 30 years?**

Seminoma. This is also the most common type of testicular neoplasm. Peak incidence is between the ages of 20 and 40 years, with a smaller peak occurring in those younger than 10 years. Ninety percent to 95% are germinal tumors. However, only 60% to 70% are germinal in children. Cryptorchidism is a significant risk factor for this cancer.

○ **What is the best tumor marker for testicular cancer?**

Placental alkaline phosphatase (PLAP). Seventy percent to 90% of patients with testicular cancer have elevated PLAP levels. Other tumor markers are α-fetoprotein and β-human chorionic gonadotropin.

○ **What is an important difference between testicular teratomas in boys and those in men?**

In boys, teratomas are benign lesions; in men, they may metastasize.

○ **What is the most common cancer in young adult men?**

Testicular cancer is 1 of the leading cancers in young adult men, with an average age of occurrence of about 32 years. There is a significantly increased incidence of carcinoma developing in cryptorchid testes.

○ **What are the main risk factors for prostate cancer?**

The main risk factors for prostate cancer include a positive family history, African American race, and being older than 50 years. Benign prostatic hyperplasia (BPH) is not a risk factor for prostate cancer.

○ **Which is the most common type of prostate cancer?**

Acinar adenocarcinoma (95%)

○ **Where in the gland is prostate cancer most commonly found?**

In the peripheral regions of the prostate

○ **What are typical presenting symptoms in men with BPH?**

Urinary hesitancy, weak stream, nocturia, incontinence, and recurrent UTIs

○ **What percentage of men with BPH have occult prostate cancer?**

10% to 30%

○ **How well does the size of the prostate in BPH correlate with the symptoms?**

Not well. Symptoms can arise because of a small fibrous prostate as well as because of a large one. Additional symptoms can develop as a result of median bar hypertrophy of the posterior vesicle neck, detrusor muscle decompensation, or instability.

○ **Which is the most common type of bladder cancer?**

Transitional cell carcinoma accounts for 90% of bladder cancers in the United States. Age, male sex, cigarette smoking, and a large number of occupational carcinogens are all risk factors.

○ **What is the most common malignant renal tumor in children?**

Wilms tumor is a highly malignant tumor of mixed histologic findings. A suspected hereditary form of Wilms tumor that is transmitted as an autosomal dominant disorder accounts for about 40% of all tumors. An abdominal mass is the presenting complaint in these children, with peak ages at diagnosis of 1 to 3 years.

○ **One percent to 2% of affected patients will have a recurrence of Wilms tumor. Where is this recurrence most likely to be?**

The chest

○ **Which treatment has both the highest cure rates and the lowest relapse rates for childhood nocturnal enuresis?**

The bed-wetting alarm has a higher success rate (75%) and a lower relapse rate (41%) than do other techniques or pharmacologic treatment.

○ **Differentiate between radiolucent and radiopaque renal calculi.**

Ninety percent of all stones are radiopaque and are composed of calcium oxalate, cystine, calcium phosphate, or magnesium ammonium phosphate. The causes of radiolucent obstruction consist of uric acid stones and/or blood clots.

○ **Name some adverse effects of alkalization of the urine.**

Hypernatremia and hyperosmolality

○ **Where is the most common site of penetrating ureteral injuries?**

In the upper one-third of the ureter

○ **How is a posterior urethral tear diagnosed in male patients?**

A high-riding, boggy prostate is indicative of this injury.

○ **What signs and symptoms are associated with an anterior urethral tear?**

Severe perineal pain with blood usually found at the meatus. A good urinary stream will be maintained.

○ **A patient has a pelvic fracture with probable bladder or ureteral injury. Which test should be performed first: cystography or IVP?**

Cystography is preferable to avoid distal ureteral dye from IVP mimicking extravasation from the bladder.

○ **What is the only absolute contraindication to performing IVP?**

Profound hypotension because the kidneys cannot be perfused. Two relative contraindications are renal insufficiency with a serum creatinine greater than 1.6 μg/dL and a history of allergic reactions.

○ **What sexually transmitted disease pathogens cause painful ulcers?**

Type 2 genital herpes and chancroid

Sexually Transmitted Disease	Ulcer	Node
Genital herpes	Painful	Painful
Chancroid	Painful	Painful
Syphilis	Painless	Less painful
Lymphogranuloma venereum	Painless	Moderately painful

○ **What arrhythmia is frequently encountered during renal dialysis?**

Hypokalemia-induced ventricular fibrillation

○ **What is the clinical name for inflammation of the foreskin?**

Balanitis or balanoposthitis

○ **What is phimosis?**

A condition in which the foreskin cannot be retracted over the glans. The preliminary treatment is a dorsal slit.

○ **What is paraphimosis?**

A condition in which the foreskin is retracted posterior to the glans and cannot be advanced over the glans

○ **What causes priapism?**

Prolonged sex; leukemia; sickle cell trait and disease; blood dyscrasias; pelvic hematoma or neoplasm; syphilis; urethritis; and drugs, including phenothiazine, prazosin, tolbutamide, anticoagulants, and corticosteroids

○ **When is postvoid residual urine considered abnormal?**

When it exceeds 200 mL

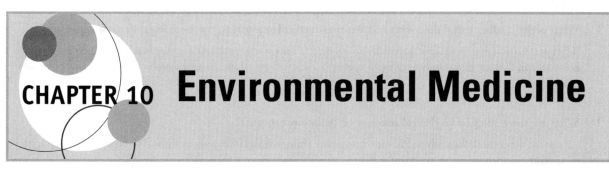

CHAPTER 10 Environmental Medicine

Miguel A. Salas, MD, MPH

○ **What is acute radiation syndrome and its main phases?**

It is the constellation of signs and symptoms occurring after exposure to ionizing radiation.

There are 4 main phases.

1. Prodromal phase: Usually occurs in the first 48 hours after exposure but may develop as long as 6 days after exposure

2. Latent phase: A short period characterized by improvement of symptoms. However, this effect is transient, lasting for several days to a month. The duration of this phase is inversely related to the dose of radiation received and may be absent at the highest, fatal doses.

3. Stage of manifest illness: May last for weeks and is characterized by intense immunosuppression. It is the most difficult to manage. If the person survives this stage, recovery is likely.

4. Death or recovery phase: Patients who recover will require close follow-up for the first year owing to the risk of unusual infections, as aberrant immune reconstitution is probable in those with significant exposure. Survivors will require lifelong follow-up to monitor for long-term complications, such as organ dysfunction and carcinogenesis.

○ **What organ is most commonly affected in a radiation accident?**

The skin. Burns may take as long as 2 weeks to become clinically apparent.

○ **What level of damage distinguishes ionizing radiation (eg, radiographs or proton beams) from nonionizing radiation (eg, microwaves or infrared light)?**

Nonionizing radiation generally causes damage through direct or indirect transfer of thermal (heat) energy, causing external damage only; sunburn and microwave heating are classic examples of such exposures. Ionizing radiation acts at the cellular level and has the potential to cause structural and chemical damage to vital targets such as nucleic acids and proteins.

○ **What is the lowest observable radiation dose in humans?**

The lowest radiation dose resulting in an observable effect in humans causes bone marrow depression, with a resultant decrease in blood cell counts, and is in the range of 10 to 50 rem (100 to 500 mSv, 0.1 to 0.5 Gy).

○ **What ionizing radiation dose is fatal in humans?**

There is virtually no chance of survival after total body exposure in excess of 10 to 12 Gy.

○ **What is the median lethal dose with and without medical support for an ionizing radiation survivor?**

3.5 to 4.0 Gy in persons without supportive care, 4.5 to 7 Gy when antibiotics and transfusion support are provided, and 10 Gy in patients with rapid access to intensive care units, reverse isolation, and hematopoietic cell transplantation

○ **What are the biologic and clinical markers of radiation exposure?**

Currently, the 3 most clinically useful markers are the time to onset of emesis, lymphocyte depletion kinetics, and chromosomal aberrations.

○ **What is the most practical method for assessing radiation dose within hours or days after radiation exposure?**

Monitoring the decrease in absolute lymphocyte count

○ **What is the first hematopoietic line depleted after radiation? What is its meaning?**

Lymphocytes. Lymphopenia is common and occurs before depression of the other cellular elements, and it may develop within the first 6 to 24 hours after exposure to a moderate or high dose of radiation. A 50% decrease in the absolute lymphocyte count within the first 24 hours after exposure, followed by a more severe decrease within 48 hours, characterizes a potentially fatal exposure in the range of 5 to 10 Gy. An absolute lymphocyte count that remains within 50% of normal during the first week after exposure suggests an exposure of less than 1 Gy and a survival probability in excess of 90%.

○ **Do hypnotics improve sleep quality with jet lag?**

Yes. Hypnotics (eg, zopiclone or zolpidem), taken before bedtime on the first few nights after flying, may reduce the effects of jet lag by improving sleep quality and duration but not other components of jet lag. However, they are associated with various adverse effects, including headache, dizziness, nausea, confusion, and amnesia, which may outweigh any short-term benefits.

○ **What recommendations do you give to a patient who is going to have a westward flight?**

It is worth staying awake while it is daylight at the destination and trying to sleep when it gets dark.

○ **What recommendations do you give to a patient who is going to have an eastward flight?**

One should stay awake but avoid bright light in the morning and be outdoors as much as possible in the afternoon. This will help adjust the body clock and turn on the body's own melatonin secretion at the right time.

○ **Is melatonin recommended to avoid jet lag? And is it safe?**

No. It is not recommended to avoid jet lag. The adverse effects of melatonin have not been systematically studied, but people with epilepsy and people taking an oral anticoagulant should probably not use it without medical supervision.

○ **What is the clinical significance of fixed, dilated pupils in a near-drowning survivor?**

Ten percent to 20% of patients presenting with coma and fixed, dilated pupils recover completely. Patients without symptoms should be observed for a minimum of 4 to 6 hours.

○ **What are the expected blood gas findings of a near-drowning survivor?**

Poor perfusion and hypoxia, resulting in metabolic acidosis

○ **Are abdominal thrusts, such as the Heimlich maneuver, indicated in a near-drowning survivor?**

No. Near-drowning survivors usually aspirate small quantities of water, and no drainage procedure is helpful.

○ **Do the Centers for Disease Control and Prevention recommend sampling for molds?**

No. It is important to understand that no indoor space is completely free from mold spores—not even an operating room. Certain molds are toxigenic, meaning they can produce toxins (mycotoxins), but the molds themselves are not toxic or poisonous. Measurements of mold in air are not reliable or representative. If mold is seen or smelled, there is a potential health risk; therefore, no matter what type of mold is present, you should arrange for its removal. Furthermore, sampling for mold can be expensive, and standards for judging what is and what is not an acceptable or tolerable quantity of mold have not been established.

○ **What type of disease does organic dust (mold) produce in humans?**

Hypersensitivity pneumonitis is a kind of lung inflammation that occurs in persons who develop immune system sensitization (similar to an allergy) to inhaled organic dust. It can be mistaken for pneumonia, but it does not get better with antibiotics for infection.

○ **What is latrodectism?**

It is the clinical syndrome caused by black widow spider envenomation and is characterized by the combination of erythema, urticaria, abdominal rigidity, localized lymph node pain, and target lesion at the site of the bite, along with agitation, difficulty speaking with salivation, diaphoresis, and convulsions. It is often mistaken for acute abdomen or appendicitis.

○ **How is latrodectism treated?**

Tetanus prophylaxis, opiates for pain control, muscle relaxants such as dantrolene, and calcium gluconate

○ **What are the distinguishing characteristics of a black widow spider?**

Most adult black widow spiders are shiny black with red markings on the body, although this is not universal. The American species has a red hourglass or anvil-shaped mark on the ventral portion of the abdomen, which can range from a perfect hourglass to 2 separated triangles to 1 triangle and a barely perceptible lower red mark.

○ **What are the indications for administering antivenom for a black widow spider envenomation?**

Severe pain; dangerous hypertension; pregnancy, with moderate to severe envenomations, and pregnancy threatening abortion in women with mild symptoms after envenomation, although black widow antivenom has been administered during pregnancy with no adverse effects. Antivenom should be avoided in patients taking β-adrenergic blocking agents because anaphylaxis will be difficult to treat if it occurs.

○ **What is the skin's appearance after a bite from a brown recluse spider?**

Initially, there is an area of erythema with a bluish target or bull's-eye lesion that is minimally tender. A black eschar forms 3 to 4 days after the bite, and necrotic ulceration develops 7 to 14 days later. Brown recluse spiders live in the Midwest and south central United States.

○ **What are the medical manifestations of a brown recluse spider bite?**

"Loxoscelism" is the term for systemic symptoms of brown recluse spider envenomation. Nonspecific symptoms (eg, malaise, nausea and vomiting, fever, and myalgia) that accompany the lesion, preferably with an identifiable spider, are essential for making the diagnosis.

○ **What is the recommended treatment for brown recluse spider envenomation?**

Benign neglect. Dapsone, 25 to 100 mg orally for 1 to 2 weeks, was previously recommended to prevent ulceration if started early, but results from recent studies have called this into question. It is especially useful if the face or the digits are involved. Dapsone is contraindicated in pregnant patients and in patients with glucose-6-phosphate dehydrogenase deficiency. Steroids, vasodilators, and antibiotics are generally not helpful. Avoid nonsteroidal anti-inflammatory drugs because they may induce bleeding. Early wide excision is ineffective, unnecessary, and expensive, and it may result in increased disability or worsen scarring.

○ **Can a scratch from a rattlesnake result in serious envenomation?**

Yes. However, as many as 25% of rattlesnake bites do not result in envenomation.

○ **Which patients, bitten by a rattlesnake, will develop serum sickness after antivenom administration? What is the treatment?**

Most patients who receive more than 5 vials of antivenom will develop serum sickness. Symptoms may range from mildly viral-like to severe urticarial rash and arthralgias. Treatment includes antihistamines, corticosteroids, and analgesics.

○ **What criteria are used to determine if a patient with a venomous snakebite should receive antivenom?**

Since most antivenoms have a high risk of causing allergic reactions, one must consider the risk-benefit ratio for each patient; however, antivenom is generally indicated when there is evidence of systemic envenomation (eg, neurotoxicity, coagulopathy, rhabdomyolysis, persistent hypotension, and/or renal failure) or when there is severe local envenomation manifested by local tissue destruction.

○ **At what point should fasciotomy be considered for a rattlesnake bite survivor?**

Only after increased compartment pressure that is unresponsive to limb elevation has been documented. Provide antivenom, 5 to 10 vials, and mannitol, 1 to 2 g/kg intravenously (IV).

○ **Which type of rattlesnake bite leads to most deaths?**

The diamondback rattlesnake accounts for nearly all lethal snake bites in the United States. However, it accounts for only 3% of the snakebites seen. Treat with 10 to 20 vials of antivenom.

○ **A color-blind, 36-year-old Texan presents with a history of snakebite. He says the snake was as big as a telephone pole, had fangs like a lion, and was striped like a zebra. At examination, you find ptosis, slurred speech, dysphagia, myalgia, and dilated pupils. What snake bit this man?**

Most likely a coral snake

○ **A young boy presents for evaluation after being bitten by a coral snake. He appears to be fine. What is appropriate treatment?**

Admit him to the intensive care unit and be ready for respiratory arrest. Coral snake venom is neurotoxic.

○ **Describe the appearance of a coral snake.**

This is a round snake with red, yellow, and black stripes and a black spot on the head. Coral snake bites typically do not cause immediate local pain, whereas viper bites do. Remember: "Red on yellow kills a fellow."

○ **How does a thrill seeker recognize a pit viper?**

If the person is close enough, he or she will observe heat-sensing pits and an elliptical pupil that looks like a football standing on end.

○ **What test can be performed in the field in a snakebite survivor to determine if the venom injected by the snake may produce coagulopathy?**

The whole blood clotting test is a useful screening test; failure of the blood to clot in a clean glass tube after 20 minutes is evidence of severe hyperfibrinogenemia.

○ **What does blood or hematuria on a urine dipstick from a snakebite survivor suggest?**

Urine dipstick tests for the presence of blood detect myoglobin and hemoglobin (as well as hematuria), and positive results are suggestive of significant rhabdomyolysis.

○ **What are the signs and symptoms of a scorpion sting?**

The site of the bite is painful but with minimal swelling; restlessness, anxiety, agitation, salivation, incontinence, muscle spasm or fasciculations, roving eye movements, and hyperthermia develop.

○ **How do you treat a scorpion sting?**

Supportive measures, with respiratory status and airway management, benzodiazepines for anxiety, and calcium gluconate for pain

○ **What are the signs and symptoms of a systemic beesting reaction?**

When severe, they are bronchospasm and shock. Local reaction may be limited to pain, edema, and erythema around sting site. If they are severe, treat the patient rapidly with epinephrine, antihistamines, corticosteroids, and airway support.

○ **A 12-year-old boy presents with fatigue, fever, headache, pruritic rash, and joint aches. Examination reveals multiple sites of lymphadenopathy. The patient cannot recall any past medical problems, but the mother points out that he was stung by a bee 2 weeks ago. What is your diagnosis?**

Serum-sickness-like delayed reaction

○ **How should a honeybee's stinger be removed?**

Scrape it out. Squeezing with tweezers or fingers may increase envenomation.

○ **In patients with a previous reaction to an insect bite, what is the risk of anaphylaxis with repeat sting?**

Individuals who are sensitized to insect venom (eg, wasps, bees, or ants) and have immunoglobulin E antibodies against it have a 60% risk of recurrent anaphylaxis at each reexposure to the venom.

○   **A 4-year-old presents with an itching lesion on the legs and waist. At examination, you find hemorrhagic puncta surrounded by urticarial and erythematous patches following a zigzag pattern. What is appropriate treatment?**

Starch baths at bedtime are used to treat pruritus from fleabites.

○   **A 6-year-old child who lives in Texas presents after being bitten by a caterpillar. The child has tense rhythmic pain. Edema and a red, blotchy rash are apparent at the site, as well as a white vesicle. Your diagnosis and treatment?**

Megalopyge opercularis larva (puss caterpillar) sting. Remove the remaining spines with sticky tape and treat with 10 mL of 10% calcium gluconate IV.

○   **A patient presents with a bite wound inflicted while he was in a psychiatric ward. What bacterium is likely?**

Eikenella corrodens is common in hospitalized and institutionalized patients. Most community-acquired human bite infections are due to *Staphylococcus aureus* or *Streptococcus*.

○   **What types of bites most commonly become infected?**

Bites by cats and humans

○   **What medical complications can occur after a cat bite?**

Deep puncture wounds are of particular concern because cats have long, slender, sharp teeth. When the hand is the target of such a puncture wound, bacteria can be inoculated below the periosteum or into a joint and result in osteomyelitis or septic arthritis. Infection with *Pasteurella multocida* characteristically develops rapidly, with erythema, swelling, and intense pain evident as early as 12 to 24 hours after the bite. Systemic signs of infection, such as fever and lymphadenopathy, are infrequent. Localized cellulitis caused by this organism can be subacute in onset, beginning 24 to 72 hours after the injury; systemic infection occurs in fewer than 20% of these cases.

○   **What is distinctive about the appearance of an adult human bite?**

If a bite mark has an intercanine distance greater than 3 cm, the bite probably came from an adult human and, if noted on a child, should raise concerns about child abuse.

○   **If a child is bitten in the scalp by a dog, what study must be performed before discharge of the patient from the emergency department?**

The jaws of large dogs can exert a force of more than 450 psi, which is sufficient to penetrate light sheet metal and can inflict serious injury, especially in young children. With a bite to the scalp, the dog's teeth may penetrate the skull, which can cause a depressed skull fracture; local infection; and, eventually, brain abscess. Thus, skull radiography or computed tomography (CT) should be performed in all patients with a dog bite to the scalp, even if the only visible injury is a puncture.

○   **What complication may result from a wound over or near the metacarpophalangeal joint?**

These wounds may develop a deep-compartment infection, with tendonitis and osteomyelitis of the metacarpophalangeal joint, and should be explored carefully in the clenched-fist position for damage to the underlying tendon sheath, fascia, joint capsule, and metacarpal head, especially if the patient has pain at finger movement. This is particularly important because these wounds typically seem trivial initially and often do not come to medical attention for 24 to 48 hours.

○ **A swimmer presents with a painful, local, linear, erythematous, urticarial lesion and symptoms of generalized back, chest, and abdominal pain; gastrointestinal symptoms; sweating; agitation; elevated blood pressure; and tachycardia after being stung while in the ocean. What is the most likely cause?**

Irukandji syndrome typically involves a mild to moderately painful local sting from a jellyfish that is followed 20 to 40 minutes later by the onset of severe generalized back, chest, and abdominal pain, gastrointestinal symptoms, sweating, agitation, hypertension, and tachycardia. Patients may develop myocardial injury and pulmonary edema 6 to 18 hours after the sting.

○ **What is the frequency of eye injuries in lightning strike survivors?**

Fifty percent develop structural eye lesions. Cataracts are the most common and develop within days to years. Unreactive dilated pupils may not indicate death because transient autonomic instability may occur.

○ **What is the most common otologic injury in lightning strike survivors?**

Tympanic membrane rupture (50%). Hemotympanum, basilar skull fracture, and acoustic and vestibular deficits may also occur.

○ **What is the most common arrhythmia in patients with hypothermia?**

Atrial fibrillation. Other electrocardiographic (ECG) findings include paroxysmal atrial tachycardia; prolongation of the PR, QRS, or QT waves; decreased P-wave amplitude; T-wave changes; premature ventricular contractions; or humped ST-wave segment adjacent to the QRS complex (Osborn wave).

○ **What is the first-line medical treatment of ventricular fibrillation for patients with hypothermia?**

Bretylium, not lidocaine

○ **An Osborn (J) wave seen at ECG is associated with what disorder?**

Hypothermia

○ **Hypothermia is defined as a core temperature below:**

35°C

○ **What months and places have the highest incidence of hypothermia?**

Cases of hypothermia occur more frequently during the summer months and in hospitalized patients. Even with modern supportive care, the in-hospital mortality of patients with moderate or severe accidental hypothermia approaches 40%.

○ **Which medications could cause hypothermia?**

The most common medications that impair thermoregulation are anxiolytics, antidepressants, antimanics, antipsychotics, and opioids. Medications that can impair a patient's ability to compensate for a low ambient temperature include oral antihyperglycemics, β-blockers, α-adrenergic agonists (eg, clonidine), and general anesthetic agents. Certain medications directly or indirectly cause hypothermia by impairing thermoregulatory mechanisms, by decreasing awareness of cold, or by clouding judgment.

○   **What risks factors are associated with lethal hypothermia?**

Risk factors associated with death from accidental hypothermia include ethanol use, homelessness, psychiatric disease, and older age.

○   **Heat loss can occur by means of radiation, convection, conduction, and evaporation. Which of these accounts for the greatest loss?**

Radiation. However, if the patient is not perspiring, convection accounts for the greatest loss. If the person is immersed, conduction does.

○   **A 4-year-old child bites into an extension cord and receives a burn on the lips. What specific concern do you have?**

Delayed rupture of the labial artery may occur 3 to 5 days after injury.

○   **Is lightning alternating current or direct current?**

Direct current. It may cause asystole and respiratory arrest.

○   **What type of arrhythmia is expected with alternating current shock?**

Ventricular fibrillation

○   **How long should a lightning strike survivor without symptoms be monitored?**

Several hours because congestive heart failure may be delayed

○   **What neurologic injury may be expected in a lightning injury?**

Lower and upper extremity paralysis due to vascular spasm

○   **What laboratory workup should be considered for a lightning strike survivor?**

Complete blood cell count, serum urea nitrogen-to-creatinine ratio, urinalysis (check myoglobin), creatine kinase-MM & MB fractions, ECG, and CT if there is a change in sensorium

○   **What are the signs and symptoms of carbon monoxide poisoning?**

Headache, nausea, vomiting, flulike symptoms, syncope, tachypnea, tachycardia, coma, circulatory vascular collapse, and respiratory failure. The manifestation depends on the degree of carbon monoxide poisoning.

○   **What is the most common cause of death in carbon monoxide poisoning?**

Cardiac arrhythmias

○   **How is topical phenol exposure treated?**

Isopropyl alcohol, glycerol, or polyethylene glycol mixture are used in the emergency department for carbolic acid exposure. Water and olive oil can be useful in the field.

○ **What laboratory test result abnormalities may be found in a patient with heatstroke?**

High elevations in aspartate aminotransferase, alanine aminotransferase, and lactate dehydrogenase levels. The serum urea nitrogen-to-creatinine ratio will also show dehydration in many cases.

○ **What distinguishes heatstroke from heat exhaustion?**

Heat exhaustion involves the progressive loss of electrolytes and body fluid. The patient needs to be rehydrated. Heatstroke occurs when the body temperature exceeds 42°C and enzyme systems cease to function normally. As a result, there is necrosis, denaturing of enzymes, and organ failure. Heatstroke requires much more aggressive treatment than simple fluid rehydration.

In patients with an altered sensorium and a core temperature higher than 42°C, always suspect heatstroke. Only half of these patients will be diaphoretic.

○ **How should a patient with heatstroke be treated?**

- Cool the patient with lukewarm water and fans.
- Pack the axillae, neck, and groin with ice.
- Administer fluids cautiously because large boluses of fluids may precipitate pulmonary edema.
- Treat shivering with chlorpromazine 25 to 50 mg IV.

○ **What complications can result from heatstroke?**

Renal failure, rhabdomyolysis, disseminated intravascular coagulation, and seizures. Antipyretics will not help.

○ **How should a jellyfish sting be treated?**

Rinse with saline. Apply 5% acetic acid (vinegar) locally to the wound for approximately 30 minutes. In addition, corticosteroid agents may be applied topically. No antibiotics are necessary. Administer tetanus prophylaxis.

○ **What are the key features in the diagnosis of trench foot?**

Trench foot is a superficial partial burn with no deep tissue damage. It results from exposure to wet and cold (above freezing) for 1 to 2 days.

○ **What are chilblains?**

Exposure of an extremity for a prolonged period of time to dry cold, but above freezing temperatures. Patients develop superficial, small, painful ulcerations over the chronically exposed areas. Sensitivity of the surrounding skin, erythema, and pruritus may also develop.

○ **Describe frostnip.**

The skin becomes numb and blanched and then cessation of discomfort occurs. A sudden loss of the cold sensation at the location of injury is a reliable sign of precipitant frostbite. Frostnip will proceed to frostbite if treatment is not initiated.

○ **How is frostnip treated?**

It is treated by warming the affected areas by using the hands, breathing on the skin, or by placing the exposed extremities in the armpits. The affected part should not be rubbed because this treatment does not thaw the tissues completely. Frostnip is the only form of frostbite that can be treated at the scene.

○   **What is appropriate treatment for frostbite?**

Do not use dry heat. The exposed extremity should be rewarmed rapidly by immersing the affected area in circulating water at 42°C for 20 minutes or until flushing is observed. Refreezing thawed tissue greatly increases damage. Remember to provide tetanus prophylaxis. Debride white or clear blisters as toxic mediators (prostaglandin and thromboxanes) may be present. However, leave hemorrhagic blisters intact. Topical antibiotics, such as silver sulfadiazine, may be used. After admission, the patient should undergo whirlpool treatments with a warm antibiotic solution at least twice a day.

○   **What are some common complications of frostbite?**

Rhabdomyolysis, permanent depigmentation of the extremity, and an increased probability of a subsequent injury caused by cold conditions. Radiography performed approximately 3 to 6 months after a frostbite injury reveals irregular, fine, punched-out lytic lesions that may appear on the metacarpophalangeal, proximal interphalangeal, and distal interphalangeal joints.

○   **What are the 4 degrees of frostbite?**

1. First degree: Erythema and edema
2. Second degree: Blister formation
3. Third degree: Necrosis
4. Fourth degree: Gangrene

○   **What is the sequence of arrhythmia development in a patient with hypothermia?**

Bradycardia to atrial fibrillation to ventricular fibrillation to asystole

○   **What animals are the most prevalent vectors of rabies in the world? In the United States?**

Worldwide, the dog is the most common carrier of rabies. In the United States, the skunk has become the primary carrier; in descending order, bats, raccoons, cows, dogs, foxes, and cats are also carriers.

○   **Describe the intracorporeal dissipation of the rabies virus.**

The virus spreads centripetally up the peripheral nerves into the central nervous system. The incubation period for rabies is usually 30 to 60 days, with a range of 10 days to 1 year. Transmission usually occurs via infected secretions, saliva, or infected tissue. Stages of the disease include upper respiratory tract infection symptoms, followed by encephalitis. The brain stem is affected last.

○   **What is the vector of malaria?**

Anopheles mosquito

CHAPTER 11

Hematology and Oncology

Brenda K. Fann, MD, FAAFP

○ **What 4 types of blood loss indicate a bleeding disorder?**

1. Spontaneous bleeding from many sites
2. Bleeding from nontraumatic sites
3. Delayed bleeding several hours after trauma
4. Bleeding into deep tissues or joints

○ **Mucocutaneous bleeding, including petechiae, ecchymoses, epistaxis, gastrointestinal (GI), genitourinary, and menorrhagia, indicate what coagulation abnormalities?**

Qualitative or quantitative platelet disorders

○ **Delayed bleeding and bleeding into joints or potential spaces, such as the retroperitoneum, suggest what type of bleeding disorder?**

Coagulation factor deficiency

○ **What is primary hemostasis?**

The platelet interaction with the vascular subendothelium that results in the formation of a platelet plug at the site of injury.

○ **What 4 components are required for primary hemostasis?**

1. Normal vascular subendothelium (collagen)
2. Functional platelets
3. Normal von Willebrand factor (connects the platelet to the endothelium via glycoprotein Ib)
4. Normal fibrinogen (connects platelets to each other via glycoprotein IIB-IIIA)

○ **What is the end product of secondary hemostasis (coagulation cascade)?**

Cross-linked fibrin

○ **What is the principal physiologic activator of the fibrinolytic system?**

Tissue plasminogen activator. Endothelial cells release tissue plasminogen activator, which converts plasminogen, adsorbed in the fibrin clot, to plasmin. Plasmin degrades fibrinogen and fibrin monomer into fibrin degradation products (once called "fibrin split products") and cross-linked fibrin into D-dimers.

○ **Below what platelet count is serious spontaneous hemorrhage likely to occur?**

Less than $10 \times 10^3/\mu L$

○ **When a platelet transfusion is indicated, how much will the platelet count be increased for each unit of platelets infused?**

One adult dose should increase the platelet level by at least $20 \times 10^3/\mu L$.

○ **What patients with thrombocytopenia are unlikely to respond to platelet infusions?**

Patients with antiplatelet antibodies: idiopathic thrombocytopenic purpura (ITP) or hypersplenism

○ **What is the only coagulation factor not synthesized by hepatocytes?**

Factor VIII

○ **Which 4 hemostatic alterations are seen in patients with liver disease?**

1. Decreased protein synthesis leading to coagulation factor deficiency
2. Thrombocytopenia
3. Increased fibrinolysis
4. Vitamin K deficiency

○ **What 5 treatments are available to bleeding patients with liver disease?**

1. Transfusion with packed red blood cells (PRBCs; maintains hemodynamic stability)
2. Vitamin K
3. Fresh frozen plasma
4. Platelet transfusion
5. Desmopressin

○ **What hemostasis test result is most often prolonged in uremic patients?**

Bleeding time

○ **What treatment options are available to patients with renal failure and coagulopathy?**

- Dialysis
- Optimizing the hematocrit level (by recombinant human erythropoietin or transfusion with PRBCs)
- Desmopressin
- Conjugated estrogens
- Cryoprecipitate and platelet transfusions if hemorrhage is life threatening

○ **What are the clinical complications of disseminated intravascular coagulation (DIC)?**

Bleeding, thrombosis, and purpura fulminans

○ **What are the most common hemostatic abnormalities in patients infected with human immunodeficiency virus (HIV)?**

Thrombocytopenia and acquired circulating anticoagulants, which causes prolongation of the partial thromboplastin time (PTT)

○ **What is the pentad of thrombotic thrombocytopenic purpura (TTP)?**

1. Fever
2. Thrombocytopenia
3. Neurologic symptoms
4. Renal insufficiency
5. Microangiopathic hemolytic anemia (MAHA)

○ **What is the leading cause of death in persons with hemophilia?**

AIDS

○ **What is the most common inherited bleeding disorder?**

von Willebrand disease

○ **Seventy percent to 80% of patients with von Willebrand disease have type 1. What is the currently approved mode of therapy for bleeding in these patients? What is the dose?**

Desmopressin, 0.3 μg/kg intravenously or subcutaneously every 12 hours for 3 to 4 doses

○ **What is the most common hemoglobin variant?**

Hemoglobin S (valine substituted for glutamic acid in the sixth position on the β-chain)

○ **Which clinical crises are seen in patients with sickle cell disease?**

1. Vasoocclusive (thrombotic)
2. Hematologic (sequestration and aplastic)
3. Infectious

○ **Which is the most common type of sickle cell crisis?**

Vasoocclusive (average of 4 attacks per year)

○ **What percentage of patients with sickle cell disease have gallstones?**

75% (only 10% have symptoms)

○ **What is the only painless type of vasoocclusive crisis?**

Central nervous system crisis (most commonly cerebral infarction in children and cerebral hemorrhage in adults)

○ **What are the 4 mainstays of therapy for a patient in sickle cell crisis?**

1. Hydration
2. Analgesia
3. Oxygen (only beneficial if patient is hypoxic)
4. Cardiac monitoring (if patient has history of cardiac disease or is having chest pain)

○ **What is the most commonly encountered sickle hemoglobin variant?**

Sickle cell trait

○ **What is the most common human enzyme defect?**

Glucose-6-phosphate dehydrogenase (G6PD) deficiency

○ **What drugs should be avoided in patients with G6PD deficiency?**

- Drugs that induce oxidation
- Sulfa
- Antimalarial
- Phenazopyridine
- Nitrofurantoin

○ **What is the most common clinical manifestation of TTP?**

Neurologic symptoms, including headache, confusion, cranial nerve palsies, coma, and seizures

○ **What syndrome is suggested in child who is 6 months to 4 years old with an antecedent urinary tract infection, fever, acute renal failure, MAHA, and thrombocytopenia?**

Hemolytic uremic syndrome

○ **What malignancy is most frequently associated with MAHA?**

Gastric adenocarcinoma

○ **What components of whole blood are used for transfusion?**

- RBCs
- Platelets
- Plasma
- Cryoprecipitate

○ **How much will the infusion of 1 U of PRBCs increase the hemoglobin and hematocrit levels in a 70-kg patient?**

- Hemoglobin: 1 g/dL
- Hematocrit: 3%

○   **What 5 factors indicate the need to type and cross-match blood in the emergency department?**

  1. Evidence of shock from any cause

  2. Known blood loss greater than 1000 mL

  3. Gross GI bleeding

  4. Hemoglobin level lower than 10 g/dL; hematocrit level lower than 30% with ongoing bleeding

  5. Potential of surgery with further significant blood loss

○   **What are the 5 contents of cryoprecipitate?**

  1. Factor VIII:C

  2. von Willebrand factor

  3. Fibrinogen

  4. Factor XIII

  5. Fibronectin

○   **What infection has the highest risk for transmission through blood transfusion?**

  Hepatitis C (1/3300 U)

○   **What is the current recommended emergency replacement therapy for massive hemorrhage?**

  Type-specific, uncross-matched blood. Type O negative, whereas immediately lifesaving in certain situations, also has the risk for life-threatening transfusion reactions.

○   **What condition should be suspected in a patient with multiple myeloma who presents with paraparesis, paraplegia, and urinary incontinence?**

  Acute spinal cord compression. This condition occurs primarily with multiple myeloma and lymphoma, but it is also encountered with carcinomas of the lung, breast, and prostate.

○   **What are the 2 most common neoplasms that cause pericardial effusion and tamponade?**

  Carcinoma of the lung and breast

○   **A 48-year-old male smoker presents with a headache, swelling of the face and arms, and a feeling of fullness in his face and neck. He is noted to have jugular venous distention at physical examination and papilledema at funduscopic examination. What is the most likely diagnosis?**

  Superior vena cava syndrome

○   **What is the most common cause of hyperviscosity syndrome?**

  Waldenstrom macroglobulinemia

○   **What should be considered in a patient who presents in a coma and with anemia and rouleaux formation in the peripheral blood smear?**

  Hyperviscosity syndrome

○ **What factors of the clotting cascade depend on vitamin K?**

X, IX, VII, and II. Remember "1972."

○ **A patient with classic hemophilia has a major head injury. What treatment should be administered?**

Factor VIII, 50 IU/kg

○ **What is von Willebrand disease?**

An autosomal dominant disorder of platelet function. It causes bleeding from mucous membranes, menorrhagia, and increased bleeding from wounds. Patients with von Willebrand disease have less (or dysfunctional) von Willebrand factor.

von Willebrand factor is a plasma protein secreted by endothelial cells and serves 2 functions: (1) It is required for platelets to adhere to collagen at the site of vascular injury, which is the initial step in forming a hemostatic plug. (2) It forms complexes in plasma with factor VIII, which are required to maintain normal factor VIII levels.

○ **What blood product is administered when coagulation abnormality is unknown?**

Fresh frozen plasma

○ **What agent can be used to treat mild hemophilia A and von Willebrand disease type 1?**

Desmopressin induces a rapid increase in factor VIII levels.

○ **Where is a parotid gland tumor most likely to develop?**

The superficial lobe, which is located just below the earlobe. Forty percent of parotid gland tumors are malignant. All tumors, benign or malignant, should be removed.

○ **What is the most common type of malignant parotid gland tumor?**

Mucoepidermoid carcinoma. Other types of malignant tumors are acinic cell carcinoma, adenocarcinoma, malignant mixed tumor, adenoid cystic carcinoma, and epidermoid carcinoma.

○ **What age and ethnic group are at greatest risk for esophageal cancer?**

Elderly African Americans. Their risk is 4 times higher than that in elderly whites. Other ethnic groups at higher risk include those who are Chinese, Iranian, or South African.

○ **Which are the most common cancer cell types of the esophagus?**

Squamous cell carcinoma, occurring most frequently in African Americans. Adenocarcinoma is most common type in whites.

○ **Which organs are the most common sites of metastasis from esophageal cancer?**

Lungs, liver, and bones

○ **Which types of cancer metastasize to bone?**

Prostate, thyroid, breast, lung, and kidney. Remember: "P.T. Barnum loves kids."

○   **A hard mass is detected in the upper outer quadrant of the right breast in a 45-year-old woman. What are the next steps?**

Mammography followed by excisional biopsy. Negative results at needle aspiration alone cannot rule out malignancy. False-negative rates for fine-needle biopsy are 3% to 30%.

○   **What is the most common histologic type of breast cancer?**

Infiltrating ductal carcinoma (70%–80%). Subtypes are colloid, medullary, papillary, and tubular.

○   **A 30-year-old woman comes to you worried that she has breast cancer in both breasts. She is concerned because of a yellowish, green discharge from her nipples, soreness in the upper outer quadrants of her breasts, what she calls a lumpy feeling at self-examination, and mild swelling that seems to come and go. Further questioning reveals that her pain begins 1 week before she menstruates and then disappears when menstruation ends. Understandably concerned, your patient wants to know when she can start chemotherapy. What do you tell her?**

Do not begin chemotherapy. She most likely has fibrocystic breast changes. Put her mind at rest and let her know that fibrocystic changes are not a premalignant syndrome.

○   **What is the most common lung cancer in nonsmokers?**

Adenocarcinoma. Smoking is a great risk factor for all lung cancers, with the exception of adenocarcinoma.

○   **What does a middle-aged man with painless jaundice likely have?**

Possible pancreatic carcinoma

○   **A 44-year-old man presents with a deep, dull pain in the center of his abdomen that radiates to his back and will not go away. He states that he has not felt like himself for a few weeks and that he has been slightly depressed. He also notes that he has lost a lot of weight—about 30 pounds in 3 weeks. At physical examination, you palpate an enlarged liver and an abdominal mass in the epigastrium. What is your diagnosis?**

Most likely pancreatic cancer. The ability to palpate a mass suggests that the disease has progressed too far to be surgically resectable. Carcinoma of the pancreas can be resected in only 20% of patients. Depression often occurs before the onset of other symptoms.

○   **Where is the most common anatomic and histologic location of pancreatic cancer?**

Head of the pancreas (80%). Pancreatic cancer is generally adenocarcinoma and located in the ducts.

○   **What sex and age group most commonly presents with pancreatic cancer?**

Middle-aged men

○   **What is the 5-year survival rate for pancreatic carcinoma?**

It is poor at 2% to 5%. Symptoms generally do not appear until the tumor has metastasized or spread to local structures.

○ **What is the most common endocrine tumor of the pancreas?**

Insulinoma. However, only 10% are malignant. Gastrinomas are the second most common and have a malignancy rate of 50%. VIPomas and glucagonomas are also endocrine tumors of the pancreas.

○ **Glucagonomas arise from which type of cells?**

Alpha cells. Most are malignant. Increased plasma glucagon is diagnostic.

○ **Pheochromocytomas produce what compounds?**

Catecholamines. This group of chemicals causes increased blood pressure, perspiration, heart palpitations, anxiety, and weight loss.

○ **Where are most pheochromocytomas located?**

Ninety percent are found in the adrenal medulla. The remainder are located in other tissues originating from neural crest cells.

○ **What is the pheochromocytoma rule of 10s?**

Ten percent are malignant, 10% are multiple or bilateral, 10% are extraadrenal, 10% occur in children, 10% recur after surgical removal, and 10% are familial.

○ **What organs are the most common sites of metastasis from primary hepatic carcinoma?**

The lungs (bronchiogenic carcinoma)

○ **Clinically, how is right-sided colon cancer differentiated from left-sided colon cancer?**

Right-sided lesions manifest as occult bleeding, weakness, anemia, dyspepsia, palpable abdominal mass, and dull abdominal pain. Left-sided lesions manifest as visible blood, obstructive symptoms, and noticeable changes in bowel habits; pencil-thin stools are also common.

○ **Adenocarcinoma develops from adenomatous polyps. What percentage of patients without symptoms have adenomatous polyps at routine colonoscopy?**

25%. Prevalence increases with age. The risk for adenomatous polyps is greater in patients with a history of breast cancer.

○ **The advancement to adenocarcinoma of the colon from adenoma depends on size. What is the risk of developing cancer if a 1.5-cm polyp is found at colonoscopy?**

10%. The risk for developing adenocarcinoma is 1% if the polyp is smaller than 1 cm, 10% if it is 1 to 2 cm, and 45% if it is larger than 2 cm.

○ **Is a villous, tubulovillous, or tubular adenoma more likely to become malignant?**

Forty percent of villous adenomas will become malignant, compared to 22% of tubulovillous adenomas and 5% of tubular adenomas. Remember: villous adenomas are "villainous."

○ **Which are more likely to turn malignant, pedunculated or sessile lesions?**

Sessile

○ **In what area of the colon are most colorectal cancers found?**

In the rectum (30%), ascending colon (25%), sigmoid colon (20%), descending colon (15%), and transverse colon (10%)

○ **Where are soft-tissue sarcomas most often found?**

In the lower extremities. They are fairly rare. The most common sarcomas are liposarcomas, leiomyosarcomas, fibrosarcomas, rhabdomyosarcomas, and malignant fibrous histiocytomas.

○ **What percentage of those with familial polyposis will develop colorectal carcinoma?**

100%. Because of the imminent development of cancer, such patients should be advised to undergo total colectomy and ileostomy.

○ **A 64-year-old man presents with jaundice, upper GI bleeding, anemia, a palpable nontender gallbladder, a palpable liver, and rapid weight loss. What is your diagnosis?**

This is the clinical picture of a tumor of the ampulla of Vater.

○ **Serum acid phosphatase was a common cell marker used to follow prostate cancer. What other diseases can cause the serum acid phosphatase level to increase?**

Benign prostatic hypertrophy, bone tumors, multiple myeloma, and urinary retention

○ **What laboratory test result abnormality can indicate metastatic disease to the bones?**

Increased alkaline phosphatase level

○ **How can you tell if an increased alkaline phosphatase level is of bony or hepatic origin?**

Isoenzyme separation

○ **What percentage of palpable prostate nodules are malignant?**

50%. Surgical cure in patients who present with asymptomatic nodules and no metastasis is attempted with radical prostatectomy or radiation therapy.

○ **Why are RBC transfusions rarely required to treat iron-deficiency anemia?**

Nucleated RBCs and reticulocytes appear in the blood stream within 72 hours after starting oral iron replacement.

○ **What are the 3 major proteins that inhibit clotting?**

1. Antithrombin III
2. Protein C
3. Protein S

292 Family Medicine Board Review ● ● ●

○ **What does deficiency of antithrombin III, protein C, or protein S increase the risk of?**

Venous thrombosis

○ **Why should warfarin be avoided as an initial treatment for venous thrombosis secondary to protein C deficiency?**

It may, by inhibiting the synthesis of protein C, lead to paradoxical hypercoagulability. Always initially concomitantly treat with both heparin and warfarin.

○ **What is the most important aspect of treating DIC?**

Attempting to correct the underlying disorder (usually septic shock)

○ **What is the characteristic bone marrow finding in ITP?**

Increased or normal number of megakaryocytes

○ **What are the potential treatment modalities for ITP?**

Gamma globulins, steroids, radioactive phosphorus, fresh frozen plasma, and plasmapheresis

○ **How do gamma globulin and steroids work in the treatment of ITP?**

They block the uptake of antibody-coated platelets by splenic macrophages.

○ **Under what circumstances is bone marrow aspirate crucial in the diagnosis and treatment of ITP?**

If treatment with steroids is planned, bone marrow aspirate must be obtained to rule out leukemia. Steroid treatment can delay the diagnosis of occult leukemia.

○ **What are the signs and symptoms of splenic sequestration crisis?**

Pallor, weakness, lethargy, disorientation, shock, decreased level of consciousness, and enlarged spleen

○ **What is the treatment for splenic sequestration crisis?**

Rapid infusion of saline and transfusion of RBCs or whole blood

○ **Increased levels of hemoglobin A2 are found in what conditions?**

Thalassemia trait and megaloblastic anemia secondary to vitamin B12 and folic acid deficiency

○ **What factors contribute to the pathophysiology of anemia of chronic disease?**

Decreased RBC life span (hyperactive reticuloendothelial system), hypoactive bone marrow, erythropoietin production inadequate for degree of anemia, and abnormal iron metabolism

○ **What is the formula for calculating the proper volume of RBCs to transfuse in an anemic patient?**

Desired hemoglobin (g/dL) = observed hemoglobin (g/dL) × weight (kg) × 3

○ **What are the most common sites for bleeding in patients with hemophilia?**

Joints, muscles, and subcutaneous tissue

○ **There is simultaneous activation of coagulation and fibrinolysis in what pathologic condition?**

DIC

○ **What are some common ischemic complications of DIC?**

Renal failure, seizures, coma, pulmonary infarction, and hemorrhagic necrosis of the skin

○ **What are the common laboratory findings in DIC?**

Decreased platelet count, increased prothrombin time (PT) and PTT, decreased fibrinogen level, and increase in fibrin split products

○ **What is the most common familial and congenital abnormality of the RBC membrane?**

Hereditary spherocytosis

○ **What are the major complications of hereditary spherocytosis?**

Hyperbilirubinemia in the newborn period, hemolytic anemia, gallstones, and susceptibility to aplastic and hypoplastic crises secondary to viral infections

○ **What can be used to treat hemosiderosis from long-term transfusion therapy for thalassemia successfully?**

Subcutaneous deferoxamine via pump

○ **What is the incompatibility risk with each of the following: typed blood, screened blood, and fully cross-matched blood?**

The risk of incompatibility of ABO/Rh-compatible blood is 0.1% if the patient has never undergone transfusion. The risk increases to 1.0% if the patient has previously undergone transfusion. Adding a negative antibody screen decreases the risk to 0.06%. Fully cross-matched blood should have a risk of less than 0.05%.

○ **What is the most common blood group in humans? What percentage of blood is Rh positive?**

The most common blood group is type O; 45% of whites, 49% of African Americans, 79% of Native Americans, and 40% of Asians have blood type O. Approximately 85% of the population is Rh positive, and 15% is Rh negative.

○ **At what hematocrit level is oxygen treatment capacity maximum?**

It occurs at a hematocrit level of 30%.

○ **What does PT measure? How is it performed?**

PT measures the extrinsic and common pathways of the coagulation system. The time to clot formation is measured after the addition of thromboplastin. If the concentration of factors V, VII, IX, and X are significantly lower than normal, PT may be prolonged.

○ **What does activated PTT measure? How is it performed?**

PTT measures the intrinsic and common pathways of the coagulation cascade. After the blood sample is exposed to celite for activation and a reagent is added, clot formation is measured. When factors II, V, VIII, IX, X, XI, or XII or fibrinogen are deficient, PTT may be prolonged.

○ **What are the indications for the administration of fresh frozen plasma?**
- Replacement of isolated factor deficiencies
- Reversal of warfarin effect
- Treatment of pathologic hemorrhage in patients who have received massive transfusion
- Use in antithrombin III deficiency
- Treatment of immunodeficiencies

○ **What are the indications for cryoprecipitate administration?**

Treatment of congenital or acquired fibrinogen and factor VIII deficiencies. Cryoprecipitate can also be administered prophylactically for nonbleeding perioperative or peripartum patients with congenital fibrinogen deficiencies or for von Willebrand disease unresponsive to desmopressin.

○ **What are the indications for platelet transfusion?**

Platelets should be administered to correct thrombocytopenia or platelet dysfunction (thrombocytopathy). Perioperative factors to consider for the transfusion of platelets for counts between $50–100 \times 10^3/\mu L$ are the type of surgery, anticipated and actual blood loss, extent of microvascular bleeding, and medications (eg, aspirin) and disorders (eg, uremia) known to affect platelet function and coagulation. Prophylactic administration of platelets is not recommended in patients with chronic thrombocytopenia caused by increased platelet destruction (eg, ITP).

○ **What is the potassium load with transfusion?**

It depends on the age of the blood. The potassium load in 1-week-old whole blood is 4.5 to 4.8 mEq/U. With the transfusion of 20 U of 1-week-old whole blood, the potassium load is 60 mEq (presuming no urinary output). If these 20 U are 21 days old, the potassium load is 110 mEq.

○ **What is the incidence of transmission of HIV types 1 and 2 with transfusion?**

The newest revised estimate for the risk of transfusion-transmitted HIV infection is 1 in approximately 2 million U. Before the implementation of testing for HIV-1 p24 antigen, 1996 estimates were 1 in 450,000 to 1 in 600,000 infected donor units.

○ **How are human T-lymphotropic virus (HTLV) types 1 and 2 transmitted, and what are the clinical implications?**

Transmission of HTLV-1 and -2 through transfusion is limited to cellular blood components. The risk for HTLV infection is estimated to be about 1 in 2 million when the older published risk estimate (1 in 641,000) is adjusted for the fact that only one-third of potentially infectious units actually transmit HTLV because viable virus is lost during blood component storage. Two diseases are associated with HTLV-1 infection: (1) a chronic degenerative neurologic disease, HTLV-1 associated myelopathy/tropical spastic paraparesis (HAM/TSP), characterized by progressive lower extremity weakness, spasticity, sensory deficits and urinary incontinence; and (2) adult T-cell leukemia or lymphoma. The lifetime risk of developing overt neurologic or neoplastic disease is thought to be less than 4%. The consequences of HTLV-2 infection are less clear but may include HAM/TSP.

○ **What is the incidence of hemolytic transfusion reaction (HTR)?**

1 in 33,000 U. HTR is potentially life threatening and is often regarded the most serious complication of transfusions. Fifty-one percent of 256 transfusion-associated deaths reported to the US Food and Drug Administration between 1976 and 1985 resulted from acute hemolysis after the transfusion of ABO-incompatible blood or plasma.

○ **What are the types of HTRs, and what is the pathophysiology of each type?**

HTRs are categorized as 1 of 2 types of reactions: (1) intravascular hemolysis and (2) extravascular hemolysis. Intravascular hemolysis occurs when the antibody-coated RBC is destroyed by the activation of the complement system. Extravascular hemolysis destroys antibody-coated RBCs by means of phagocytosis by macrophages in the reticuloendothelial system. In most HTRs, some RBCs are probably destroyed by both mechanisms.

○ **What is the treatment for HTRs?**

First, any transfusion should be stopped immediately. Hypotension should be treated with fluids, inotropes, or other blood, as appropriate. Renal output should be maintained with crystalloids, diuretics, or dopamine, as necessary. Component therapy should be used if DIC develops.

○ **What causes febrile reactions to blood, and what are the incidences?**

The febrile reaction is the most common mild transfusion reaction and occurs in 0.5% to 4% of transfusions. It is caused by alloantibodies (leukoagglutinins) to white blood cell, platelet, or other donor plasma antigens. Fever is presumably caused by pyrogens liberated from lysed cells. It occurs more commonly in patients who have previously undergone transfusion.

○ **What is transfusion-related acute lung injury (TRALI)?**

TRALI is a form of noncardiogenic pulmonary edema that occurs within 2 to 4 hours after a transfusion. This reaction should be suspected in any patient who develops pulmonary edema after a transfusion in which volume overload is thought to be unlikely. Clinical signs of respiratory distress vary from mild dyspnea to severe hypoxia. It usually resolves within 48 hours in response to oxygen, mechanical ventilation, and other forms of supportive treatments.

○ **What is the MOPP regimen of drugs used to treat?**

Hodgkin lymphoma
Mechlorethamine
Oncovin (vincristine)
Prednisone
Procarbazine

○ **After a course of chemotherapy, your patient has had a course of fever, neutropenia, and granulocytopenia for more than a week, despite antibiotic use. What should you do now?**

Add amphotericin B for a presumed fungal infection while continuing your search for the source of the infection

○ **A patient receiving chemotherapy for Burkitt lymphoma is found to be hyperkalemic, hypocalcemic, hyperphosphatemic, and hyperuricemic. What is the presumptive diagnosis?**

Tumor lysis syndrome

○ **What percentage of children with acute lymphoblastic leukemia (ALL) are cured with conventional chemotherapy?**

70%

○ **What is graft-vs-host disease (GVHD)?**

Engraftment of immunocompetent donor cells into an immunocompromised host, resulting in cell-mediated cytotoxic destruction of host cells if an immunologic incompatibility exists.

○ **When does acute GVHD manifest, and what are the typical manifestations?**

Acute GVHD typically occurs around day 19 (median), just as engraftment begins, and is characterized by erythroderma, cholestatic hepatitis, and enteritis.

○ **What is the clinical definition of chronic GVHD?**

As early as 60 to 70 days after engraftment, the patient exhibits signs of a systemic autoimmune process, manifesting as Sjögren syndrome, systemic lupus erythematosus, scleroderma, and primary biliary cirrhosis, and commonly experiences recurrent infection with encapsulated bacteria, fungi, or viruses.

○ **How long is immunosuppressive treatment required for bone marrow transplant recipients?**

Usually 6 to 12 months or until a state of tolerance is attained

○ **What agent may be a treatment alternative for patients with high-risk GVHD or with refractory chronic GVHD?**

Thalidomide has a 59% response rate, with a 76% survival rate for those with refractory GVHD and a 48% survival rate for those with high-risk chronic GVHD.

○ **List the significant toxic adverse effects of cyclosporine therapy.**

- Neurotoxic: Tremors, paresthesia, headache, confusion, somnolence, seizures, and coma
- Hepatotoxic: Cholestasis, cholelithiasis, and hemorrhagic necrosis
- Endocrine: Ketosis, hyperprolactinemia, hypertestosteronemia, gynecomastia, and impaired spermatogenesis
- Metabolic: Hypomagnesemia, hyperuricemia, hyperglycemia, hyperkalemia, and hypocholesterolemia
- Vascular: Hypertension, vasculitic hemolytic uremic syndrome, and atherogenesis
- Nephrotoxic: Oliguria, acute tubular damage, fluid retention, interstitial fibrosis, and tubular atrophy

○ **What drugs may exacerbate the nephrotoxicity of cyclosporine?**

Aminogylcosides, amphotericin B, acyclovir, digoxin, furosemide, indomethacin, and trimethoprim

○ **What are the long-term effects of corticosteroid treatment?**

Growth failure, cushingoid appearance, hypertension, cataracts, GI bleeding, pancreatitis, psychosis, hyperglycemia, osteoporosis, aseptic necrosis of the femoral head, and suppression of the pituitary-adrenal axis

○ **What are the most common types of infections seen after transplant engraftment (day 0–30)?**

Oral thrush, bacterial sepsis, catheter infections, fungal infections, pneumonia, and sinusitis

○ **What are the most common types of infections seen after transplant engraftment (day 30–100)?**

Cytomegalovirus and Epstein-Barr virus infection, viral hepatitis, toxoplasmosis, diffuse interstitial pneumonia, and cystitis

○ **What are the most common types of infections seen after transplant engraftment (day 100–365)?**

Varicella, herpes, cytomegalovirus, toxoplasmosis, *Pneumocystis carinii* pneumonia, viral hepatitis, and common bacterial infections

○ **What are the most common cancers of the small bowel?**

Adenocarcinoma, followed by carcinoid, lymphoma, and leiomyosarcoma. The small bowel is not a common site for malignancy and accounts for only 2% of all GI malignancies.

○ **Where are most benign tumors of the small bowel located?**

Sixty percent are in the ileum, 25% are in the jejunum, and 15% are in the duodenum.

○ **What carcinoid tumors have the highest rate of metastasis?**

Ileal carcinoids. Malignancy is highly dependent on tumor size: only 2% of tumors smaller than 1 cm in diameter are malignant, whereas 80% to 90% of tumors larger than 2 cm are malignant.

○ **What is the most common childhood malignancy?**

ALL. Leukemia accounts for one-third of all cancers diagnosed in the pediatric population. ALL accounts for 75% of all acute leukemias, and acute myelogenous leukemia (AML) accounts for 25%.

○ **What do ALL and AML stand for?**

Acute lymphoblastic leukemia and acute myelogenous leukemia

○ **When is ALL most common?**

ALL peaks between ages 3 and 5 years and again around 30 years.

○ **What are some signs and symptoms of leukemia?**

Fatigue, petechiae, bleeding, purpura, lymphadenopathy, hepatosplenomegaly, bone and joint pain, low-grade fever, and pallor

○ **Petechiae and bruising occur with platelet counts lower than what number? Internal hemorrhage occurs with counts lower than what number?**

Less than $20 \times 10^3/\mu L$ and less than $10 \times 10^3/\mu L$, respectively

○ **What are some metabolic complications of leukemia?**

Hypercalcemia, hyperuricemia, and syndrome of inappropriate antidiuretic hormone

○ **What is the malignant cell in Hodgkin disease?**

The Reed-Sternberg cell

○ **What are the peak age groups for Hodgkin disease?**

13 to 35 years and 50 to 75 years

○ **What are the signs and symptoms of Hodgkin disease?**

Painless supraclavicular or cervical lymphadenopathy, hepatomegaly, splenomegaly, unexplained fever, and night sweats

○ **What are indications for lymph node biopsy?**

Nodes that continue to enlarge after 2 to 3 weeks, that do not return to normal size after 5 to 6 weeks, or that are associated with mediastinal enlargement at chest radiography

○ **How are childhood cases of non-Hodgkin lymphoma different from adult cases?**

They grow rapidly, are rarely nodular, and are as likely to be T-cell lymphomas as B-cell lymphomas.

○ **What is the most common manifestation of B-cell lymphomas?**

Abdominal masses

○ **Excluding skin cancer, what are the 4 most common malignancies in descending order?**

1. Prostate
2. Breast
3. Lung
4. Colon/rectum

○ **Name the top 3 malignancies in women in descending order.**

1. Breast
2. Lung
3. Colorectal

○ **Name the top 3 malignancies in men in descending order.**

1. Prostate
2. Lung
3. Colorectal

○ **Name the top 3 causes of cancer mortality in descending order for women?**

1. Lung
2. Breast
3. Colorectal

○ **Name the top 3 causes of cancer mortality in descending order for men.**

1. Lung

2. Prostate

3. Colorectal

○ **Which group of patients, younger patients or those older than 70 years, present with colorectal cancer at an earlier stage?**

Those older than 70 years present at an earlier stage. Younger patients typically have more aggressive disease.

○ **A patient with a family history of colon cancer has what percentage lifetime risk of colon cancer?**

5% to 10%

○ **Do colorectal cancers arise most commonly from adenomatous polyps or from sessile adenomas?**

Seventy percent to 90% of colorectal cancers are from adenomatous polyps; 10% to 30% are from sessile adenomas.

○ **Explain lead-time bias as it specifically relates to prostate cancer.**

In the era of prostate-specific antigen (PSA) screening, prostate cancer is being diagnosed earlier, which provides a longer time between the diagnosis and death. PSA screening results in a lead time of 3 to 5 years. This results in an increased survival rate, which may be the result of earlier diagnosis rather than earlier treatment.

○ **In which group of women, premenopausal or postmenopausal, is breast cancer more aggressive?**

Although breast cancer is less common in premenopausal women, it is more aggressive in this group. Breast cancer is the leading cause of cancer death in premenopausal women.

○ **What percentage of breast cancers is thought to be familial?**

Between 20% and 30% of women with breast cancer have at least 1 relative with the disease, but only 5% to 10% have a true hereditary predisposition.

○ **One-third of familial breast cancers are attributed to mutations of which 2 inherited cancer-susceptibility genes?**

BRCA1 and *BRCA2*. *BRCA1* is a tumor suppressor gene on chromosome 17, and *BRCA2* is on chromosome 13.

○ **What percentage of women who are younger than 29 years and who have breast cancer have a *BRCA1* or *BRCA2* mutation?**

Approximately 33%. In contrast, only 2% of women aged 70 to 79 years with breast cancer have a mutation in *BRCA1* or *BRCA2*.

○ **Women of what ethnicity have a higher percentage of *BRCA1* or *BRCA2* mutations?**

In women with breast cancer, *BRCA1* mutations are found in 0.3%. In women in the general population, *BRCA1* mutations are found in 0.12%. However, in Ashkenazi Jewish women, *BRCA1* and *BRCA2* mutations are found in 1%; most Jewish people in the United States are of this origin.

○ **A patient complaining of early satiety and nausea with a palpable left supraclavicular node is suspected of having what kind of cancer?**

Gastric carcinoma

○ **Which ethnic groups are twice as likely as whites to have gastric carcinoma?**

Native Americans, Hispanic Americans, and African Americans are twice as likely as whites to have gastric carcinoma.

○ **What are the peak age groups for gastric carcinoma?**

Between the ages of 40 and 70 years

○ **In which sex is gastric carcinoma more common?**

Men, with a male:female ratio of 1.7:1

○ **Ninety-five percent of all malignant gastric carcinomas are of what pathologic type?**

Adenocarcinoma

○ **List the definite risk factors for gastric carcinoma.**

Definite risk factors for gastric carcinoma are as follows: familial adenomatous polyposis, gastric adenomas, gastric biopsy with high-grade dysplasia or metaplasia, chronic atrophic gastritis, *Helicobacter pylori* infection, or hereditary nonpolyposis colorectal cancer (Lynch syndrome II).

○ **Name the lifestyle factors implicated as causal risk factors for gastric carcinoma.**

Tobacco use, dietary factors (such as a high intake of salted, smoked, or pickled foods and low intake of fruits and vegetables), and excess ethanol consumption

○ **A high intake of which vitamin may be protective against gastric carcinoma?**

Vitamin C

○ **As many as 80% of patients have no symptoms in the early stages of gastric carcinoma. What are some of the symptoms and signs associated with late-stage gastric carcinoma?**

Symptoms include early satiety, weight loss, abdominal pain, nausea, and vomiting. Signs can include an enlarged palpable stomach, a mass, Virchow node, Sister Mary Joseph node, or Blumer shelf (metastatic tumor felt at rectal examination).

○ **What are Virchow node and Sister Mary Joseph node?**

Virchow node is an enlarged left supraclavicular node, and Sister Mary Joseph node is a periumbilical node. Both may be found in gastric carcinoma.

○ **What is the most commonly used cancer staging system created by the American Joint Committee on Cancer?**

TNM: Tumor, node, metastasis

○ **A patient who presents with back pain, fatigue, hypercalcemia, renal insufficiency, and anemia would likely have what type of cancer?**

Multiple myeloma

○ **What is the most common primary bone malignancy?**

Multiple myeloma

○ **What would be the first tests to order in a patient with a likelihood of multiple myeloma?**

Serum and urine protein electrophoresis

○ **In what age group, sex, and race is multiple myeloma most common?**

The median age at diagnosis is 70 years, and multiple myeloma incidence increases with age; men are more likely than women to have multiple myeloma; the rate in African Americans is nearly twice that in whites.

○ **Describe 3 pathophysiologic abnormalities of the plasma cells in multiple myeloma and their resulting clinical consequences.**

1. Overproliferation and overproduction of M protein, causing hyperviscosity leading to arterial infarctions or venous thrombosis
2. Abnormal light-chain production, either κ or λ, causing end-organ damage, particularly in the kidneys
3. Cytokine production, causing the stimulation of osteoclasts and the suppression of osteoblasts, causing bone pain, osteoporosis, and hypercalcemia

○ **What is the most common presenting symptom in patients with multiple myeloma?**

Bone pain, especially back pain, with an incidence of 58%. The long bones, ribs, skull, and pelvis are common sites of involvement. Most patients have multiple lytic lesions.

○ **What protein abnormality is found in most patients with symptomatic multiple myeloma?**

M protein is found in either the serum or the urine in 97% of patients presenting with multiple myeloma.

○ **What is Bence Jones myeloma?**

Increased urine excretion of light chains, either κ or λ

○ **What is the standard treatment for patients younger than 65 years with symptomatic multiple myeloma and for older patients who are physically able to tolerate the treatment?**

Autologous stem cell transplant

○ **What is the treatment for iron-deficiency anemia?**

Iron-deficiency anemia symptoms are treated with iron. The correct answer is that iron-deficiency anemia is a sign of a disease and that the treatment for iron-deficiency anemia is to treat the disease that is causing the anemia. Anemia should always be considered a sign, not a disease.

○ **What are 4 primary causes of normocytic anemia?**

1. Decreased production of RBCs (ie, aplastic anemia)
2. Increased destruction or loss of RBCs (ie, hemorrhage)
3. Uncompensated increase in plasma volume (ie, fluid overload, pregnancy)
4. Combination of conditions that cause microcytic and macrocytic anemias

○ **What is the most common type of anemia?**

Iron-deficiency anemia

○ **What is the most common cause of hemolytic normocytic anemia in children?**

Homozygous sickle cell disease

○ **List at least 5 types of hemolytic anemia.**

1. Alloimmune hemolytic anemia due to Rh or ABO incompatibility in the newborn
2. Sickle cell disease
3. Hereditary spherocytosis
4. G6PD deficiency
5. Paroxysmal nocturnal hemoglobinuria
6. DIC
7. Hemolytic uremic syndrome
8. TTP

○ **What is the differential diagnosis for microcytic anemia?**

Iron-deficiency anemia, thalassemia, sideroblastic anemia, and lead poisoning

○ **What is the most accurate initial diagnostic test for iron-deficiency anemia?**

Serum ferritin test. If the serum ferritin level is less than 25 ng/mL, there is a high probability of iron deficiency. Ferritin can be used to differentiate anemia of chronic disease from iron-deficiency anemia in 70% of patients.

○ **In which patients would a high ferritin level be interpreted other than as an indication of adequate iron stores?**

In patients with inflammatory diseases, liver injury, cirrhosis, or some types of tumor. Ferritin is an acute-phase reactant and can increase to normal levels even during iron deficiency.

○ **Is the transferrin saturation level increased or decreased in iron-deficiency anemia? What about the total iron-binding capacity?**

The transferrin saturation level is decreased and the total iron-binding capacity is increased in iron-deficiency anemia.

○ **How many weeks of oral iron therapy is required to increase the hemoglobin level by 1 g/dL in a patient with iron-deficiency anemia?**

2 to 3 weeks

○ **What 2 factors increase the GI absorption of iron? What factor decreases the absorption of iron?**

Iron absorption is increased in an acidic gastric environment, which can be accomplished through the simultaneous intake of (1) ascorbic acid (vitamin C) and (2) iron on an empty stomach, which unfortunately increases the chance of stomach upset. If an acidic environment increases absorption, then medications that decrease the acidic environment will decrease absorption. Such medications would include antacids, H2 blockers and proton pump inhibitors.

○ **What is the life span of an RBC?**

120 days

○ **What are the 2 mechanisms of hemolysis? Give examples of each kind.**

1. Intravascular hemolysis, such as from infectious agents or mechanical trauma from damaged endothelium

2. Extravascular hemolysis, which is from the portal and splenic destruction of RBCs with altered membranes as in hereditary spherocytosis

○ **What are 2 signs of the increased unconjugated bilirubin found in hemolysis?**

1. Jaundice

2. Dark urine

○ **If there is no bone marrow disease, how soon should there be reticulocytosis after a decrease in the hemoglobin?**

Reticulocytosis should be seen within 3 to 5 days.

○ **Autoimmune hemolytic anemia is caused by autoantibodies that maximally bind RBCs at either higher or lower temperatures (ie, warm hemolysis and cold hemolysis). What 2 infectious diseases can have cold autoimmune hemolytic anemia with immunoglobulin M autoantibodies (cold agglutinins)?**

1. Infectious mononucleosis

2. *Mycoplasma pneumoniae*

HIV can cause both warm and cold autoimmune hemolytic anemia.

○ **What is the best blood test for autoimmune hemolytic anemia?**

The direct Coombs test, which is infrequently called the "direct antiglobin test." This test shows the presence of antibodies or complement on RBC surfaces.

○ **Describe the signs and symptoms of alloimmune (transfusion) hemolytic anemia.**

This is a serious acute transfusion reaction caused by ABO incompatibility during RBC transfusion. Signs and symptoms include fever, chills, dyspnea, hypotension, and shock.

○ **What is the most common enzymopathy causing hemolysis? Which sex does it predominantly affect and why?**

G6PD deficiency. It is predominantly found in men because it is an X-linked disorder.

○ **What is the most common cause of anemia in the elderly?**

Anemia of chronic disease causes 30% to 45% of cases. Iron-deficiency anemia is the second most common cause at 15% to 30%.

○ **Name at least 5 diseases associated with anemia of chronic disease.**

1. Chronic infections, such as <u>tuberculosis</u> or <u>infective endocarditis</u>
2. Chronic inflammatory disorders, such as <u>osteoarthritis</u>, <u>rheumatoid disease</u>, <u>collagen vascular disease</u>, <u>polymyalgia rheumatica</u>, and <u>acute and chronic hepatitis</u>
3. Malignancy, such as <u>metastatic carcinoma</u>, <u>hematologic malignancies</u>, <u>leukemia</u>, <u>lymphoma</u>, and <u>myeloma</u>

○ **In the elderly, what is the most common cause of iron-deficiency anemia?**

Chronic GI blood loss

○ **Is vitamin B12 deficiency or folate deficiency the result of inadequate intake?**

Folate deficiency is usually due to inadequate intake. Vitamin B12 deficiency is usually due to reduced intestinal absorption.

○ **How does aspirin inhibit platelet activation?**

It inhibits platelet cyclooxygenase and thromboxane production.

○ **Which drug, aspirin or the thienopyridine derivatives (ticlopidine and clopidogrel), causes less GI hemorrhage?**

Thienopyridine derivatives

○ **What is the most common cancer in boys and men aged between 15 and 34 years?**

Testicular cancer

○ **What are the risk factors for testicular cancer?**

White race, cryptorchidism, testicular atrophy or dysgenesis, and family history

○ **What is the most common histologic variant of testicular cancer?**

Germ cell tumors, accounting for approximately 95% of testicular cancers

○ **What serum tumor marker levels are commonly increased in testicular cancer?**

Human chorionic gonadotropin and α-fetoprotein. Lactate dehydrogenase is also increased in 50% of patients with testicular cancers.

○ **What are the typical signs and symptoms of ITP in early childhood?**

Bruising, petechiae, and isolated thrombocytopenia

○ **If the same child has a fever, and the child's clinical condition is poor, what other diseases should you consider?**

Meningococcal disease, leukemia, and Henoch-Schönlein purpura

○ **What drugs most frequently cause thrombocytopenia?**

Quinidine, gold, and trimethoprim-sulfamethoxazole

○ **Should antibiotics be used for acute chest syndrome in patients with sickle cell crisis?**

No. There is no evidence from randomized controlled trials that antibiotics are effective in acute chest syndrome.

○ **Fifty percent of patients with ITP have had what in the preceding 4 weeks?**

An acute infection, usually viral, or measles, mumps, and rubella vaccination

○ **What are the American College of Rheumatology 1990 criteria for Henoch-Schönlein purpura?**

At least 2 of the following: palpable purpura, age younger than 20 years at onset, bowel angina (diffuse abdominal pain, worse after eating) or bowel ischemia (usually manifests as bloody diarrhea), or wall granulocytes at biopsy of the arteriole or venule. Two of the 4 has a sensitivity of 87.1% and a specificity of 87.7%.

○ **Which malignant neoplasm has the highest rate of spontaneous regression?**

Neuroblastoma. This neoplasm occurs predominantly in children younger than 6 years. Although the rate of spontaneous regression is high, the overall survival rate is only 30% because the disease tends to be widespread before it is detected.

○ **What malignancy is most commonly associated with AIDS?**

Kaposi sarcoma, followed by non-Hodgkin lymphoma

○ **What therapy should be used for a patient with hemophilia A who has a head injury?**

Cryoprecipitate. Maintain a low total volume, if possible. Cryoprecipitate has a higher concentration of factor VIII complex than does fresh frozen plasma.

○ **What therapy should be initiated for a bleeding patient who is receiving warfarin and has a high PT?**

Discontinue the warfarin, and then administer a water-soluble form of vitamin K; prescribe subcutaneous administration and consider a test dose. If bleeding is severe or in a dangerous location (ie, the brain), fresh frozen plasma containing active factors X, IX, VII, and II should be administered. Remember "1972."

○ **What electrolyte abnormality is commonly associated with the transfusion of PRBCs?**

Hypocalcemia secondary to citrate toxicity (the anticoagulant used in blood products). Citrate, when rapidly infused, binds ionized calcium and therefore decreases the calcium level. Hyperkalemia may also develop, especially if the patient has renal failure or if the blood products are old.

○ **What are the common manifestations of a transfusion reaction?**

Myalgia, dyspnea, fever associated with hypocalcemia, hemolysis, allergic reactions, hyperkalemia, citrate toxicity, hypothermia, coagulopathy, and altered hemoglobin function

○ **What is the universal type of blood donor?**

Type O Rh-negative blood with anti-A and anti-B titers of less than 1:200 in saline

○ **RBC basophilic stippling occurs with what 2 disorders?**

1. Thalassemia
2. Lead poisoning

○ **What are some signs and symptoms of TTP?**

Thrombocytopenia, purpura, and MAHA. Patients with TTP present with fever, fluctuating neurologic signs, and renal complications. If the disease goes untreated, it is almost uniformly fatal. Therapy includes steroids, splenectomy, plasmapheresis and exchange, and administration of antiplatelet agents.

○ **Which type of blood test is used to determine if a patient needs Rho(D) immune globulin therapy?**

A Kleihauer-Betke test is used to check for fetomaternal bleeding.

○ **Dysphagia occurs when the esophageal intraluminal diameter is reduced to what size?**

Smaller than 10 mm. This is a common problem in esophageal cancer. Palliation is achieved by widening the esophageal intraluminal diameter through photoablation of the tumor.

○ **What are the clinical signs of cerebrospinal fluid leakage?**

Raccoon eyes, bruises behind the ears (Battle sign), otorrhea, and rhinorrhea

○ **What is the most common type of brain tumor in adults?**

Glioblastoma multiforme (40%). Meningiomas account for 15% to 20% of brain tumors in adults, and metastatic tumors account for 5% to 10%.

○ **Which type of brain tumor occurs most frequently in pediatric patients?**

Medulloblastoma

○ **What is the most common tumor in a child's first year of life?**

Wilms tumor. Hepatoma is the second most common tumor in this age range.

○ **One percent to 2% of patients with Wilms tumor will develop secondary malignancies. Which types are most common?**

Hepatocellular carcinoma, leukemia, lymphoma, and soft-tissue sarcoma

○ **What does a high cathepsin D level indicate in a woman with breast cancer?**

A high risk of metastasis

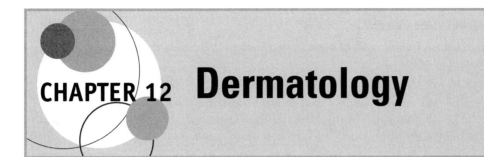

CHAPTER 12 Dermatology

Carrie E. Nelson, MD, MS, FAAFP

○ **A 76-year-old, slender woman with no history of diabetes or other endocrine problem has acanthosis nigricans at routine examination. What is a probable diagnosis?**

Underlying malignancy. Acanthosis nigricans is often a marker for malignancy, especially of the gastrointestinal tract. It is the velvety brown hyperpigmentation and thickening of the flexures common in the axilla and the groin. It is also associated with obesity, diabetes, and endocrine disorders. In younger age groups, it is more likely to be associated with obesity, insulin resistance, or diabetes mellitus.

○ **What is the most common skin malignancy?**

Basal cell carcinoma accounts for 75% of all skin cancers. Eighty percent to 90% of these lesions are found on the head and neck. Basal cell carcinoma appears as a pearly telangiectasia with a central ulceration. It may spread locally but rarely metastasizes.

○ **What are Beau lines?**

Transverse grooves in the nail bed that are caused by the disruption of the nail bed matrix secondary to systemic illness. These lines can be used to date illnesses because nails grow 1 mm per month.

○ **What type of scalp hair loss manifests as patches of balding but without scarring?**

Alopecia areata.

○ **Alopecia areata can be differentiated from tinea capitis as the source of patchy hair loss in what way?**

Tinea capitis hair loss is often characterized by the presence of tiny stumps of hair at the base of the bald area that is caused by the hairs breaking off.

○ **In what areas are *Candida albicans* infections of the skin most commonly located?**

The intertriginous areas (ie, in the folds of the skin, axilla, groin, or under the breasts). *C albicans* appears as a beefy, red rash with satellite lesions.

○ **How should an uncomplicated skin abscess be treated?**

With incision and drainage only

○ **What is folliculitis?**

Folliculitis is an infection of the hair follicles usually caused by *Staphylococcus aureus*.

○ **When should folliculitis be treated with oral antibiotics?**

When it involves the beard (sycosis barbae) or when it is deep or widespread. The drug of choice is a first-generation cephalosporin.

○ **A father is worried that his 5-year-old will contract chicken pox because she was playing with a neighborhood friend who has chicken pox. The neighbor child had crusty lesions all over his body. If this was the only day she played with the neighbor, will she develop chicken pox, too?**

No. Chicken pox is contagious only from 48 hours before the rash breaks out until the vesicles have crusted over.

○ **What are the most common causes of allergic contact dermatitis?**

Poison ivy, poison sumac, poison oak, ragweed, topical medications, nickel, chromium, rubber, glue, cosmetics, and hair dyes

○ **A mother brings her 14-year-old boy to you a week after you prescribed ampicillin for his pharyngitis. She says he developed a rash over his torso, arms, legs, and even the palms of his hands. At examination, the patient has an erythematous, maculopapular rash. What might he have other than pharyngitis?**

Infectious mononucleosis. In almost 95% of patients with Epstein-Barr viruses that are treated with ampicillin, a rash will develop. The rash and subsequent desquamation will last about a week.

○ **Ecthyma most commonly manifests on what body parts?**

The lower legs. Ecthyma is similar to impetigo but can also be associated with a fever and lymphadenopathy. The most common infecting agent is *S aureus*. This infection is most prevalent in moist warm climates.

○ **What is the most common bullous disease?**

Erythema multiforme. The typical erythema multiforme lesion is the iris lesion (a gray center with a red rim). These lesions are symmetrical and most frequently found on the distal extremities spreading proximally. Patients may also develop plaques, papules, and bullous lesions. The disease is most common in children and young adults.

○ **What is the most common cause of erythema multiforme?**

Repetitive minor herpes simplex infections (90%). Drug reactions are the second most common cause of erythema multiforme. The rash generally erupts 7 to 10 days after a bout of herpes.

○ **Where is the most common location of erythema nodosum?**

The shins. It can also be found on the extensor surfaces of the forearms. Erythema nodosum is erythematous subcutaneous nodules that result from inflammation of subcutaneous fat and small vessels.

○ **A patient presents with a raised, red, small, and painful plaque on the face. At examination, a distinct, sharp, advancing edge is noted. What is the cause?**

Erysipelas, which is caused by group A streptococci. When the face is involved, the patient should be admitted to the hospital and treated with intravenous antibiotics.

○ **What type of reaction is erythema multiforme?**

Hypersensitivity. Bullae are subepidermal, the dermis is edematous, and a lymphatic infiltrate may be present around the capillaries and venules. In children, infections are the most important cause; in adults, drugs and malignancies are common causes. Erythema multiforme is often noted during epidemics of adenovirus, atypical pneumonia, and histoplasmosis.

○ **What are the causes of exfoliative dermatitis?**

Chemicals, drugs, and cutaneous or systemic diseases. Usually, scaly erythematous dermatitis involves most or all of the surface skin. It can be recognized by means of erythroderma, with epidermal flaking or scaling. Acute signs and symptoms include low-grade fever, pruritus, chills, and skin tightness. The chronic condition may produce dystrophic nails, thinning of body hair, and patchy hyperpigmentation or hypopigmentation. Cutaneous vasodilation may result in increased cardiac output and high-output cardiac failure. Splenomegaly suggests leukemia or lymphoma.

○ **What is a furuncle?**

A deep inflammatory nodule (boil) that results from an infection of the entire hair follicle.

○ **What is lichen simplex chronicus?**

Lichen simplex chronicus is a localized skin thickening that arises from intense local scratching. The areas most involved are the posterior neck, anus, vulva, extremities, and scrotum.

○ **What are the classic findings of lichen planus lesions on the skin?**

Lichen planus is an inflammatory condition involving the skin and mucous membranes. The skin lesions are classically described as follows: **p**ruritic, **p**olygonal, **p**lanar (flat-topped), **p**urple **p**apules, and **p**laques. Lesions also can appear on the oral mucosa in a white, lacy, reticular pattern.

○ **What is hidradenitis suppurativa?**

Chronic suppurative abscesses located in the apocrine sweat glands of the groin and/or axilla. *Proteus mirabilis* overgrowth is common.

○ **Your neighbor brings her 4-year-old girl to you because she has a terrible rash. The child's face is patched with vesiculopustular lesions covered in a thick, honey-colored crust. Just 2 days ago, these lesions were small red papules. What is your diagnosis?**

Impetigo contagiosa. This is most common in children and usually occurs on exposed areas of skin. Treat the child by removing the crusts, cleansing the bases, and prescribing systemic antibiotics (erythromycin, cephalosporin, or dicloxacillin).

○ **Which organism is probably responsible for the above child's infection?**

Fifty percent to 90% of impetigo contagiosa cases are caused by *S aureus*. β-Hemolytic streptococci are the second most common infecting agent. This latter organism is the sole agent in 10% of cases and can cause blistering. It can also be coinfecting with *S aureus*.

○ **What is the Koebner phenomenon?**

The development of plaques in areas where trauma has occurred. Just a scratch can trigger the development of a plaque. This condition is most common in patients with psoriasis and lichen planus.

○ **What are the ABCDEs of melanomas?**

Asymmetry
Border irregularity
Color variation
Diameter greater than 6 mm
Elevation above skin

○ **What age group has the highest incidence of melanoma?**

Sixty-two percent of melanomas are diagnosed in persons younger than 65 years.

○ **A melanoma that is only in the epidermis is at what level in the Clark classification?**

Level I

The Clark classification is based on the invasiveness of the tumor.

- Level I: Epidermis
- Level II: Loose papillary zone of dermis
- Level III: Expands the papillary dermis
- Level IV: Reticular dermis
- Level V: Subcutaneous tissue

○ **A patient has dysplastic nevus syndrome and is concerned because her aunt has just received a diagnosis of melanoma. What is the patient's risk of also developing melanoma?**

100%

○ **What is the risk of a congenital melanocytic nevus undergoing malignant transformation?**

Less than 1%

○ **What are the most common locations of melanomas in African Americans? In whites?**

- African Americans: Hands, feet, and nails
- Whites: Back and lower legs

○ **Differentiate between pigmented and dysplastic nevi.**

Pigmented nevi are benign moles that are uniform in appearance. They are most common in sun-exposed areas and warrant biopsy if they grow suddenly, change color, bleed, develop satellite lesions, or begin to hurt.

Dysplastic nevi are not uniform in appearance and are frequently as large as 5 to 12 mm in diameter; 50% of malignant melanomas originate from the melanocytes in moles.

○ **What is a pilonidal abscess?**

An abscess that occurs just above the gluteal fold resulting from an acquired sinus that develops from hair, skin scales, and debris becoming trapped in the subcutaneous tissue. Treatment is incision and drainage. Pilonidal abscess recurs easily, and the best way to prevent recurrence is with good local hygiene. Recurrence should prompt referral to a surgeon for definitive excision.

○ **Where does a perirectal abscess originate?**

In anal crypts burrowing through the ischiorectal space. They may be perianal, perirectal, supralevator, or ischiorectal. Perianal abscesses that involve the supralevator muscle, ischiorectal space, or rectum require surgical drainage.

○ **How should steroids be dosed in patients with poison ivy?**

Prednisone, 40 to 60 mg/d tapered over 2 to 3 weeks. Short courses may result in rebound.

○ **How quickly will people react to the *Toxicodendron* (poison ivy) antigen?**

Contact dermatitis typically develops within 2 days after exposure. Cases have been reported from 8 hours to 10 days after exposure. Lesions appear in a linear arrangement of papulovesicles or erythema. Fluid from vesicles does not contain the antigen and cannot transmit the dermatitis.

○ **What is the most common cause of secondary pyoderma?**

Similar to impetigo and ecthyma, this superinfection (ie, of eczematous lesions) of the skin is caused predominantly by *S aureus* (80%–85%). Other responsible organisms are *Streptococcus, Proteus, Pseudomonas,* and *Escherichia coli.*

○ **A 17-year-old girl has a rash on her elbows and knees. At examination, you find several clearly demarcated erythematous plaques covered with silvery scales that can be removed with scraping. These lesions are on her extensor surfaces only in the areas previously mentioned. Examination of her nails reveals pitting in the nail bed. What is the diagnosis?**

Psoriasis. This is an intermittent disease that may either spontaneously disappear or be lifelong. There may be associated arthritis in the distal interphalangeal joints; otherwise, the disease is limited to the skin and nails. Treat with skin hydration therapy and topical midpotency steroids. Remember "Silvery scales and pitting nails."

○ **A 12-year-old girl complains of intense itching in the webs between her fingers and other skin folds that worsens at night. Her skin examination shows a papular rash with excoriations. What is the most likely diagnosis?**

Scabies. Scabies is due to the mite *Sarcoptes scabiei hominis.* A single application of 5% permethrin cream is curative in children older than 2 months. Scabies is spread through close contact; therefore, all household contacts should also be treated. Diagnosis can be confirmed through skin scrapings, but the sensitivity is low.

○ **How are head lice best diagnosed?**

Head lice can be diagnosed accurately in patients presenting with an intensely pruritic scalp by looking closely at the hair shaft while separating the hairs. Nits are usually found within 1 cm of the scalp, attached to the hair shaft. Lice inspection can be aided with a bright light and a magnifying lens. Combing through the hair with a louse comb and examining the teeth of the comb for living lice also aids in detecting cases.

○ **A 50-year-old patient presents with mild greasy, scaling of the scalp and red, scaly, plaques in the nasolabial folds. What is the most likely diagnosis?**

Seborrheic dermatitis. Several factors contribute to the development of this common condition, including hormonal, immunologic, neurogenic, and nutritional factors. *Malassezia* yeast species are also strongly associated. The infant form of the disease is "cradle cap."

○ **What are the treatment options for seborrheic dermatitis?**

Effective treatment options for seborrheic dermatitis include anti-inflammatory agents (such as topical steroids), keratolytic agents, and antifungals.

○ **A 72-year-old woman has a painful red rash with crops of blisters on erythematous bases in a bandlike distribution on the right side of her lower back that has spread down and out toward her hip. What is the diagnosis?**

Shingles or herpes zoster disease. This is due to the reactivation of a dormant varicella virus in the sensory root ganglia in a patient with a history of chicken pox. The rash is in the distribution of the dermatome, in this case, L5. It is most common in the elderly population or in patients who are immunocompromised. Treatment is antiviral medications such as acyclovir, valacyclovir, or famciclovir and oral analgesics. Concomitant oral steroid use can speed the rate of cutaneous healing but does not appear to affect the risk of postherpetic neuralgia.

○ **Where is the most common site of herpes zoster eruption?**

The thorax. Unlike chicken pox, shingles can recur.

○ **A patient with shingles extending to the tip of his nose is at risk for what complication?**

Corneal ulceration and scarring. Lesions on the tip of the nose indicate that the nasociliary branch of the ophthalmic nerve is affected and the cornea is at risk. This is a medical emergency and needs immediate care.

○ **Which of the following is the premalignant lesion that can lead to squamous cell carcinoma: seborrheic keratosis or actinic keratosis?**

Actinic keratosis. The 2 can be differentiated.

- Actinic keratosis: An isolated red-brown macule or papule with a rough yellow-brown scale over it
- Seborrheic keratosis: A benign, well-circumscribed, brownish papule with a greasy, warty appearance

○ **What is the most common type of drug hypersensitivity reaction?**

An exanthematous rash is the most common type of drug hypersensitivity reaction. It is most often symmetrical in distribution but can vary in appearance significantly. If the only reaction is an exanthematous rash, a drug can be tried again with caution. If fever or rash appear, it must be stopped immediately.

○ **What drugs are most often implicated in toxic epidermal necrolysis?**

Sulfas, penicillins, cephalosporins, anticonvulsants, allopurinol, phenylbutazone, sulfonylureas, barbiturates, and NSAIDs

○ **What areas does staphylococcal scalded skin syndrome (SSSS) usually affect?**

The face around nose and mouth, neck, axillae, and groin. The disease commonly occurs after upper respiratory tract infections or purulent conjunctivitis. The Nikolsky sign is present when lateral pressure on the skin results in epidermal separation from the dermis.

○ **What is the treatment for SSSS?**

Oral or intravenous penicillinase-resistant penicillin, baths of potassium permanganate or dressings soaked in 0.5% silver nitrate, and fluids. Corticosteroids and silver sulfadiazine are contraindicated.

○ **A patient presents with fever, myalgia, malaise, and arthralgia and has bullous lesions of the lips, eyes, and nose. The patient indicates that eating is painful. What is the diagnosis?**

Stevens-Johnson syndrome. This syndrome has a mortality rate of 5% to 10% and may have significant complications, including corneal ulceration, panophthalmitis, corneal opacities, anterior uveitis, blindness, hematuria, renal tubular necrosis, and progressive renal failure. Scarring of the foreskin and stenosis of the vagina can occur. Treatment in a burn unit is supportive. Steroids may provide relief of symptoms; however, they are not of proven value and may be contraindicated.

○ **What is the most common cause of Stevens-Johnson syndrome (also called "erythema multiforme major")?**

Drugs—most commonly sulfa drugs. Other causes are responses to infections with *Mycoplasma pneumoniae* and herpes simplex virus. The disease is self-limiting but severely uncomfortable.

○ **A patient who was born with a diffuse capillary hemangioma in the distribution of the ophthalmic division of the trigeminal nerve will have what neurologic findings?**

Epilepsy (usually generalized seizures), mental retardation, and/or hemiparesis. This is Sturge-Weber syndrome. The patient has a hemangioma of the ophthalmic nerve and ipsilateral angiomas of the pia mater and cortex, most commonly in the parietooccipital area.

○ **Tinea capitis most commonly occurs in what age group?**

Children aged 4 to 14 years. Tinea capitis is a fungal infection of the scalp that begins as a papule around one hair shaft and then spreads to other follicles. The infection can cause the hairs to break off, leaving little black dot stumps and patches of alopecia. *Trichophyton tonsurans* is responsible for 90% of cases. The Wood lamp examination will indicate only *Microsporum* infections, which are responsible for the remaining 10% of cases; this is also called "ringworm of the scalp."

○ **What are the 4 most common causes of acute urticaria?**

1. Medicine
2. Hymenoptera stings
3. Infection
4. Idiopathic causes

Urticaria, also known as "hives" or "weals," is a rash characterized by areas of localized swelling ranging in size from 1 mm to large confluent areas. The weals are caused by a cytokine-mediated increase in vascular permeability, and a single lesion lasts less than 24 hours.

○ **Where is the most common location of verruca vulgaris?**

The back of the hands or fingers. Common warts are caused by human papillomavirus.

○ **Xanthomas are associated with which metabolic disorder?**

Hyperlipidemia. Xanthomas are yellow plaques surrounded by erythematous rings. They are most common on the extensor surfaces of the extremities; however, eruptive xanthomas are most common on the buttocks.

○ **How can the development of decubitus ulcers be prevented?**

Change the patient's position every 2 hours, keep the skin clean and dry, use protective padding at potential sites of ulceration (ie, heel pads or ankle pads), and keep patients on egg crate mattresses or the equivalent. For diabetic patients, encourage daily foot examination.

○ **A pressure sore that is a skin defect limited to the epidermis or dermis is classified as what stage?**

This would be a stage 2 pressure sore. The staging of pressure sores is based on the extent of tissue injury and is classified as follows:

- Stage 1: Nonblanching erythema on intact skin
- Stage 2: Skin defect limited to the epidermis or dermis
- Stage 3: Injury penetrating the whole dermis into subcutaneous tissue, demarcating in the underlying fascia
- Stage 4: Skin defect with tissue destruction or necrosis, penetrating into muscle, bone, or connective tissue

○ **What rash is classically associated with a herald patch?**

Pityriasis rosea. Most cases begin with a single large, oval patch (herald patch); then a secondary eruption of small oval scaly patches on the trunk in a Christmas tree pattern appear. Mild pharyngitis and malaise may accompany the rash.

○ **What is the treatment for pityriasis rosea?**

Reassurance. The rash is self-limited.

○ **What are the skin care recommendations for preventing atopic dermatitis?**

Daily use of skin emollients, avoidance of irritants (ie, wool clothing, household cleansers), bathing with warm or lukewarm (not hot) water, using small amounts of mild soap for cleansing

○ **What are the medical treatment options for atopic dermatitis?**

Topical steroids, calcineurin inhibitors (pimecrolimus and tacrolimus). The calcineurin inhibitors should not be used in children younger than 2 years, those who are immunosuppressed, or as long-term therapy in any patient. Oral antihistamines are effective for pruritis.

○ **What are the 2 main organisms responsible for tinea capitis?**

1. *Microsporum canis*
2. *T tonsurans*, which is the more contagious

○ **How do you diagnose tinea versicolor?**

Examination under a Wood lamp shows yellow fluorescence. Also, potassium hydroxide preparation is useful in confirming the diagnosis.

○   **What is the recommended therapy for tinea capitis?**

Griseofulvin is considered the treatment of choice and appears to be superior to terbinafine for treating *Microsporum* infections. Griseofulvin is dosed at 250 mg twice daily for adults and 20 mg/kg per day for children, with a duration of treatment of 6 to 8 weeks for both groups. Alternatively, terbinafine, itraconazole, or fluconazole are equally effective for the treatment of *Trichophyton* infections. Each of these agents allows a shorter course of treatment than with griseofulvin, but they are typically more expensive, and, therefore, should be reserved for resistant cases or for patients who cannot tolerate griseofulvin. Itraconazole can be used in children as continuous therapy at a dose of 3 to 5 mg/kg daily for 4 to 6 weeks or as pulse therapy at a dose of 5 mg/kg daily for 1 week each month for 2 to 3 months. Terbinafine treatment schedules are based on weight: 10 to 20 kg, 62.5 mg daily for 4 weeks; 20 to 40 kg, 125 mg daily for 4 weeks; more than 40 kg, 250 mg daily for 4 weeks). A 6-week course of fluconazole may also be used: 6 mg/kg per day for 3 to 6 weeks in adults and 6 mg/kg per day for 6 weeks in children. Tinea capitis is not responsive to topical treatments alone, although infected patients and potential asymptomatic carriers should be instructed to shampoo twice a week with 2.5% selenium sulfide.

○   **What is the causative agent of tinea versicolor?**

Tinea versicolor, also known as "pityriasis versicolor," is not a true tinea infection because it is not caused by a dermatophyte. After adolescence, increased sebum production may allow the proliferation of *Pityrosporum ovale* or *Pityrosporum orbiculare* (*Malassezia furfur*), which can cause a brown, pink, or reddish discoloration of the skin. Over time, the *Pityrosporum* species can block the conversion of tyrosine to melanin, leading to hypopigmented patches instead of increased coloration.

○   **Patients with what conditions are more likely to develop vitiligo?**

Diabetes mellitus, Addison disease, thyroid disorders, and pernicious anemia. Vitiligo results from an immune-mediated destruction of melanocytes and is found in 1% of the general population.

○   **Which areas of the body are normally most affected by vitiligo?**

Common sites of involvement include the face, neck, dorsal sides of the hands, genitalia, body folds, and axillae. Perioral, periorbital, periumbilical, and perianal lesions also occur.

○   **What is the treatment for vitiligo?**

The most important treatment is protection from the sun with sunscreen, hats, and other garment coverage. Treatment may also involve cosmetics and topical steroids. Less common forms of treatment include immune modifiers, topical and oral psoralens, psoralen plus long-wave ultraviolet A therapy, narrow-band ultraviolet B therapy, depigmentation therapy, and surgical grafting techniques.

○   **A patient presents with red and tender lateral nail folds on his ring finger with a small adjacent abscess. What is the diagnosis?**

Paronychia

○   **What is the drug of choice for head lice?**

Permethrin

○   **A 31-year-old woman presents with a maculopapular rash on her trunk and upper legs. The rash is in lines along the long axis of the ovoid lesions. The patient states that 1 week ago, she had only 1 lesion, which was round and about as wide as a golf ball. What is the diagnosis?**

Pityriasis rosea

○ **Patients receiving which antibiotics are most likely to have a photoallergic drug reaction?**

Tetracycline and sulfonamides

○ **An obese 18-year-old man with a history of diabetes mellitus reports dark patches in the groin and axilla. What is the most likely diagnosis?**

Acanthosis nigrans, which may be caused by insulin resistance

○ **What is the treatment for scalp lesions of seborrheic dermatitis?**

Therapies include anti-inflammatories (ie, steroid shampoo, tacrolimus ointment), keratolytics (ie, salicylic acid or tar shampoo), and antifungal preparations (ie, ketoconazole or selenium sulfide shampoo).

○ **A patient with AIDS presents with a grayish-white plaque on the lateral borders of her tongue that do not scrape off. What is the diagnosis?**

Hairy leukoplakia

○ **Describe the skin lesions found in a patient with disseminated gonococcemia.**

Umbilicated pustules with red halos

○ **Describe the skin lesions associated with a *Pseudomonas aeruginosa* infection.**

Pale, erythematous lesions 1 cm in size with an ulcerated necrotic center

○ **Describe the rash associated with exanthem subitum (roseola infantum).**

The rash is usually found on the trunk and the neck and is maculopapular.

○ **Erythema nodosa is associated with which type of gastroenteritis?**

Yersinia

○ **What are the complications of impetigo?**

Streptococcal impetigo can result in poststreptococcal glomerulonephritis. However, it is not associated with rheumatic fever. Treat with erythromycin, dicloxacillin, or cephalexin to help eliminate the skin lesions. There is no conclusive proof that treatment prevents glomerulonephritis.

○ **Where are the 3 most common locations of malignant melanomas?**

1. Skin

2. Eye

3. Anal canal

CHAPTER 13 Obstetrics/Gynecology

Maria I. Brown, DO

○ **Define the normal menstrual cycle.**

The normal menstrual cycle is 28 days, with a flow lasting 2 to 7 days. The variation in cycle length is set at 21 to 35 days.

○ **In a normal menstrual cycle, when does ovulation typically occur?**

Ovulation in a 28-day cycle typically occurs on day 14. The luteal phase of the cycle is normally 14 days long. The estrogenic (proliferative) phase of the cycle can be variable.

○ **Name the hormones, and their sources, that are involved in maintaining a normal menstrual cycle.**
- From the ovary: Estrogen and progesterone
- From the pituitary: Follicle-stimulating hormone (FSH) and luteinizing hormone (LH)
- From the hypothalamus: Gonadotropin-releasing hormone (GnRH)

Prolactin and thyrotropin are also vital in maintaining a normal menstrual cycle.

○ **Describe the effect of estrogen on the endometrium.**

Estrogen causes growth of the endometrium. The endometrial glands lengthen, and the glandular epithelium becomes pseudostratified. Mitotic activity is present in both the glands and the stroma.

○ **When does implantation of the fertilized ovum typically occur?**

At approximately postovulatory day 9 (day 23)

○ **What is the life span of a normal corpus luteum in the absence of pregnancy?**

Approximately 14 days

○ **In a woman of reproductive age, what is the first step in the evaluation of abnormal uterine bleeding after obtaining the history and performing a physical examination?**

A pregnancy test

○ **What is the action of oxytocin?**

It stimulates uterine contractions during labor and elicits milk ejection by myoepithelial cells of the mammary ducts.

○ **What is the function of FSH?**

It stimulates maturation of the graafian follicle and its production of estradiol.

○ **What is the function of LH?**

It causes follicular rupture, ovulation, and establishment of the corpus luteum.

○ **The ovarian luteal phase corresponds to what phase of the uterus?**

The secretory phase. The luteal phase begins after ovulation. At this time, the expelled follicle is called the "corpus luteum." The corpus luteum secretes estradiol and progesterone, which cause secretory ducts to develop in the endometrial lining.

○ **What does a biphasic curve on a basal body temperature chart of a 25-year-old woman indicate?**

Normal ovulation and the effect of progesterone. A monophasic basal body temperature curve indicates an anovulatory cycle. A temperature that remained elevated after a normal biphasic curve would indicate pregnancy.

○ **What is the most accurate test of ovulation?**

Endometrial biopsy. This will show if there is a secretory phase, thereby indicating ovulation.

○ **What is the cause of midcycle spotting or light bleeding?**

The decrease in estrogen that occurs immediately before the LH surge

○ **Decrease in which hormone heralds the onset of menses?**

Normal menses occurs because of progesterone withdrawal.

○ **What levels of FSH and LH would you expect in a 63-year-old woman who is not receiving estrogen replacement therapy?**

High levels of both FSH and LH. The ovarian response to FSH and LH is decreased in menopause. Consequently, less estrogen and progesterone are being produced, there is no negative feedback to inhibit the increasing levels of FSH and LH.

○ **What is the function of prolactin?**

It initiates and sustains lactation by the breast glands, and it may influence synthesis and release of progesterone by the ovary and testosterone by the testis.

○ **What is the main physiologic stimulus for prolactin release?**

Suckling of the breast

○ **What is the most common presenting symptom of a prolactinoma in a woman?**

Secondary amenorrhea

○ **Match the words with their definitions.**

1. Menorrhagia	**a.** Bleeding between menstrual periods
2. Metrorrhagia	**b.** Excessive amount of vaginal bleeding or duration of bleeding
3. Menometrorrhagia	**c.** Excessive amount of blood at irregular frequencies
4. Polymenorrhea	**d.** Menstrual periods more than 35 days apart
5. Oligomenorrhea	**e.** Menstrual periods fewer than 21 days apart

Answers: (1) b, (2) a, (3) c, (4) e, and (5) d

○ **What is secondary amenorrhea?**

No menstruation for 6 months or more in a woman who previously had regular menses

○ **What is the most common cause of secondary amenorrhea?**

Pregnancy. The second most common cause is hypothalamic hypogonadism, which can be due to weight loss, anorexia nervosa, stress, excessive exercise, or hypothalamic disease.

○ **What are some causes of premature menopause?**

Smoking, radiation, chemotherapy, and anything else that limits the ovarian blood supply

○ **A 26-year-old woman with secondary amenorrhea and essentially normal workup results receives an intramuscular injection of 100 mg of progesterone and responds with a normal menstrual period. What does this tell you?**

She has a functional endometrium and a normal production of estrogen. Patients producing less than 40 pg/mL of estrogen will not bleed. This test is called the "progesterone challenge."

○ **What are the 2 major differential diagnoses in the above patient?**

1. Premature ovarian failure

2. Hypothalamic dysfunction

Premature ovarian failure can be diagnosed if the serum LH level is greater than 25 mIU/mL; otherwise, the diagnosis is most likely hypothalamic dysfunction.

○ **A patient with secondary amenorrhea fails the progesterone challenge and has a high FSH level. What is the problem?**

Gonadal failure. A low FSH level would be more indicative of hypothalamic dysfunction.

○ **In hyperprolactinemia, the serum prolactin level is higher than _____.**

400 ng/mL. Hyperprolactinemia is caused by pituitary adenomas, hypothyroidism, or drugs, such as reserpine, methyldopa, phenothiazine, or the oral contraceptive pill (OCP). Clinically, patients do not menstruate, and they have galactorrhea.

○ **What is the most frequent gynecologic disease of children?**

Vulvovaginitis, and the cause is poor perineal hygiene

○ **List the differential diagnosis of persistent vaginal bleeding in a preadolescent girl.**
- Neoplasia
- Precocious puberty
- Ureteral prolapse
- Trauma
- Sexual assault
- Vulvovaginitis
- Exposure to exogenous estrogen
- *Shigella* infection
- Group A and β-hemolytic streptococcal infection
- Foreign body in vagina

○ **Without therapy, approximately 50% of girls with precocious puberty will not reach what height?**

5 ft

○ **What blood tests would be appropriate in the evaluation of a female child with precocious puberty?**

Serum levels of FSH, LH, prolactin, thyrotropin, estradiol, testosterone, dehydroepiandrosterone sulfate, and human chorionic gonadotropin (hCG)

○ **Breast hyperplasia is a normal physiologic phenomenon in the neonatal period and may persist for how many months?**

As long as 6 months

○ **Retrospective historical data derived from adults imply that what percentage of women are believed to have been sexually abused as children?**

15% to 25%. Eighty percent of all cases of sexual abuse of children involve a family member.

○ **What is the most common cause of vaginal bleeding in childhood?**

A foreign body. Patients will have a bloody, foul-smelling discharge.

○ **What is the median age for menopause?**

51 years

○ **A 37-year-old woman, gravida 2, para 2 presents with a history of lengthening menses and acquired dysmenorrhea. This problem had been subtly going on for 2 years and now is a quality-of-life issue. Examination reveals a globular uterus, at the upper limits of normal in size. What is the most likely diagnosis?**

Adenomyosis

○ **What is the most common cause of postmenopausal bleeding?**

Atrophic endometrium and/or atrophic vaginitis

○   **What is Halban syndrome?**

This is the persistence of a corpus luteum. Patients commonly present with delayed menses, pelvic mass, and negative pregnancy test. Clinically, this is often confused with an ectopic pregnancy.

○   **In women of reproductive age, what is the most common cause of estrogen-induced excess bleeding?**

Chronic anovulation associated with polycystic ovaries

○   **How does progesterone work at the cellular level to control dysfunctional uterine bleeding when prescribed in pharmacologic doses?**

Progestins are powerful antiestrogens. They stimulate 17β-hydroxysteroid dehydrogenase and sulfotransferase activity. This results in conversion of estradiol to estrone sulfate, which is rapidly excreted in the urine. Progestins also inhibit augmentation of estrogen receptors. In addition, progestins suppress estrogen-mediated transcription of oncogenes.

○   **A 27-year-old woman presents with secondary amenorrhea of 6 months' duration. What should appropriate initial evaluation include?**

Pelvic examination, Papanicolaou (Pap) smear screening, pregnancy test, prolactin and progestin challenges, and measurement of thyrotropin level

○   **What are the common changes associated with estrogen depletion?**

Menstrual cycle changes, cardiovascular disease, osteoporosis, genitourinary atrophy, and vasomotor and psychological symptoms

○   **What are the expected changes in gonadotropin levels after menopause?**

FSH increases 10- to 20-fold and LH increases threefold, reaching a maximum 1 to 3 years after menopause.

○   **Which hormones decrease as a result of menopause?**

Estrogen and androstenedione

○   **What happens to progesterone production in menopause?**

Progesterone is no longer produced.

○   **What hormone is secreted more by the postmenopausal ovary than by the premenopausal ovary?**

Testosterone. Before menopause, the ovary contributes 25% of circulating testosterone, and in menopause the ovary contributes 40% of circulating testosterone.

○   **What is the cause of mild hirsutism in menopause?**

Increased free androgen:estrogen ratio as a result of decreased levels of sex hormone-binding globulin and estrogen

○   **What is the leading cause of death for women?**

Heart disease, followed by malignancies, cerebrovascular disease, and motor vehicle accidents

○   **How many deaths are attributed to cardiovascular disease in women older than 50 years?**

More than 50%

○   **How much does the risk of coronary heart disease increase after menopause?**

It doubles.

○   **After menopause, what is the percentage of bone loss per year?**

2.5% for the first 4 years, then 1% to 1.5% annually

○   **What risk factors are associated with bone loss and osteoporosis?**

White or Asian race, thinness, sedentary lifestyle, smoking, coexisting endocrine disease, and age at menopause

○   **How does estrogen therapy help maintain bone mass?**

Estrogen has a direct effect on osteoblasts, improves intestinal absorption of calcium, and decreases renal excretion of calcium.

○   **Why does vaginitis increase during the postmenopausal years?**

Because of estrogen deficiency, vaginal pH increases from 3.5 to 4.5 up to 6.0 to 8.0, predisposing the woman to colonization by bacterial pathogens

○   **What is the origin of breakthrough bleeding during continuous hormone replacement therapy (HRT)?**

Progestational dominance resulting in an atrophic endometrium

○   **What effect does estrogen therapy have on colorectal cancer?**

It significantly decreases the risk of colorectal cancer.

○   **What are contraindications to estrogen therapy?**

Estrogen-sensitive cancers, chronically impaired liver function, undiagnosed genital bleeding, acute vascular thrombosis, neurophthalmologic vascular disease, and known or suspected pregnancy

○   **A patient using OCP is concerned about the added risk of gynecologic cancers. What should you tell her?**

Combined estrogen and progesterone OCP is not associated with a significant risk for breast cancer. In fact, OCP use decreases the risk of ovarian and endometrial cancers. OCP use increases the risk for thromboembolism, myocardial infarction, cerebrovascular accident, hypertension, amenorrhea, cholelithiasis, and benign hepatic tumors, but it helps regulate the menstrual cycle; decrease cramping; and curb the progression of endometriosis, ovarian cysts, and benign breast disease. OCP use also decreases the incidence of ectopic pregnancy, salpingitis, and anemia, and it is therapeutic against rheumatoid arthritis.

○   **What effect does estrogen have on Alzheimer disease?**

Alzheimer disease is less frequent among HRT users, and cognitive function in affected individuals is improved.

○ **What predisposes a woman to yeast infections?**

Diabetes, OCP use, and antibiotics

○ **What is the most common cause of vaginitis?**

Candida albicans

○ **What causes a greenish gray frothy vaginal discharge with mild itching?**

Trichomonas vaginalis. At physical examination, the cervix will have a strawberry appearance 20% of the time.

○ **Describe the presentation of a patient with *Gardnerella vaginalis*.**

At physical examination, there is a frothy, grayish white, fishy-smelling vaginal discharge. Wet-mount examination may show clue cells (clusters of bacilli on the surface of epithelial cells).

○ **A patient presents with a 2-day history of vaginal itching and burning. At examination, you note a thin, yellowish green, bubbly discharge and petechiae on the cervix (also known as a "strawberry" cervix). What test do you perform, and what do you expect to find?**

Mix the discharge with saline and view under a microscope. If you see *T vaginalis* (mobile, pear-shaped protozoa with flagella), then the patient and her partner should be treated with metronidazole.

○ **A 20-year-old sexually active woman presents to your office complaining of a heavy thin discharge with an unpleasant odor. Adding 10% potassium hydroxide to the discharge produces a fishy odor. What would you expect to see at microscopic examination?**

Clue cells that indicate bacterial vaginosis

○ **What is the most common bacterial cause of urinary tract infections?**

Escherichia coli. Other causative agents are also gram negative.

○ **What is the normal pH of the vagina?**

3.8 to 4.4. Vaginal pH greater than 4.9 indicates bacterial or protozoal infection.

○ **What causes condylomata acuminata (venereal warts)?**

Human papillomavirus (HPV) types 6 and 11

○ **What subtypes of HPV are associated with cervical cancer?**

HPV types 16, 18, and 31 are risk factors for cervical dysplasia, which can lead to cervical cancer. Multiple sexual partners and early onset of sexual activity are risk factors for cervical cancer because of HPV infection.

○ **When should you avoid treating a woman with metronidazole?**

During the first trimester of pregnancy, metronidazole may have teratogenic effects. Clotrimazole may be used instead. Adverse effects of metronidazole include nausea, vomiting, and metallic tastes; it acts similarly to disulfiram and therefore should not be taken with ethanol.

○ **A 30-year-old woman complains of a painful vulval sore that resembled a pimple at first. At examination, you find an ulcer with vague borders and a gray base. What is the probable diagnosis?**

Gram stain, culture, and biopsy (used in combination because of the high false-negative rates) should show that *Haemophilus ducreyi* has caused a chancroid. Treatment is erythromycin or ceftriaxone.

○ **Condylomata acuminata frequently occur in combination with what other sexually transmitted disease?**

T vaginalis

○ **What is the most common cause of septic arthritis in young adults?**

Disseminated gonococcal infection

○ **What is the treatment for gonorrhea?**

Ceftriaxone and doxycycline. The latter is administered because half of the patients infected with gonorrhea are simultaneously infected with chlamydia.

○ **What is the predominant organism in a healthy woman's vaginal discharge?**

Lactobacilli (95%)

○ **A 34-year-old woman presents with a maculopapular rash on her palms and soles and states that she had a strange vaginal lesion about a month and a half ago. She complains of headaches and general weakness. At examination, you find she has multiple condyloma lata and lymphadenopathy. What is the diagnosis?**

Secondary syphilis. This develops 6 to 9 weeks after the syphilitic chancre, which will have resolved by this time. If it goes untreated, tertiary syphilis will develop, which can affect all the tissues in the body, including the central nervous system and the heart. Treatment is with penicillin G.

○ **Is polycystic ovary syndrome a unilateral or a bilateral phenomenon?**

Bilateral. Both ovaries are cystic and enlarged with a thickened and fibrosed tunica. Patients are often infertile, obese, and hirsute.

○ **What are the risk factors for pelvic inflammatory disease (PID)?**

- Age younger than 20 years
- Multiple sexual partners
- Nulliparity
- Previous history of PID

○ **True/False: A woman with PID is likely to have an exacerbation of symptoms when she menstruates.**

True. The breakdown of the cervical mucous antibacterial barrier allows bacteria to ascend from the lower tract to the upper tract. Pelvic examination, intercourse, and exercise can all exacerbate symptoms.

○ **What 2 organisms cause most cases of PID?**

1. *Neisseria gonorrhoeae*
2. *Chlamydia trachomatis*

○ **Describe lesions associated with chlamydia.**

Painless, shallow ulcerations; papular or nodular lesions; and herpetiform vesicles that wax and wane

○ **Which patients with PID should be admitted to the hospital?**

Admit patients who are pregnant, have a temperature higher than 100.4°F, are nauseated or vomiting (which prohibits use of oral antibiotics), have pyosalpinx or tubo-ovarian abscess peritoneal signs, have an intrauterine device (IUD), show no response to oral antibiotics, or for whom diagnosis is uncertain.

○ **What are the criteria for diagnosing PID?**

All of the following must be present: (1) adnexal tenderness, (2) cervical and uterine tenderness, and (3) abdominal tenderness. In addition, 1 of the following must be present: (1) temperature higher than 100.4°F, (2) endocervix positive for gram-negative intracellular diplococci, (3) leukocytosis greater than $10 \times 10^3/\mu L$, (4) inflammatory mass at ultrasonography or pelvic examination, or (5) white blood cells (WBCs) and bacteria in the peritoneal fluid.

○ **What percentage of patients with PID become infertile?**

10%

○ **When does ectopic pregnancy most commonly manifest?**

6 to 8 weeks into the pregnancy. Patients usually present with amenorrhea and sharp, generally unilateral abdominal or pelvic pain. Rupture of an ampullary ectopic pregnancy typically occurs at 8 to 12 weeks, allowing adequate time for early diagnosis and treatment before rupture in most cases. Isthmic ectopic pregnancies may rupture earlier at 6 to 8 weeks.

○ **What percentage of pregnancies are ectopic?**

1.5%. Ectopic pregnancies are the leading cause of death in the first trimester.

○ **What is the risk of a repeat ectopic pregnancy?**

10% to 15%

○ **What is the most common site of implantation in ectopic pregnancy?**

The ampulla of the fallopian tube (95%). Less common are ectopic pregnancies in the abdomen, uterine cornu, cervix, and ovary.

○ **What are the risk factors for ectopic pregnancy?**

Prior scarring of the fallopian tubes from infection (ie, PID or salpingitis), IUDs, a previous ectopic pregnancy, tubal ligation, sexually transmitted diseases, changes in circulating levels of hormones, use of fertility medications, and previous abdominal surgery

○ **How often is an adnexal mass found in women with ectopic pregnancy?**

Fifty percent of women with ectopic pregnancy have an adnexal mass at examination.

○ **How do hCG levels differ in women with ectopic pregnancies versus intrauterine pregnancies?**

In 85% of women with ectopic pregnancy, the hCG level is lower than expected.

○ **Which is most common sign of ectopic pregnancy at transvaginal ultrasonography: adnexal mass or absence of intrauterine pregnancy?**

The absence of intrauterine pregnancy at an hCG level higher than 2000 mIU/mL is highly predictive of ectopic pregnancy. An adnexal mass or gestational sac in the adnexal region is a less reliable finding and is not always seen early in ectopic pregnancies.

○ **Does the presence of a thick endometrial stripe at ultrasonography indicate intrauterine pregnancy?**

The endometrium can be thickened due to the hormonal stimulation associated with either ectopic or intrauterine pregnancy, so this is not a consistent sign of normal pregnancy

○ **Does the presence of a gestational sac always rule out an ectopic pregnancy?**

As many as 15% of women with ectopic pregnancy can have a pseudosac or fluid area (representing blood and mucus) within the uterine cavity. Therefore, it is critical with women at high risk for ectopic pregnancy to confirm intrauterine pregnancy with follow-up ultrasonography, which can be used to identify the yolk sac (double ring sign) or fetal pole within the gestational sac.

○ **What are the indications for laparotomy for treatment of ectopic pregnancy?**

Common indications for laparotomy include an unstable patient, large hemoperitoneum, cornual pregnancy, and lack of appropriate surgical tools for laparoscopy. Additionally, a large ectopic pregnancy (>6 cm) and fetal heart tones in the adenexa are also indications for laparotomy.

○ **Who is eligible for methotrexate treatment for ectopic pregnancy?**

Patients who are hemodynamically stable with unruptured gestations smaller than 4 cm in diameter at ultrasonography.

○ **What is the mode of action of methotrexate?**

Methotrexate is a folic acid antagonist.

○ **What criteria are used for ensuring the success of methotrexate?**

With single-dose therapy, the hCG levels should decrease by 15% between days 4 and 7 after therapy and continue to decrease weekly until undetectable.

○ **Why is the Rh status of a pregnant patient important?**

If the mother is Rh negative and the fetus is Rh positive, there is a risk of developing Rh isoimmunization and fetal anemia and hydrops, and fetal loss can result. Rh immunoglobulin should be administered in all Rh-negative patients. The standard dose of Rho(D) immune globulin is 300 mg.

○ **Should Rh-negative women with ectopic pregnancies receive Rho(D) immune globulin?**

Most experts recommend administration of a smaller dose of Rho(D) immune globulin (50 μg) with any failed pregnancy during the first 12 weeks, with administration of a full dose after 12 weeks.

○ **The standard 300-mg dose of Rho(D) immune globulin protects against how much fetomaternal hemorrhage?**

Approximately less than 30 mL of whole blood. After trauma, fetomaternal hemorrhage should always be considered. Rho(D) immune globulin can be administered as long as 14 days afterward.

○ **When can an intrauterine gestational sac be identified at abdominal ultrasonography?**

In the fifth week. A fetal pole can be identified in the sixth week, and an embryonic mass with cardiac motion can be identified in the seventh.

○ **What is the most common nongynecologic condition manifesting as lower abdominal pain?**

Appendicitis

○ **Is appendicitis more common during pregnancy?**

No. The rate is 1 in 850 pregnancies. However, the outcome is worse. Prompt diagnosis is important because the incidence of perforation increases from 10% in the first trimester to 40% in the third.

○ **How is the appendix displaced during pregnancy?**

Superiorly and laterally. Diagnosis of appendicitis in pregnant patients may be further complicated by the fact that a normal pregnancy can itself cause an increase in WBCs. The WBC count usually does not increase beyond the normal value of 12,000/μL to 15,000/μL. In a pregnant patient, pyuria with no bacteria suggests appendicitis. Pregnant patients may lack gastrointestinal (GI) distress, and fever may be absent or low grade.

○ **A patient presents with pain in her eyes, canker sores in her mouth, and sores and scars in her genital area. What is the diagnosis?**

Behcet disease. This is a rare disease involving ocular inflammation, oral aphthous ulcers, and destructive genital ulcers (generally on the vulva). No cure is known, but remission may occur with high estrogen levels.

○ **A patient who is 3 months pregnant presents to your office with pelvic pain. At examination, a retroverted and retroflexed uterus is found. What is the diagnosis?**

Incarceration of the uterus. Patients typically complain of rectal and pelvic pressure. Urinary retention may occur, and the knee-chest position or rectal pressure may correct the problem.

○ **What is Sheehan syndrome?**

Anterior pituitary necrosis after postpartum hemorrhage and hypotension. It results in amenorrhea, decreased breast size, and decreased pubic hair.

○ **What surgical treatment should be performed in patients with testicular feminization due to androgen insensitivity?**

The undescended testicles should be excised because of the increased risk of testicular cancer.

○ **What condition usually causes female pseudohermaphroditism?**

Congenital adrenal hyperplasia. The defective adrenal glands cannot produce normal amounts of cortisol. These patients have normal XX chromosomes, but an excess of endogenous adrenal steroids has virilizing effects.

○ **What causes toxic shock syndrome (TSS)?**

An exotoxin composed of certain strains of *Staphylococcus aureus*. Other organisms that cause TSS are group A streptococci, *Pseudomonas aeruginosa*, and *Streptococcus pneumoniae*. Tampons, IUDs, septic abortions, sponges, soft-tissue abscesses, osteomyelitis, nasal packing, and postpartum infections can all house these organisms.

○ **What dermatologic changes occur with TSS?**

Initially, the patient will have a blanching erythematous rash that lasts for 3 days; 10 days after the start of the infection, there will be a full-thickness desquamation of the palms and soles.

○ **What criteria are necessary to diagnose TSS?**

All of the following must be present: temperature higher than 102°F, rash, systolic blood pressure (BP) lower than 90 mm Hg with orthostasis, involvement of 3 organ systems (GI, renal, musculoskeletal, mucosal, hepatic, hematologic, or central nervous system), and negative serologic test results for diseases such as Rocky Mountain spotted fever, hepatitis B, measles, leptospirosis, and VDRL test.

○ **How should a patient with TSS be treated?**

Fluids, pressure support, fresh frozen plasma or transfusions, vaginal irrigation with iodine or saline, and antistaphylococcal penicillin or cephalosporin with anti-β-lactamase activity (nafcillin or oxacillin). Rifampin should be considered to eliminate the carrier state.

○ **What is the most common type of urinary fistula?**

Vesicovaginal fistulas. They most commonly occur after surgical procedures, but they can also occur with invasive cervical carcinoma or radiotherapy for cervical cancer.

○ **What is the most common cause of pelvic pain in an adolescent girl?**

Ovarian cysts

○ **What is the most common complication of ovarian cysts?**

Torsion of the ovary. Torsion is more common in small to medium cysts and tumors. Emergency surgery is required.

○ **What are the indications for performing dilation and curettage?**

- Removal of endometrial polyp or hydatidiform mole
- Termination of pregnancy or incomplete abortion
- Removal of retained placental tissue
- Relief of profuse uterine hemorrhage

○ **What major complication is associated with the performance of dilation and curettage?**

Perforation of the uterus

○ **What are the most common indications for hysterectomy?**

The most common indications were leiomyomata (26.8%), prolapse (20.8%), endometriosis (14.7%), cancer (10.7%), and endometrial hyperplasia (6.2%). The remaining 20.7% were performed for abnormal bleeding; diseases of the parametrium and pelvic peritoneum; infections and other diseases of the cervix, tubes, and ovaries; obstetric catastrophe; and other benign neoplasms.

○ **What is the correct terminology regarding hysterectomies (ie, total, subtotal, vaginal, and abdominal)?**

The word "hysterectomy" may be modified by the words "total" or "subtotal" to denote whether the cervix is removed or retained and by "vaginal" or "abdominal" to specify the route of removal. More recently, the nomenclature has been modified to include "laparoscopic hysterectomy" and "laparoscopic-assisted vaginal hysterectomy."

○ **What are the indications for cesarean hysterectomy?**

The most common indications are severe, life-threatening intrauterine infection; an unrepairable uterine scar; laceration of major uterine vessels; uterine atony unresponsive to oxytocin, prostaglandins, and massage; large leiomyomata; severe cervical dysplasia or early cervical cancer; and placenta accreta. Uterine rupture and uterine inversion may also require hysterectomy.

○ **What is the most frequent complication of hysterectomy?**

Infection. The most common organisms are those found in normal vaginal flora. Because the vagina is difficult to cleanse, most experts recommend antibiotic prophylaxis for all patients undergoing vaginal hysterectomy.

○ **What must be identified and located before clamping the infundibulopelvic ligament?**

The ureter

○ **What percentage of the female population has endometriosis?**

More than 15%. Seven percent of these women have it during their reproductive years.

○ **What is the most common site of endometriosis?**

The ovaries (60%)

○ **What is the drug of choice for treating endometriosis?**

Danazol

○ **What is a nabothian cyst?**

A mucous inclusion cyst of the cervix (usually asymptomatic and harmless)

○ **How long after the removal of implanted etonogestrel should patients wait to become pregnant?**

Ovulation usually occurs within 3 months.

○ **What chemical changes may predispose patients using OCP to weight gain?**

Increases in low-density lipoproteins, decreases in high-density lipoproteins, and sodium retention

○   **At what level of smoking does the risk of using OCP exceed the risks of having a baby for a 35-year-old woman?**

35 cigarettes per day. Women who smoke more than 15 cigarettes per day and are older than 35 years should not use OCP.

○   **How much is menstrual blood flow decreased by OCP use?**

By 60% or more. This results in fewer cases of iron-deficiency anemia.

○   **By how much is the incidence of functional cysts reduced by OCP use?**

80% to 90%. OCP use suppresses FSH and LH ovarian stimulation.

○   **For women using OCP for 4 years or fewer, what is their reduction in risk of ovarian cancer?**

30%. For 12 or more years of use, the risk is decreased by 80%.

○   **For women using OCP for at least 2 years, what is the reduction in risk of endometrial cancer?**

40%. This increases to 60% for 4 or more years of use.

○   **What are the estrogen-mediated adverse effects of OCP use?**

Headache, nausea, breast enlargement or tenderness, fluid retention, chloasma, and telangiectasia

○   **What are the progestin/androgen-mediated adverse effects of OCP use?**

Depression, fatigue, acne, oily skin, and increased appetite

○   **What is the incidence of venous thrombosis in OCP users?**

10 to 20 per 100,000 users

○   **How long do sperm stay in the vagina after coitus?**

At least 72 hours. However, sperm are motile for only 6 hours. When using a rape kit, it is important to test for acid phosphatase. This enzyme is present for 24 hours and confirms that ejaculation has occurred.

○   **How effective is breastfeeding alone in preventing pregnancy?**

98% for the first 6 months in women who have not resumed their menses and who breastfeed exclusively

○   **Are women more likely to gain or lose weight with OCP use?**

Both are equally likely. Rarely does OCP use cause a gain of 10 to 20 pounds or more.

○   **How does medroxyprogesterone acetate work?**

By suppressing FSH and LH levels and eliminating the LH surge, which inhibits ovulation

○   **What is the effect of progestin on the uterus?**

It results in a shallow atrophic endometrium and thick cervical mucus. These both result in decreased sperm transport.

○ **What is the average delay in return to fertility after cessation of medroxyprogesterone acetate?**

6 months to 1 year

○ **What is the risk of an ectopic pregnancy with an IUD in place?**

More than 5%

○ **How long after exposure can emergency oral contraception be administered?**

As long as 72 hours. It is most effective if initiated within 12 to 24 hours. Emergency contraception provides a 75% reduction in the risk of pregnancy. Patients should have negative pregnancy test results before treatment.

○ **What is the total dose of estrogen that should be used in emergency oral contraception?**

200 μg of ethinyl estradiol; 2 doses of 100 μg administered 12 hours apart

○ **What is the rationale for multiphasic OCP?**

A lower total dose of steroid is administered.

○ **What is the association between OCP use and gallbladder disease?**

They accelerate the development of symptoms without increasing the overall incidence of cholelithiasis.

○ **What effect does OCP use have on the risk of developing cervical cancer?**

OCP users as a group are at higher risk for cervical neoplasia. This increased risk may be secondary to sexual habits rather than OCP use itself.

○ **A 21-year-old woman requests counseling because she was using OCP without knowing she was pregnant. Should she abort the pregnancy?**

No. Results from recent studies indicate that exposure to progestins and estrogens (as in OCP) is not associated with any specific structural abnormalities in the exposed offspring. Results from earlier studies had indicated an increased incidence of a pattern of malformations called the vertebral, anal, cardiac, tracheoesophageal, renal, and radial (VACTERR) association, but these were retrospective studies that were later found to be inaccurate.

○ **What are the differences among spontaneous, threatened, incomplete, complete, and missed abortions?**

- Spontaneous abortion is loss of the fetus before the 20th week of gestation.
- Threatened abortion is uterine cramping or bleeding in the first 20 weeks of gestation without the passage of products of conception or cervical dilatation.
- Incomplete abortion is a partial abortion in which part of the products of conception are aborted and part remain within the uterus. The cervix is dilated at examination, and dilation and curettage is necessary to remove the remainder of tissue.
- Complete abortion is when all the products of conception have been passed, the cervix is closed, and the uterus is firm and nontender.
- Missed abortion is defined as no uterine growth, no cervical dilation, no passage of fetal tissue, and minimal cramping or bleeding. Diagnosis is made because of the absence of fetal heart tones and an empty sac at ultrasonography.

○ **What percentage of pregnancies result in spontaneous abortions?**

20% to 25%

○ **What is the most common cause of spontaneous abortion?**

Chromosomal abnormality or genetic defect (50%)

○ **How do spontaneous abortions most commonly manifest?**

Abdominal pain followed by vaginal bleeding

○ **Before what gestational age do most spontaneous abortions occur?**

8 to 9 weeks

○ **During spontaneous abortion, pain is most often midline and crampy. During ectopic pregnancy, pain is acute, unilateral, and severe. Does pain caused by threatened abortion occur before or after bleeding has begun?**

After

○ **Spontaneous labor will occur within 3 weeks after fetal death in what percentage of patients?**

80%. It may be helpful to induce labor with vaginal suppositories because of the psychological effects of carrying a dead fetus.

○ **What is the chance of spontaneous abortion once fetal cardiac activity is established at 8 weeks of gestation?**

3% to 5%

○ **Suction or vacuum curettage is used to terminate pregnancies at which gestational ages?**

7 to 13 weeks

○ **What is the most common cause of postabortal pain, bleeding, and low-grade fever?**

Retained gestational tissue or clot

○ **Name 3 independent risk factors for spontaneous abortion.**

1. Increasing parity
2. Maternal age
3. Paternal age

○ **What is the effect of smoking and drinking on the abortion rate?**

Those who smoke more than 14 cigarettes daily have a 1.7 times greater chance of spontaneous abortion. Those who drink ethanol at least 2 days a week have a twofold greater risk for spontaneous abortion.

○ **What percentage of American couples is infertile?**

15%. Twenty percent of women in the United States older than 35 years are infertile.

○ **What are the numbers for a normal semen analysis result?**

More than 1 mL in volume (>20,000,000 sperm) with more than 50% motility

○ **What percentage of infertility is due to male infertility?**

40%. Problems with the cervix, uterus, fallopian tubes, peritoneum, or ovulation account for the remaining 60%.

○ **Endometriosis is responsible for what percentage of infertility in women?**

25% to 50%

○ **Where is the most common site of endometriosis?**

The ovaries (60%). Other sites include the cul-de-sac, uterosacral ligaments, broad ligaments, fallopian tubes, uterovesical fold, round ligaments, vermiform appendix, vagina, rectosigmoid colon, cecum, and ileum.

○ **At what gestational age does hCG peak?**

8 to 10 weeks

○ **Name 4 physiologic actions of hCG.**

1. Maintenance of corpus luteum and continued progesterone production

2. Stimulation of fetal testicular testosterone secretion promoting male sexual differentiation

3. Stimulation of the maternal thyroid by binding to thyrotropin receptors

4. Promotion of relaxin secretion by the corpus luteum

○ **What secretes β-hCG? Why?**

Placental trophoblasts secrete β-hCG to maintain the corpus luteum, which in turn maintains the uterine lining. The corpus luteum is maintained through the sixth to eighth week of pregnancy, by which time the placenta begins to produce its own progesterone to maintain the endometrium.

○ **How soon after implantation can β-hCG be detected?**

2 to 3 days

○ **In a healthy pregnancy, how often does β-hCG double in the first 12 weeks?**

Every 72 hours

○ **True/False: During pregnancy, the uterus can grow to be 500 times its prepregnant capacity.**

True. The uterus can grow to be 1000 times its prepregnant capacity.

○ **A mother can feel fetal movement by which week of gestation?**

The 16th to 20th week

○ **When can one auscultate the fetal heart?**

Ultrasonography: 6 weeks
Doppler imaging: 10 to 12 weeks
Stethoscope: 18 to 20 weeks

○ **What WBC count is expected during pregnancy?**

WBC counts of 15,000/μL to 20,000/μL are considered normal during pregnancy.

○ **Why should pregnant women rest in the left lateral decubitus position?**

To avert supine hypotension syndrome due to compression of the inferior vena cava by the uterus

○ **Your 28-year-old pregnant patient expresses concerns about the ultrasonographic examination you have prescribed. How do you counsel her?**

Diagnostic ultrasonography is safe. Resonance (mechanical vibration of tissue) does not occur, and most of the sound energy is converted to heat that is distributed into the tissues. A safe level of tissue ultrasonographic exposure is equal to or greater than 100 mW/cm^2. Most commercial machines produce energies of 10 to 20 mW/cm^2, which is low. At present, there are no known examples of damage to target tissues from conventional usage.

○ **What is pica?**

Pica is a craving for eating nonfoods such as laundry starch and clay during pregnancy. If severe, it can result in nutritional deficiencies and anemia. The agent ingested also may be toxic to the developing fetus.

○ **What immunizations are contraindicated during pregnancy?**

In general, live virus vaccines are contraindicated during pregnancy. These include measles, mumps, rubella, oral polio, and varicella. On the other hand, all toxoids, immunoglobulins, and killed virus vaccines are considered safe during pregnancy and should not be withheld, if indicated.

○ **A progesterone level of 25 ng/mL or higher indicates what about a pregnancy?**

A viable uterine pregnancy. Serum progesterone is produced by the corpus luteum in the pregnant patient and remains constant for the first 8 to 10 weeks of pregnancy.

○ **Teenage pregnancies are associated with increased risks of what?**

Maternal complications such as gonorrhea, syphilis, toxemia, anemia, malnutrition, low birth weights, and perinatal mortality.

○ **When does the corpus luteum stop producing progesterone during pregnancy?**

7 to 8 weeks of gestation

○ **At what gestational age does the uterus rise out of the pelvis?**

About 12 weeks

○ **What are the normal physical changes in the cervix during pregnancy?**

Softening and cyanosis

○ **What are the changes in cervical mucus that occur during pregnancy?**

Thick tenacious mucus forms a plug blocking the cervical canal. Increased cervical and vaginal secretions result in thick, white, odorless discharge. The pH is between 3.5 and 6.0 because of increased production of lactic acid from the action of *Lactobacillus acidophilus*.

○ **What is the average weight gain in pregnancy?**

25 lbs. Only 30% of maternal weight gain is attributed to the placenta and fetus. Another 30% is attributed to blood, amniotic fluid, and extravascular fluid. Another 30% is attributed to maternal fat.

○ **In general terms, what is the physiology of the maternal immune system during pregnancy?**

Pregnancy represents a 50% allograft from the paternal contribution. As a result, there is a general suppression of immune function.

○ **What are the normal changes in the auscultative heart examination during pregnancy?**

Exaggerated split S1 with increased loudness of both components is heard, systolic ejection murmurs heard at the left sternal border are present in 90% of patients, soft and transient diastolic murmurs are heard in 20% of patients, and continuous murmurs from breast vasculature are heard in 10% of patients. The significance of murmurs during pregnancy must be carefully evaluated and clinically correlated. Harsh systolic murmurs and all diastolic murmurs should be taken seriously and worked up before being attributed to pregnancy.

○ **A pregnant patient complains that her contact lenses have become painful to wear. Is this normal?**

Yes. Corneal thickness increases during pregnancy and can cause discomfort in wearing lenses fitted before pregnancy.

○ **What is the most common presentation of twins?**

Vertex-vertex. If the first twin is vertex and the second breech, it is still possible to attempt a vaginal delivery because the extra space afforded after the birth of the first baby allows room to manipulate the position of the second.

○ **The average gestational age for singletons is 39 weeks. What is the average gestational age for twins?**

35 weeks. Prematurity is a large risk factor for respiratory distress syndrome. Half of perinatal deaths involving twins are due to respiratory distress syndrome.

○ **Describe the effect pregnancy has on (1) cardiac output, (2) BP, (3) heart rate, (4) coagulation, (5) sedimentation rate, (6) leukocyte levels, (7) blood volume, (8) tidal volume, (9) bladder position, (10) ratio of serum urea nitrogen to creatinine, and (11) GI function.**

    1. Cardiac output: Increases due to moving the uterus off of the inferior vena cava

    2. BP: Decreases during second trimester; returns to normal during third trimester

    3. Heart rate: Increases

    4. Coagulation: Factors VII, VIII, IX, and X and fibrinogen increase; others remain unchanged

    5. Sedimentation rate: Increases

    6. Leukocyte levels: Increase (as high as $18,000/\mu L$)

    7. Blood volume: Increases; no change in red blood cell count; dilutional anemia is physiologic

    8. Tidal volume: Increases 40%

    9. Bladder position: Displaces superiorly and anteriorly

    10. Ratio of serum urea nitrogen to creatinine: Decreases because of increased glomerular filtration rate and renal blood flow

    11. GI function: Gastric emptying and GI motility decrease; alkaline phosphatase level increases; peritoneal signs such as rigidity and rebound are diminished or absent

○ **What kind of changes occur in the cardiovascular system of a pregnant patient?**

Cardiac output increases by 30% during the first trimester and then by 50% during the second trimester, plasma volume increases 50%, pulse increases 12 to 18 beats per minute, systolic and diastolic BP decrease by 10 to 15 mm Hg during the second trimester and then gradually return to prepregnant levels during the third trimester, stroke volume increases 25%, and hematocrit level decreases because of hemodilution.

○ **When does labor begin?**

Labor begins with the onset of regular, rhythmic contractions that lead to serial dilatation and effacement of the cervix; thus, to say labor has begun, one must observe changes in the cervix. The presence of contractions alone does not qualify as the onset of labor.

○ **What are the 4 stages of labor and delivery?**

    1. First stage: Onset of labor to complete dilatation of the cervix

    2. Second stage: Cervical dilatation to birth

    3. Third stage: Birth to delivery of the placenta

    4. Fourth stage: Placenta delivery to stability of the mother (about 6 hours)

○ **How long is the average latent (First) phase of labor?**

In a nulliparous patient, the average is 6.4 hours; in the multiparous patient, the average is 4.8 hours.

○ **What are the 6 movements of delivery?**

1. Descent

2. Flexion

3. Internal rotation

4. Extension

5. External rotation

6. Expulsion

○ **How long may a patient push once the cervix is fully dilated?**

Provided that the fetal heart pattern is good and maternal expulsive forces remain effective, a second stage may last as long as 2 hours in the nulliparous patient; as long as 3 hours is appropriate if the patient has regional analgesia or anesthesia. Beyond these time limits, one sees an increase in fetal acidosis and lower Apgar scores, as well as a greater risk of maternal postpartum hemorrhage and febrile morbidity. In the nulliparous patient, the average second stage is approximately 40 minutes; in the multiparous patient, it is about 20 minutes

○ **What complications are seen with precipitous labor?**

There is a higher incidence of fetal trauma (intracranial hemorrhage and fractured clavicle) and long-term neurologic injury. The mother is at higher risk for pelvic lacerations and postpartum hemorrhage (including, somewhat paradoxically, from uterine atony.)

○ **What is effacement of the cervix?**

"Effacement" refers to the foreshortening and thinning of the cervix as it is drawn upward intraabdominally. It is usually expressed in percentages by which cervical length has been reduced: from 0% (uneffaced) to 100% (fully effaced).

○ **What agents may be used to ripen the cervix?**

Both chemical and physical agents have been used. Oxytocics, prostaglandins (especially prostaglandin E2), progesterone antagonists (mifepristone), and dehydroepiandrosterone are such pharmacologic agents. *Laminaria* and Foley catheter balloons are examples of physical dilators.

○ **What is oxytocin?**

Oxytocin is a decapeptide synthesized by the posterior pituitary gland. It is a powerful uterotonic agent; that is, it causes the uterus to contract. In nature, it is secreted in pulsatile fashion throughout labor. The fetus also produces oxytocin and at least some traverses the placenta, escaping enzymatic breakdown.

○ **What other uterotonic agents are there besides oxytocin?**

Vasopressin (antidiuretic hormone), prostaglandins (prostaglandin E2 and prostaglandin F2α), and thromboxane are natural oxytocics. Ergot alkaloids (eg, methylergonovine maleate) and the synthetic prostaglandin 15-methyl prostaglandin F2α are used clinically to increase uterine contractions, especially for postpartum uterine atony.

○ **Does epidural analgesia affect the course of labor?**

Study results have shown that epidural analgesia does not slow the progress of labor during the first stage. However, the second stage of labor appears to be prolonged an average of 20 to 25 minutes. There is no evidence that this prolongation is harmful to the fetus.

○ **What is a "walking epidural?"**

An intrathecal opioid or epidural opioid plus an ultralow dose of local anesthetic, followed by continuous infusion of opioid and local anesthetics, for labor analgesia. These regimens cause no or minimal motor block on the lower extremities and allow the mother to ambulate in the early first stage of labor.

○ **What is the first step in evaluation of a protraction or arrest disorder of labor?**

Assess fetopelvic size. If disproportion is suspected, augmentation should not be undertaken.

○ **What pelvic type is the most common in women?**

Gynecoid. Approximately 50% of women are estimated to have this type of pelvis. In reality, most women have intermediate pelvic shapes rather than true gynecoid, anthropoid, android, or platypelloid shapes.

○ **What is the average gestational age at delivery for twins, triplets, and quadruplets?**

- Twins: 35 to 37 weeks
- Triplets: 33 to 34 weeks
- Quadruplets: 30 to 31 weeks
- 3 or more fetuses reduced to twins: 35 to 36 weeks

○ **At term, what percentage of fetuses are in vertex presentation?**

95%

○ **What is the greatest risk for breech presentation?**

Prematurity. Most breech fetuses at 28 weeks are cephalic by term.

○ **What are the 3 types of breech presentation?**

1. Frank breech: Thighs flexed, legs extended
2. Complete breech: At least 1 leg flexed
3. Incomplete (footling) breech: At least 1 foot below the buttocks, with both thighs extended

○ **What is the most common breech position?**

Frank breech

○ **What is the modified Ritgen maneuver?**

The modified Ritgen maneuver describes the elevation of the fetal chin achieved by placement of the delivering hand between the maternal coccyx and perineal body, while the other hand guides the crowning vertex. This technique assists in extension of the fetal head and allows the obstetrician to control delivery.

○ **What are high forceps, midforceps, and low forceps deliveries?**
- High forceps: Use of forceps when a baby is not yet in the birth canal (rarely used)
- Midforceps: Baby in the birth canal and within reach (used in cases of fetal distress)
- Low forceps: Refers to the outlet and is used when the baby's head is at the pelvic floor (most often used to shorten labor when the mother is tiring or to control normal labor)

○ **What is the most common cause of a prolonged active phase of labor?**
Cephalopelvic disproportion caused by contraction of a narrowed midpelvis

○ **What is the immediate treatment for cord prolapse?**
Displace the head cephalad

○ **How can ruptured membranes be diagnosed?**
Nitrazine paper will turn blue and a ferning pattern will be seen under the microscope in the presence of amniotic fluid. Also, look for pooling of amniotic fluid in the posterior fornix.

○ **Describe the different types of perineal tears that can occur with delivery.**
- First degree: Perineal skin or vaginal mucosa
- Second degree: Submucosa of vagina or perineum
- Third degree: Anal sphincter
- Fourth degree: Rectal mucosa

○ **What are the advantages of mediolateral episiotomy?**
Mediolateral episiotomy allows for greater room without lacerating the external anal sphincter or rectum. However, these episiotomies are associated with greater blood loss and postpartum pain and greater likelihood for suboptimal healing and subsequent dyspareunia.

○ **What are the advantages of midline (median) episiotomy?**
This type is easier to repair, is associated with less blood loss, usually heals better (less postpartum discomfort and better cosmetic result), and is associated with less subsequent dyspareunia. The principal disadvantage to such an episiotomy, compared to a mediolateral episiotomy, is a greater propensity to extend into the external anal sphincter or rectum.

○ **What effect on the bony pelvis does the McRoberts maneuver have?**
This maneuver, which consists of maximal maternal hip flexion onto her abdomen, results in a straightening of the sacrum relative to the lumbar vertebrae and ventral rotation of the pubic symphysis and maternal pelvis. This may increase the size of the posterior outlet thus allowing easier disimpaction of the anterior fetal shoulder.

○ **How common is shoulder dystocia?**
Although reports vary from 0.15% to 1.7%, most accept a rate of 1 in 100 to 1 in 200. However, this complication is clearly weight dependent. The risk is approximately 0.2% if the fetus weighs 2500 to 3000 g but increases to about 10% if the fetus is between 4000 and 5000 g and as much as 20% if the fetus weighs more than 4500 g. In diabetic patients, these latter weight-associated risks are approximately doubled. Permanent neurologic damage results in 1% to 3% of cases.

○ **What are risk factors for shoulder dystocia?**

Diabetes, maternal obesity, postterm delivery, and excessive maternal weight gain. Intrapartum risk factors include a prolonged second stage of labor, oxytocin use (augmentation or induction), and midforceps deliveries.

○ **What percentage of women can have vaginal births after low transverse incision cesarean sections?**

75%. Vaginal birth is contraindicated after a classic cesarean section.

○ **What is the average blood loss for vaginal delivery and for cesarean section?**

400 to 600 mL for vaginal delivery and 800 to 1000 mL for cesarean section

○ **Why is rapid cesarean delivery an important part of maternal resuscitation?**

- Removing the fetus relieves aortocaval compression.
- With uterine contraction after delivery, some blood may enter the circulation and may help increase venous return.
- Cardiac output produced by chest compression may be more adequate without the fetus.

○ **How long after delivery should a postpartum tubal ligation be performed? Why?**

It is common practice to wait 8 to 12 hours post partum before inducing anesthesia for tubal ligation. This interval is useful to allow the patient to reach cardiovascular stability and increase the likelihood of gastric emptying.

○ **How can fetal lung maturity be assessed?**

Ratio of lecithin to sphingomyelin. If the ratio of lecithin to sphingomyelin is greater than 2:1, then the fetal lungs are mature.

○ **What is the normal fetal heart rate?**

120 to 160 beats per minute. If bradycardia is detected, position the mother on her left side and administer oxygen and an intravenous (IV) fluid bolus.

○ **Are accelerations in fetal heart rate normal?**

Yes and no. Rapid heart rate can indicate fetal distress, whereas 2 accelerations every 20 minutes are normal. An acceleration must be at least 15 beats per minute above baseline and last at least 15 seconds.

○ **What causes variable decelerations?**

Transient umbilical cord compression, which often changes with maternal position

○ **A baby is born with a pink body, blue extremities, and a heart rate of 60 beats per minute. She is mildly irritable (grimaces) and has weak respiration and no muscle tone. What is this child's Apgar score?**

$1 + 1 + 1 + 1 + 0 = 4$

Apgar Points	0	1	2
Color	Blue	Extremities blue	All pink
Heart rate	None	Less than 100 beats per minute	More than 100 beats per minute
Irritability	None	Mild grimace	Strongly irritable
Respiratory effort	None	Weak	Cry
Muscle tone	Flaccid	Weak	Strong

○ **What is the puerperium?**

The puerperium refers to the time just after birth and lasts about 6 weeks. It is the time it takes the uterus to return to the nonpregnant state.

○ **How common are postpartum blues?**

Fifty percent to 70% of mothers will have postpartum blues.

○ **How common is postpartum depression?**

Only 4% to 10% of mothers will have true postpartum depression.

○ **What happens if some placenta or fetal membranes are left inside the uterus?**

Retained tissue or products of conception may lead to postpartum hemorrhage and also increases the risk of postpartum endometritis.

○ **What is lochia?**

Lochia refers to the uterine discharge that follows delivery. It consists of necrotic decidua, blood, inflammatory cells, and bacteria. This discharge lasts about 5 weeks.

○ **When does ovulation resume post partum?**

In nonlactating women, ovulation may occur as early as 27 days post partum. The average is 10 weeks. In women exclusively breastfeeding, ovulation may be delayed for the duration of active breastfeeding, although the mean is 6 months.

○ **Why is the risk of a thromboembolic event increased post partum?**

Although immediate platelet count changes are variable, there is clearly an increase by 2 weeks. Fibrinogen levels remain high for at least 1 week, as do factors VII, VIII, IX, and X. In addition, there is clearly greater vessel trauma and less mobility.

○   **How does colostrum differ from breast milk?**

Colostrum is more cellular and has more minerals but is lower in calories. True milk has more fat and carbohydrate (especially lactose) but less protein.

○   **When does breast milk production typically begin?**

Colostrum secretion usually persists for 3 to 4 days after which the fluid begins to change in composition. Mature milk is usually present by 1 to 2 weeks post partum.

○   **How many extra calories above baseline does a woman need when breastfeeding?**

About 500 calories per day

○   **How much daily dietary calcium intake is recommended for lactating women?**

1200 to 1500 mg/d

○   **Why does lactation not occur during pregnancy even though prolactin levels are elevated?**

The receptor sites in the breast are competitively bound by estrogen and progesterone, preventing prolactin from activating lactation. When the placenta is delivered, these levels of estrogen and progesterone rapidly decrease, and prolactin floods the receptors.

○   **What is the proper postpartum care for a mother who chooses not to breastfeed?**

A firmly fitting (but not binding) bra, ice packs as needed, and decreased stimulation to the nipples such as loose clothes rubbing across the breast or direct contact from a shower. Pharmacologic suppression is frequently ineffective because it is improperly prescribed and/or used. Bromocriptine is no longer indicated because of severe maternal adverse effects and should not be prescribed. Use of 35 μg or higher OCP within 2 weeks after delivery may inhibit lactation in some women and may be of use in decreasing milk production.

○   **A 2-week-old infant cries and wants to be put to the breast every 1 to 2 hours around the clock. After 5 minutes at the breast, he falls asleep, so the mother puts him down. She is now exhausted and thinking of bottle-feeding. What can you do to save this breastfeeding experience? What is wrong?**

This mother needs information, guidance, and reassurance. Her infant is not nursing long enough with each episode. The infant is receiving only the foremilk, which is high in proteins, carbohydrates, and water. He falls asleep before getting the hindmilk, which is high in fat and satiates the appetite and takes longer to digest. This infant should be stimulated when he dozes off, changed to the opposite breast, and not put down immediately. If this fails, the mother can pump or express the hindmilk at that time, and it can be given by another caregiver later so the mother can rest. This process is only a temporary measure because decreased contact time at the breast will ultimately lead to decreased milk production.

○   **All vitamins are found in human breast milk except which one?**

Vitamin K. This is why vitamin K is administered in newborns. Formula is also deficient in vitamin K.

○   **How does human milk differ from bovine milk?**

Although the 2 are similar in calories, human milk has more lactose, less protein (and different protein constitution), and slightly more fat (especially more polyunsaturated fatty acids and cholesterol, which are needed for brain development). There is significantly more calcium, phosphorous, and iron in bovine milk.

○ **A breastfeeding mother presents to your office complaining of fever, chills, and a swollen red breast. What is the most likely causative organism?**

S aureus is the most common cause of mastitis. Mastitis is seldom present in the first week post partum. It is most often seen 3 to 4 weeks post partum.

○ **What is the treatment for the above patient?**

Warm compresses to the breast, analgesics, and dicloxacillin or a penicillinase-resistant cephalosporin

○ **Can a breastfeeding mother with mastitis continue to breastfeed?**

Yes, as long as there is no abscess formation. Nursing facilitates the drainage of the infection, and the infant will not be harmed because he or she is already colonized.

○ **What postpartum immunizations are part of standard care?**

Rubella and rubeola immunizations should be administered in all susceptible postpartum women. In theory, diphtheria and tetanus toxoid boosters may also be administered if indicated. The nonisoimmunized Rh-negative patient should also receive Rho(D) immune globulin if her child is Rh positive.

○ **When may coitus resume after delivery?**

Most physicians instruct their patients to abstain from coitus for 6 weeks. From a physiologic standpoint, once uterine involution and perineal healing are complete, coitus may resume.

○ **What factors predispose one to uterine atony?**

Fetal macrosomia, polyhydramnios, abnormal labor progress, amnionitis, oxytocin stimulation, and multiple gestations

○ **What are the common signs of uterine rupture?**

Fetal distress, unrelenting pain, hypotension, tachycardia, and vaginal bleeding. Fetal distress is usually the first sign of uterine rupture.

○ **What causes uterine rupture?**

Oxytocin stimulation, cephalopelvic disproportion, grand multiparity, abdominal trauma, prior hysterotomy, cesarean section, myotomy, curettage, or manual removal of the placenta

○ **What 2 findings at physical examination indicate uterine rupture?**

1. Loss of uterine contour
2. Palpable fetal part

○ **What is the number 1 risk factor for uterine rupture?**

Previous cesarean section

○ **How should a diagnostic peritoneal lavage be performed in a pregnant patient?**

Use an open supraumbilical approach. Always make sure a nasogastric tube and Foley catheter are in place.

○   **What does painless third trimester vaginal bleeding likely represent?**

Placenta previa

○   **What does painful third trimester vaginal bleeding likely represent?**

Placenta abruptio

○   **Describe the appearance of placenta previa.**

Painless, bright red vaginal bleeding

○   **Describe the appearance of placenta abruptio.**

Painful, dark red vaginal bleeding

○   **What physical examination findings may be discovered with placenta abruptio?**

Rapidly increasing fundal height secondary to bleeding into the uterus or a higher than expected fundal height

○   **What is the difference between placenta previa and placenta abruptio.**

Placenta previa is the implantation of the placenta in the lower uterine segment thus covering the cervical os. Manifestation is painless vaginal bleeding with a soft nontender uterus. Placenta abruptio is the premature separation of the placenta from the uterine wall. Placenta abruptio causes painful uterine bleeding. Both are complications of the third trimester of pregnancy.

○   **A patient presents in her third trimester of pregnancy complaining of vaginal bleeding but no pain or contractions. What is the diagnosis?**

Use transabdominal ultrasonography. Because 95% of cases of placenta previa can be diagnosed this way, vaginal examination should be avoided until placenta previa has been ruled out by means of ultrasonography. Placenta abruptio is generally accompanied by pain, shock, or an expanding uterus and is not easily diagnosed at ultrasonography.

○   **What are the risk factors for placenta previa?**

Previous cesarean section, previous placenta previa, multiparity, multiple induced abortions, maternal age older than 40 years, and multiple gestations

○   **What causes dependent and nondependent edema in pregnant women?**

Compression of veins by the growing uterus causes dependent edema, whereas hypoalbuminemia can cause nondependent edema.

○ **Name 7 risk factors for placenta abruptio.**

1. Smoking
2. Trauma
3. Cocaine
4. Hypertension
5. Ethanol
6. Premature rupture of membranes
7. Retroplacental fibroids

○ **Why is ephedrine usually the first choice to treat maternal hypotension?**

Ephedrine does not produce significant uterine vascular constriction, so it does not decrease uterine blood flow.

○ **What viral or protozoal infections require extensive workup during pregnancy?**

ToRCH
Toxoplasma gondii
Rubella
Cytomegalovirus
Herpes genitalis

○ **True/False: According to results from some studies, highly active antiretroviral therapy initiated at 14 weeks of pregnancy can reduce the risk of transmission of human immunodeficiency virus to the fetus to less than 1%.**

True

○ **A patient presents 3 days post partum with a fever, malaise, and lower abdominal pain. At examination, a foul lochia and tender, boggy uterus are present. What is the diagnosis?**

Endometritis. This typically occurs 1 to 3 days post partum. The mechanism of infection is thought to be from ascending cervicovaginal flora.

○ **Is endometritis more common after vaginal delivery or after cesarean section?**

The rate of endometritis is 5 to 10 times greater after cesarean section.

○ **What is the treatment for endometritis?**

Admission and IV broad-spectrum antibiotics

○ **What are the most common causes of immediate postpartum hemorrhage?**

Uterine atony, followed by vaginal or cervical lacerations and retained placenta or placental fragments

○ **What is routinely performed to decrease the risk of postpartum hemorrhage?**

Uterine massage and oxytocin administration. Lacerations are sutured. In severe cases, if bleeding cannot be stopped, the hypogastric vessels are ligated or hysterectomy is performed.

○ **What are some common causes of polyhydramnios?**

Maternal causes include diabetes, Rh incompatibility, and other hematologic diseases. Fetal causes are anencephaly, duodenal atresia, tracheoesophageal fistula, and pulmonary disorders.

○ **What are the baseline congenital anomaly risks in the general population?**

Regardless of family history or teratogenic exposure, the background risk for major congenital anomalies is 3% to 5%. These include abnormalities that, if uncorrected, affect the health of the individual. Some examples are pyloric stenosis, cleft lip and palate, and neural tube defects. The background rate for minor congenital anomalies is 7% to 10%. These include anomalies such as strabismus, polydactyly, and misshapen ears. If uncorrected, they do not significantly affect the health of the individual.

○ **Which women today are most at risk for mercury poisoning?**

Fish eaters. The only real human exposure to organic mercury is through consumption of fish, primarily from predatory fish such as the shark, swordfish, pike, and bass. Fish consumption by pregnant women should be limited to 350 g/wk. Fetuses are more susceptible to the toxic effects of mercury than are their mothers. Large exposures to methyl mercury have resulted in infants with microcephaly, mental retardation, cerebral palsy, and blindness.

○ **Is working as a medical resident harmful during pregnancy?**

Overall, residency training has not been shown to cause spontaneous abortion, preterm birth, or low birth weight. However, results from 1 study of women working more than 100 h/wk indicated that preterm births increased. Mild preeclampsia that was not associated with adverse pregnancy outcome also increased in women residents.

○ **How does cocaine adversely affect pregnancy?**

Cocaine is especially toxic during pregnancy. The most common complication caused by cocaine during pregnancy is placenta abruptio, which may result in fetal death. In addition, brain anomalies, intestinal atresia, and limb reduction defects have been described. Investigators have also reported increases in congenital heart defects in exposed infants. Cocaine may cause these effects by means of vasoconstriction and subsequent infarction.

○ **Is methadone as bad for pregnancy as cocaine is?**

No. Methadone is not nearly as bad as cocaine. In 1 study in which investigators compared women who abused cocaine with women being treated with methadone, they found a much higher complication rate in the cocaine-abuse group. Methadone is not thought to be a teratogen.

○ **What are the signs and symptoms of fetal alcohol syndrome?**

Infants have intrauterine growth restriction and mental retardation, and they develop a characteristic facies that consists of short palpebral fissures, flat midface, thin upper lip, and hypoplastic philtrum. Ethanol abuse is the most common preventable cause of mental retardation during pregnancy.

○ **At what time during gestation is the fetus most susceptible to ethanol toxicity?**

Probably in the second and third trimesters. In a study of 60 women, those who were heavy drinkers but stopped after the first trimester had children with normal mentation and behavioral patterns.

○ **In general, which time during pregnancy is the fetus most susceptible to teratogens?**

During the embryonic period, which lasts from 2 to 8 weeks after conception. This is the time of organogenesis.

○ **What are the major adverse effects of smoking during pregnancy?**

Smoking causes intrauterine growth restriction and increases the incidence of preterm delivery in a dose-dependent manner. The incidence of placenta previa, placenta abruptio, and spontaneous abortion also appears to be increased by smoking.

○ **Folic acid deficiency is associated with what in pregnancy?**

Folate deficiency is associated with neural tube defects (ie, spina bifida, anencephaly).

○ **What is the neonatal abstinence syndrome, and what agents cause it?**

It is caused by maternal heroin addiction or maternal methadone treatment during pregnancy. It results from neonatal withdrawal and consists of tremulousness, hyperreflexia, high-pitched cry, sneezing, sleepiness, tachypnea, yawning, sweating, fever, and seizures. The onset of symptoms is at birth.

○ **What are the drug-labeling categories for use during pregnancy?**

The US Food and Drug Administration lists 5 categories of labeling:

- Category A: The drug is safe for use during pregnancy.
- Category B: Results from animal studies have demonstrated the drug's safety, and results from human studies do not reveal any adverse fetal effects.
- Category C: The drug is a known animal teratogen, but no data are available about human use; or there are no data in either humans or animals.
- Category D: There is positive evidence of human fetal toxicity, but benefits in selected situations makes use of the drug acceptable despite its risks.
- Category X: The drug is a definite human and animal teratogen and should not be used during pregnancy.

○ **What are the benefits of antepartum corticosteroids in premature babies?**

Increased lung compliance, increased surfactant production, and less respiratory distress syndrome; less intraventricular hemorrhage; less necrotizing enterocolitis; less neonatal mortality

○ **When is the critical period of organogenesis?**

Between 15 and 56 days of gestation, or day 31 to day 71 after the first day of the last menstrual period

○ **What radiation dose increases the risk of inhibited fetal growth?**

10 rad. Typical abdominal and pelvic radiography delivers 100 to 350 mrad. Shielded chest radiography should deliver less than 10 mrad to the fetus. Do not withhold necessary radiography.

○ **Can iodinated radiodiagnostic agents be used in pregnant patients?**

No. They should be avoided because concentration in the fetal thyroid gland can cause permanent loss of thyroid function. Nuclear medicine scanning, pulmonary angiography with pelvic shielding, and impedance plethysmography are preferred.

○ **What are the indications for cardiotocographic monitoring in a pregnant trauma patient?**

All women past 20 weeks of gestation with indirect or direct abdominal trauma require 4 hours of monitoring. Loss of beat-to-beat variability, uterine contractions, or fetal bradycardia or tachycardia demands immediate obstetric care.

○ **What percentage of pregnant women get morning sickness?**

50% to 70%. It generally occurs in the first trimester.

○ **How should morning sickness be treated?**

Frequent small meals, carbohydrates, and IV hydration and antiemetics

○ **What is hyperemesis gravidarum?**

Excessive vomiting during pregnancy that results in starvation (ketonuria), dehydration, and acidosis

○ **Define pregnancy-induced hypertension.**

An increase in the systolic pressure greater than 30 mm Hg or an increase in diastolic pressure greater than 15 mm Hg over baseline, measured on 2 separate occasions at least 6 hours apart.

○ **Define preeclampsia.**

Hypertension (ie, systolic pressure >160 mm Hg or diastolic pressure >110 mm Hg) and proteinuria occurring most commonly in the last trimester of pregnancy (after 20 weeks estimated gestational age). In severe cases, patients can have edema, oliguria, headache, visual acuity changes, abdominal pain, pulmonary edema, thrombocytopenia and elevated liver function test results, and intrauterine growth retardation.

○ **Who is more likely to have preeclampsia; primiparous or multiparous women?**

Primiparous women. Other risk factors include pregnancies associated with a large placenta, patients with a history of hypertension, renal disease, family history of preeclampsia, being older, having multiple gestations, and prior vascular disease.

○ **What medications should be used to treat preeclampsia and eclampsia?**

Magnesium and hydralazine

○ **How should hydralazine be dosed for preeclampsia?**

Hydralazine should be administered in 5-mg boluses every 20 minutes until adequate BP control is achieved or a total of 20 mg is reached.

○   **What are the signs and symptoms of preeclampsia?**

Upper abdominal pain, headache, visual complaints, cardiac decompensation, creatinine level greater than 2 mg/dL, proteinuria greater than 100 mg /dL, and BP greater than 160 mm Hg systolic or 110 mm Hg diastolic. Preeclampsia is most common in nulliparous women late in pregnancy, typically after 20 weeks of gestation. Look for edema, hypertension, and proteinuria to diagnose preeclampsia.

The emergency department treatment for preeclampsia is IV hydralazine titrated to diastolic BP of 90 to 110 mm Hg by using 5-mg boluses every 20 to 30 minutes. BP must be lowered slowly to avoid compromising the uteroplacental blood flow. Patients with moderate to severe preeclampsia need IV magnesium (though its true usefulness is not well demonstrated).

○   **Should BP be lowered quickly in a preeclampsia patient?**

No. Dangerous hypertension (>170/110 mm Hg) should be lowered gradually with hydralazine, 10 mg IV followed by IV drip. Definitive treatment for preeclampsia and eclampsia is delivery.

○   **How long should treatment continue after delivery in a woman with preeclampsia?**

24 hours. The cure for preeclampsia is delivery. Antihypertensive and antiseizure medications (IV magnesium sulfate) should be continued until there is no longer a risk to the mother.

○   **Define eclampsia.**

Preeclampsia plus grand mal seizures or coma

○   **What does HELLP stand for?**

Hemolysis, elevated liver enzymes, and low platelet levels. The HELLP syndrome is a severe form of preeclampsia. Signs and symptoms include right upper quadrant pain or tenderness, nausea, vomiting, edema, jaundice, GI bleeding, and hematuria, in addition to the symptoms of preeclampsia.

○   **What is the major cause of death in women with eclampsia?**

Intracranial hemorrhage

○   **What are the warning signs of impending seizure in a patient with preeclampsia?**

Headache, visual disturbances, hyperreflexia, and abdominal pain

○   **What is the treatment for eclampsia?**

Delivery. Until you are able to deliver the baby, you can use magnesium sulfate, diazepam, and hydralazine. Phenytoin can be used for seizures resistant to magnesium therapy.

○   **At what point does magnesium become toxic?**

Respiratory arrest occurs at levels higher than 12 mEq/L. Loss of reflexes occurs at levels higher than 8 mEq/L and can therefore be used as a treatment guide.

○   **What is the antidote for magnesium toxicity?**

Calcium gluconate (1-g IV push). Magnesium should be stopped if deep tendon reflexes disappear.

○ **What are the risk factors for placenta abruptio?**

Smoking, hypertension, multiparity, trauma, and previous placenta abruptio

○ **What are the presenting signs and symptoms of placenta abruptio?**

Placental separation before delivery is associated with vaginal bleeding (78%) and abdominal pain (66%), as well as with tetanic uterine contractions, uterine irritability, and fetal death.

○ **What is the most likely diagnosis in a patient whose uterus is larger than expected from the history of gestation, has vaginal bleeding, and passes grapelike tissue from the vagina?**

Hydatidiform mole

○ **A patient presents to your office for a regular prenatal checkup. She is in the first trimester of pregnancy. You note that she has a BP of 160/94 mm Hg. What is the probable diagnosis?**

Hypertension in the first half of pregnancy indicates hydatidiform mole. Patients most commonly complain of painless vaginal bleeding. The uterus is enlarged; no fetal heart tones are present. Theca lutein cysts are visible at ultrasonography. The growths should be removed by means of suction curettage. The patient should be treated weekly with β-hCG titers to ensure there is no remaining tissue or distant metastasis.

○ **Is the hCG level high or low in a molar pregnancy?**

High

○ **With what endocrine abnormalities are moles and other gestational trophoblastic neoplasms associated?**

Hyperthyroidism

○ **Describe the characteristics of an invasive mole.**

Invasive moles are pathologically similar to complete hydatidiform moles but invade beyond the normal placentation site into the myometrium. Penetration into the venous system can result in venous metastases to the lower genital tract and lungs.

○ **Describe the characteristics of gestational choriocarcinoma.**

Gestational choriocarcinomas contain both cytotrophoblastic and syncytiotrophoblastic elements. Chorionic villi are absent but, if present, represent an invasive molar pregnancy. Gestational choriocarcinomas readily invade the maternal venous system, producing metastasis by means of hematogenous dissemination. Metastases tend to outgrow their blood supply, resulting in central necrosis and often massive hemorrhage.

○ **How does age influence the incidence of hydatidiform moles?**

Compared with women aged 25 to 29 years, women older than 50 years have a 300- to 400-fold increase in risk, and girls younger than 15 years have a sixfold increase. Similarly, increased paternal age (older than 45 years) also confers an increased risk of a complete molar pregnancy, although the increase is only 4.9 times (2.9 when adjusted for maternal age).

○ **Why is induction of labor with oxytocin or prostaglandins not recommended for the evacuation of molar pregnancies?**

Uterine contraction against an undilated cervix theoretically has an increased risk for the dissemination of trophoblasts throughout the systemic circulation.

○ **What is the leading type of cancer in women?**

Breast cancer (32%)

○ **What is the leading cause of cancer deaths in women?**

Lung cancer. Breast cancer is second.

○ **What is the most common type of benign breast tumor?**

Fibroadenoma. These are usually solitary, mobile masses with distinct borders. They are more prevalent in women younger than 30 years.

○ **A 53-year-old woman presents with a hard, barely palpable lump in the upper, outer quadrant of her left breast. The lump is mobile and causes no pain. The patient has noted blood oozing from her nipple. What is the probable diagnosis?**

Benign intraductal papilloma. Intraductal papillomas are the most common cause of bleeding from the nipple. Growths usually develop just before or during menopause, and they are rarely palpable.

○ **Are most breast cancers in the ducts or in the lobes?**

Invasive ductal tumors account for 90% of all breast cancers. Only 10% are lobular.

○ **What is the most common invasive ductal tumor?**

Nonspecific infiltrating ductal carcinoma

○ **What are the American Cancer Society's 1996 recommendations for when to perform mammography?**

Every 1 to 2 years after age 40 years; annually after age 50 years

○ **What are the risk factors for breast cancer, and how do they compare with the risk factors for endometrial cancer?**

Risk factors for both cancers include nulliparity; early menarche; late menopause; significant amounts of unopposed estrogen; and prior ovarian, endometrial, or breast cancer. Unopposed estrogen is a much greater risk in endometrial cancer than in breast cancer. Risk factors specific to breast cancer include family history, being older than 40 years, high fat intake, radiation of the breast, or cellular atypia in fibrocystic disease.

○ **Geographically, where is breast cancer most common?**

North America and northern Europe have an incidence and mortality rate 5 times that of most Asian and African countries. However, although Asians and Africans who immigrate to North America or northern Europe maintain a lower rate of incidence, their offspring quickly assume a higher rate, which indicates the importance of environmental and dietary factors.

○ **What is the surgical treatment of choice for breast cancer?**

Modified radical mastectomy: removal of the breast tissue, pectoralis minor, and axilla. Radical mastectomy includes the pectoralis major. For small primary tumors, partial mastectomy may be performed. This procedure is local lumpectomy with axillary node dissection and postoperative irradiation of the breast. It has not been shown whether radiation after modified radical mastectomy affects survival.

○ **Who has higher incidences of estrogen receptor-positive tumors: premenopausal women or postmenopausal women?**

Postmenopausal women (60%). If the tumors are both estrogen and progesterone sensitive, then the antiestrogen drug tamoxifen is 80% effective. Otherwise, it is 40% to 50% effective.

○ **What is the most accurate prognostic indicator of breast cancer?**

Axillary node involvement, which is related to the size of the tumor, not the location. Forty percent to 50% of patients have axillary node involvement when the cancer is diagnosed.

○ **A patient presents with crusty erosion of the nipple and no discharge. What is the possible diagnosis?**

Paget disease. This rare cancer occurs in 3% of breast cancer patients. It involves the excretory ducts of the breast.

○ **What is peau d'orange?**

French for "skin of the orange," it is the dimpling and thickening of the breast in breast cancer.

○ **What are the American Cancer Society's recommendations for when to perform Pap smear screening?**

Pap smear screening should be performed annually for 3 years starting at age 18 or when the patient becomes sexually active and every 1 to 3 years thereafter.

○ **Is there an increased risk of breast cancer associated as hormone and estrogen replacement therapy?**

There may be a slightly increased risk of breast cancer especially with long duration of use (10 or more years).

○ **What neoplastic marker is associated with ovarian cancer?**

Cancer antigen 125

○ **What is the treatment for stage IA or IB ovarian cancer?**

Surgical excision alone (abdominal hysterectomy and bilateral salpingo-oophorectomy)

○ **What is the treatment for all other stages of ovarian cancer?**

Surgical resection followed by adjuvant chemotherapy or radiation

○ **If a woman has ascites, what is the most likely tumor to be found?**

Ovarian carcinoma. This is part of Meigs syndrome.

○ **What is Meigs syndrome?**

Ascites in the presence of an ovarian tumor

○ **The squamocolumnar junction is the junction between the columnar epithelium and the squamous epithelium, and it moves progressively throughout a woman's life. Where does it move, and why is this area important?**

This junction moves closer to the endocervical canal. The squamous epithelium of the ectocervix and the vagina invades the columnar epithelium of the endocervix. This is called the "transformation zone," and it is this squamous epithelium that is most likely to become dysplastic.

○ **What are the risk factors for carcinoma of the cervix?**
- Multiple sexual partners
- Early age at first intercourse
- Early first pregnancy

○ **Most cervical cancers are of what type?**

Eighty percent are squamous cell and arise from the squamocolumnar junction of the cervix.

○ **When performing radical hysterectomy for cervical cancer, is it also necessary to perform oophorectomy?**

No. Early cervical cancer rarely spreads to the ovaries.

○ **How effective has Pap smear screening been in reducing the incidence of cervical cancer?**

Since the development of cytologic screening in the 1940s, the incidence of cervical cancer in the United States has decreased by almost 80%. In contrast, cervical cancer remains a major cause of cancer-related deaths among women in many poorer countries where Pap smear screening is not routinely performed.

○ **What is the most common presenting symptom in patients with cervical cancer?**

As many as 80% of patients present with abnormal vaginal bleeding, most commonly postmenopausally. Only 10% note postcoital bleeding. Less frequent symptoms include vaginal discharge and pain.

○ **Colposcopically directed cervical biopsy in a 25-year-old woman, gravida 0, para 0 reveals a small focus of invasive squamous cell carcinoma. What is the next step in this patient's care?**

Cervical cone biopsy to establish the full extent of invasion

○ **What are the advantages of radical hysterectomy relative to radiation therapy for stage I cervical cancer?**
- Ovarian preservation is possible
- Unimpaired vaginal function
- Extent of disease can be established

○ **What clinical triad strongly indicates cervical cancer extension to the pelvic wall?**
1. Unilateral leg edema
2. Sciatic pain
3. Ureteral obstruction

○ **A 66-year-old woman presents with vaginal bleeding. What is your provisional diagnosis?**

Endometrial cancer. Fifteen percent of women with postmenopausal bleeding have endometrial cancer; 30% of these tumors are due to exogenous estrogens, 30% are due to atrophic endometriosis or vaginitis, 10% are due to cervical polyps, and 5% are due to endometrial hyperplasia. Most tumors are found at stage I.

○ **Describe the initial office evaluation in a woman whose history is suspicious for endometrial cancer.**

Pelvic examination, Pap smear screening, biopsy of any abnormal cervical or vaginal lesion, and endometrial biopsy

○ **What percentage of women with endometrial cancer will have abnormal Pap smear results?**

Approximately 50%

○ **What is the most common symptom of endometrial cancer?**

Abnormal perimenopausal or postmenopausal bleeding

○ **What is the risk of endometrial cancer in postmenopausal women using unopposed estrogen compared with those not using estrogen replacement therapy?**

2 to 10 times higher, depending on dose and duration of exposure

○ **What is the most common clinical condition associated with the development of endometrial hyperplasia?**

Polycystic ovary syndrome

○ **What is Lynch syndrome type II?**

A hereditary predisposition for the development of colon, breast, ovarian, and endometrial cancer

○ **What is the most common neoplasm in women of reproductive age?**

Benign leiomyomata. The most frequent presenting symptom for patients with leiomyosarcoma is vaginal bleeding, which occurs in more than three-fourths of patients.

○ **Why is it unlikely that you will find a uterine myoma in a 65-year-old woman?**

Uterine myomas are benign smooth muscle growths that are responsive to hormones and grow primarily during the reproductive years. They are the most common type of gynecologic pelvic neoplasm.

○ **What type of myoma is symptomatic?**

Submucosal myomas, though small, can cause profuse bleeding, potentially requiring hysterectomy. Most other myomas are asymptomatic.

○ **What is the rate of spontaneous abortion in women with polycystic ovaries?**

20% to 40%

○ **Is it acceptable to administer emergency contraception in a woman who is breastfeeding and has migraines?**

Yes. The advantages of emergency contraception outweigh the risks.

○ **How do you try to prevent transmission of herpes to the fetus in a woman with a history of recurrent genital herpes?**

Suppressive antiviral therapy should be administered at 36 weeks of gestation through delivery.

○ **Is it safe to administer acyclovir during the first trimester of pregnancy?**

Yes. Acyclovir is safe during pregnancy, including during the first trimester.

○ **Which drugs for gestational hyperglycemia are not diet controlled?**

Insulin and glyburide

○ **What is the most common cause of vaginal discharge in women of childbearing age?**

Bacterial vaginosis (40%–50%)

○ **True/False: Bacterial vaginosis is caused by 1 type of bacteria.**

False. It is polymicrobial.

○ **What is the most common cause for early discontinuation of implanted etonogestrel?**

Irregular bleeding

○ **How long post partum should you wait to begin ethinyl estradiol 0.75 mg and norelgestromin 6 mg in a breastfeeding woman?**

4 weeks

○ **Are Word catheter placement and marsupialization similarly effective for the treatment of Bartholin gland abscess?**

Yes. Both lead to less than a 20% chance of recurrence.

○ **Which method causes less postoperative discomfort: Word catheter placement or marsupialization of a Bartholin gland abscess?**

Marsupialization

○ **True/False: Biopsy should be performed for neoplasm in Bartholin gland cysts in women older than 40 years.**

True

○   **What is the appropriate response to finding atypical glandular cells on a Pap smear?**

Colposcopy. Ten percent to 40% of cases will be associated with a premalignant or malignant lesion of the endocervix or endometrium.

○   **What percentage of women of reproductive age have polycystic ovary syndrome?**

5% to 7%

○   **In which trimester of pregnancy are urinary tract infection and pyelonephritis most common?**

Third

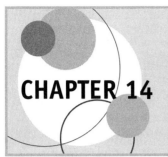

CHAPTER 14

General Surgery and Trauma

Scott H. Plantz, MD

○ **How many days should sutures remain in the following areas: face; scalp; trunk; hands, back, and extremities?**

- Face: 3 to 5 days
- Scalp: 5 to 7 days
- Trunk: 7 to 10 days
- Hands, back, and extremities: 10 to 14 days

○ **Which type of needle should be used for skin sutures? Which type should be used for deep tissue sutures?**

For skin, use cutting needles (or reverse cutting needles). For deeper tissues, use taper needles. Taper needles are less likely to cut blood vessels and delicate tissue.

○ **What are lines of Langerhans?**

Lines of tension in the skin that incisions should follow when possible for the best cosmetic results. In the forehead, these lines run horizontally, whereas in the lower face they run vertically.

○ **Which is more painful to the patient: plain lidocaine or lidocaine with epinephrine?**

Lidocaine with epinephrine because it has a low pH. To avoid this pain, buffer the solution with sodium bicarbonate. The injection should be administered slowly and subdermally.

○ **Can lidocaine with epinephrine be used on the arm?**

Yes. Lidocaine with epinephrine should not be used on fingers, toes, ears, nose, or the penis because the limited vascularity in these regions might be compromised.

○ **Why is epinephrine added to local anesthesia?**

To increase the duration of the anesthesia. Epinephrine also causes vasoconstriction and therefore decreases bleeding. However, epinephrine weakens tissue defenses and increases the incidence of wound infection.

○ **Where is local anesthetic injected for an ulnar nerve block?**

On the anterior side of the wrist in the proximal volar skin crease between the ulnar artery and the flexor carpi ulnaris

○ **Where is local anesthetic injected for a median nerve block?**

On the anterior side of the wrist in the proximal volar skin crease between the tendon of the palmaris longus and the flexor carpi radialis

○ **What nerve block is used to anesthetize of the sole of the foot?**

Tibial nerve block. Tibial nerve block does not provide anesthesia to the lateral aspect of the heel and foot.

○ **What is the preferred route for anesthesia for deep lacerations of the anterior portion of the tongue?**

Lingual nerve block

○ **How should hair be removed before wound repair?**

Clip the hair around the wound. Razor preparation can increase the infection rate.

○ **What is the rate of wound infection in the average surgical service?**

4% to 7%. The clean wound infection rate is 2%; clean-contaminated wounds, 3% to 4%; contaminated wounds, 10% to 15%; and dirty wounds, 25% to 40%. The wound infection rate depends on the degree of contamination, viability of tissue, blood supply to the tissue, dead space, amount of foreign material, patient age, concomitant infections, nutrition, and immune system status.

○ **How long can a clean wound closure be delayed before proliferation of infection-causing bacteria develops?**

6 hours, though the high vascularity of the face and scalp can allow for longer delays in these areas

○ **What mechanisms of injury create wounds that are most susceptible to infection?**

Compression or tension injuries. They are 100 times more susceptible to infection.

○ **What factors increase the likelihood of wound infection?**

Dirty or contaminated wounds, stellate or crushing wounds, wounds longer than 5 cm, wounds older than 6 hours, and infection-prone anatomic sites

○ **A mountain bike racer comes to your office after stepping on a nail that went right through her favorite, oldest pair of riding shoes. What gram-negative organism might infect her puncture wound?**

Pseudomonas aeruginosa

○ **Which has greater resistance to infection: sutures or staples?**

Staples

○ **Which 2 factors determine the ultimate appearance of a scar?**

Static and dynamic tension on surrounding skin

○ **Can tetanus develop after surgical procedures?**

Yes. Although most cases of tetanus in the United States develop after minor trauma, there have also been numerous reports of tetanus after general surgical procedures, especially those involving the gastrointestinal (GI) tract.

○ **Characterize wounds prone to tetanus.**

- Age of wound: More than 6 hours
- Configuration: Stellate
- Depth: More than 1 cm
- Mechanism of injury: Missile, crush, burn, frostbite
- Signs of infection: Present
- Devitalized tissue: Present
- Contaminants: Present
- Denervated and/or ischemic tissue: Present

○ **How long should one wait before delayed primary closure of a wound?**

4 days. Delayed primary closure will decrease the infection rate. It is used for severely contaminated wounds.

○ **How long does an area of abraded skin or a laceration have to be kept out of the sun?**

For at least 6 months. Abraded skin can develop permanent hypopigmentation when exposed to the sun.

○ **What organisms are most common in wound infections?**

Staphylococci

○ **A patient who develops a reddish brown exudate within 6 hours after appendectomy most likely has a wound infected with what?**

Clostridium. Necrotizing fasciitis, dehiscence, and sepsis may result if it is not treated promptly.

○ **What is the most likely cause of a postoperative fever that occurs: (1) the day of the operation, (2) 1 to 2 days postoperatively, (3) 3 to 5 days postoperatively, (4) 5 to 7 days postoperatively, and (5) 2 weeks postoperatively?**

1. Metabolic abnormalities
2. Atelectasis
3. Urinary tract infection
4. Wound infection
5. Deep vein thrombosis or pulmonary embolism

Remember "What—Wind—Water—Wound—Walk—Wonder drugs."

○ **What gas is used to create pneumoperitoneum during laparoscopy? Why is this gas used? What are the associated risks?**

Carbon dioxide. Carbon dioxide is noncombustible and has a high rate of diffusion, which results in a low risk of gas embolism. The use of carbon dioxide also can result in tachycardia; increased central venous pressure; hypertension; decreased cardiac output; and, occasionally, transient arrhythmias because of its rapid rate of absorption into the systemic circulation, which increases the partial pressure of carbon dioxide and decreases pH.

○ **A 32-year-old woman is under general anesthesia for a cholecystectomy. Partway into surgery, her body tenses up and she develops tachycardia and a fever of 101.8°F. What should you do?**

Administer dantrolene. This patient has malignant hyperthermia, a muscular response to general anesthetics that causes the release of calcium. Dantrolene will help prevent renal failure and will inhibit the release of calcium.

○ **What is the maintenance intravenous (IV) fluid rate for a child weighing 30 kg?**

100 mL/kg per day for the first 10 kg, plus 50 mL/kg per day for the next 10 kg, plus 20 mL/kg per day for the next 10 kg. This child should receive 1700 mL/d.

○ **What is the appropriate bolus for a dehydrated child weighing 15 kg?**

300 mL (20 mL/kg)

○ **Normal saline and Ringer lactate have how many milliequivalents of sodium per liter, respectively?**

- Normal saline: 154 mEq/L
- Ringer lactate: 130 mEq/L

○ **What are the laboratory criteria for using mechanical ventilation?**

- Partial pressure of oxygen lower than 70 mm Hg, with use of 50% oxygen.
- Partial pressure of oxygen lower than 55 mm Hg, with the patient breathing room air
- Partial pressure of carbon dioxide higher than 50 mm Hg
- pH lower than 7.25

However, a patient's clinical status is still the primary consideration.

○ **What negative pressure must be generated by an intubated patient for weaning to be successful?**

At least 20 cm of water. Other important factors include partial pressure of arterial oxygen, arterial oxygen saturation, pH, respiratory rate, minute volume, tidal volume, alveolar arterial oxygen gradient, and ratio of dead space to tidal volume.

○ **What is the Whipple procedure?**

Pancreaticoduodenectomy. The procedure involves resection of the distal portion of the stomach, pylorus, duodenum, proximal portion of the pancreas, and the gallbladder, plus truncal vagotomy. The jejunum is then anastomosed to the stomach, biliary, and pancreatic ducts. This procedure is used for treating cancer of the pancreatic, duodenal, ampulla of Vater, and common bile duct.

○ **What are the Billroth I and II procedures?**

The Billroth I anastomosis is gastroduodenostomy, and the Billroth II procedure is gastrojejunostomy.

○ **What is the Roux-en-Y operation?**

Formation of an end-to-side anastomosis between the distal segment of small bowel and the stomach or esophagus. This forms a Y shape. This procedure is used to treat reflux of bile and pancreatic secretions into the stomach.

○ **Matching:**

1. Autograft
2. Heterotrophic
3. Isograft
4. Orthotopic
5. Allograft
6. Xenograft

    a. Donor and recipient are genetically same
    b. Donor and recipient are same person
    c. Donor and recipient are same species
    d. Donor and recipient are different species
    e. Transplant to a normal anatomic position
    f. Transplant to a different anatomic position

Answers: (1) b, (2) f, (3) a, (4) e, (5) c, and (6) d

○ **What fungal infection is most common in transplant patients?**

Candida albicans

○ **What transplant organ can be preserved the longest?**

The kidney. Kidneys can be preserved in cold storage for as long as 48 hours, the pancreas and liver for 8 hours, and the heart for 4 hours. Viability can be extended by using cold storage solutions, such as Collins solution and Belzer solution.

○ **Differentiate between visceral and parietal pain.**

- Visceral pain: Diffuse and poorly localized pain caused by the stretching of a hollow viscus. It is frequently associated with autonomic nervous system responses.
- Parietal pain: Sharp and localized pain due to irritation or inflammation of a parietal surface and associated with guarding, rebound, and a rigid abdomen.

○ **What is the most common cause of postoperative bleeding?**

Poor hemostasis at the surgical site.

○ **A patient is burned over both legs, his entire back, and his right arm. What percentage of his body is burned?**

63%. Follow the rule of "9's": face, 9%; arms, 9% each; front, 18%; back, 18%; and legs, 18% each.

○ **A patient who has been burned over the entire top of his body (arms and torso, front, and back) develops severe difficulty breathing and appears to be starting respiratory arrest. What should you do?**

Perform escharotomy. The patient most likely has ventilatory restriction due to the circumferential eschar about his chest, resulting in constriction of the chest cavity. Escharotomy need not be performed with use of anesthesia, not even local anesthesia. Third-degree burns destroy the nervous tissue, so the tissue is insensitive to pain.

○ **What is the caloric requirement of a 100-kg firefighter who was burned over 20% of his body?**

3300 kcal. 25 kcal/kg of body weight plus 40 kcal per 1% burnt surface

○ **What is the 24-hour fluid resuscitation requirement for the above patient?**

4 L in the first 8 hours (500 mL/h) and 4 L in the next 16 hours (250 mL/h). The Parkland formula gives the requirement as 4 mL × body weight (kg) × percentage burned (4 mL × 100 kg × 20% = 8 L). Administer half the volume in the first 8 hours and the other half in the next 16 hours. Treatment after this should be based on clinical judgment. Urine output should be maintained at 50 mL/h in adults and 0.5 to 1 mL/kg per hour in children.

○ **What does an increase in pulmonary arterial wedge pressure indicate?**

Fluid overload. Normal pulmonary wedge pressure is 4 to 12 mm Hg. Higher levels can indicate left ventricular failure, constrictive pericarditis, or mitral regurgitation with stenosis.

○ **A trauma patient has blood at the urinary meatus. What test should be performed?**

Retrograde urethrography. Ten milliliters of radiocontrast solution should be injected into the urinary meatus.

○ **What are the 2 most commonly injured genitourinary organs?**

1. Kidneys
2. Bladder

○ **In blunt trauma, what is the most common renal pedicle injury?**

Renal artery thrombosis

○ **A trauma patient presents with a "rocking horse" type of ventilation. What is the diagnosis?**

Probable high spinal cord injury with intercostal muscle paralysis

○ **What should be checked before inserting a chest tube in an intubated patient with respiratory distress and decreased breath sounds on 1 side?**

Position of the endotracheal (ET) tube

○ **A trauma patient presents with subcutaneous emphysema. What is the diagnosis?**

Pneumothorax or pneumomediastinum. If the emphysema is severe, consider a major bronchial injury.

○ **What rib fracture has the worst prognosis?**

The first rib. First and second rib fractures are associated with bronchial tears, vascular injury, and myocardial contusions.

○ **A patient presents to the emergency department after a motor vehicle accident with hematuria and fractures of the tenth and eleventh ribs. What internal organ is most likely damaged?**

The spleen is the most commonly injured organ in blunt trauma. However, the spleen is injured in only 10% of penetrating trauma incidents. Be especially suspicious of splenic trauma if the tenth or eleventh ribs are fractured and the patient has hematuria.

○ **For a trauma patient, what test is most helpful for evaluating retroperitoneal organs?**

Computed tomography (CT)

○ **A patient presents with fever and shoulder pain 4 days after splenectomy. What is the most probable postoperative complication?**

Subphrenic abscess. This condition can cause fever and irritation to the diaphragm and to the branch of the phrenic nerve that innervates it.

○ **What organisms are most commonly responsible for overwhelming postsplenectomy sepsis?**

Encapsulated organisms: pneumococcal, 50%; meningococcal, 12%; *Escherichia coli*, 11%; *Haemophilus influenzae*, 8%; staphylococcal, 8%; and streptococcal, 7%

○ **What is a sentinel loop?**

A distended loop of bowel detected at radiography that lies near a localized inflammatory process. The possibility of pancreatitis or appendicitis should be considered.

○ **What is a delphian node?**

A palpable node on the trachea just above the thyroid isthmus. It indicates thyroid malignancy or thyroiditis.

○ **Which types of nodules are more likely to be malignant at thyroid scanning: hot or cold?**

Cold. This procedure should not be considered confirmatory. Cysts and benign adenomas can also appear cold. Some types of thyroid cancers will appear warm and thus be dismissed. Use caution when interpreting results.

○ **What test should be performed to distinguish a benign cystic nodule from a malignant nodule?**

Fine-needle aspiration biopsy and cytologic evaluation

○ **Are epidural hematomas and subdural hematomas more or less common among elderly patients?**

Subdural hematomas are more common. Epidural hematomas are less common.

○ **When does a subdural hematoma become isoattenuating?**

1 to 3 weeks after bleeding. However, it may not be detectable at CT unless contrast material is used.

○ **What percentage of cervical spinal fractures can be identified on a lateral radiograph?**

90%

○ **Name the function and spinal innervation level of the biceps, triceps, flexor digitorum, interossei, quadriceps, extensor hallucis, biceps femoris, soleus and gastrocnemius, and rectal sphincter.**

Muscle	Action	Spinal Level
Biceps	Forearm flexion	C5–C6
Triceps	Forearm extensor	C7
Flexor digitorum	Finger flexion	C8
Interossei	Finger adduction/abduction	T1
Quadriceps	Knee extension	L3–L4
Extensor hallucis	Hallux dorsiflexion	L5
Biceps femoris	Knee flexion	S1
Soleus and gastrocnemius	Foot plantar flexion	S1–S2
Rectal sphincter	Sphincter tone	S2–S4

○ **What is the sensory innervation to the nipple, umbilicus, and perianal region?**

- Nipple: T4
- Umbilicus: T10
- Perianal: S2-S4

○ **What is a solitary thyroid nodule most likely to be?**

A nodular goiter (50%). Other possibilities to consider include cancer (20%), adenoma (20%), cyst (5%), or thyroiditis (5%).

○ **Which nerves must be located and then avoided when performing thyroidectomy?**

The recurrent laryngeal nerves that lie in the transesophageal grooves. Failure to avoid these nerves could result in damage to the voice.

○ **What is the most common type of thyroid carcinoma?**

Papillary carcinoma (60% to 70% of tumors). Papillary carcinoma has the best prognosis; the 10-year survival rate is 89%. Other thyroid carcinomas are follicular (10% to 20%, common in older patients), anaplastic (3% to 5%), and medullary (2% to 5%, often occurring with familial multiple endocrine neoplasia).

○ **A 44-year-old woman comes to your office complaining of a mass in the center of her neck near the hyoid bone. It is tender and raises if she sticks her tongue out. What is the diagnosis?**

An infected thyroglossal duct cyst. This is a remnant from the embryologic descent of the thyroid in the neck. Thyroid tissue is found in 10% to 45% of these cysts. Treatment includes antibiotics, drainage, and then excision once the inflammation subsides. If the cyst were found in a noninfected state, elective surgery would be the treatment of choice because most of these cysts eventually become infected.

○ **Inability to pass a nasogastric tube in a trauma patient suggests damage to what organ?**

Diaphragm, usually on the left

○ **What type of contrast medium should be used to evaluate the esophagus if a traumatic injury is suspected?**

Diatrizoate meglumine and diatrizoate sodium solution

○ **Dysphagia occurs when the esophageal intraluminal diameter is reduced to what size?**

Smaller than 10 mm. This is a common problem in esophageal cancer. Palliation is achieved by widening the esophageal intraluminal diameter through photoablation of the tumor.

○ **What age and ethnic group is at greatest risk for esophageal cancer?**

Elderly African Americans. Their risk is 4 times higher than that for elderly whites. Other ethnic groups at higher risk include those who are Chinese, Iranian, or South African.

○ **Cancer occurs more frequently in which third of the esophagus?**

The middle third (50%), followed by the distal third (30%) and the proximal third (20%)

○ **Which are the most common cancer cell types of the esophagus?**

Squamous cell carcinoma occurs most frequently in African Americans, whereas adenocarcinoma is most common type in whites.

○ **What is Hamman sign?**

Air in the mediastinum after esophageal perforation. This condition produces a crunching sound over the heart during systole.

○ **What is the most common site of rupture in Boerhaave syndrome?**

The posterior distal esophagus. Boerhaave syndrome is a rupture of the esophagus that occurs after binge drinking and vomiting. Patients experience sudden, sharp pain in the lower part of the chest and epigastric area. The abdomen becomes rigid, and shock may follow.

○ **What is the most common acute surgical condition of the abdomen?**

Acute appendicitis

○ **What is the most common cause of appendicitis?**

Fecaliths. Fecaliths are found in 40% of uncomplicated appendicitis cases, 65% of cases involving gangrenous appendices that have not ruptured, and 90% of cases involving ruptured appendices. Other causes of appendicitis include lymphoid tissue hypertrophy, inspissated barium, foreign bodies, and strictures.

○ **How does retrocecal appendicitis most commonly manifest?**

Dysuria and hematuria due to the proximity of the appendix to the right ureter. Poorly localized abdominal pain, anorexia, nausea, vomiting, diarrhea, mild fever, and peritonitis are also common signs.

○ **What percentage of patients with a preoperative diagnosis of appendicitis actually have appendicitis?**

85%. Other postoperative diagnoses commonly include acute mesenteric lymphadenitis, pelvic inflammatory disease, epiploic appendicitis, ruptured Graafian follicle, acute gastroenteritis, and twisted ovarian cysts.

○ **Differentiate between the McBurney point, Rovsing sign, obturator sign, and psoas sign.**
- McBurney point: Point of maximal tenderness in a patient with appendicitis. The location is two-thirds of the way between the umbilicus and the iliac crest on the right side of the abdomen.
- Rovsing sign: Palpation of left lower quadrant causes pain in the right lower quadrant.
- Obturator sign: Internal rotation of a flexed hip causes pain.
- Psoas sign: Extension of the right thigh causes pain.
- These signs are all indicative of an inflamed appendix.

○ **Which type of antibiotic should be administered in a patient with a perforated appendix before surgery?**

A broad-spectrum antibiotic effective on both aerobic and anaerobic enteric organisms. Intraoperative cultures can guide further antibiotic therapy. Antibiotics may be continued for 7 days postoperatively. If the patient has uncomplicated appendicitis (ie, no perforation or gangrene), then 1 preoperative dose of a broad-spectrum antibiotic such as cefoxitin or cefotetan is sufficient.

○ **Who has a higher rupture rate in appendicitis: the very young or the very old?**

The very old. The rupture rate for geriatric patients is 65% to 90%; the associated mortality rate is 15%. The pediatric population has a rupture rate of 15% to 50%, with an associated mortality rate of 3%.

○ **What kind of wound closure should be used in a patient with a perforated appendix?**

Delayed primary closure with direct drainage of the infection. Wound infection occurs in 20% of patients with perforated appendices.

○ **What is the most common site of intracranial aneurysms?**

The circle of Willis (most common in the anterior communicating artery). A ruptured aneurysm manifests as a headache followed by altered consciousness.

○ **What are the clinical signs of cerebrospinal fluid (CSF) leakage?**

Raccoon eyes, bruises behind the ears (Battle sign), otorrhea, and rhinorrhea

○ **A hard mass is detected in the upper outer quadrant of the right breast in a 45-year-old woman. What are the next steps?**

Mammography followed by excisional biopsy. A negative result at fine-needle aspiration biopsy alone cannot be used to rule out malignancy. False-negative rates for fine-needle aspiration biopsy are 3% to 30%.

○ **What is the most common histologic type of breast cancer?**

Infiltrating ductal carcinoma (70% to 80%). Subtypes are colloid, medullary, papillary, and tubular.

○ **A 30-year-old woman comes to you worried that she has breast cancer in both breasts. She is concerned because of a yellowish green discharge from her nipples, soreness in the upper outer quadrants of her breasts, what she calls a lumpy feeling at self-examination, and mild swelling that seems to come and go. Further questioning reveals that her pain begins 1 week before she menstruates and then disappears when menses ends. Understandably concerned, your patient wants to know when she can start chemotherapy. What should you tell her?**

Do not begin chemotherapy. She most likely has fibrocystic breast changes. Put her mind at rest, and let her know that fibrocystic changes are not a premalignant syndrome.

○ **Which is the most common type of noncystic breast tumor?**

Fibroadenoma is most common in women younger than 25 years. These tumors are painless, small, mobile, and round.

○ **What is the most common lung cancer in nonsmokers?**

Small cell carcinoma. Smoking is a great risk factor for all lung cancers, with the exception of adenocarcinoma.

○ **What is Westermark sign?**

Decreased vascular markings at chest radiography, indicative of pulmonary embolism

○ **What do muffled heart tones, hypotension, and distended neck veins indicate?**

Pericardial tamponade. This is the Beck triad.

○ **What are Grey Turner and Cullen signs?**

- Cullen sign: Periumbilical ecchymosis indicative of pancreatic hemorrhage
- Grey Turner sign: Flank ecchymosis indicative of pancreatic hemorrhage

Both are caused by dissection of blood retroperitoneally.

○ **Serum amylase level is frequently elevated in acute pancreatitis. What other conditions can cause a similar increase in the level of amylase?**

Bowel infarction, cholecystitis, mumps, perforated ulcer, and renal failure. Lipase level is more specific. A 2-hour urine amylase test is more accurate for pancreatitis.

○ **What are the most common causes of acute pancreatitis?**

Alcoholism (40%) and gallstone disease (40%). The remaining cases of acute pancreatitis are due to familial pancreatitis, hypoparathyroidism, hyperlipidemia, iatrogenic pancreatitis, and protein deficiency.

○ **Name some abdominal radiographic findings associated with acute pancreatitis.**

Sentinel loop (of the jejunum, transverse colon, or duodenum), colon cutoff sign (an abrupt cessation of gas in the middle or left transverse colon caused by inflammation of the adjacent pancreas), or calcification of the pancreas. About two-thirds of patients with acute pancreatitis have radiographic abnormalities.

○ **What are the Ranson criteria?**

A means of estimating the prognosis for patients with pancreatitis.

At initial presentation, developing within 24 hours

- Older than 55 years
- Lactate dehydrogenase level higher than 700 IU/L
- White blood cell count higher than 16,000/μL
- Aspartate aminotransferase level higher than 250 U/L
- Serum glucose level higher than 200 mg/dL

48 hours later

- Hematocrit level decreasing more than 10%
- Increase in serum urea nitrogen level greater than 5 mg/dL
- Serum calcium level lower than 8 mg/dL
- Partial pressure of arterial oxygen lower than 60 mm Hg
- Base deficit higher than 4 mEq/L
- Fluid sequestration greater than 6 L
- 0 to 3 criteria = 3% mortality
- 3 to 6 criteria = 15% mortality
- 5 to 6 criteria = 40% mortality
- 7 to 8 criteria = 100% mortality

(Editor's note: These are the classic mortality percentages. Current treatment has decreased these rates.)

○ **What is the most common cause of pancreatic pseudocysts in children? In adults?**
- Children: Trauma
- Adults: Chronic pancreatitis

Pseudocysts are generally filled with pancreatic enzymes and are sterile. They manifest about 1 week after the patient has a bout with acute pancreatitis manifested as upper abdominal pain with anorexia and weight loss. Forty percent of pseudocysts will regress on their own.

○ **What is the treatment for pancreatic pseudocysts?**

Initial therapy is to wait for regression (4 to 6 weeks). If no improvement occurs, or if superinfection occurs, surgical drainage or excision is required.

○ **A 44-year-old man presents with a deep, dull pain in the center of his abdomen that radiates to his back and will not go away. He states he has not felt like himself for a few weeks and that he has been depressed. He also notes that he has lost a lot of weight, about 30 pounds in 3 weeks. At physical examination, you palpate an enlarged liver and an abdominal mass in the epigastrium. What is the diagnosis?**

Most likely pancreatic cancer. The ability to palpate a mass suggests that the disease has progressed too far for surgical removal. Carcinoma of the pancreas can be resected in only 20% of patients. Depression often occurs before the onset of other symptoms.

○ **What is the most common anatomic and histologic location of pancreatic cancer?**

Head of the pancreas (80%). Pancreatic cancer is generally adenocarcinoma and located in the ducts.

○ **What sex and age group most commonly presents with pancreatic cancer?**

Middle-aged men

○ **Is there a genetic marker for adenocarcinoma of the pancreas?**

Yes. Ninety percent of patients with adenocarcinoma of the pancreas have a mutation of the Ki-ras oncogene on codon 12.

○ **What is the 5-year survival rate for pancreatic carcinoma?**

2% to 5%. Symptoms generally do not appear until the tumor has metastasized or spread to local structures.

○ **What is the Courvoisier law?**

The gallbladder is smaller than its normal size if a gallstone is blocking the common bile duct and larger than its normal size if the bile duct is blocked by something else, most commonly cancer of the pancreas.

○ **What is the most common endocrine tumor of the pancreas?**

Insulinoma. However, only 10% are malignant. Gastrinomas are the second most common and have a malignancy rate of 50%. VIPomas and glucagonomas are also endocrine tumors of the pancreas.

○ **Glucagonomas arise from which type of cells?**

α Cells. Most are malignant. Increased plasmin glucagon is diagnostic.

○ **Which type of surgery is associated with a higher incidence of common bile duct injury: laparoscopic cholecystectomy or conventional cholecystectomy?**

Laparoscopic

○ **What is the most common benign liver tumor?**

Cavernous hemangioma

○ **All types of hepatomas are associated with underlying liver disease except for 1 of them. Which is it?**

Fibrolamellar hepatomas. These are single nodules in noncirrhotic livers.

○ **Where does hepatic cancer most commonly metastasize?**

The lungs (bronchiogenic carcinoma)

○ **What is the 2-year survival rate for patients with liver cancer who have a liver transplant?**

25% to 30%

○ **Where will colorectal cancer most commonly metastasize?**

The liver

○ **α-Fetoprotein will be elevated in which types of tumors?**

Primary hepatic neoplasms and endodermal sinus or yolk sac tumors of the ovaries and testes. α-Fetoprotein is present in 30% of patients with primary liver cancer. It is not associated with metastatic tumors to the liver, but it is used as a cellular marker in the above-mentioned tumors.

○ **What is the most common cause of portal hypertension?**

Intrahepatic obstruction (90%), which is most often due to cirrhosis. Other causes of portal hypertension are increased hepatic flow without obstruction (ie, fistulas) and extrahepatic outflow obstruction.

○ **What are the most commonly isolated organisms in pyogenic hepatic abscesses?**

E coli and other gram-negative bacteria. The source of such bacteria is most likely an infection in the biliary system.

○ **Which has a higher mortality rate: amebic or pyogenic liver abscesses?**

Pyogenic. The mortality rate for a singular pyogenic abscess is 25%,; for multiple abscesses, to the mortality rate can be as high as 70%. Amebic abscesses have mortality rates of only 7% if uncomplicated by superinfection. Amebic abscesses are more likely to be singular, whereas pyogenic abscesses can be singular or multiple.

○ **What clinical sign can assist in the diagnosis of cholecystitis?**

Murphy sign: pain at inspiration with palpation of the right upper quadrant. As the patient breathes in, the gallbladder is lowered in the abdomen and comes in contact with the peritoneum just below the examiner's hand. This will aggravate an inflamed gallbladder, causing the patient to discontinue breathing deeply.

○ **What is the difference between cholelithiasis, cholangitis, cholecystitis, and choledocholithiasis?**

• Cholelithiasis: Gallstones in the gallbladder
• Cholangitis: Inflammation of the common bile duct, often secondary to bacterial infection or choledocholithiasis
• Cholecystitis: Inflammation of the gallbladder secondary to gallstones
• Choledocholithiasis: Gallstones that have migrated from the gallbladder to the common bile duct

○ **What percentage of people with gallstones will develop symptoms?**

Only 50%

○ **Which ethnic group has the largest proportion of people with symptomatic gallstones?**

Native Americans. By the age of 60 years, 80% of Native Americans with previously asymptomatic gallstones will develop symptoms, as compared with only 30% of whites and 20% of African Americans.

○ **What percentage of patients with cholangitis also have sepsis?**

50%. Chills, fever, and shock can occur.

○ **What percentage of gallstones can be seen at ultrasonography?**

95%. Ultrasonography is the diagnostic procedure of choice in patients suspected of having cholecystitis.

○ **How much bile can be held within a distended gallbladder?**

50 mL

○ **What is the Charcot triad?**

1. Fever
2. Jaundice
3. Abdominal pain

This is the hallmark of acute cholangitis.

○ **What is the Reynolds pentad?**

The Charcot triad plus shock and mental status changes. This is the hallmark of acute toxic ascending cholangitis.

○ **What are most gallstones composed of?**

Cholesterol (75% to 95%). The rest are made of pigment.

○ **What are most kidney stones made of?**

Calcium oxalate (60%). The remainder of kidney stones are made of uric acid, calcium oxalate and calcium phosphate, struvite, and cystine.

○ **What percentage of patients with cancer of the gallbladder also have cholelithiasis?**

90%

○ **What is the diagnostic test of choice for acute cholecystitis?**

Hepatic iminodiacetic acid scanning (technetium-99–labeled N-substituted iminodiacetic acid scanning). Hepatic iminodiacetic acid scanning involves a gamma-ray–emitting isotope that is selectively extracted by the liver into bile. The labeled bile can then be used to determine if there is cystic duct obstruction or extrahepatic bile duct obstruction, depending on whether the bile fills the gallbladder or enters the intestine. For practical reasons, cholecystitis is frequently diagnosed by using clinical impressions, complete blood cell count, and ultrasonography.

○ **How effective is oral dissolution therapy with bile acids for those with symptomatic gallstones?**

Oral therapy with bile acids can dissolve as many as 90% of stones. However, therapy works only on stones smaller than 0.5 mm, made of cholesterol, and floating in a functioning gallbladder. Patients are then treated for 6 to 12 months, and 50% have recurrence of gallstones within 5 years.

○ **What are the contraindications to lithotripsy?**

Stones larger than 2.5 cm, more than 3 stones, calcified stones, stones in the bile duct, and poor overall condition of the patient

○ **Laparoscopic cholecystectomy is the procedure of choice for removal of gallstones. What is the most common major complication associated with this surgery?**

Injury to the bile duct

○ **Can gallstones reform after cholecystectomy?**

Yes. They can recur in the bile ducts.

○ **What is the most common site for fibromuscular dysplasia?**

The right renal artery. Fibromuscular dysplasia is an arterial disease that causes areas of stenosis and dilatation; the artery looks like a link of sausage. Women are more commonly affected than men.

○ **Where are most hernias located?**

In the groin (75%). Incisional and ventral hernias account for 10% of case, and umbilical hernias account for 3%.

○ **Are most inguinal hernias in infants and children direct or indirect?**

Indirect

○ **Differentiate between reducible, incarcerated, strangulated, Richter, and complete hernias.**
- Reducible: Contents of hernia sac return to the abdomen spontaneously or with slight pressure when the patient is in a recumbent position.
- Incarcerated: Contents of the hernia sac are irreducible and cannot be returned to the abdomen.
- Strangulated: Sac and its contents become gangrenous.
- Richter: Only part of the hernia sac and its contents becomes strangulated. This hernia may spontaneously reduce and be overlooked.
- Complete: This is an inguinal hernia that passes all the way into the scrotum.

○ **What are the boundaries of the Hesselbach triangle?**

The triangle is medial to the inferior epigastric artery, superior to the inguinal ligament, and lateral to the rectus sheath. The Hesselbach triangle is the site through which direct hernias pass.

○ **A direct hernia is due to a weakness in what tissue?**

The transversalis fascia that makes up the floor of the Hesselbach triangle. Direct hernias do not pass through the inguinal canal and are often called "pantaloon hernias."

○ **Indirect inguinal hernias occur secondary to what defect?**

A failure of the processus vaginalis to close. The resulting hernia can then pass through the inguinal ring.

○ **Which type of hernia is most common in women?**

Direct hernia, which is the most common hernia in both women and men. Although femoral hernias are more common in women than in men, they are still less common than direct hernias.

○ **Of all hernias in the groin area, which is most likely to strangulate?**

A femoral hernia. Femoral hernias occur in the femoral canal, an unyielding space between the lacunar ligament and the femoral vein.

○ **Which are more common: sliding or paraesophageal hiatal hernias?**

Sliding hiatal hernias account for 95% of hiatal hernias.

○ **In paraesophageal hiatal hernias, does the stomach herniate to the left or to the right of the esophagus?**

Most frequently to the left. Paraesophageal hiatal hernias have a high rate of strangulation that can quickly lead to death. These hernias should be repaired surgically. Treat sliding hernias with antacids, hydrogen ion blockers, and changes in eating and sleeping habits; surgery should be used only as a last resort.

○ **What is the most common site of duodenal ulcers?**

The duodenal bulb (95%). Surgery is indicated only if perforation, gastric outlet obstruction, intractable disease, or uncontrollable hemorrhage occur.

○ **What is the most common site for gastric ulcers?**

The lesser curvature of the stomach. Surgery is considered earlier for gastric ulcers because of the higher recurrence rate after medical treatment and because of the higher potential for malignancy.

○ **What are the signs and symptoms of intestinal obstruction in the newborn?**

Maternal polyhydramnios, abdominal distension, failure to pass meconium, and vomiting

○ **What amount of residual volume suctioned from the stomach of a newborn is diagnostic of obstruction?**

More than 40 mL.

○ **A newborn's vomit will be stained with bile if the obstruction is distal to what anatomic structure?**

Ampulla of Vater

○ **What are the common causes of neonatal intestinal obstruction?**

Annular pancreas, Hirschsprung disease, intestinal atresia, malrotation, volvulus, peritoneal bands, meconium plug, small left colon syndrome, and stenosis

○ **What is the most prevalent location for atresia of the bowel?**

Duodenum (40%), jejunum (20%), ileum (20%), and colon (10%)

○ **What is the double bubble sign?**

The appearance of a distended stomach and duodenum at radiography in a patient with duodenal obstruction. This is classically seen in duodenal atresia of the newborn.

○ **What is the most common cause of bowel obstruction in children?**

Hernia

○ **What are the most common causes of small bowel obstruction in adults?**

Adhesions (70%), followed by strangulated groin hernia and neoplasm of the bowel. Twenty percent of acute abdominal surgical admissions are due to obstructions.

○ **Volvulus of the colon most frequently involves which segment?**

Sigmoid (65%), cecum (30%), transverse colon (3%), and splenic flexure (2%). Volvulus is the cause of 5% to 10% of all large bowel obstructions.

○ **What is the most common site of intestinal obstruction secondary to gallstones?**

The terminal ileum. Fifty-five percent to 60% of cases have associated air in the biliary tree.

○ **What is the differential diagnosis for a 65-year-old man who has abdominal pain and bloody diarrhea a few days after the repair of an abdominal aortic aneurysm?**

Ischemic colitis is most probable. This condition occurs secondary to decreased blood flow to the inferior mesenteric artery during the operation. Other differential diagnoses include pseudomembranous colitis (if the patient was receiving antibiotics) and aortoenteric fistulas (generally a later development).

○ **Is colovesical fistula between the colon and the urinary tract more common among men or women?**

Men (3:1) more than women because a woman's uterus lies between her colon and bladder.

○ **How much blood must be lost in the GI tract to cause melena?**

50 mL. Healthy patients normally lose 2.5 mL/d.

○ **What are the most common causes of upper GI bleeding?**

Peptic ulcer disease (45%), esophageal varices (20%), gastritis (20%), and Mallory-Weiss syndrome (10%)

○ **What percentage of patients with upper GI bleeding will stop bleeding within hours after hospitalization?**

85%. About 25% of these patients will bleed again within the first 2 days of hospitalization. If bleeding does not recur in 5 days, the chance of bleeding again is only 2%.

○ **What are the most common causes of rebleeding in patients with upper GI bleeding?**

Peptic ulcer disease or esophageal varices

○ **What percentage of patients with peptic ulcer disease bleed from their ulcers?**

20%

○   **Bleeding ulcers are more predominant in patients with which blood type?**

Type O. The reason is not known.

○   **Where are bleeding duodenal ulcers most commonly located?**

On the posterior surface of the duodenal bulb

○   **How soon after an episode of bleeding has occurred can a patient with an ulcer eat?**

12 to 24 hours after the bleeding has stopped

○   **Which type of ulcer is more likely to bleed again?**

Gastric ulcers are 3 times more likely to bleed again than are duodenal ulcers.

○   **What is the surgical treatment of choice for a bleeding peptic ulcer?**

Oversewing the ulcer combined with bilateral truncal vagotomy and pyloroplasty. Other treatments are proximal gastric vagotomy and Billroth II gastrojejunostomy. The decision to perform surgery is based on the rate of bleeding, not on the location of the bleeding.

○   **What percentage of patients with large intestinal bleeding will stop bleeding before transfusion requirements exceed 2 U?**

90%

○   **If blood is recovered from the stomach after a nasogastric tube is inserted, what is the most likely location of bleeding?**

Above the ligament of Treitz

○   **Where do most Mallory-Weiss tears occur?**

In the stomach (75%), esophagogastric junction (20%), and distal esophagus (5%)

○   **Where is angiodysplasia most frequently found?**

In the cecum and proximal ascending colon. Lesions are generally singular, and bleeding is intermittent and seldom massive.

○   **What is the major cause of death in patients with Hirschsprung disease?**

Enterocolitis

○   **Is Hirschsprung disease more common in male or female patients?**

Male patients (5:1)

○   **Are tumors located in the jejunum and ileum more likely malignant or benign?**

Benign. Tumors of the jejunum and ileum are only 5% of all GI tumors. Most are asymptomatic.

○　**What is the most common remnant of the omphalomesenteric duct?**

Meckel diverticulum

○　**What is the Meckel diverticulum rule of 2s?**

Two percent of the population has it, it is 2 inches long, it is 2 ft from the ileocecal valve, it occurs most commonly in children younger than 2 years, and is symptomatic in 2% of patients.

○　**What is the most likely cause of rectal bleeding in a patient with Meckel diverticulum?**

Ulceration of ileal mucosa adjacent to the diverticulum lined with gastric mucosa

○　**What is the most likely cause of cellulitis of the umbilicus in a pediatric patient with acute abdomen?**

Perforated Meckel diverticulum

○　**What is the difference in the prognosis between familial polyposis and Gardner disease?**

Although both are inheritable conditions of colonic polyps, Gardner disease rarely results in malignancy, whereas familial polyposis virtually always results in malignancy.

○　**Clinically, how is right-sided colon cancer differentiated from left-sided colon cancer?**

Right-sided lesions manifest with occult bleeding, weakness, anemia, dyspepsia, palpable abdominal mass, and dull abdominal pain. Left-sided lesions manifest with visible blood, obstructive symptoms, and noticeable changes in bowel habits. Pencil-thin stools are also common.

○　**Adenocarcinoma develops from adenomatous polyps. What percentage of patients without symptoms have adenomatous polyps at routine colonoscopy?**

25%. Prevalence increases with age: 50 years, 30%; 60 years, 40%; 70 years, 50%; and 80 years, 55%. The risk for adenomatous polyps is greater in patients with a history of breast cancer.

○　**The advancement to adenocarcinoma of the colon from adenoma depends on size. What is the risk of developing cancer if a 1.5-cm polyp is found at colonoscopy?**

10%. The risk for developing adenocarcinoma is 1% if the polyp is smaller than 1 cm, 10% if it is 1 to 2 cm, and 45% if the polyp is larger than 2 cm.

○　**Is a villous, tubulovillous, or tubular adenoma more likely to become malignant?**

Forty percent of villous adenomas will become malignant, compared to 22% of tubulovillous adenomas and 5% of tubular adenomas.

○　**Which are more likely to turn malignant: pedunculated or sessile lesions?**

Sessile

○　**Where are most colorectal cancers found?**

In the rectum (30%), ascending colon (25%), sigmoid colon (20%), descending colon (15%), and transverse colon (10%)

○ **What is the surgical treatment of choice for cecal cancer?**

Colonic resection from the vermiform appendix to the junction of the ascending and transverse colon

○ **What is the treatment of choice for plantar warts?**

Cryosurgery with liquid nitrogen. First, the callus should be shaved off with a razor. If possible, the keratin plug should be removed. Lastly, liquid nitrogen should be applied. The wart will fall off in 3 to 4 weeks.

○ **Where are soft-tissue sarcomas most often found?**

In the lower extremities. They are fairly rare. The most common sarcomas are liposarcomas, leiomyosarcomas, fibrosarcomas, rhabdomyosarcomas, and malignant fibrous histiocytomas.

○ **A 41-year-old man complains of severe but short rectal spasms but has not noticed any bleeding. He is stressed and overtaxed at work. What is the diagnosis?**

Proctalgia fugax. These short rectal spasms last less than 1 minute and occur infrequently. They are associated with people who are anxious or overworked or have a history of irritable bowel syndrome. No cause is known. Treatment is with analgesic suppositories, heating pads, and relaxation techniques.

○ **A patient complains of severe pain when defecating. He is constipated and has blood-streaked stools and a bloody discharge after bowel movements. What is the diagnosis?**

Anal fissure. Ninety percent of anal fissures are located in the posterior midline. If fissures are found elsewhere in the anal canal, then anal intercourse, tuberculosis, carcinoma, Crohn disease, and syphilis should be considered.

○ **Differentiate between mucosal rectal prolapse, complete rectal prolapse, and occult rectal prolapse.**

- Mucosal rectal prolapse: Involves only a small portion of the rectum protruding through the anus and has the appearance of radial folds
- Complete rectal prolapse: Involves all the layers of the rectum protruding through the anus and appears as concentric folds
- Occult rectal prolapse: Does not involve protrusion through the anus but rather intussusception

○ **Which are more painful: internal or external hemorrhoids?**

External. The nerves above the pectinate or dentate line are supplied by the autonomic nervous system and have no sensory fibers. The nerves below the pectinate line are supplied by the inferior rectal nerve and have sensory fibers.

○ **Differentiate between first, second, third, and fourth degree hemorrhoids.**

- First degree: Appear in the rectal lumen but do not protrude past the anus
- Second degree: Protrude into the anal canal if the patient only strains
- Third degree: Protrude into the anal canal but can be reduced manually
- Fourth degree: Protrude into the anal canal and cannot be reduced manually

Treatment for the first and second degrees is a high-fiber diet, sitz baths, and good hygiene. The treatment of choice for third or fourth degree hemorrhoids is rubber band ligation. Other treatments are photocoagulation, electrocauterization, and cryosurgery.

○ **Diverticular disease is most common in which part of the colon?**

The sigmoid colon, which accounts for 95% of diverticular disease

○ **What percentage of patients with diverticula have symptoms?**

20%

○ **What are the signs and symptoms of diverticulitis?**

Abdominal pain, generally in the left lower quadrant, a low-grade fever, change in bowel habits, nausea, and vomiting. If there is perforation, patients may have peritoneal signs and appear toxic.

○ **What is the treatment for diverticulitis?**

Bowel rest and antibiotics. Treatment can be outpatient unless there are signs of systemic infection or perforation.

○ **Kultschitzsky cells are the precursors to what tumor?**

Carcinoid. A carcinoid tumor can arise anywhere in the GI tract, but its most frequent site of involvement is the appendix.

○ **What is the probable cause of colovesical fistulas?**

Sigmoid diverticulitis. Other causes are radiation enteritis, colon carcinoma, and bladder carcinoma. Colovesical fistulas are diagnosed by means of cystoscopic examination.

○ **A 47-year-old man complains of impotence, as well as pain and coldness in both legs after exercise. What would you expect to find at examination?**

This patient probably has Leriche syndrome, caused by occlusion of the abdominal aorta secondary to atherosclerosis. Physical examination should reveal weak or absent femoral and pedal pulses, bruit, thrill, pallor with elevation of the limb, dependent rubor, and high blood pressure (BP). Treatment is either bypass or thromboendarterectomy.

○ **What is the most commonly obstructed artery in the lower extremity?**

Superficial femoral artery. It is a branch of the common femoral artery, which is a branch of the external iliac artery.

○ **A 64-year-old man presents with jaundice, upper GI bleeding, anemia, a palpable nontender gallbladder, a palpable liver, and rapid weight loss. What is the diagnosis?**

This is the clinical picture of a tumor of the ampulla of Vater.

○ **Testicular torsion occurs most commonly in what age group?**

Teens

○ **What is the maximum amount of time a testicle can remain in torsion without being irreversibly damaged?**

4 to 6 hours

○ **What is definitive treatment for testicular torsion?**

Emergency surgical scrotal exploration

○ **What percentage of palpable prostate nodules are malignant?**

50%. Surgical cure in patients who present with asymptomatic nodules and no metastasis is attempted with radical prostatectomy or radiation therapy.

○ **What are mycotic aneurysms?**

Mycotic aneurysms are true aneurysms that have become infected or false aneurysms that have occurred because of an arterial infection. The femoral artery is the most common site for such aneurysms.

○ **Where is mesenteric ischemia more serious: in the small bowel or the large bowel?**

The small bowel. Embolization in the superior mesenteric artery affects the entire small bowel. The mortality rate from ischemia in the small bowel is 60%. Embolization to the large bowel is not as serious because of collateral circulation. Ischemia of the large bowel rarely result in a full-thickness injury or perforation.

○ **Where do glomus tumors develop?**

In the hands, more specifically under the fingernails. These tumors are composed of blood vessels and unmyelinated nerves. Benign yet painful, they should be removed surgically.

○ **What is an ABI, and why is it significant?**

Ankle-brachial index. The ankle systolic pressure (numerator) is compared to the higher of the 2 brachial arterial pressures (denominator). It is used to determine if arterial obstruction is present.

○ **What technical factors can affect the accuracy of the ABI?**

Probe pressure, rapid deflation of the BP cuff, arterial wall calcifications, and probe placement, which should be longitudinal to the vessel and at a 30° to 60° angle to the skin surface

○ **What percentage of cervical fractures are visible on lateral, odontoid, and anteroposterior radiographs of the neck?**

- Lateral: 90%
- Odontoid: 10%
- Anteroposterior: Just a few

○ **At lateral radiography of the cervical spine, how much soft-tissue prevertebral swelling is normal from C1 through C4?**

As much as 4 mm is normal, but more suggests a fracture.

○ **How much anterior subluxation is normal in an adult lateral cervical spine?**

3.5 mm

○ **How much angulation is normal in an adult lateral cervical spine, measured across a single interspace?**

As much as 10°

○ **In the lateral cervical spine, what does fanning of the spinous processes suggest?**

Posterior ligamentous disruption

○ **What are the 3 most unstable cervical spine injuries?**

  1. Transverse atlantal ligament rupture

  2. Dens fracture

  3. Burst fracture with posterior ligament disruption

○ **Describe a Jefferson fracture.**

A burst ring of C1, usually the result of a vertical compression force. It is best detected by using an odontoid view.

○ **Describe a hangman fracture.**

A C2 bilateral pedicle fracture. It is usually caused by hyperextension.

○ **What is a clay-shoveler fracture?**

In order of frequency, C7, C6, or T1 avulsion fractures of the spinous process. They can be caused by either flexion or a direct blow.

○ **Describe the key features of spinal shock.**

Sudden areflexia that is transient and distal, with a duration of hours to weeks. BP is usually 80 to 100 mm Hg, with paradoxical bradycardia.

○ **A trauma patient presents with a decreasing level of consciousness and an enlarging right pupil. What is the diagnosis?**

Probable uncal herniation with oculomotor nerve compression

○ **What nerves does the corneal reflex test?**

The ophthalmic branch (V1) of the trigeminal (fifth) nerve (afferent) and the facial (seventh) nerve (efferent)

○ **Name 5 clinical signs of basilar skull fracture.**

  1. Periorbital ecchymosis (raccoon eyes)

  2. Retroauricular ecchymosis (Battle sign)

  3. Otorrhea or rhinorrhea

  4. Hemotympanum or bloody ear discharge

  5. First, second, seventh, and eighth cranial nerve deficits

○ **A trauma patient presents with anisocoria, neurologic deterioration, and/or lateralizing motor findings. What should be the immediate treatment?**

Immediate intubation and hyperventilation. Unless the patient is hypovolemic, infuse mannitol 1 g/kg rapidly. Elevate the head of the bed 30°. Some experts still recommend dexamethasone, 10 mg, and phenytoin, 18 mg/kg at 20 mg/min.

○ **How is posterior column function tested? Why is it significant?**

Position and vibration sensation are carried in the posterior columns and are usually spared in anterior cord syndrome. Light touch sensation may also be spared. Pain and temperature sensation cross near the level of entry and are carried in the more posterior spinothalamic tract.

○　**Define increased intracranial pressure.**

Intracranial pressure higher than 15 mm Hg

○　**What is the most common site of a basilar skull fracture?**

Petrous portion of the temporal bone

○　**What cardiovascular injury is commonly associated with sternal fracture?**

Myocardial contusions (blunt myocardial injury)

○　**Which valve is most commonly injured during blunt trauma?**

Aortic valve

○　**What is the most likely cause of a new systolic murmur and electrocardiographic (ECG) infarct pattern in a patient with chest trauma?**

Ventricular septal defect

○　**What plain film radiographic finding most accurately indicates traumatic rupture of the aorta?**

Deviation of the esophagus more than 2 cm right of the spinous process of T4

○　**What is the differential diagnosis of distended neck veins in a trauma patient?**

Tension pneumothorax, pericardial tamponade, air embolism, and cardiac failure. Neck vein distension may not be present until hypovolemia has been treated.

○　**What is the most sensitive indicator of shock in children?**

Tachycardia

○　**What initial fluid bolus should be administered in children in shock?**

20 mL/kg

○　**Radial pulse at examination indicates BP of at least what level?**

80 mm Hg

○　**Femoral pulse at examination indicates BP of at least what level?**

70 mm Hg

○　**Carotid pulse at examination indicates BP of at least what level?**

60 mm Hg

○　**Do posttraumatic seizures occur more frequently in children or adults?**

Children

○ **What is the most common complaint of patients with traumatic aortic injury?**

Retrosternal or intrascapular pain

○ **Amputation is often required after vascular injury to what artery?**

Popliteal artery. Injuries to arteries below the adductor hiatus lead to a loss of limb more frequently than do injuries elsewhere.

○ **How long does it take to prepare fully cross-matched blood?**

30 to 60 minutes

○ **Should a chest tube be placed into a bullet hole apparent in the fourth lateral interspace?**

No. The tube might follow the bullet track into the diaphragm or lung.

○ **Why do simple through-and-through wounds of the extremities fare better regardless of the velocity of the bullet?**

The bullet's short path in the tissue results in (1) little or no deformation of the type seen with slower bullets and (2) less time to yaw, which results in less tissue damage, because the bullet is traveling at higher velocity.

○ **Is the heat of firing significant enough to sterilize a bullet and its wound?**

No. Contaminants from the body surface and viscera can be carried along the bullet's path.

○ **What anatomic locations of bullets or pellets are associated with lead intoxication?**

Bursa, joints, and disk spaces

○ **Other than lead intoxication, why should intraarticular bullets be removed?**

There is a potential for lead synovitis leading to severe damage of articular cartilage.

○ **What artery is usually involved in epidural hematoma?**

Middle meningeal artery

○ **Where are epidural hematomas located?**

Between the dura and inner table of the skull

○ **Where are subdural hematomas located?**

Beneath the dura, over the brain, and in the arachnoid mater. They are caused by tears of pial arteries or of bridging veins. Subdural hematomas typically become symptomatic 24 hours to 2 weeks after injury.

○ **What risk is associated with not treating a septal hematoma of the nose?**

Aseptic necrosis followed by absorption of the septal cartilage, resulting in septal perforation

○   **What organ is most commonly injured as a result of a blunt trauma?**

The spleen. Generalized abdominal pain with radiation to the left shoulder subsequent to blunt trauma indicates splenic rupture (Kehr sign). Splenic rupture can also occur after infectious mononucleosis.

○   **When performing a neurologic examination in a patient suspected of having anterior dislocation of the shoulder, what sign should be monitored and documented?**

Sensation over the lateral deltoid. In anterior dislocations of the shoulder, the radial nerve can be torn easily. Intact sensation to the lateral deltoid will indicate an intact radial nerve.

○   **A patient who was recently hit in the eye during a barroom brawl complains of diplopia when looking up. The injured eye does not appear able to look up. What is the diagnosis?**

Orbital blowout fracture with entrapment of the inferior rectus or inferior oblique muscle. Always test extraocular movements in patients with blunt trauma to the eye.

○   **What is the most common joint dislocation?**

Anterior shoulder dislocations account for half of all joint dislocations. They occur with abduction and external rotation.

○   **What organism is commonly found in infected wounds caused by animal bites?**

Pasteurella multocida. The second most common organism is *Staphylococcus aureus*.

○   **Is succinylcholine a depolarizing or a nondepolarizing neuromuscular blocking agent?**

Depolarizing. Succinylcholine is the only commonly used depolarizing agent. It binds to postsynaptic acetylcholine receptors, thereby causing depolarization. The material is enzymatically degraded by pseudocholinesterase (serum cholinesterase). Onset is within 1 minute; paralysis lasts 7 to 10 minutes.

○   **What is the rationale for pretreating a patient with a subpolarizing (defasciculating) dose of a nondepolarizing agent before treatment with succinylcholine?**

Attenuates fasciculations from succinylcholine-induced depolarization. This may decrease subsequent muscle pain. Increased intragastric and intraocular pressure is associated with the administration of succinylcholine.

○   **What dosage of midazolam causes a loss of consciousness and amnesia during rapid sequence induction?**

0.1 mg/kg. Five milligrams is effective for most people.

○   **What dosage of thiopental should be prescribed during rapid sequence induction?**

Approximately 4 mg/kg

○   **Loss of consciousness usually occurs within 15 seconds after thiopental is administered. What is the usual duration of action?**

2 to 30 minutes, depending on the source. Less than 5 minutes commonly occurs.

○ **What is the defasciculating or the priming dose of vecuronium?**

Approximately 0.01 mg/kg

○ **What dosage of vecuronium should be administered for paralysis (no priming)?**

0.15 to 0.20 mg/kg

○ **What is the defasciculating or the priming dose of pancuronium?**

0.015 mg/kg. About 1 mg is a common adult dose.

○ **A laryngeal fracture is suggested by noting the hyoid bone elevated above what cervical level at radiography?**

C3

○ **Describe the mechanism and cause of boutonniere deformity.**

It occurs secondary to rupture of the extensor apparatus of the proximal interphalangeal joint. The cause of the injury is a proximal interphalangeal joint that is flexed and a distal interphalangeal joint that is hyperextended. Treatment is splinting the proximal interphalangeal joint in full extension.

○ **What is the most common foot fracture?**

Calcaneus (60%). Talus fracture is a distant second.

○ **Where does a metatarsal fracture most commonly occur?**

At the base of the fifth metatarsal and is called a "Jones fracture."

○ **What is the most common form of anorectal abscess?**

Perianal abscess. Anorectal abscesses are usually mixed infections (ie, both gram-negative and anaerobic organisms). Fistula formation is a frequent complication.

○ **What concerns are associated with anterior dislocation of the shoulder?**

Axillary nerve injury, axillary artery injury (geriatric patients), compression fracture of the humeral head (Hill-Sachs deformity), rotator cuff tear, fractures of the anterior glenoid lip, and fractures of the greater tuberosity

○ **Describe the Galeazzi fracture-dislocation.**

A radial shaft fracture with dislocation of the distal radioulnar joint

○ **What formula should be used to calculate the fluid requirements for resuscitation of a burn patient?**

Parkland formula: 2 to 4 mL/kg per percentage of area burned per day. One-half of this is administered in the first 8 hours, and the second half is administered over the next 16 hours.

○ **How should you treat a patient who has been bitten by a wild raccoon?**

Wound care; tetanus prophylaxis; rabies immune globulin, 20 IU/kg (one-half at the bite site and one-half intramuscularly); and human diploid cell (rabies) vaccine, 1 mL intramuscularly

○ **Describe the intracorporeal dissipation of the rabies virus.**

The virus spreads centripetally up the peripheral nerve into the central nervous system. The incubation period for rabies is usually 30 to 60 days, with a range of 10 days to 1 year. Transmission usually occurs via infected secretions, saliva, or infected tissue. Stages of the disease include upper respiratory tract infection symptoms, followed by encephalitis. The brain stem is affected last.

○ **What animals are the most prevalent vectors of rabies in the world? In the United States?**

Worldwide, the dog is the most common carrier of rabies. In the United States, the skunk has become primary carrier. In descending order, bats, raccoons, cows, dogs, foxes, and cats are also sources.

○ **Describe the signs and symptoms of spinal shock.**

Flaccid paralysis, complete sensory loss, areflexia, and loss of autonomic function. Patients usually have bradycardia, hypotension, hypothermia, and vasodilation.

○ **Active adduction of the thumb tests which nerve?**

Ulnar nerve

○ **An elderly woman presents with pain in the knee and medial aspect of the thigh. What GI diagnosis should be considered?**

Obturator hernia

○ **What is the most common site of volvulus?**

Sigmoid colon

○ **Describe the location of an indirect inguinal hernia.**

Lateral to the epigastric vessels, protruding through the inguinal canal

○ **Describe the location of a femoral hernia.**

Protruding through the femoral canal and below the inguinal ligament

○ **Describe the location of a spigelian hernia.**

3 to 5 cm above the inguinal ligament

○ **What is a pantaloon hernia?**

A hernia with both direct and indirect inguinal hernia components

○ **What is a sliding hernia?**

A hernia in which 1 wall of the hernia sac includes viscus

○ **Describe a Richter hernia.**

An incarceration containing only one wall of viscus

○ **Which is the most common type of hernia in children?**

Indirect. Direct inguinal hernias are more common in the elderly.

○ **What is the most common cause of painless lower GI bleeding in an infant or child?**

Meckel diverticulum

○ **A 16-month-old child presents with bilious vomiting, a distended abdomen, and blood in the stool. What is the diagnosis?**

Malrotation of the midgut

○ **A child presents with periodic abdominal cramps, currant jelly stools, and a sausage-like tumor in the right lower quadrant. Contrast material–enhanced radiography shows a coil-spring sign. What is the diagnosis?**

Intussusception

○ **What is the most common anatomic source of a subdural hematoma?**

Bridging veins

○ **What is the most common source of subarachnoid bleeding?**

Saccular aneurysm

○ **If a lesion is in the right hemisphere, which way will the eyes deviate?**

Toward the lesion

○ **If a lesion is in the brain stem, which way will the eyes deviate?**

Away from the lesion in the brain stem

○ **What is the most common intraparenchymal site of intracranial bleeding?**

Putamen

○ **In the pediatric esophagus, where is a foreign body most commonly lodged?**

The cricopharyngeal narrowing

○ **What is the most commonly injured area of the mandible?**

The angle

○ **What is the most reliable method of diagnosing posterior shoulder dislocation?**

Performing physical examination. Y-view radiography may be helpful.

○ **What is the mortise view of the ankle important in the diagnosis of?**

Medial (deltoid) ligament disruption of the ankle

○ **What is the best radiographic view for diagnosing lunate and perilunate dislocations?**

Lateral views of the wrist

○ **A baby is brought to the emergency department because of vomiting and persistent crying. At examination, a testicle is tender and enlarged. What is the diagnosis?**

Testicular torsion

○ **In a humeral shaft fracture, what nerve is most commonly injured?**

Radial nerve

○ **Which type of hip dislocation is most common: anterior, posterior, lateral, or medial?**

Posterior

○ **Of the following, which is not a common cause of large bowel obstruction: diverticulitis, adhesion, sigmoid volvulus, or neoplasm?**

Adhesion

○ **Fracture of the acetabulum may be associated with damage to what nerve?**

Sciatic nerve

○ **What is the adult dose of epinephrine for acute anaphylactic shock?**

0.3 to 0.5 mg of 1:10,000 IV

○ **How should neurogenic shock be managed?**

With replacement of the volume deficit, followed by vasopressors

○ **What medication is most appropriate for hypertensive patients with acute aortic dissections?**

Nitroprusside and β-blockers

○ **What is the most common cause of sigmoid volvulus in the elderly?**

Constipation

○ **The anterior drawer test of the ankle is used to test what ligament?**

Anterior talofibular ligament

○ **Which type of injury should be suspected in a patient with a shortened, internally rotated right leg as the result of an accident?**

Posterior hip dislocation

○ **Describe mallet finger deformity.**

Deformity produced by forced flexion of the distal interphalangeal joint when finger is in full extension. It is a result of either a rupture of the distal extensor tendon or an avulsion fraction of the tendon insertion on the distal phalanx with a dorsal plate avulsion.

○ **A patient has a fracture of the proximal third of the ulna. Which type of injury should be ruled out?**

Dislocation of the radial head, also known as "Monteggia fracture." An anterior dislocation is most common.

○ **What therapy should be used for a patient with hemophilia A who has a head injury?**

Cryoprecipitate. Maintain a low total volume, if possible. Cryoprecipitate has a higher concentration of factor VIII complex than does fresh frozen plasma.

○ **Describe a patient with sigmoid volvulus.**

Sigmoid volvulus usually affects psychiatric patients and elderly patients with severe chronic constipation. Symptoms include intermittent cramping, lower abdominal pain, and progressive abdominal distension.

○ **Describe a typical patient with intussusception.**

It usually occurs in children aged 3 months to 2 years, although most are 5 to 10 months old. It is more common in boys.

○ **A patient has a rotational knee injury and hears a pop. Within 90 minutes, hemarthrosis develops. What is the suspected location of injury?**

Anterior cruciate ligament

○ **What are the radiologic and laboratory test results indicating duodenal injury?**

Retroperitoneal air and increased serum amylase level

○ **What is the most common cause of airway obstruction in trauma?**

Central nervous system depression

○ **What wound is most commonly associated with pericardial tamponade?**

Right ventricular injury

○ **What are the signs and symptoms of acute pericardial tamponade?**

Triad of hypotension, elevated central venous pressure, and tachycardia. Muffled heart tones may be auscultated.

○ **What ECG result is pathognomonic of pericardial tamponade?**

Total electrical alternans. Pulsus paradoxus is nonspecific. Muffled heart tones are a subjective finding and are difficult to hear.

O   **What cause of death is secondary to untreated tension pneumothorax?**

Decreased cardiac output. The vena cava is compressed, which lowers blood return to the right side of the heart and severely compromises stroke volume, BP, and cardiac output.

O   **How does chronic pericardial effusion appear at chest radiography?**

Gradual pericardial sac distension results in a "water bottle" appearance of the heart.

O   **What are the key features of anterior spinal cord syndrome?**

Compression of the anterior cord causes complete motor paralysis and loss of pain and temperature sensation distal to the lesion. Posterior columns are spared; light touch and proprioception are preserved.

O   **Describe the presentation of placenta abruptio.**

Painful, dark red vaginal bleeding

O   **What is the most common growth plate (Salter class) injury?**

Salter II fracture

O   **What signs of tension pneumothorax appear at physical examination?**

Tachypnea, unilateral absent breath sounds, tachycardia, pallor, diaphoresis, cyanosis, tracheal deviation, hypotension, and neck vein distension

O   **What is the most common cause of abdominal pain in children?**

Constipation

O   **What is the most frequent carpal fracture?**

Navicular fracture

O   **In the wrist, what bone is dislocated most often?**

Lunate. It is also the second most commonly fractured bone in the wrist.

O   **What is the worst way to confirm diagnosis of delayed pericardial injury after blunt trauma?**

Autopsy

O   **Which is the most common type of hepatitis transmitted through blood transfusions?**

Hepatitis C

O   **What is the best method to open an airway while maintaining cervical spine precautions?**

Jaw thrust

○ **What is the formula for determining the appropriate ET tube size for children older than 1 year?**

ET size = (age + 16) / 4 mm

○ **What is the correct ET tube size for a 1- to 2-year-old child?**

4.0 to 4.5 mm

○ **What is the correct ET tube size for a 6-month-old baby?**

3.5 to 4.5 mm

○ **What is the correct ET tube size for a newborn?**

3.0 to 3.5 mm. For a premature newborn, use a 2.5- to 3.0-mm ET tube.

○ **What is the average distance from the mouth to 2 cm above the carina in men and in women?**

- Men: 23 cm
- Women: 21 cm

○ **What deficits can result from ocular motor nerve paralysis?**

Ptosis, which is caused by levator palpebrae superioris/cranial nerve III injury. Lateral nerve gaze is controlled by cranial nerve VI, and corneal reflex is controlled by cranial nerve V. The superior oblique muscle moves the gaze downward and laterally. It is controlled by cranial nerve IV.

○ **Describe the signs and symptoms of pressure on the first sacral root (S1).**

Symptoms of S1 injury include pain radiating to the midgluteal region, posterior thigh, and posterior calf and down to the heel and sole of the foot. Sensory signs are localized to the lateral aspects of the toes. S1 root compression typically involves the plantar flexor muscles of the foot and toes. The ankle reflex is decreased or absent.

○ **What are common entities in the differential diagnosis of pinpoint pupils?**

Narcotic overdose; clonidine overdose; and sedative hypnotic overdose, including ethanol; cerebellar pontine angle infarct; and subarachnoid hemorrhage

○ **When should blood products be supplemented with fresh frozen plasma for a trauma patient receiving multiple units of transfused blood?**

For each 5 U of transfused blood, 1 U fresh frozen plasma should be administered.

○ **What is the universal donor blood type?**

Type O Rh-negative blood with anti-A and anti-B titers less than 1:200 in saline

○ **What are the common manifestations of transfusion reaction?**

Myalgia, dyspnea, fever associated with hypocalcemia, hemolysis, allergic reactions, hyperkalemia, citrate toxicity, hypothermia, coagulopathy, and altered hemoglobin function

○   **What are the signs of the Cushing reflex?**

Increased systolic BP and bradycardia secondary to neurologic event

○   **Surgery is curative for liver cancer in what percentage of resectable, asymptomatic tumors?**

In more than 70% of children without cirrhosis and more than 40% of adults without cirrhosis. If patients have cirrhosis and a tumor smaller than 2 cm, surgery is curative 70% of the time. The cure rate for patients with cirrhosis and a tumor larger than 3 cm is only 10%.

○   **What is the most common anatomic abnormality in the arterial blood supply to the liver?**

The right hepatic artery branches from the superior mesenteric artery instead of the common hepatic artery, which arises from the proper hepatic artery in 15% to 20% of the population.

○   **What is the Kehr sign?**

Pain in the left shoulder made worse in the Trendelenburg position, which indicates splenic injury. However, it is present in only 50% of such cases. In addition to the patient's history and physical examination results, peritoneal lavage will help to determine if the spleen is bleeding.

○   **What spinal level innervates the diaphragm?**

C3, C4, C5. Remember: "3, 4, and 5 keep the diaphragm alive."

○   **What are the most common causes of shock in patients who have received blunt chest trauma?**

Pelvic or extremity fractures

○   **Technetium-99m–labeled studies of the gallbladder are viewed every 10 minutes for 1 hour. If the gallbladder is not visible at the 1-hour interval, what does this signify?**

Either complete obstruction of the cystic duct because of inflammation and stones (acute cholecystitis) or partial obstruction with a slow filling rate because of scarring (chronic cholecystitis). Images delayed as long as 4 hours are obtained to rule out the latter possibility.

○   **What percentage of distal tibial (medial malleolus) fractures that are treated closed result in nonunion?**

10% to 15%

○   **What is the most common thoracolumbar wedge fracture in the elderly?**

L1

○   **What is the significance of the fat pad sign with an elbow injury?**

It indicates effusion or hemarthrosis of the elbow joint, which suggests occult fracture of the radial head.

○   **Which test is more sensitive when used to determine anterior cruciate ligament tear in the knee: the anterior drawer test or the Lachman test?**

Lachman test. While the knee is held at 20° flexion and the distal femur is stabilized, the lower leg is pulled forward. More than 5 mm of anterior laxity compared to the other knee is evidence of an anterior cruciate ligament tear.

○ **If medical management fails to relieve symptoms of gastroesophageal reflux after a 1-year trial, what surgical methods might be attempted?**

Hill gastropexy, Nissen fundoplication, Angelchik antireflux prosthesis placement, or Belsey Mark IV operation. Surgical correction provides a 90% cure rate.

○ **How many points are possible in the Glasgow Coma Scale by measuring eye-opening response?**

4

Remember: "I've got an eye 4 U."

○ **How many points equal the best verbal response in the Glasgow Coma Scale?**

5

○ **How many points is the best motor response in the Glasgow Coma Scale?**

6

○ **What results are normal in the oculocephalic reflex?**

Conjugate eye movement is opposite to the direction of head rotation.

○ **When testing a patient's oculovestibular reflex, which direction of nystagmus is anticipated in response to cold water irrigation: toward or away from the irrigated ear?**

Away from the irrigated ear. Nystagmus is defined as the direction of the fast component of saccadic eye movement.

Remember: COWS = Cold Opposite, Warm Same.

○ **What does tonic eye movement toward an irrigated ear in response to warm caloric testing signify in a comatose patient?**

Life

○ **How long should sutures remain in the face? In the scalp or trunk? In the extremities? In the joints?**

Facial sutures: 3 to 5 days
Scalp or trunk: 7 to 10 days
Extremities:10 to 14 days
Joints: 14 days

○ **What are the signs and symptoms of uncal herniation?**

An uncal herniation typically compresses the ipsilateral third cranial nerve, resulting in ipsilateral pupil dilation. Contralateral weakness occurs because the pyramidal tract decussates below this level. Occasionally, a shift will be great enough to cause compression of both sides, leading to a combination of ipsilateral or contralateral pupillary dilatation and weakness.

○ **What common finding at sinus radiography suggests basilar skull fracture?**

Blood in the sphenoid sinus

○   **What is the best view of the zygomatic arch at radiography of the face ?**

Modified basal view. This is also called the "jug-handle," "submental-occipital," or "submental-vertical" view.

○   **What radiographic view should be used to evaluate the maxilla, maxillary sinus, orbital floor, inferior orbital rim, or zygomatic bones?**

Waters view

○   **What are the normal values on a pediatric cervical spine radiograph?**

The predental space in a child is smaller than 5 mm; in an adult, it is smaller than 3 mm. The posterior cervical line attaching the base of the spinous process of C1 to C3 should be considered. If the base of the C2 spinous process lies less than 2 mm behind the posterior cervical line, hangman fracture should be suspected. The distance from the anterior border of C2 to the posterior wall of the fornix is less than 7 mm. Finally, the distance from the anterior border of C6 to the posterior wall of the trachea is 14 mm in children younger than 15 years; it is smaller than 22 mm in an adult.

○   **Injury to what cervical area results in Horner syndrome (ptosis, miosis, and anhidrosis)?**

Disruption of the cervical sympathetic chain at C7 to T2

○   **What spinal level corresponds to the dermatomal innervation of the following: perianal region, nipple line, index finger, knee, and lateral aspect of the foot?**

- Perianal region: S2-S4
- Nipple line: T4
- Index finger: C7
- Knee: L4
- Lateral aspect of the foot: S1

○   **Describe central cord syndrome.**

Injury to the ligamentum flavum and to the cord, which causes an upper extremity neurologic deficit greater than the lower extremity deficit.

○   **Describe the presentation of a patient with Brown-Séquard syndrome.**

Ipsilateral motor paralysis, ipsilateral loss of proprioception, and a vibratory sensation. Contralateral loss of pain and temperature sensation are also exhibited.

○   **Describe the presentation of a patient with anterior cord syndrome.**

Complete motor paralysis and loss of pain and temperature sensations distal to the lesion. Posterior column sparing results in intact proprioception and vibration sense. The cause is attributed to occlusion of the anterior spinal artery or the protrusion of fracture fragments into the anterior canal.

○   **What is the most common site of penetrating ureteral injuries?**

Upper third of the ureter

○   **What is the most common cause of coagulopathy in patients who require massive transfusions?**

Thrombocytopenia

○ **What percentage of individuals with ureteral injuries present without hematuria?**

33%

○ **How is posterior urethral tear diagnosed in men?**

A high-riding, boggy prostate indicates this injury.

○ **What signs and symptoms are associated with anterior urethral tear?**

Severe perineal pain with blood, usually found at the meatus. A good urinary stream will be maintained.

○ **A patient has pelvic fracture with probable bladder or ureteral injury. Which test should be performed first: cystography or IV pyelography?**

Cystography should be performed so that distal ureteral dye from the IV pyelography will not mimic extravasation from the bladder.

○ **What is the half-life of carboxyhemoglobin?**

6 hours for 21% fraction of inspired oxygen, 1.5 hours for 100% fraction of inspired oxygen, and 0.5 hours in 3 atm for hyperbaric 100% fraction of inspired oxygen

○ **What is the best method for transporting an amputated extremity?**

Wrap the extremity in sterile gauze moistened with saline. Place it in a waterproof plastic bag and then immerse it in ice water.

○ **What neighboring structures may be injured with supracondylar distal humeral fracture?**

The anterior interosseous nerve (a branch of the median nerve) and the brachial artery

○ **What ligament is commonly injured after inversion ankle sprain?**

Anterior talofibular ligament

○ **How is a perilunate dislocation diagnosed?**

Anteroposterior and lateral radiography. The lunate remains in alignment with the radial fossa, while the other carpal bones appear displaced.

○ **What organ is most severely affected in a blast injury?**

The lungs

○ **What organ is most commonly affected in a blast injury?**

The ears

○ **A patient with dementia contracts a wound infection. Is it true that such a patient can present with a severe decrease in mental status?**

Yes. Normal minor insults can cause drastic changes in the neurologic functioning of patients with preexisting deficits.

○ **What is the most serious transfusion reaction?**

Hemolytic. Treat with aggressive fluid replacement and furosemide.

○ **What is the most common transfusion reaction?**

Febrile

○ **A patient has xanthochromic CSF with a low protein count. What is the most likely cause?**

Subarachnoid hemorrhage

○ **A patient has xanthochromic CSF with a high protein count (>150 g/dL). What is the most likely cause?**

Traumatic tap

○ **What are the classic findings of shaken baby syndrome?**

- Failure to thrive.
- Lethargy
- Seizures
- Retinal hemorrhages
- Subarachnoid hemorrhage or subdural hematoma from torn bridging veins visible at CT

○ **What is the immediate treatment for cord prolapse?**

Displace the head cephalad

○ **What nerve may be injured in distal femoral fracture?**

Peroneal nerve

○ **Which types of anorectal abscesses can be drained in the emergency department?**

Perianal, submucosal, and pilonidal abscesses. Ischiorectal and supralevator abscesses must be drained in the operating room.

○ **Describe a patient with intussusception.**

Patients are most likely young. Seventy percent of patients have intussusception within the first year of life. In children, the cause is thought to be secondary to lymphoid tissue at the ileocecal valve; in adults, it is thought to be caused by local lesions, Meckel diverticulum, or tumor. At examination, bowel sounds are usually normal. Intussusception typically involves the terminal ileum. Meckel diverticulum is the single most common intrinsic bowel lesion involved.

○ **What is painful, bright red rectal bleeding most often caused by?**

Anal fissure. External hemorrhoids manifest with acute painful thrombosis and are not typically associated with constant, bright red bleeding. Internal hemorrhoids manifest with painless bright red bleeding, usually with defecation.

○ **What is the most common site of lumbar disk herniation?**

Ninety-eight percent of clinically important lumbar disk herniations are at the L4-L5 or L5-S1 intervertebral levels. Evaluate these patients by checking for weakness of ankle and hallux dorsiflexors (L5). Also check pinprick sensation over the medial aspect of the foot (L5) and the lateral portion of the foot (S1).

○ **What white blood cell count is expected during pregnancy?**

White blood cell counts of 15,000/μL to 20,000/μL are considered normal during pregnancy.

○ **When monitoring a pregnant trauma patient, whose vital signs are the most sensitive: those of the mother or those of the fetus?**

The fetal heart rate is more sensitive to inadequate resuscitation. Remember that the mother may lose 10% to 20% of her blood volume without a change in vital signs, whereas the fetus's heart rate may increase or decrease above 160 or below 120 beats per minute, indicating significant fetal distress. The most common pitfall is failure to adequately resuscitate the mother.

○ **What 2 findings at physical examination indicate uterine rupture?**

1. Loss of uterine contour

2. Palpable fetal part

○ **What physical examination findings may be discovered in placenta abruptio?**

Rapidly increasing fundal height secondary to bleeding into the uterus or a higher than expected fundal height

○ **What is the number 1 risk factor for uterine rupture?**

Previous cesarean section

○ **What size tracheostomy tube is appropriate for a woman and for a man?**

A woman generally requires a number 4 tracheostomy tube, and a man generally requires a number 5 tracheostomy tube.

○ **You are having a hard time remembering which anesthetics are amides and which anesthetics are esters. What is a fairly easy way of telling these 2 classifications apart?**

With the exception of the suffix "-caine," only the anesthetics in the amide classification include the letter "i."

Amides
• Lidocaine
• Bupivacaine
• Mepivacaine

Esters
• Procaine
• Cocaine
• Tetracaine
• Benzocaine

○   **An elderly patient presents with sudden onset of severe abdominal pain followed by a forceful bowel movement. What is the probable diagnosis?**

Acute mesenteric ischemia. Results of abdominal series may be normal early in acute mesenteric ischemia. Possible late radiographic findings include absent bowel gas, ileus, gas in the intestinal wall, and thumbprinting of the intestinal mucosa. In most cases, radiographs are normal or not specifically suggestive. Expect heme-positive stools. Patients especially prone to mesenteric ischemia include those with congestive heart failure and chronic heart disease.

○   **What is the most commonly missed hip fracture?**

Femoral neck fracture

○   **Which is more common: a medial or a lateral tibial plateau fracture?**

The lateral tibial plateau is most commonly fractured. If anteroposterior and lateral radiographs are negative for fracture, follow up with oblique views if you suspect the patient has tibial plateau fracture.

○   **What is the most commonly missed fracture in the elbow region?**

Radial head fracture. As with the navicular fracture, radiographic signs of a radial head fracture may not appear for days after the injury. A positive fat pad sign may be the only finding suggestive of this injury.

○   **What are the 2 most common errors made in the intubation of a neonate?**

1. Placing the neck in hyperextension; this moves the cords even more anteriorly.

2. Inserting the laryngoscope too far.

○   **What are the National Institutes of Health's recommendations for treating spinal cord injuries?**

Administer high-dose methylprednisolone, 30 mg/kg bolus over 15 minutes, followed by 45 minutes of normal saline drip. Over the subsequent 23 hours, the patient should receive an infusion of 5.4 mg/kg per hour of methylprednisolone.

○   **What is the most common cause of obstruction of the small bowel in the surgically virgin abdomen?**

Incarcerated hernia

○   **A straight (Miller) blade is preferred for intubation in children younger than what age?**

4 years

○   **What is the Parkland formula for treating a pediatric burn patient?**

Ringer lactate, 4 mL per percentage of body surface area per kilogram over 24 hours, with half administered in the first 8 hours. Large burns in children younger than 5 years may require colloid (5% albumin or fresh frozen plasma) at 1 mL per percentage of body surface area per kilogram per day. The same formula is used for adults.

○   **How much fluid is required for maintenance of pediatric patients?**

100 mL/kg per day for each kilogram up to 10 kg, 50 mL/kg per day for each kilogram from 10 to 20 kg, and 20 mL/kg per day for each kilogram thereafter

○ **When examining a lateral adult cervical spine radiograph, the predental space looks particularly wide. What width is normal for an adult?**

Normal is 2.5 to 3 mm. If it is greater than 3 mm, consider that the transverse ligament has ruptured or is at least lax.

○ **How is a laryngeal fracture diagnosed at plain film radiography?**

At lateral soft-tissue radiography of the cervical spine, check for retropharyngeal air and elevation of the hyoid bone. The hyoid bone is usually at the level of C3 if there is no evidence of a laryngeal fracture. Elevation of the hyoid bone above C3 suggests a laryngeal fracture.

○ **In a trauma patient, what is dimpling of the cheek associated with?**

Zygomatic arch fracture

○ **What radiographic views should be used to diagnose fracture of the zygoma?**

Jug-handle view, Waters view, or submental view

○ **Blood is originating from a tooth after trauma. What is the Ellis classification?**

3

○ **What is the most common site of cervical disk herniation?**

C5-C6. The patient will complain of bilateral shoulder pain.

○ **What nerve is located in the tarsal tunnel?**

Tibial nerve

○ **A patient has difficulty squatting and standing. What is the most likely spinal disease?**

L4 root compression with involvement of the quadriceps

○ **Absent knee-jerk reflex involves which spinous level?**

L4

○ **Absent Achilles reflex involves which spinous level?**

S1

○ **Paresthesia of the hallux involves which spinous level?**

L5

○ **Paresthesia of the little toe involves which spinous level?**

S1

○ **What is the most common site of compartment syndrome?**

The anterior compartment of the leg

○   **Describe the leg position associated with anterosuperior hip dislocation.**

The leg is externally rotated with a slight abduction. In the pubic type, the hip is extended; in the iliac type, it is slightly flexed.

○   **Describe the leg position associated with obturator hip dislocation.**

External rotation, flexion, and abduction

○   **Describe the leg position associated with posterior hip dislocation.**

Internal rotation, flexion, and adduction

○   **A patient in the emergency department cannot recall ever having had a tetanus shot. The nurse administers a tetanus shot. Later, he develops a hypersensitivity reaction and recalls that he recently had had a tetanus shot. Which type of reaction does he have?**

Type III (Arthus reaction), which is caused by immune complexes or antigen-antibody complexes that activate complement and platelets that form aggregates and complexes with immunoglobulin E.

○   **What is the initial dose of blood administered in children?**

10 mL/kg of packed red blood cells

○   **Other than laparotomy, what invasive examination can be used to confirm suspected mesenteric ischemia?**

Angiography

○   **What is the most common cause of painless upper GI bleeding in an infant or child?**

Varices from portal hypertension

○   **With brain-stem herniation, is decorticate or decerebrate posturing expected?**

Decerebrate posturing (hyperextension). Decorticate posturing is flexion of the upper extremities and extension of the lower extremities.

○   **A patient presents after experiencing trauma to the head. He has an elevated systolic BP and bradycardia. What is this reflex?**

Cushing reflex

○   **What is the name for a flexion mechanism fracture through the anterior aspect of a vertebral body that is associated with ligamentous damage and anterior cord syndrome?**

Teardrop fracture

○   **What nerves control the corneal reflex?**

The ophthalmic branch of the fifth nerve and the afferent branch of the facial (seventh) nerve

○ **Name the most unstable cervical spine injuries.**

In order, from most unstable to least: rupture of transverse atlantal ligament, dens fracture, burst fracture (flexion teardrop), and bilateral facet dislocation

○ **What is the eponym for a C1 burst fracture from vertical compression?**

Jefferson fracture

○ **A patient in a motor vehicle accident sustains a hyperextension injury to the neck. Plain film radiography reveals a C2 bilateral facet fracture through the pedicles. You describe this fracture in consultation with the neurosurgeon. Which type of fracture have you described?**

Hangman fracture

○ **A patient has avulsion fracture of the spinous process of C7 with a history of a hyperflexion mechanism. What is the diagnosis?**

Clay-shoveler fracture, which involves the spinous process of C6, C7, or T1. The mechanism is usually flexion or a direct blow.

○ **A patient has bilateral interfacetal dislocation. What is your concern?**

Injury occurs as a result of flexion, and the cervical spine is unstable with ligament disruption.

○ **Stable or unstable: clay shoveler fracture.**

Stable

○ **Stable or unstable: fracture of the posterior arch of C1.**

Stable

○ **Name the 4 stable cervical spine fractures.**

1. Simple wedge
2. Clay shoveler
3. Pillar
4. C1 posterior neural arch

All other cervical spine fractures are unstable or potentially unstable.

○ **A patient presents after receiving a blow to the forehead. Her neck is hyperextended, and she complains of weakness in her arms and minimal weakness in her lower extremities. What is the diagnosis?**

Central cord syndrome

○ **You see a patient with an obvious traumatic spinal cord lesion. At physical examination, he has motor paralysis, loss of gross proprioception, loss of vibratory sensation on 1 side, and loss of pain and temperature sensation on the opposite side. What is the diagnosis?**

Brown-Séquard syndrome

○ **What is the most common cause of shock in patients with blunt chest trauma?**

Pelvic (or extremity) fracture concomitant with massive bleeding

○ **What is the most common site of traumatic aortic laceration?**

Just distal to the left subclavian artery

○ **A patient presents with high-speed traumatic injury to the chest. A systolic murmur over the precordium is auscultated. The patient has a slightly hoarse voice, and her pulse is stronger in the upper extremities. What is the diagnosis?**

Traumatic rupture of the aorta

○ **What is the most common radiographic finding in traumatic rupture of the aorta?**

Widening of the superior mediastinum

○ **What is the most accurate radiographic finding in traumatic rupture of the aorta?**

Rightward deviation of the esophagus greater than 1 to 2 cm

○ **A patient who has been involved in a motor vehicle accident has radiographic findings of retroperitoneal air seen on a flat plate of the abdomen. What is a likely diagnosis?**

Duodenal injury. A tentative test is a contrast material–enhanced study with diatrizoate meglumine and diatrizoate sodium solution. Extravasation is used to confirm duodenal injury.

○ **At radiography of the hand, the anteroposterior view shows a triangular lunate bone. What is the diagnosis?**

Lunate dislocation. Lateral radiographs will reveal what resembles a cup spilling water.

○ **What radiographic view is required to diagnose perilunate dislocation?**

Lateral

○ **A patient presents with a snapping sensation in the wrist and a click. Radiography of the patient's hand reveals a 3-mm space between the scaphoid and lunate bones. What is the diagnosis?**

Scaphoid dislocation

○ **In a boxer fracture, how much angulation of the fifth metacarpal neck is acceptable?**

50°

○ **What ligament in the hand is commonly injured in a fall while skiing?**

Thumb metacarpophalangeal joint ulnar collateral ligament rupture (gamekeeper thumb)

○ **Posterior dislocation of the shoulder is often missed with a standard radiographic shoulder series. What radiographic view aids in this diagnosis?**

Scapular Y view

○ **Name the 4 muscles of the rotator cuff.**

1. Supraspinatus

2. Infraspinatus

3. Teres minor Subscapularis

Patients with a rotator cuff tear will not be able to fully abduct or internally or externally rotate the arm.

○ **What is the usual mechanism of injury in a supracondylar fracture?**

A fall on the outstretched arm

○ **What artery is commonly injured with a supracondylar fracture?**

Brachial

○ **What nerve is commonly injured with a supracondylar fracture?**

Anterior interosseous nerve, which is a branch of the median nerve

○ **At radiography of the elbow, you find a posterior fat pad sign. What is the diagnosis?**

Occult fracture, such as a supracondylar fracture of the humerus. Posterior fat pad seen on a lateral radiograph of the flexed elbow is usually due to hemarthrosis caused by a fracture.

○ **What nerve injury is associated with a medial epicondyle fracture?**

Ulnar nerve

○ **About how many liters of blood can a patient lose in the retroperitoneal space?**

6 L

○ **Which type of pelvic fracture has the greatest amount of bleeding?**

Vertical sheer

○ **What nerve may be injured with a knee dislocation?**

Peroneal nerve

○ **Where are the most common sites of stress fractures in the foot?**

Second and third metatarsals

○ **What are the radiographic findings in ischemic bowel disease?**

Thumbprinting at plain film radiography, with a ground-glass appearance and absence of bowel gas

○ **How common is dumping syndrome?**

Ten percent to 20% of patients develop dumping syndrome after gastric resection. The syndrome consists of crampy abdominal pain, nausea, vomiting, diarrhea, flushing, and diaphoresis after eating. These symptoms are caused by an osmotic shift in the small intestine, which is caused by the quick entry of a bolus of hypertonic food. Dumping syndrome is resolved in most patients without treatment.

○ **A patient opens his eyes when he hears a voice, makes incomprehensible sounds, and withdraws from painful stimulus. What is his Glasgow Coma Scale score?**

9

Eye Opening	Best Verbal Response	Best Motor Response
1 No opening	1 No response	1 No response
2 Open to pain	2 Groans to pain	2 Extends arm to pain
3 Open on request	3 Words spoken	3 Flexes either arm
4 Open spontaneously	4 Confused conversation	4 Localizes pain stimulus
5 Oriented x 3		5 Obeys commands

○ **A near-drowning survivor is comatose and intubated. Severe pulmonary edema is diagnosed. What specific pulmonary treatment should be provided in the emergency department?**

It is important to administer positive end-expiratory pressure early to decrease intrapulmonary shunting and prevent terminal airway closure.

○ **Under what conditions does neurogenic pulmonary edema occur?**

Neurogenic pulmonary edema is commonly associated with increased intracranial pressure. It is commonly seen with head trauma, subarachnoid hemorrhage, and even with seizures.

○ **A patient had a severe headache 2 days ago. The headache is now subsiding, and physical examination results are normal. Should the possibility of a subarachnoid hemorrhage still be evaluated, and if so, how?**

Yes. Use CT. A significant percentage of scans will be negative 48 hours after intracranial hemorrhage. However, lumboperitoneal CT performed 2 to 3 days after bleeding should be positive, and xanthochromia typically persists for 7 to 10 days.

○ **A patient is in anaphylactic shock. She is taking β-blockers. She is not responding to epinephrine. What alternative agents might you consider?**

Norepinephrine, diphenhydramine, and glucagon

○ **A young man was found on the street by police and is brought to the emergency department. He has a fever of 105°F, altered mental status, and muscle rigidity. You find a bottle of thioridazine in his pocket. What conditions should be considered?**

Neuroleptic malignant syndrome should be considered first. Meningitis, encephalitis, hyperthyroidism, anticholinergic agents, strychnine poisoning, and heat stroke are also possible. He may also have hypotension, hypertension, or tachycardia.

○ **How should a patient with neuroleptic malignant syndrome be treated?**

- Ice packs to the groin and axilla
- Cooling blankets
- Fan
- Water mist evaporation
- Dantrolene, 0.8 to 3 mg/kg IV every 6 hours to a total of 10 mg/kg

○ **When does dysbaric air embolism typically occur?**

Dysbaric air embolism develops within minutes of surfacing after a dive. Symptoms are sudden and dramatic; they include loss of consciousness, focal neurologic symptoms (such as monoplegia, convulsions, blindness, and confusion), and sensory disturbances. Sudden loss of consciousness or other acute neurologic deficits immediately after surfacing are due to dysbaric air embolism unless proven otherwise. Treatment includes high-flow oxygen and rapid transport for hyperbaric oxygen treatment.

○ **A patient presents with a history of chest trauma, systolic murmur, and infarct pattern at ECG. What is the diagnosis?**

Traumatic ventricular septal defect

CHAPTER 15 Ophthalmology

William A. Schwer, MD

○ **What are cotton-wool spots?**

White patches on the retina that are observed at funduscopic examination. These patches are due to ischemia of the superficial nerve layer of the retina. They are most commonly associated with hypertension but also occur in patients with diabetes, anemia, collagen vascular disease, leukemia, endocarditis, and AIDS.

○ **Do visual changes in patients with chronic open-angle glaucoma begin centrally or peripherally?**

Peripherally. Patients with chronic glaucoma experience a gradual and painless loss of vision. Those with acute or subacute angle glaucoma have dull or severe pain, blurry vision, lacrimation, and even nausea and vomiting. The pain may be more severe in the dark.

○ **Which is more common: chronic open-angle glaucoma or acute closed-angle glaucoma?**

Chronic open-angle glaucoma (90%). Four percent of the population older than 40 years has glaucoma.

○ **What is the most common cause of chronic open-angle glaucoma?**

Outflow obstruction through the trabecular meshwork. Other causes are obstruction of the Schlemm canal and excess secretion of aqueous fluid.

○ **What is the normal range of intraocular pressure?**

10 to 23 mm Hg. Patients with acute closed-angle glaucoma generally have pressures elevated to 40 to 80 mm Hg.

○ **Topical steroids for the eyes are absolutely contraindicated in what cases?**

If the patient has a herpetic infection, herpetic lesions in the eye are often seen as dendritic patterns of fluorescein uptake at slitlamp examination.

○ **What is the most common finding at funduscopic examination in a patient with AIDS?**

Cotton-wool spots due to disease of the microvasculature. Other findings are hemorrhage, exudate, or retinal necrosis.

○ **A patient presents with an itching, tearing, right eye. At examination, large cobblestone papillae are found under the upper lid. What is the probable diagnosis?**

Allergic conjunctivitis

○   **A patient is seen with herpetic lesions on the tip of the nose. Why is this a problem?**

The tip of the nose and the cornea are both supplied by the nasociliary nerve. Thus, the cornea may also be involved. This is an ophthalmologic emergency.

○   **A patient presents with conjunctiva and lid margin inflammation. Slitlamp examination reveals a greasy appearance of the lid margins with scaling, especially around the base of the lashes. What is the diagnosis?**

Blepharitis. This is often caused by a staphylococcal infection of the oil glands and skin next to the lash follicles. Treatment consists of scrubbing with baby shampoo and, after consultation with an ophthalmologist, sulfacetamide drops and steroids.

○   **A patient presents with a painful red eye. Slitlamp examination reveals a localized, white, flocculent infiltrate in the anterior chamber. What is this?**

Hypopyon, which is an accumulation of white inflammatory exudate in the anterior chamber

○   **A welder presents with severe eye pain. What is the expected finding at slitlamp examination?**

Diffuse punctate keratopathy (welder flash), which manifests as a multiple pinpoint area of fluorescein uptake representing ruptured corneal epithelial cells

○   **A patient presents with a pustular vesicle at the lid margin. What is the diagnosis and treatment?**

Hordeolum (sty). An acute inflammation of the meibomian gland, most commonly of the upper lid. Treat with topical antibiotics and warm compresses. Surgical drainage may be necessary.

○   **A patient presents with a chronic, nontender, uninflamed nodule of the upper lid. What is the diagnosis?**

Chalazion. Treat with surgical curettage.

○   **A patient presents with the sensation of a foreign body in the eye. Slitlamp examination reveals a dendritic (branchlike) pattern. What is the treatment?**

Antiviral agents and cycloplegics. This is most probably herpes simplex keratitis. Steroids are strongly not advised. Emergency ophthalmologic consultation is indicated.

○   **A patient presents with sudden onset of vision loss in 1 eye that quickly returns. What is the diagnosis?**

Amaurosis fugax. It is usually caused by central retinal artery emboli from extracranial atherosclerosis.

○   **A patient presents with painless vision loss in 1 eye described as a wall slowly developing in the visual field. What finding do you expect at examination?**

A gray, detached retina. The patient may also complain of flashing lights in the peripheral visual field or spiderwebs in the visual field. Inferior detachment is treated with the patient sitting up. Superior detachment is treated with the patient lying flat.

○   **A patient was hit in the eye during a drunken brawl. He presents 8 hours after the incident with proptosis and visual loss. Examination reveals an intact globe and an afferent pupillary defect. What is the problem?**

Retro-orbital hematoma with ischemia of the optic nerve or retina. The pressure of the blood in the orbit exceeds the perfusion pressure, resulting in a lack of blood flow and loss of function. Treatment is to release the pressure by means of lateral canthotomy. A similar situation can occur with orbital emphysema.

○ **What 5 lid lacerations should be referred to an ophthalmologist?**

1. Near the lacrimal canaliculi (between the medial canthus and the punctum)
2. Near the levator (transverse lacerations of the upper lid)
3. Near the orbital septum (upper lid deep wounds, between the tarsus and the superior orbital rim)
4. Canthal tendons (wounds penetrating the lateral and medial canthi)
5. Lid margins (wounds through the tarsal plate and lid margins)

○ **What are the 4 Ss of hyphema complications?**

1. **S**taining of the cornea due to hemosiderin deposits
2. **S**ynechiae, which interfere with iris function
3. **S**econdary rebleeding, which usually occurs between the second and fifth day after the injury (since this is the time of clot retraction) and tend to be worse than the initial bleeding
4. **S**ignificantly increased intraocular pressure, which can lead to acute glaucoma, chronic late glaucoma, and optic atrophy

○ **Why do patients with sickle cell anemia and hyphema require special consideration when presenting with ophthalmologic concerns?**

Increased intraocular pressure can occur if the cells sickle in the trabecular network, preventing aqueous humor from leaving the anterior chamber. Some medications, such as hyperosmotics and acetazolamide, increase the likelihood of sickling.

○ **A patient presents with a history of trauma to the orbit with dull ocular pain, decreased visual acuity, and photophobia. An examination reveals a constricted pupil and ciliary flush. What will be found at slitlamp examination?**

Flare and cells in the anterior chamber are present with traumatic iritis.

○ **What are causes of a subluxed or dislocated lens?**

- Trauma
- Marfan syndrome
- Homocystinuria
- Weill-Marchesani syndrome

○ **Physiologically, what causes flare?**

Flare is caused by inflammatory proteins resulting in the "dust in the movie projector lights" or "fog in the headlights" phenomena at slitlamp examination.

○ **Which is worse: acid or alkali burns of the cornea?**

Alkali, because of deeper penetration than acid burns. A barrier is formed from precipitated proteins with acid burns. The exception is hydrofluoric acid and acids containing heavy metal that can penetrate the cornea.

○ **When should an eye not be dilated?**

When there is known narrow-angle glaucoma or an iris-supported intraocular lens

○ **Why should topical ophthalmologic anesthetics not be prescribed?**

The anesthetics inhibit healing and decrease the patient's ability to protect the eye because of the lack of sensation.

○ **What is the most common organism in contact lens–associated corneal ulcers?**

Pseudomonas

○ **How can cyanoacrylate be removed if a patient has stuck the eyelids together?**

Copious irrigation immediately and then mineral oil. Acetone and ethanol are unacceptable in the eyes. Surgical separation must be performed with extreme care to prevent laceration of the lids or globe. Often the patient will have corneal abrasion, which should be treated in the usual manner.

○ **A 24-year-old woman presents with blurred vision that becomes worse when looking at objects far away. At examination, the eyes converge, the pupils constrict, and accommodation is at a maximum. What is the diagnosis?**

Spasm of accommodation. Treat anxiety. A short-acting cycloplegic may stop the cycle.

○ **An anxious 16-year-old boy presents with vision he describes as similar to looking down a gun barrel. How do you clinically differentiate between physiologic and hysterical scotoma?**

- Physiologic: Doubling the distance between the patient and tangent screen (visual screen test) results in doubling of the size of the central visual field.
- Hysterical: The visual field remains the same when the distance between the patient and tangent screen is doubled.

○ **What test can a physician use to determine if blindness is of a hysterical origin?**

An optokinetic drum can be used. If nystagmus eye movements occur, the patient is seeing the stripes. Prisms may also be used.

○ **Three hours ago, a patient experienced sudden, painless visual loss in her right eye. Central retinal artery occlusion is suspected. What findings are expected at eye examination? What is the prognosis?**

Afferent pupillary defect, pale gray retina, and a small cherry red dot near the fovea. This dot is the choroidal vasculature being seen at the macula where the retina is the thinnest. After 2 hours, the prognosis is extremely poor for visual recovery. Digital massage or anterior chamber paracentesis may dislodge the clot. Immediate ophthalmic consultation is necessary.

○ **What conditions have been associated with central retinal vein occlusion?**

Hyperviscosity syndromes, diabetes, and hypertension. Funduscopic examination shows a chaotically streaked retina with congested dilated veins. There are superficial and deep retinal hemorrhages, cotton-wool spots, and macular edema.

○ **A patient presents with atraumatic pain behind the left eye, a left pupil afferent defect, central visual loss, and a left swollen disc. What are the diagnosis and potential causes?**

Optic neuritis. This may be idiopathic or associated with multiple sclerosis, Lyme disease, neurosyphilis, lupus, sarcoid, alcoholism, toxins, or drug abuse.

○ **After entering a dark bar, a patient developed eye pain, nausea, vomiting, and blurred vision. He also sees halos around lights. Why would this patient receive mannitol, pilocarpine, and acetazolamide?**

This patient has acute narrow-angle glaucoma. The goal of treatment is to decrease intraocular pressure.

- Decrease the production of aqueous humor with carbonic anhydrase inhibitor
- Decrease intraocular volume by making the plasma hypertonic to the aqueous humor with glycerol or mannitol
- Constrict the pupil with pilocarpine, allowing increased flow of the aqueous humor out through the previously blocked canals of Schlemm

○ **A patient presents with multiple vertical linear corneal abrasions. What should be suspected?**

A foreign body under the upper lid. This pattern is sometimes called an "ice rink" sign.

○ **How can a physician estimate if the anterior chamber of the eye is narrow?**

Tangential light (as with a penlight) is shone perpendicular to the line of vision across the anterior chamber. If the entire iris is in the light, then the chamber is most likely a normal depth. If part of the iris is in a shadow, the chamber is narrow. This can occur with narrow-angle glaucoma and with perforating corneal injuries.

○ **What is the difference between a sympathomimetic and a cycloplegic medication when dilating the eye?**

A sympathomimetic stimulates the iris's dilator muscle. The cycloplegic inhibits the parasympathetic stimulation, which constricts the iris and inhibits the ciliary muscle. Thus, cycloplegics will cause blurred near vision.

○ **A patient felt something fly into his eye while mowing the lawn. At examination, there is a brown foreign body on the cornea and a teardrop iris pointing toward the foreign body. What is the diagnosis?**

Perforated cornea with extruded iris. A similar foreign body may appear black on the sclera with scleral perforation.

○ **A patient's cornea fluoresces before instillation of fluorescein. What should be considered?**

Pseudomonal infection. Several species fluoresce on their own.

○ **How can one determine if a pupil is dilated by pharmacologic agents?**

Pharmacologic dilatation should be suspected if the pupil does not constrict at 0.125% pilocarpine instillation. The pupil can be further tested with 1% pilocarpine.

○ **A patient presents with a physical finding of chaotically blood-streaked retina with congested and dilated veins. What is the diagnosis?**

Central retinal vein occlusion. Patients often complain of a painless unilateral decrease of vision.

○ **Which anesthetic works the fastest, and which lasts the longest: proparacaine or tetracaine?**

- Proparacaine has a rapid onset and duration of 20 minutes.
- Tetracaine has a delayed onset and duration of 1 hour.

○ **Place the following mydriatic-cycloplegic medications in order of duration of activity: tropicamide, homatropine, atropine, and cyclopentolate.**

1. Tropicamide (onset in 15 to 20 minutes, brief duration)

2. Cyclopentolate (onset in 30 to 60 minutes, duration <24 hours)

3. Homatropine (long lasting, 2 to 3 days)

4. Atropine (very long lasting, 2 weeks)

○ **How can you test vision in children younger than 3 years?**

Young children can be observed to follow objects. The Cardiff Acuity Test can be used in 1- to 3-year-old children. This is a preferential looking test based on the finding that children prefer to look at complex rather than plain objects.

○ **A 3-month-old baby has continuous tearing from the left eye. What is the likely diagnosis?**

Partial lacrimal duct obstruction. Treatment is observation because most resolve by 8 months of age. If not, the duct can be probed by an ophthalmologist.

○ **What is the most common finding at fluorescein angiography in diabetes mellitus?**

Leakage of the dye from abnormal blood vessels

○ **What are the advantages of rigid versus soft contact lenses?**

Rigid contact lenses are gas permeable and reduce the risk of corneal damage from hypoxia. Proteinaceous materials are less likely to adhere to rigid lenses.

○ **What is the most common bacterial cause of orbital cellulitis?**

Haemophilus influenzae

○ **When should a periorbital capillary hemangioma be treated?**

If the size or portion obstructs the visual axis because amblyopia may develop. Treatment is local injection of steroids.

○ **What is the most common orbital tumor in children?**

Rhabdomyosarcoma of the external eye muscles. Treatment is chemotherapy if the tumor is confined to the orbital space.

○ **What are the causes of ectropion (eversion of the lid away from the globe)?**

• Age-related orbicularis muscle laxity
• Seventh nerve palsy
• Scarring of the periorbital skin

○ **What are the causes of entropion (turning in of the lid toward the globe)?**

• Age-related orbicularis muscle laxity
• Conjunctival scarring

○ **What is the treatment for entropion and ectropion?**

Definitive treatment is surgery.

○ **What is a xanthelasma?**

A lipid-containing bilateral lesion, which, in youth, may be related to hypercholesterolemia

○ **What are the causes of dry eye (keratoconjunctivitis sicca)?**
- Deficiency of tear quantity
- Excessive evaporation
- Change in mucous composition of the tears

○ **What are the causes for change in mucous composition of tears (loss of goblet cells)?**
- Erythema multiforme
- Chemical burns of the eye (especially alkaline)
- Trachoma
- Vitamin A deficiency

○ **What are the infective causes of ophthalmia neonatorium?**
- Gram-positive bacteria (staphylococci, streptococci)
- *Neisseria gonorrhoeae*
- Herpes simplex virus
- *Chlamydia*

○ **What is the name of a white, ring-shaped lipid deposit separated from the limbus by a clear interval?**

Lipid arcus. In patients younger than 50 years, it may be associated with hypercholesterolemia. In patients older than 50 years, it is called "arcus senilis."

○ **Which is more worrisome: episcleritis or scleritis?**

Scleritis. It can cause glaucoma, cataracts, uveitis, scleral thinning, and keratitis. It must be treated aggressively with steroids or cytotoxins. Episcleritis is usually self-limiting.

○ **True/False: The most common cause of a bacterial corneal ulcer in the developed world is contact lens wearing.**

True. Other causes are trauma, prolonged steroid use, dry eye, and herpetic eye disease.

○ **What is the most common cause of treatable blindness in the world?**

Cataracts that cause a painless loss of vision, glare, and refractive error

○ **What are possible complications of cataract surgery?**

Iris prolapse, vitreous loss, cystoid macular edema, capsule opacification, and endophthalmitis

○ **Cataracts may be associated with and caused by what?**

Hypocalcemia, diabetes mellitus, trauma, steroids, and myotonic dystrophy

○ **With which types of injuries is Purtscher retinopathy associated?**

Thoracic injuries and broken bones. Findings include retinal hemorrhage and cotton-wool spots.

○ **A patient presents with eye pain. She has a constricted pupil, ciliary flush, and red injected sclera at the limbus. What is the diagnosis?**

Acute iritis

○ **What is a pinguecula?**

It is a yellowish nodule, particularly on the nasal aspect of the eye, but it may be on the lateral aspect. It is often caused by wind and dust.

○ **What is a pterygium?**

It is a chronic growth over the medial or lateral aspect of the cornea approaching the pupil. It is much thicker than a pinguecula.

○ **What nerves control the corneal reflex?**

The ophthalmic branch of the fifth nerve and the afferent branch of the facial (seventh) nerve.

○ **At funduscopic examination, what are microaneurysms and soft exudates typical of?**

Hypertension

○ **At funduscopic examination, what are macular microaneurysms and hard exudates typical of?**

Diabetes

○ **What organisms are typically responsible for causing bacterial conjunctivitis?**

Staphylococcal. The second most common are streptococcal.

○ **What is the appropriate treatment of hyphema?**

Elevate the head. Other treatments are controversial; however, most ophthalmologists recommend hospitalization for patients. Treatment may include a double eye patch, topical cortisone, and cycloplegics.

○ **Differentiate between strabismus, esotropia, and exotropia.**
- Strabismus: Lack of parallelism of the visual axis of the eyes
- Esotropia: Medial deviation
- Exotropia: Lateral deviation

CHAPTER 16 Ear, Nose, and Throat

David A. Stewart, MD

○ **What percentage of the elderly are hard of hearing?**

Twenty-nine percent of people older than 65 years and 36% of people older than 75 years have hearing loss sufficient to interfere with normal conversation.

○ **What is the most common type of hearing loss in the elderly?**

Presbycusis. This is an idiopathic, insidious, symmetric decrease in hearing that is associated with aging.

○ **What is the prognostic significance of vertigo in a patient with sudden sensorineural hearing loss?**

Vertigo is a poor prognostic sign. Patients younger than 40 years regain their normal hearing in 50% of cases. Recovery correlates to the degree of hearing loss and the length of time hearing has been altered. Hearing loss lasting more than 1 month is most likely permanent.

○ **What systemic sexually transmitted disease is associated with sensorineural hearing loss?**

Syphilis. Seven percent of patients with idiopathic hearing loss test positive for treponemal antibodies.

○ **Acute tinnitus is associated with toxicity of what medication?**

Salicylates. Other causes of tinnitus are vascular abnormalities, mechanical abnormalities, and damaged cochlear hair cells. Unilateral tinnitus is associated with chronic suppurative otitis, Ménière disease, and trauma.

○ **Hairy leukoplakia is characteristic of which 2 viruses?**

1. Human immunodeficiency virus
2. Epstein-Barr virus

Hairy leukoplakia is usually found on the lateral aspect of the tongue. Oral thrush may also be associated with human immunodeficiency virus.

○ **What is the most common cause of odontogenic pain?**

Carious tooth. When percussed with a tongue blade, the tooth will produce a sharp pain felt in the ear, throat, eyes, temple, or other side of the jaw.

○ **A child presents after falling and knocking out his front tooth. How would treatment differ if the child were aged 3 years versus 13 years?**

With primary teeth, no reimplantation should be attempted because of the risk of ankylosis or fusion to the bone. However, with permanent teeth, reimplantation should occur as soon as possible. Remaining periodontal ligament fibers are a key to success. Therefore, the tooth should not be wiped dry, because this may disrupt the fibers still attached.

○ **What is the best transport medium for an avulsed tooth?**

Hanks solution, a pH balanced cell culture medium, which may even help restore cell viability if the tooth has been avulsed for more than 30 minutes. Milk is an alternative. The patient may place the tooth underneath the tongue if aspiration can be prevented.

○ **A patient presents 3 days after tooth extraction with severe pain and a foul mouth odor and taste. What is the appropriate diagnosis and treatment?**

Alveolar osteitis (dry socket) results from loss of the blood clot and local osteomyelitis. Treat with irrigation of the socket and application of a medicated dental packing or iodoform gauze moistened with camphor-phenol topical or eugenol.

○ **A patient presents with gingival pain and a foul mouth odor and taste. At examination, fever and lymphadenopathy are present. The gingiva is bright red, and the papillae are ulcerated and covered with a gray membrane. What is the diagnosis and treatment?**

Acute necrotizing ulcerative gingivitis. Treat with antibiotics (tetracycline or penicillin) and a topical anesthetic. A possible complication of this disease is the destruction of alveolar bone.

○ **What is the most common oral manifestation of AIDS?**

Oropharyngeal thrush. Some other AIDS-related oropharyngeal diseases are Kaposi sarcoma, hairy leukoplakia, and non-Hodgkin lymphoma.

○ **A 47-year-old woman presents complaining of excruciating pain described as an electric shock sensation that waxes and wanes in her right cheek. What are the diagnosis and treatment?**

Trigeminal neuralgia, also known as "tic douloureux." The most significant finding is that the pain follows the distribution of the trigeminal nerve. Minor trigger zone stimulation will often reproduce the pain. Treat with carbamazepine, 100 mg twice a day as the starting dose and increasing to 1200 mg daily, if needed. Refer the patient to a neurologist and a dentist to rule out cerebellopontine angle tumors, multiple sclerosis, nasopharyngeal carcinoma, cluster headaches, polymyalgia rheumatica, temporal arteritis, and oral disease.

○ **A 3-year-old child presents with unilateral purulent rhinorrhea. What is the probable diagnosis?**

Nasal foreign body

○ **What potential complications of nasal fracture should always be considered at physical examination?**

Septal hematoma and cribriform plate fractures. Septal hematoma appears as a bluish mass on the nasal septum. If not drained, aseptic necrosis of the septal cartilage and septal abnormalities may occur. Cribriform plate fracture should be considered in a patient who has clear rhinorrhea after trauma.

○ **What 4 physical examination findings would make posterior epistaxis more likely than anterior epistaxis?**

1. Inability to see the site of bleeding. Anterior epistaxis usually originates at the Kiesselbach plexus and is easily seen on the nasal septum.

2. Blood from both sides of the nose. In posterior epistaxis, the blood can more easily pass to the other side because of the proximity of the choanae.

3. Blood trickling down the oropharynx

4. Inability to control bleeding with direct pressure

○ **A patient returns to the emergency department with fever, nausea, vomiting, and hypotension 2 days after having nasal packing placed for anterior epistaxis. What potential complication of nasal packing should be considered?**

Toxic shock syndrome

○ **A child with a sinus infection presents with proptosis; a red, swollen eyelid; and an inferolaterally displaced globe. What is the diagnosis?**

Orbital cellulitis and abscess associated with ethmoid sinusitis

○ **A patient with frontal sinusitis presents with a large forehead abscess. What is the diagnosis?**

Pott puffy tumor. This is a complication of frontal sinusitis in which the anterior table of the skull is destroyed, allowing the formation of the abscess.

○ **A patient who appears ill presents with a fever of 103°F, bilateral chemosis, third nerve palsies, and untreated sinusitis. What is the diagnosis?**

Cavernous sinus thrombosis. This life-threatening complication occurs from direct extension through the valveless veins. Complications of sinusitis may be local (osteomyelitis), orbital (cellulitis), or within the central nervous system (meningitis or brain abscess).

○ **Retropharyngeal abscesses are most common in what age group? Why?**

6 months to 3 years. Retropharyngeal lymph nodes regress in size after age 3 years.

○ **Describe the overall appearance of a child with retropharyngeal abscess.**

These children are often appear ill, febrile, stridorous, drooling, and in an opisthotonic position. They may complain of difficulty swallowing or may refuse to eat.

○ **What radiographic sign indicates retropharyngeal abscess?**

Widening of the retropharyngeal space, which is normally 3 to 4 mm, or less than half the width of the vertebral bodies. False widening may occur if the radiograph is not obtained during inspiration and with the patient's neck extended. Occasionally, an air-fluid level may be noted in the retropharyngeal space.

○ **Retropharyngeal abscesses are most commonly caused by which organisms?**

β-*Hemolytic Streptococcus*

○ **Where is the most common origin of Ludwig angina?**

The lower second and third molar. Ludwig angina is a swelling in the region of the submandibular, sublingual, and submental spaces, which may cause upward and posterior displacement of the tongue. It is most commonly caused by hemolytic streptococci, staphylococci, and mixed anaerobic and aerobic bacteria.

○ **Can a patient lose more of the upper or lower lip without cosmetic problems?**

As much as one-third of the lower lip can be avulsed or debrided while still may maintaining acceptable cosmetic appearance. The upper lip is more problematic because of its relationship with the columella, alar bases, and philtrum.

○ **What are the signs and symptoms of mandibular fracture?**

Malocclusion, pain, opening deviation or abnormal movement, decreased range of motion, bony deformity, swelling, ecchymosis, and lower lip (mental nerve) anesthesia

○ **A patient was yawning during a lecture and is now unable to close his mouth. He is having difficulty talking and swallowing. What is the diagnosis?**

Bilateral dislocation of the mandibular condyles, which can occur if the mouth is opened excessively widely. Radiography can be used to rule out bilateral condyle fractures, which can have a similar clinical appearance.

○ **A 42-year-old woman presents with dull pain in her right ear and jaw and a burning sensation on the roof of her mouth. The pain is worse in the evening. She also hears a popping sound when opening and closing her mouth. Further examination reveals tenderness of the joint capsule. What are the diagnosis and treatment?**

Temporomandibular joint syndrome. Treat with physiotherapy, analgesia, a soft diet, muscle relaxants, and occlusive therapy. Apply warm, moist compresses 4 to 5 times daily for 15 minutes for 7 to 10 days.

○ **In internal derangement of the temporomandibular joint because of meniscal displacement, in which direction is the meniscus displaced?**

Anteromedially, which may cause the joint to lock in a closed position. The jaw may deviate toward the affected side. The articular disk may become displaced owing to tears, perforation, or stretching of the posterior ligamentous attachments.

○ **What are the signs and symptoms of a fracture of the zygomaticomaxillary complex?**

Subcutaneous emphysema; edema; ecchymosis; facial flattening; subconjunctival hemorrhage; unilateral epistaxis; anesthesia of the cheek, upper lip, and gum from infraorbital nerve injury; step deformity; decreased mandibular movement; and diplopia

○ **What 2 findings are most commonly associated with orbital floor fractures?**

1. Diplopia
2. Globe lowering

○ **What radiographic findings might suggest orbital blowout fracture?**

- Fracture lines or bony fragments in the maxillary sinus
- Subcutaneous or orbital emphysema
- Air-fluid level in the maxillary sinus
- A teardrop sign where a soft-tissue mass protrudes into the maxillary sinus

○ **What plain radiographic views are most helpful in evaluating facial fractures?**
- Waters view: Useful for evaluating the zygomaticomaxillary complex, orbital blowout, and Le Fort fractures
- Modified basal view of the skull: Useful for evaluating zygomatic arch fractures
- Panoramic views: Useful for evaluating mandibular fractures

○ **A 48-year-old presents with pain, itching, and discharge from the right ear. The tympanic membrane is intact. What is the diagnosis?**

Otitis externa. Suction the ear and prescribe antibiotic steroid otic solution for 1 week. An ear wick may improve delivery of the antibiotic. Consider malignant otitis externa if the patient is diabetic.

○ **A patient presents with ear pain and fluid-filled blisters on the tympanic membrane. What is the diagnosis?**

Bullous myringitis, commonly caused by *Mycoplasma* or a virus. Treat with erythromycin or another macrolide.

○ **A 16-year-old boxer presents with right ear pain and swelling after receiving a blow to the ear. What is the treatment?**

The ear should be aseptically drained by means of incision or aspiration and a mastoid-conforming dressing should be applied. Follow-up with an ear, nose, and throat (ENT) specialist is mandatory. If the ear is not treated appropriately, a cauliflower deformity may result.

○ **A patient presents with a swollen, tender, red left auricle. What is the diagnosis?**

Perichondritis. This is most often caused by *Pseudomonas*.

○ **What is the most common cause of hearing loss?**

Cerumen impaction

○ **Describe the physical finding of unilateral sensory hearing loss.**

The patient lateralizes and has air conduction greater than bone conduction (ie, normal Rinne test results) indicating no conductive loss. Weber test results indicate lateralization to the normal ear. The most common cause of unilateral sensory hearing loss is viral neuritis.

○ **Which causes should be suspected in a patient with bilateral sensory hearing loss?**

Noise or ototoxins (eg, certain antibiotics, loop diuretics, or antineoplastics)

○ **What is the most common neuropathy associated with acoustic neuroma?**

The corneal reflex may be lost due to trigeminal nucleus involvement.

○ **Name some causes of tympanic membrane perforation.**
- Air or water blast injuries
- Foreign bodies in the ear (particularly cotton-tip swabs)
- Lightning strikes
- Otitis media
- Associated temporal bone fractures

○ **A young man who was involved in a barroom brawl complains of ear pain, significantly decreased hearing, and vertigo. Tympanic membrane rupture is determined at examination. What is of concern?**

Injury to the ossicles, temporal bone, or labyrinth. Urgent consultation with an ENT specialist is necessary.

○ **A diver on vacation decided to go scuba diving despite having a cold. While descending, she had acute ear pain followed by vertiginous symptoms and vomiting. What happened?**

Middle ear squeeze. Pressure from the middle ear could not be equalized because of abnormal eustachian tube function resulting from the illness. The middle ear volume decreased until the tympanic membrane retracted to the point of rupture. The inrush of cold water caused vestibular stimulation. This is the most common form of barotrauma in amateur scuba divers. Similar problems may occur on planes.

○ **What organism usually causes pediatric acute otitis media?**

Streptococcus pneumoniae, followed by *Haemophilus influenzae* and *Moraxella catarrhalis*. Viruses are the cause of otitis media in approximately 15% of cases.

○ **Why are preschool children more susceptible to acute otitis media?**

Children have shorter, more horizontal eustachian tubes, which may prevent adequate drainage and allow aspiration of nasopharyngeal bacteria into the middle ear, particularly with upper respiratory infections.

○ **What is a Bezold abscess?**

A complication of acute mastoiditis. Infection spreads to the soft tissues below the ear and sternocleidomastoid muscle.

○ **What is the most common cause of sialadenitis?**

Mumps

○ **A patient presents with trismus, fever, and an erythematous, tender parotid gland. Pus is expressed from the Stensen duct. What conditions predisposes the patient to bacterial parotitis?**

Any situation that decreases salivary flow, including irradiation, phenothiazines, antihistamines, parasympathetic inhibitors, dehydration, and debilitation. As many as 30% of cases occur postoperatively.

○ **Where do salivary gland stones most frequently develop?**

Eighty percent are submandibular. The least likely location is the sublingual gland.

○ **What is the most common benign salivary gland tumor?**

Salivary pleomorphic adenoma

○ **Where is a parotid gland tumor most likely to develop?**

The superficial lobe, which is located just below the earlobe. Forty percent of parotid gland tumors are malignant. All tumors, benign or malignant, should be removed.

○ **What is the most common type of malignant parotid gland tumor?**

Mucoepidermoid carcinoma. Other types of malignant tumors are acinic cell carcinoma, adenocarcinoma, malignant mixed tumor, adenoid cystic carcinoma, and epidermoid carcinoma.

○ **What does grunting versus inspiratory stridor indicate?**

Grunting is specific to lower respiratory tract diseases, such as pneumonia, asthma, and bronchiolitis. Stridor localizes respiratory obstruction to the level at or above the larynx.

○ **A patient presents with well-demarcated swelling of the lips and tongue. She started using an antihypertensive agent 3 weeks ago. What is the most likely agent?**

Angiotensin-converting enzyme inhibitor. Although angioneurotic edema may occur anytime during therapy, it is most likely to occur within in the first month of using an angiotensin-converting enzyme inhibitor.

○ **A patient is seen with herpetic lesions on the tip of the nose. Why is this a problem?**

The tip of the nose and the cornea are both supplied by the nasociliary nerve. Thus, the cornea may also be involved. This is an ophthalmologic emergency.

○ **Peritonsillar abscess is most common in what age group?**

Adolescents and young adults. Symptoms may include ear pain, trismus, drooling, and alteration of voice.

○ **What is Spanierman sign?**

Blood under the nails, which indicates epistaxis due to nose picking. Bleeding in such cases is generally from the Kiesselbach plexus.

○ **Where in the airway are foreign bodies usually lodged in children older than 1 year?**

In the lower airway

○ **What is the most common complication of acute otitis media?**

Tympanic membrane perforation. Other complications include mastoiditis, cholesteatoma, and intracranial infections.

○ **Describe the key features of Ménière disease, also known as "endolymphatic hydrops."**

Vertigo, hearing loss, and tinnitus. Ménière disease typically manifests with the rapid onset of vertigo, nausea, and vomiting that lasts for hours to 1 day. Nystagmus may be spontaneous during the critical stage. Tinnitus may be present and is louder during attacks, and sensorineural hearing loss may occur. There also may be an aura with a sensation of fullness in the ear during an attack. Symptoms are unilateral in more than 90% of patients, and recurring attacks are typical.

○ **What are the key features of viral labyrinthitis or vestibular neuritis?**

Severe vertigo (usually lasting 3 to 5 days), with nausea and vomiting. Symptoms generally regress over 3 to 6 weeks. Nystagmus may be spontaneous during the severe stage.

○ **A patient presents with hearing loss, nystagmus, facial weakness, and diplopia. Vertigo is provoked with sudden movement. Results from lumbar puncture reveal elevated levels of central nervous system protein. What diagnosis is suspected?**

Acoustic neuroma

○ **Describe the signs and symptoms of acoustic neuroma.**

Unilateral high-tone sensorineural hearing loss and tinnitus. Decreased corneal sensitivity, diplopia, headache, facial weakness, and positive radiographic findings may occur. Vertigo usually appears late, is more often exhibited as a progressive feeling of imbalance, and can be provoked by changes in head movement. Nystagmus is frequently present and is usually spontaneous. The cerebrospinal fluid may have elevated protein levels.

○ **What is the most common cause of Ludwig angina?**

Odontogenic abscess of a lower molar

○ **What is the most serious complication associated with dental infection, besides possible respiratory compromise, from Ludwig angina?**

Septic cavernous sinus thrombosis

○ **What are the key features of Ellis class I, II, and III dental fractures?**

- Class I: Enamel only
- Class II: Enamel and dentin
- Class III: Enamel, dentin, and pulp

○ **What is the best emergency treatment of an Ellis class III dental fracture in an adult?**

Cover the tooth with moist cotton and then dry aluminum foil, and refer the patient immediately to an orthodontist.

○ **What is the presentation of a patient with postextraction alveolitis?**

Dry socket pain occurs on the second or third day after extraction.

○ **How does an adult with epiglottitis present?**

Pharyngitis and dysphagia are prominent symptoms. Adenopathy is uncommon. The patient may have a muffled voice and speak softly; however, hoarseness is rare. Pain is out of proportion to objective findings.

○ **What are the 2 most common pathogens in adult acute sinusitis?**

1. *S pneumoniae*
2. *H influenzae*

○ **What is a frequent complication of ethmoid sinusitis?**

Orbital cellulitis

○ **What is rhinocerebral phycomycosis?**

Rhinocerebral phycomycosis, also known as mucormycosis, is a fungal infection typically seen in diabetic patients with ketoacidosis and in immunocompromised patients. The disease is rapidly fatal if not recognized and treated quickly. Treatment includes antifungal drugs and surgical debridement.

○ **A 2-year-old girl has jammed a pencil into the lateral portion of her soft palate. What complication might develop?**

Ischemic stroke is a complication of soft-palate pencil injuries and can result in contralateral hemiparesis.

○ **What nerve supplies taste to the anterior two-thirds of the tongue and the lacrimal and salivary glands?**

Cranial nerve VII

○ **What are the advantages of pacifier use in newborns and infants?**

Benefits of pacifiers include analgesic effects during minor medical procedures such as heel sticks, immunizations, and venipuncture; shorter hospital stays for preterm infants; and reduction in the risk of sudden infant death syndrome.

○ **What are the risks associated with pacifier use in newborns and infants?**

Potential complications of pacifier use, particularly with prolonged use, include a negative effect on breastfeeding, dental malocclusion, and otitis media. Adverse dental effects can be evident by 2 years of age but mainly after 4 years. Pacifier use should be stopped or limited in the second 6 months of life to reduce the risk of otitis media.

○ **Can use of clinical decision rules for diagnosing group A β-hemolytic streptococcal pharyngitis improve quality of care while reducing unwarranted treatment and overall cost?**

Yes. In a patient presenting with a sore throat, assign 1 point each for (1) absence of cough, (2) swollen and tender anterior cervical lymph nodes, (3) temperature higher than 100.4 F°, and (4) tonsillar exudates or swelling. One additional point is given for patients aged 3 to 14 years, and one point is subtracted for age 45 years or older. Scoring is as follows:

• 0: No further testing or antibiotics is needed.
• 1: Further testing is optional.
• 2 to 3: Perform throat culture or rapid antigen detection test and treat based on results.
• 4 to 5: Consider empiric treatment with antibiotics.

○ **What are treatment options for acute group A β-hemolytic streptococcal pharyngitis?**

Penicillin (oral for 10 days or a single intramuscular injection of benzathine penicillin) remains the drug of choice for group A β-hemolytic streptococcal pharyngitis, although an increase in treatment failure with penicillins is beginning to be seen. Alternative treatments include amoxicillin, which is equally effective and more palatable. Erythromycins and first-generation cephalosporins are options for patients allergic to penicillins.

○ **How is recurrent group A β-hemolytic streptococcal pharyngitis managed?**

For patients presenting with recurrent sore throat within 28 days of a previously diagnosed and treated group A β-hemolytic streptococcal pharyngitis, a rapid streptococcal antigen detection test should be performed. If the result is positive, treatment with the usual antistreptococcal antibiotics is warranted. Intramuscular penicillin G is an option when oral antibiotics were initially prescribed.

○ **What is the most common presenting symptom in a patient with Hodgkin lymphoma?**

Painless lymphadenopathy, often involving cervical, supraclavicular, or axillary nodes. The nodes tend to be freely movable with a rubbery consistency. In Hodgkin lymphoma, lymphadenopathy generally has a contiguous spread.

○   **What ENT manifestations may be associated with atypical manifestations of gastroesophageal reflux diseases?**

Laryngitis, hoarseness, chronic sore throat, globus sensation, sinusitis, nasal polyps, halitosis, and dental erosions. Asthma, chronic cough, aspiration pneumonia, and noncardiac chest pain may also be manifestations of atypical gastroesophageal reflux disease.

○   **What are the most common causes of primary otalgia?**

Otitis media and otitis externa are the most common primary causes of ear pain (otalgia). Primary otalgia is defined as pain arising directly from the ear, and the cause is usually evident at physical examination.

○   **What are the most common causes of secondary otalgia?**

Secondary, or referred, otalgia, usually has normal ear examination results, with the pain referred from a variety of possible sites. Dental disease, temporomandibular joint disorders, cervical spine disorders, and neuralgias are the most common causes of secondary otalgia, accounting for approximately 30% to 50% of diagnoses in patients presenting with ear pain.

○   **What are appropriate diagnostic interventions for evaluation of secondary otalgia without a clear cause at physical examination?**

Magnetic resonance imaging and referral for nasolaryngoscopy should be considered for patients with otalgia with normal examination results and risk factors for tumor, such as smoking, ethanol abuse, or being older than 50 years. Patients aged 40 years and younger with normal ear examination results can have their symptoms treated. Referral is indicated for persistent symptoms of otalgia.

○   **What vascular cause of secondary otalgia should be considered in patients older than 50 years?**

Temporal arteritis should be considered in patients aged 50 years or older who present with unexplained ear pain. The erythrocyte sedimentation rate should be measured to help rule out temporal arteritis.

○   **What is the most common deep infection of the head and neck?**

Peritonsillar abscess. It occurs in all age groups but with the highest incidence in adults aged 20 to 40 years. Patients present with peritonsillar abscess most frequently between November and December and in April and May, coinciding with the peak incidence of streptococcal and exudative pharyngitis.

○   **What is the clinical presentation of a patient with peritonsillar abscess?**

Symptoms of peritonsillar abscess include fever, malaise, severe sore throat (worse on the affected side), dysphagia, and ipsilateral otalgia. Physical examination findings include a swollen, erythematous soft palate and anterior tonsils; a swollen tonsil, often displaced inferiorly and medially, with deviation of the uvula to the contralateral side; trismus; drooling; muffled "hot potato voice"; rancid breath; and cervical lymphadenitis.

○   **What is the most common pediatric infection for which antibiotics are prescribed in the United States?**

Acute otitis media, either viral or bacterial. Acute otitis media is most commonly diagnosed in children between ages 6 and 24 months. More than 80% of children have had a diagnosis of otitis media by age 3 years.

○ **What are the diagnostic criteria for acute otitis media?**

Acute onset of symptoms, with signs and symptoms of middle ear inflammation, including erythema of the tympanic membrane or otalgia affecting sleep and/or normal activity. Signs of middle ear effusion, such as bulging tympanic membrane, air-fluid level behind the membrane, or abnormal findings at pneumatic otoscopy or tympanometry, should be sought to confirm the diagnosis.

○ **What is the recommended treatment for acute otitis media?**

Since 70% to 90% of children with acute otitis media with have spontaneous resolution within 7 to 14 days, observation without antibiotic treatment is an option. If antibiotics are used, amoxicillin at a dosage of 80 to 90 mg/kg per day should be the first-line antibiotic for most children. Patients who do not respond to initial therapy should be reassessed within 48 to 72 hours. If the diagnosis is confirmed, antibiotic therapy should be initiated or adjusted. Antihistamines and decongestants should not be prescribed for children with acute otitis media.

○ **What is the rationale for universal newborn hearing screening?**

A critical period for optimal language development exists. Earlier intervention improves outcomes, and treatment of hearing deficits improves communication skills. Approximately 20% to 40% of children with profound hearing impairment will be missed if risk factor screening alone is used.

○ **What is a pregnancy oral tumor?**

A pregnancy oral tumor is a soft-tissue mass that occurs most commonly at the gum line but that also may develop on the lip, tongue, or buccal mucosa. It can develop in as many as 5% of pregnancies. It is indistinguishable from pyogenic granuloma. Unless it is complicated by bleeding, observation is appropriate because it has a high recurrence rate after excision, and resolution after delivery often occurs.

○ **What is the most common oral cancer in the United States?**

Squamous cell carcinoma, which accounts for approximately 90% of oral cancers in the United States. Incidence increases with age. Tobacco use and heavy ethanol use are principal risk factors and are associated in 75% of cases. Sixty percent of oral cancers are advanced at time of diagnosis, and another cancer in such sites as the larynx, esophagus, or lung are found in approximately 15% of patients.

○ **What agents cause otitis externa?**

Acute otitis externa is generally bacterial in origin, with *Pseudomonas aeruginosa* accounting for approximately 50% of cases, followed in incidence by *Staphylococcus aureus*, and then various other aerobic and anaerobic bacteria. Chronic otitis media, in which symptoms last 3 months or more, are more likely to be fungal or allergic in origin.

○ **When should antibiotics be used to treat acute sinusitis?**

The diagnosis of acute bacterial sinusitis should be considered in patients with symptoms of viral upper respiratory infections (rhinorrhea, daytime cough, fever, purulent nasal discharge, facial pain) that do not improve after 10 days or worsen after 5 to 7 days. Additional symptoms indicating the diagnosis of bacterial sinusitis include increasing facial pressure or pain, especially if unilateral or focused over a particular sinus; hyposmia; anosmia; maxillary dental pain; and ear pressure or fullness. Nearly all cases of acute bacterial sinusitis resolve spontaneously, so antibiotics should be limited to use in patients with moderate symptoms not improving after 10 days, those worsening in 5 to 7 days, or those with severe symptoms.

○   **What percentage of palpable thyroid nodules are malignant?**

Approximately 5% of palpable thyroid nodules are malignant. The main objective in evaluating thyroid nodules is to exclude malignancy.

○   **What is the recommended evaluation for solitary thyroid nodule?**

Serologic testing, including evaluation of thyrotropin level, should be performed to differentiate thyrotoxic nodules from euthyroid nodules. Fine-needle aspiration is the modality recommended by the American Association of Clinical Endocrinologists for initial evaluation of solitary nodules. Radionuclide scanning is reserved for nodules with indeterminate cytologic findings at fine-needle aspiration and for patients with thyrotoxicosis. Fine-needle aspiration is recommended for cold nodules. Patients with hot nodules at scanning should undergo radioactive iodine therapy or surgery.

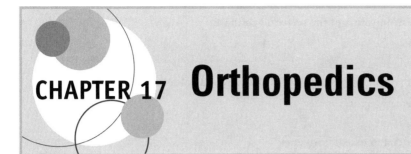

CHAPTER 17 Orthopedics

Krystian Bigosinski, MD; Deepak S. Patel, MD, FAAFP

○ **How do you differentiate clinically between acute compartment syndrome, neuropraxia, and arterial occlusion?**

The patient will have normal pulses in neuropraxia, decreased pulses in compartment syndrome (though this is a rare finding that is not sensitive), and no pulses in arterial occlusion. Stretching the muscles will cause great pain in compartment syndrome but not in neuropraxia.

○ **What is the Finkelstein test?**

A test used to determine whether a patient has de Quervain disorder (an entrapment syndrome caused by tenosynovitis of the abductor pollicis longus and extensor pollicis brevis). If pain is elicited when the patient grasps his or her thumb with the fingers of the same hand and deviates that wrist in the ulnar direction, the test result is positive.

○ **What is the most common type of peripheral nerve compression?**

Carpal tunnel syndrome. This syndrome is more often diagnosed in female patients than in male patients. Clinically, the patient will have pain and weakness that worsen at night. Moderate relief is obtained by shaking the hands. Wrist supports or hydrocortisone and lidocaine injections may provide relief. If conservative measures do not work, surgical decompression can be performed.

○ **What fingers are most often affected by carpal tunnel syndrome?**

The third and fourth digits. The sensory nerves to these digits are closest to the volar carpal ligament, which compresses the structures in the carpal tunnel.

○ **Describe the Tinel and Phalen tests.**

Both tests are for carpal tunnel syndrome.
- Tinel test: Tapping the volar aspect of the wrist over the median nerve produces paresthesias that extends along the index and long finger.
- Phalen test: Full flexion at the wrist for 1 minute leads to paresthesia along distribution of median nerve.

○ **What long bone is most commonly fractured?**

Tibia

○ **What is the most common site of osteomyelitis of the vertebral column?**

Lumbar spine

○ **What is the most common cause of pyogenic osteomyelitis of the vertebral column?**

Staphylococcus aureus, secondary to hematogenous spread

○ **What population is most likely to develop osteoid osteoma?**

Male patients younger than 30 years. Osteoid osteoma is a benign musculoskeletal tumor. It is characterized by intense localized pain that is relieved by using aspirin. Definitive treatment is surgery.

○ **What are the 4 muscles of the rotator cuff?**

1. Supraspinatus
2. Infraspinatus
3. Teres minor
4. Subscapularis

○ **What is the cause of boutonniere deformity?**

Disruption of the extensor hood at the proximal interphalangeal (PIP) joint of the finger

○ **Describe gamekeeper thumb.**

Disruption of the ulnar collateral ligament of the metacarpophalangeal joint of the thumb. If stress tests show an opening larger than 20°, surgical repair is indicated.

○ **What is the treatment for a felon?**

A felon is a subcutaneous infection in the pulp space of the fingertip, usually caused by *S aureus*. Treat by incising the pulp space.

○ **A 43-year-old woman complains that her left knee hurts when she walks down stairs or when she bends her knee too far. There has been no trauma or new exercise. What is the probable diagnosis?**

Patellofemoral syndrome, suspected to be caused by alterations in patellar tracking and compression against the femur. Treatment consists of strengthening of the quadriceps muscle.

○ **Describe a typical patient with a slipped capital femoral epiphysis.**

An obese boy, 10 to 16 years old, with groin or knee discomfort increasing with activity. He may also have a limp. The slip can occur bilaterally and is best observed with a lateral view of the hip.

○ **What is the most significant complication of a proximal tibial metaphyseal fracture?**

Arterial involvement, especially when there is a valgus deformity

○ **What is the most common ankle injury?**

Sprains account for 75% of all ankle injuries. Of these, 90% involve the lateral complex. Ninety percent of lateral ligament injuries are anterior talofibular.

○ **What is the most helpful physical test for anterior talofibular ligament injuries?**

Anterior drawer test. More than 3 mm of excursion might be significant (compare sides); more than 1 cm is always significant.

○ **How are sprains classified?**
- First degree: Ligament is stretched; radiograph is normal.
- Second degree: Ligament is severely stretched with partial tear, marked tenderness, swelling, and pain; radiograph is normal.
- Third degree: Ligament is completely ruptured, there is marked tenderness, and the joint is swollen and/or obviously deformed; radiograph may show an abnormal joint.

○ **A 21-year-old woman complains of pain and a clicking sound located at the posterior lateral malleolus. A fullness beneath the lateral malleolus is found. What is the diagnosis?**

Peroneal tendon subluxation with associated tenosynovitis

○ **Which bone is most often fractured in the baby during childbirth?**

Clavicle

○ **What is the most common shoulder dislocation?**

Anterior (95%)

○ **A patient cannot actively abduct her shoulder. What injury does this suggest?**

Rotator cuff tear.

○ **Why is a displaced supracondylar fracture of the distal humerus in a child considered an emergency?**

This fracture often results in injury to the brachial artery or the median nerve. It can also cause compartment syndrome.

○ **What are the signs and symptoms of compartment syndrome involving the anterior compartment of the leg?**

Pain during active and passive dorsiflexion and plantar flexion of the foot, and hypoesthesia (paresthesia) of the first web space of the foot

○ **How is a scaphoid fracture diagnosed?**

Typically, a history of injury caused by a fall on an outstretched hand. The initial radiograph frequently appears normal. If the patient has tenderness in the anatomical snuffbox or pain with axial loading of the thumb, a scaphoid (navicular) fracture should be presumed and the hand splinted. A follow-up radiograph should be obtained 10 to 14 days after the injury and may reveal the fracture.

○ **What is the most feared complication of scaphoid fracture?**

Avascular necrosis. The more proximal the fracture, the more commonly avascular necrosis occurs due to retrograde blood flow.

○ **Which type of Salter-Harris fracture has the worst prognosis?**

Type V (compression injury of the epiphyseal plate)

○ **What metatarsal fracture is often associated with a disrupted tarsometatarsal joint?**

Fracture of the base of the second metatarsal. Treatment may require open reduction and internal fixation.

○ **What fracture is frequently missed when a patient complains of ankle injury?**

Fracture at the base of the fifth metatarsal, caused by plantar flexion and inversion. Radiographs of the ankle may not include the fifth metatarsal.

○ **Describe the leg position of a patient with femoral neck fracture.**

Shortened, abducted, and slightly externally rotated

○ **Describe the leg position of a patient with anterior hip dislocation.**

Hip is abducted and externally rotated. This accounts for 10% of hip dislocations. The mechanism of injury is forced abduction.

○ **Describe the leg position of a patient with posterior hip dislocation.**

Shortened, adducted, and internally rotated. This accounts for 90% of hip dislocations. The mechanism of injury is force applied to a flexed knee directed posteriorly. This dislocation is associated with sciatic nerve injury (10%) and avascular necrosis of the femoral head.

○ **Describe the leg position of a patient with intertrochanteric hip fracture.**

Shortened, externally rotated, and abducted

○ **What is the Young classification system for pelvic fractures?**

The Young system divides pelvic fractures into 4 categories according to the type and direction of force.

1. Lateral compression
2. Anteroposterior compression
3. Vertical sheer
4. Combination mechanical-mixed

○ **Describe lateral compression pelvic fracture.**

This fracture is usually caused by a motor vehicle collision in which the car and patient are broadsided. The frequency for this type of fracture is 50%. The lateral force from the collision causes a sacral fracture, iliac wing fracture, or a sacroiliac ligamentous injury and a transverse fracture of the pubic rami. There is no ligamentous injury at the pubic symphysis.

○ **Describe anteroposterior compression pelvic fracture.**

This fracture account for about 20% of pelvic fractures and is usually caused by a head-on motor vehicle collision. They always include a disruption of the pubic symphysis and usually involve a disruption (of different degrees) of the sacroiliac joint.

○ **Describe vertical sheer pelvic fracture.**

This fracture accounts for about 6% of pelvic fractures and is usually caused by a fall. They involve (1) an injury of the sacroiliac ligaments and (2) either a disruption of the pubic symphysis or vertical fractures through the pubic rami. The iliac wing is vertically displaced.

○ **What life-threatening injury is associated with pelvic fractures?**

Severe hemorrhage, usually retroperitoneal. As much as 6 L of blood can be accommodated in this space.

○ **Which pelvic fracture is most likely to involve severe hemorrhage?**

Vertical sheer fracture (75%)

○ **Which pelvic fracture is most likely to involve bladder rupture?**

Lateral compression fracture (20%)

○ **Which pelvic fracture is most likely to involve urethral injury?**

Anteroposterior compression fracture (36%)

○ **Which fracture is associated with avascular necrosis of the femoral head?**

Femoral neck fracture. Avascular necrosis occurs with 15% of nondisplaced femoral neck fractures and with nearly 90% of displaced femoral neck fractures.

○ **What is stress fracture?**

A stress or fatigue fracture is caused by small, repetitive forces that usually involve the metatarsal shafts, the distal tibia, and the femoral neck. These fractures may not be seen on initial radiographs.

○ **What is nursemaid elbow?**

Subluxation of the radial head. During forceful retraction, fibers of the annular ligament that encircle the radial neck become trapped between the radial head and the capitellum. At presentation, children hold the arm in slight flexion and pronation.

○ **Why tap a knee with acute hemarthrosis?**

Tapping the knee relieves pressure and pain for the patient and will allow you to ascertain whether fat globules are present, indicating a fracture.

○ **What is the most common site of compartment syndrome?**

Anterior compartment of the leg

○ **What type of patient most commonly develops Achilles tendon rupture?**

Middle-aged men. It occurs most commonly on the left side.

○ **What are the most common lower extremity bone injuries in children?**

Tibial and fibular shaft fractures, usually secondary to twist forces

○   **What radiograph is best for suspected patellar fracture in a child?**

Standard radiographs, including patellar or sunrise views, plus comparison radiographs of the uninvolved knee

○   **What are the differences between avulsion of the tibial tubercle and Osgood-Schlatter disease?**

Both occur at the tibial tubercle. Avulsion manifests with an acute inability to walk. A lateral view of the knee is most diagnostic; treatment is surgical. Osgood-Schlatter disease has a vague history of intermittent pain, is bilateral 25% of the time, and is painful with range of motion but not with rest; treatment is for symptoms and is not surgical.

○   **What is toddler fracture?**

A spiral fracture of the tibia without fibular involvement. This type of fracture in toddlers is a common cause of limping or refusal to walk.

○   **What is the most commonly fractured carpal bone?**

Scaphoid (navicular) bone

○   **What is Kienbock disease?**

Avascular necrosis of the lunate bone, with its collapse secondary to fracture. As with a navicular (scaphoid) fracture, initial wrist radiographs may not demonstrate the fracture. Therefore, tenderness over the lunate bone warrants immobilization.

○   **A stress fracture of the second or third metatarsal is suspected but not detected at initial radiography. How many days after the initial examination should radiography be performed again?**

14 to 21 days

○   **After a fracture, what are the 3 stages of healing?**

1. Union
2. Consolidation
3. Remodeling

○   **How long after fracture does callus start to form?**

5 to 7 days

○   **Which type of Salter-Harris fracture is most common?**

Type II (triangular fracture involving the metaphysis and an epiphyseal separation)

○   **Which tarsal bone is most commonly fractured?**

Calcaneus (60%). Calcaneal fractures are commonly associated with lumbar compression injuries (10%).

○   **What is the tarsometatarsal joint also called?**

Lisfranc joint

○ **The second metatarsal is the locking mechanism for the middle part of the foot. A fracture at the base of the second metatarsal should raise suspicion of what?**

A disrupted joint. Treatment may require open reduction and internal fixation.

○ **What is a Jones fracture?**

A fracture at the base of the fifth metatarsal (distal to avulsion fractures), usually secondary to plantar flexion and inversion, it is the most common metatarsal fracture. It requires more aggressive treatment (fixation or prolonged nonweight-bearing immobilization) because of a high risk of complications.

○ **A pneumatic tourniquet can be inflated on an extremity to more than a patient's systolic blood pressure for how long without damaging underlying vessels or neurons?**

2 hours

○ **What basic disorder contributes to the pathophysiology of compartment syndrome?**

Increased pressure within closed tissue spaces compromising blood flow to muscle and nerve tissue. There are 3 prerequisites to the development of compartment syndrome:

1. Limiting space
2. Increased tissue pressure
3. Decreased tissue perfusion

○ **What are the 2 basic mechanisms for elevated compartment pressure?**

1. External compression by burn eschar, circumferential casts, dressings, or pneumatic pressure garments
2. Volume increase within the compartment because of hemorrhage into the compartment, intravenous infiltration, or edema secondary to injury or due to postischemic (postischial) swelling

○ **Which 2 fractures are most commonly associated with compartment syndrome?**

1. Tibia, resulting most often in anterior compartment involvement
2. Supracondylar humerus fractures

○ **What are the early signs and symptoms of compartment syndrome?**
- Tenderness and pain out of proportion to the injury
- Pain during active and passive motion
- Hypoesthesia (paresthesia)
- Abnormal 2-point discrimination

○ **What are the late signs and symptoms of compartment syndrome?**
- Tense, indurated, and erythematous compartment
- Slow capillary refill
- Pallor and pulselessness

○   **What are the 6 Ps of compartment syndrome?**

1. Pain
2. Pallor
3. Pulselessness
4. Paresthesia
5. Poikilothermia
6. Paralysis

○   **What 4 Cs determine muscle viability?**

1. Color
2. Consistency
3. Contraction
4. Circulation

○   **What are the 4 compartments of the leg?**

1. Anterior
2. Lateral
3. Deep posterior
4. Superficial posterior

○   **What intracompartmental pressure raises concern?**

Normal pressure less than 10 mm Hg. Pressure higher than 30 mm Hg mandates emergency fasciotomy. The treatment for compartment pressures between 20 and 30 mm Hg is controversial and may require surgical consultation, especially if the patient is unreliable because of an altered level of consciousness.

○   **With complete rupture of medial or collateral ligaments of the knee, how much laxity can be expected at examination?**

More than 1 cm without endpoint, as compared with an uninjured knee

○   **Which ligament in the knee is the most commonly injured?**

Anterior cruciate ligament, usually from a noncontact injury

○   **What are valgus deformity and varus deformity?**

- Valgus deformity is angulation of an extremity at a joint with the more distal part angled away from the midline.
- Varus deformity is angulation of an extremity at a joint with the more distal part angled toward the midline.

○   **Are dislocations and sprains more common in children or in adults?**

Dislocations and ligamentous injuries are uncommon in prepubertal children because the ligaments and joints are strong as compared to the adjoining growth plates. Excessive force applied to a child's joint is more likely to cause fracture through the growth plate than to cause dislocation or sprain.

○ **What is the order of ossification centers in the elbow?**

CRITOE

Capitellum

Radial head

Internal (medial) epicondyle

Trochlea

Olecranon

External (lateral) epicondyle

These ossify at ages 3, 5, 7, 9, 11, and 13 years, in that order.

○ **What is sciatica?**

A type of radiculopathy due to compression or irritation of the sciatic nerve. Typically, the pain radiates from the buttocks to the leg, below the knee. Sciatica is also known as "lumbago."

○ **What is the most common cause of low back pain?**

More than 97% (lumbar sprain or strain, 70%) is due to mechanical causes. Although commonly feared, herniated disks cause only 4%.

○ **When is imaging appropriate for low back pain?**

- Most low back pain (85%) is considered nonspecific and does not require imaging. Imaging may be considered for persistent or refractory low back pain; radicular symptoms; or suspicion of vertebral compression fracture, spinal stenosis, vertebral infection, cauda equina syndrome, or cancer.
- Magnetic resonance imaging should be considered for radiculopathy or spinal stenosis only if surgery is considered.
- Emergency imaging is suggested for symptoms of cauda equina syndrome.
- Cauda equina syndrome (saddle anesthesia, fecal incontinence, or urinary retention)

○ **What are the most effective treatments for nonspecific low back pain?**

- Encourage activity and avoid bed rest.
- Use nonsteroidal anti-inflammatory drugs (NSAIDs) or acetaminophen as first-line treatment.
- Muscle relaxants are beneficial for short-term use.
- Local heat is safe and offers some benefit.
- Spinal manipulation and exercise therapy may be considered if the above provide limited relief.
- Exercises have some benefit in subacute low back pain and definite benefit in chronic back pain.
- Massage therapy (when combined with education and exercise) may relieve subacute and chronic nonspecific low back pain.

○ **What symptoms suggest lumbar disk herniation?**

Ninety-nine percent of symptomatic lumbar disk herniations have sciatica (radicular) symptoms, but only 4% of patients with sciatica have disk herniation.

○ **What are the best physical examinations for lumbar disk herniation?**

- The straight leg raise test is the most sensitive (73%–98%).
- The crossed straight leg raise test is the most specific (88%–98%).
- Lower extremity motor/sensory/deep tendon reflex abnormalities have a specificity of 86% to 94%.

○ **How accurate is imaging for lumbar disk herniation?**

When no obvious problems are present, imaging should be delayed during an initial 6-week conservative trial period. Disk herniations are also common in individuals without symptoms (22%–40%). Imaging should be delayed during the initial 6 week conservative trial period unless red flags are present, as it adds little to treatment. Magnetic resonance imaging is the preferred modality but must be correlated with clinical findings for appropriate validity (sensitivity: 60%–100%; specificity: 43%–97%).

○ **What is the treatment for lumbar disk herniation?**

- Although not studied specifically for disk herniation, NSAIDS/Acetaminophen analgesics (and muscle relaxants) are effective in nonspecific low back pain, and may provide some pain relief.
- There is also limited evidence of benefit from physical therapy.
- More than 90% of cases resolve nonsurgically without surgical intervention; the remaining small percentage of patients not responding to conservative therapy cases may benefit from surgical intervention.
- Steroids have no proven benefit.
- There is little benefit of to bed rest

○ **What is the most important nonpharmacologic treatment for knee osteoarthritis?**

Aerobic, strengthening, and range of motion exercises. Weight loss is also effective.

○ **When is arthroscopy effective for treatment of knee osteoarthritis?**

Results from 2 studies indicate that there is no benefit from arthroscopy for moderate to severe knee osteoarthritis.

○ **Is glucosamine helpful in treating osteoarthritis?**

Studies have shown conflicting results on glucosamine's effectiveness in treating osteoarthritis; however, a trial of glucosamine may be considered.

○ **Are viscosupplements (hyaluronic acids) better than steroid injections for knee osteoarthritis?**

Corticosteroid injections have greater short-term benefits, but hyaluronic acids have greater long-term benefits.

○ **What sign should be monitored and documented during the performance of a neurologic examination in a patient suspected of having anterior dislocation of the shoulder?**

Sensation over the lateral deltoid. In anterior dislocations of the shoulder, the radial nerve may be torn easily. Intact sensation to the lateral deltoid indicates an intact radial nerve.

○ **What is the most common joint dislocation?**

Anterior shoulder dislocations account for half of all joint dislocations. They occur with abduction and external rotation.

○ **What nerve is usually injured in glenohumeral dislocation?**

Axillary nerve

○ **Describe the mechanism and cause of a boutonniere deformity.**

It is secondary to a rupture of the extensor apparatus of the PIP joint. The cause of the injury is a flexed PIP joint and a hyperextended DIP joint. The deformity is treated by splinting the PIP joint in full extension.

○ **What tendons are involved in de Quervain tenosynovitis?**

The abductor pollicis longus and the extensor pollicis brevis.

○ **Describe the Dupuytren contracture.**

A contraction of the longitudinal bands of the palmar aponeurosis

○ **Describe the Galeazzi fracture-dislocation.**

A radial shaft fracture with dislocation of the distal radioulnar joint

○ **What are Kanavel's 4 cardinal signs of infectious digital flexor tenosynovitis?**

1. Tenderness along the tendon sheath
2. Finger held in flexion
3. Pain during passive extension of the finger
4. Finger swelling

○ **Active adduction of the thumb tests which nerve?**

Ulnar nerve

○ **What is the mortise view of the ankle important for diagnosing?**

Medial (deltoid) ligament disruption of the ankle

○ **What is the best radiographic view for diagnosing lunate and perilunate dislocations?**

Lateral radiographic views of the wrist

○ **What nerve is most commonly injured in a humeral shaft fracture?**

Radial

○ **Describe mallet finger deformity.**

It is a deformity produced by forced flexion of the distal interphalangeal joint when the finger is in full extension. It is a result of either a rupture of the distal extensor tendon or an avulsion fraction of the tendon insertion on the distal phalanx with a dorsal plate avulsion.

○ **What nerve provides sensations to both the dorsal and volar aspects of the hand?**

The ulnar nerve provides sensations to both the dorsal and volar aspects of the hand. The radial nerve primarily innervates the dorsum of the hand, and the median nerve primarily innervates the volar aspect.

○ **A patient has rotational knee injury and hears a pop. Within 90 minutes, hemarthrosis develops. What is the suspected location of injury?**

Anterior cruciate ligament

○ **What bone is dislocated most often in the wrist?**

Lunate. It is also the second most commonly fractured bone in the wrist.

○ **Describe the signs and symptoms of pressure on the first sacral root (S1).**

Symptoms of S1 injury include pain radiating to the midgluteal region, posterior thigh, and posterior calf and down to the heel and sole of the foot. Sensory signs are localized to the lateral toes. S1 root compression typically involves the plantar flexor muscles of the foot and toes. The ankle reflex is decreased or absent.

○ **What is the significance of the fat pad sign with an elbow injury?**

It indicates effusion or hemarthrosis of the elbow joint and suggests an occult fracture of the radial head.

○ **What neighboring structures may be injured with a supracondylar distal humeral fracture?**

The anterior interosseous nerve (a branch of the median nerve) and the brachial artery

○ **What ligament is commonly injured after inversion ankle sprain?**

Anterior talofibular ligament

○ **Define spondylolisthesis.**

The forward movement of 1 vertebral body on the vertebra below it

○ **What nerve may be injured in a distal femoral fracture?**

Peroneal nerve

○ **Describe the signs and symptoms of chondromalacia patella.**

Chondromalacia patella typically occurs in young, active women. The pain is localized to the knee. There is no effusion and no history of trauma. Patellar compression test results are usually positive.

○ **Describe the signs and symptoms of tarsal tunnel syndrome.**

Insidious onset of paresthesia, as well as burning pain and numbness on the plantar surface of the foot. Pain radiates superiorly along the medial side of the calf. Rest decreases pain.

○ **A patient presents with back pain and complaints of incontinence. At examination, loss of anal reflex and decreased sphincter tone is noted. What is the diagnosis?**

Cauda equina syndrome. The most consistent finding is urinary retention. At physical examination, you should expect saddle anesthesia—that is, numbness over the posterior superior thighs, the buttocks, and the perineum.

○ **What is the most common site of lumbar disk herniation?**

Ninety-eight percent of clinically important lumbar disk herniations are at the L4-L5 or L5-S1 intervertebral levels. Evaluate these patients by checking for weakness of ankle and hallux dorsiflexors (L5). Also check pinprick sensation over the medial aspect of the foot (L5) and the lateral portion of the foot (S1).

○ **Which tendon is most commonly affected in calcific tendonitis?**

Supraspinatus

○ **Which epicondyle is involved in tennis elbow?**

Lateral

○ **A patient has difficulty squatting and standing. What is the most likely spinal disease?**

L4 root compression with involvement of the quadriceps

○ **A patient presents with a complaint of pain at the site of the deltoid insertion with radiation into the back of the arm (C5 distribution). At examination, there is increased pain with active abduction from 70° to 120°. Radiographs reveal calcification at the tendinous insertion of the greater tuberosity. What is the diagnosis?**

Supraspinatus tendonitis

○ **Name the 4 stable cervical spine fractures.**

1. Simple wedge
2. Clay-shoveler
3. Pillar
4. C1 posterior neural arch

All other cervical spine fractures are unstable or potentially unstable.

CHAPTER 18 Sports Medicine

Krystian Bigosinski, MD; Deepak S. Patel, MD, FAAFP

○ **How long should an athlete be kept from contact activities after concussion?**

Current guidelines recommend keeping an athlete out of all activities (physical and cognitive) from onset of the concussion to at least 24 hours after symptoms resolve. Before returning to play, the athlete must be cognitively and neurologically back to preconcussion baseline. In a setting in which a physician is skilled in concussion care and has ample support and resources, a more rapid return to play may be possible. Children and adolescents require a longer time than do adults.

○ **How should a player be returned to play after concussion?**

After concussion, a graded return to play should be started 24 hours after the athlete has no symptoms at rest. The level of exercise should be advanced every 24 hours if no symptoms arise. The stages include light aerobic exercise, sport-specific exercise, noncontact training drills, full-contact practice, and then returning to full play.

○ **What is second-impact syndrome?**

Although rare, this is the most serious risk for premature return to play after concussion. Even a minor repeat trauma to the head, after an initial concussion, can lead to rapid cerebral edema and possible herniation due to a loss of autoregulation in the brain's blood supply.

○ **What is postconcussion syndrome?**

This is a collection of symptoms that persist after a concussion. Postconcussion syndrome is characterized by headaches, blurry vision, difficulty concentrating, anxiety, fatigue, and labile mood.

○ **When should magnetic resonance imaging (MRI) or further workup be considered in an athlete who has had a concussion?**

If an athlete is experiencing prolonged concussion symptoms (>1–2 weeks) or if an intracerebral lesion is suspected, imaging such as MRI or neuropsychologic evaluation should be considered.

○ **How should an athlete suspected of having a concussion be evaluated on the sidelines?**

After cervical spine and emergency conditions have been excluded, a neurologic examination including orientation, memory (immediate, long-term, and delayed recall), concentration (and/or calculation), balance, and coordination should be performed. The athlete should be monitored closely and not left alone for the first few hours after the injury, and the examination should be repeated. The athlete should not be allowed to return to play on the same day of the concussion.

○ **What is female athlete triad?**

This is described as the combination of amenorrhea, disordered eating, and decreased bone density.

○ **What is the best way to screen for female athlete triad?**

Screening questions during the preparticipation physical examination can be used to dentify athletes at risk for female athlete triad. Screening questions should include diet history; amount of time spent training, both in and out of the sport; history of prior injuries, especially fractures; menstrual history; and satisfaction with current weight and history of recent weight gain or loss.

○ **What are effective treatment strategies for female athlete triad?**

A combination of relative rest (decrease training load by 1 day per week or 10%–20%) and increase in caloric consumption with the help of a sports nutritionist is an effective strategy. A multidisciplinary approach with a physician, nutritionist, and mental health provider is recommended.

○ **Are oral contraceptives effective in preventing bone loss in athletes with amenorrhea?**

There is conflicting and lacking evidence on whether or not oral contraceptives are effective in preventing bone loss.

○ **What is a therapeutic use exemption?**

If an athlete has a medical condition that necessitates the use of a medication that is prohibited by the governing body of the sport in which the athlete participates, a therapeutic use exemption gives the athlete the authorization to use the medication in question.

○ **Is there evidence to support the use of dietary supplements for athletes?**

Evidence is lacking for improvements in athletic endeavors through the use of dietary supplements. However, there are well-documented cases that these supplements may be tainted with banned substances, which may put the athlete at risk of inadvertently being disqualified from his or her sport or experiencing health consequences.

○ **What are some commonly used ergogenic aids?**

Some of these include anabolic steroids, diuretics (for rapid weight loss and as masking agents), β-agonists, blood doping agents (such as erythropoietin), and stimulants such as ephedra and methamphetamines.

○ **What are the signs and symptoms of exercise-induced bronchospasm?**

The signs and symptoms of exercise-induced bronchospasm include wheezing, shortness of breath or coughing, decreased endurance, chest pain or tightness, sore throat, and upset stomach or stomachache. These must occur during or after exercise and must be at least 5 minutes in duration.

○ **What is the most effective therapy for an asthmatic child with exercise-induced bronchospasm?**

The most effective pharmacologic treatment of exercise-induced bronchospasm is the use of short-acting β-agonists. The next most effective therapies are mast cell stabilizers and anticholinergic agents. It is also important to address the underlying asthma in children with exercise-induced bronchospasm.

○ **Should extensive cardiologic testing, such as electrocardiogram, exercise stress electrocardiogram, or echocardiogram, be part of preparticipation physical examinations?**

Although cardiac issues in the athletic population are of grave concern, there is no evidence at this time to show that these tests provide effective screening for cardiac abnormalities. These tests often produce false-positive results and are not cost-effective as screening tools. Although controversial, these additional tests are not recommended for the screening of all athletes. Electrocardiogram and echocardiogram may be considered part of the evaluation in athletes with abnormalities on the cardiovascular portion of history and physical examination.

○ **What elements of the history and physical examination are recommended for cardiovascular screening during preparticipation examinations?**

- Personal history: Exertional chest pain or discomfort, unexplained syncope or near syncope, excessive exertional and unexplained dyspnea or fatigue associated with exercise, prior recognition of heart murmur, and elevated systemic blood pressure
- Family history: Premature death (sudden and unexpected or otherwise) before age 50 years because of heart disease in a first-degree relative, disability from heart disease in a close relative younger than 50 years, specific knowledge of certain cardiac conditions in family members (hypertrophic or dilated cardiomyopathy, long QT syndrome or other ion channelopathies, Marfan syndrome, or clinically important arrhythmias)
- Physical examination: Heart murmur, femoral pulses, physical findings indicative of Marfan syndrome, and brachial artery blood pressure

○ **What are the most common causes of sudden cardiac death in athletes?**

- Hypertrophic cardiomyopathy (36%)
- Coronary artery anomalies (17%)
- Indeterminate left ventricular hypertrophy, possible hypertrophic cardiomyopathy (8%)

○ **What type of murmur is suggestive of hypertrophic cardiomyopathy?**

A systolic murmur accentuated with Valsalva maneuver. The murmur also becomes louder with standing and softens with squatting or lying supine.

○ **Should laboratory tests such as complete blood cell count, fasting lipid profile, spirometry, ferritin test, or chemistry profile be part of preparticipation screening?**

There is no evidence to support laboratory testing of any type during preparticipation athletic screening.

○ **What are the evidence-supported elements of athletic preparticipation screening?**

A detailed medical history by the athlete (or parent) is effective in identifying 75% of issues that may affect participation. A 90-second musculoskeletal test in athletes with no prior injuries can be used to identify 90% of musculoskeletal injuries. The examination should also include a cardiovascular examination with auscultation of the heart in standing, sitting, and supine positions and with Valsalva maneuvers to screen for hypertrophic cardiomyopathy.

○ **A 14-year-old baseball player is removed from the field complaining of light-headedness, headache, nausea, and vomiting. At examination, the patient has a heart rate of 110 beats per minute, respiratory rate of 22 breaths per minute, and blood pressure of 90/60 mm Hg. The patient is afebrile but profusely sweating. What is the diagnosis?**

Heat exhaustion. Treat with intravenous fluid.

○ **A 27-year-old marathon runner presents confused and combative. Her temperature is 105°F. Why must renal function be monitored?**

This patient has heatstroke. Rhabdomyolysis may occur 2 to 3 days after injury. In heatstroke, volume depletion and dehydration may not always occur.

○ **What is the treatment for heatstroke?**

Cool sponging, ice packs to the groin and axilla, fanning, and iced gastric lavage. Antipyretics are not useful.

○ **At what altitude does acute mountain sickness (AMS) typically develop?**

8000 ft. This may seem low, when the death zone is higher than 25,000 feet.

○ **What are the signs and symptoms of AMS?**

AMS symptoms include headache, nausea, vomiting, difficulty sleeping, malaise, anorexia, and other generalized symptoms. Many mistake for these for a hangover. It usually happens at around 9000 ft but can happen at lower altitudes (6000 ft).

○ **What is the treatment for AMS?**

Slow acclimatization to altitude is key. Once illness has started, care is largely supportive but can include acetazolamide both prophylactically and after onset. Dexamethasone can also be used. If AMS is persistent or worsens, descent is the mainstay of therapy.

○ **What are signs and symptoms of high altitude cerebral edema (HACE)?**

HACE can be thought of as a more severe form of AMS. AMS is not life threatening and is self-limited. HACE is progressive and can be fatal. Signs include ataxia, hallucinations, confusion, upper motor neurologic signs, obtundation, and finally coma.

○ **What is the treatment for HACE?**

Treatment is similar to that for AMS, but the need for support (eg, oxygen) is often more urgent. The need for descent is also urgent because HACE is a life-threatening condition. The same medications used for AMS can be used for HACE (ie, dexamethasone and acetazolamide).

○ **What are signs/symptoms of high altitude pulmonary edema (HAPE)?**

HAPE may be preceded by AMS. It usually starts with cough, then increased dyspnea that worsens, and then pink frothy sputum, lethargy, coma, and death. Physical examination may reveal tachypnea, tachycardia, and crackles throughout the lungs. HAPE usually only occurs above 9000 ft and is responsible for most deaths due to altitude illness.

○ **What is the treatment for HAPE?**

Prevention with slow acclimatization is crucial. Nifedipine, tadalafil, sildenafil, and inhaled salmeterol can be helpful. Avoid diuretics because these patients are often dehydrated. As with all altitude illness, descent or hyperbaric therapy is critical and is the mainstay of treatment.

○ **What is herpes gladiatorum?**

Herpes gladiatorum is a herpes simplex virus 1 infection of the skin. Most commonly, it occurs in wrestlers, but it can be seen in other contact-sport participants.

○ **How is herpes gladiatorum treated?**

Oral acyclovir, 200 to 400 mg 5 times per day, or valcyclovir 1g twice daily for 7 to 10 days should be initiated at the first sign of symptoms. The earlier the treatment is initiated, the more effective it is. There is no role for topical antivirals.

○ **What are the return-to-play considerations for herpes gladiatorum?**

The guidelines for return to play vary state by state, with some states having no well-defined guidelines. An excellent resource for guidance is the National Collegiate Athletic Association (NCAA) Sports Medicine Handbook. The NCAA guidelines include the following:

- The wrestler must be free from systemic symptoms of viral infection (fever, malaise, and so on).
- The wrestler must have developed no new blisters for 72 hours before the examination.
- The wrestler must have no moist lesions, and all lesions must be dried and surmounted by a firm adherent crust.
- The wrestler must have been using an appropriate dosage of systemic antiviral therapy for at least 120 hours before and at the time of the meet or tournament.
- Active herpetic infections shall not be covered to allow participation.

○ **What are the return-to-play considerations for staphylococcal skin infections (ie, methicillin-resistant *Staphylococcus aureus*, impetigo)?**

- The NCAA mandates that wrestlers must be without any new skin lesions for 48 hours before participation.
- There must be no moist purulent lesions at the time of the meet or tournament.
- Results of gram-stain examination of exudate from any questionable lesions should be provided.
- It is inappropriate to cover purulent lesions to allow for participation.

○ **What are the return-to-play considerations for tinea infections (ie, athlete's foot, jock itch, and so on)?**

Again, the NCAA guidelines can be helpful in making return-to-play decisions:

- A minimum of 72 hours of topical therapy is required for skin lesions.
- A minimum of 2 weeks of systemic antifungal therapy is required for scalp lesions.
- Wrestlers with extensive and active lesions will be disqualified. Activity of treated lesions can be judged either by use of potassium hydroxide preparation or a review of therapeutic regimen. Wrestlers with solitary or closely clustered, localized lesions will be disqualified if lesions are in a body location that cannot be properly covered.

○ **What are some absolute and relative contraindications to exercise during pregnancy?**

- Absolute: Ruptured membranes, premature labor, undiagnosed vaginal bleeding, intrauterine growth restriction, severe maternal heart disease, multiple pregnancy (ie, twins), pregnancy-induced hypertension or preeclampsia, and incompetent cervix
- Relative: Hypertension, anemia, being overweight, being underweight, heavy smoking, pulmonary disease such as asthma, breech presentation, and mild valvular heart disease

○ **What exercises are suggested during pregnancy?**

Women should focus on aerobic activities with a duration of 15 to 60 minutes daily and a target heart rate of 60% to 75% of maximal heart rate. Any exercise that puts the mother or fetus at risk owing to direct trauma, heat exhaustion, hypothermia, or hypoxia should be avoided.

○ **What is Osgood-Schlatter disease?**

This is a common cause of knee pain in active children and adolescents. It often manifests as pain at the tibial tubercle or the distal patellar tendon with squatting, running, or jumping.

○ **What is the treatment for Osgood-Schlatter disease?**

Most patients respond well to conservative therapy (analgesics and nonsteroidal anti-inflammatory drugs [NSAIDs], ice, and activity modification) and time. In advanced cases, bony ossicle excision may relieve symptoms. Corticosteroid injections are not recommended.

○ **What is Sever disease?**

This is a common cause of heel pain in active children and adolescents. It is apophysitis caused by microtrauma from mechanical overuse at the insertion of the Achilles tendon at the calcaneus.

○ **What physical examination finding is suggestive of Sever disease?**

A distinguishing feature at examination is pronounced heel pain during squeezing of the posterior one-third of the calcaneus.

○ **How is Sever disease treated?**

Patients with Sever disease respond well to the use of a compression shoe orthotic, and they can almost always continue full activity. Patients may also respond well to activity modification, ice, stretching, and analgesics and anti-inflammatories.

○ **What is Little Leaguer shoulder?**

This condition is a stress or mechanical overuse injury to the proximal humeral epiphysis. It occurs in throwing or overhead athletes (volleyball, tennis) with immature growth plates.

○ **How does Little Leaguer shoulder manifest?**

Patients present with shoulder pain and tenderness over the lateral and proximal humerus. Plain radiographs of the shoulder may demonstrate physeal widening.

○ **How is Little Leaguer shoulder treated?**

The mainstay of therapy is to rest the arm from throwing. The usual time is 3 months of rest. During this time, ice and analgesics and anti-inflamatory medication may be used as adjuncts to therapy. Patients should continue cardiovascular conditioning and consider evaluation of throwing mechanics once they are pain free.

○ **What is Little Leaguer elbow?**

This is apophysitis of the medial epicondyle of the elbow affecting throwing athletes, usually between the ages of 9 and 12 years.

○ **How does Little Leaguer elbow manifest?**

Athletes experience pain at the medial aspect of the elbow during throwing and may also have a decrease in throwing distance or velocity. Radiographs may be normal or may reveal widening of the epiphysis, bony fragments, or calcification.

○ **How is Little Leaguer elbow treated?**

Complete rest from throwing is the key to treatment and should continue for about 4 to 6 weeks. Ice and analgesics and anti-inflammatories may be used for comfort. During this time, conditioning, stretching, and core strengthening may be initiated.

○ **What is a specific musculoskeletal concern that should be screened for in athletes with Down syndrome?**

Athletes with Down syndrome should be screened radiographically for atlantoaxial instability, which is excessive movement at the junction between the atlas (C1) and axis (C2) as a result of either a bony or a ligamentous abnormality.

○ **What is a jersey finger?**

This is a rupture of the flexor digitorum profundus, often caused by catching a finger on the jersey of another player, resulting in forceful extension against a flexed finger.

○ **How does jersey finger manifest?**

Athletes have tenderness at the volar aspect of the distal interphalangeal (DIP) joint and have an inability to flex at the DIP joint.

○ **Jersey finger occurs most commonly on which finger?**

The ring finger is the weakest finger on the hand and accounts for 75% of jersey finger cases.

○ **How should jersey finger be treated?**

All patients should have the finger splinted and be referred to an orthopedic surgeon for emergency evaluation.

○ **What is mallet finger?**

This is an injury to the extensor tendon at the DIP joint. It is usually caused by an object striking the fingertip and forcing a flexed DIP joint.

○ **How does mallet finger manifest?**

Athletes have tenderness at the dorsal aspect of the DIP joint and an inability to extend at the DIP joint.

○ **How should mallet finger be treated?**

The patient should have the finger put in a splint in full extension or slight hyperextension for 6 weeks. The splint should be worn at all times, and patients should be monitored closely for compliance to ensure extension is maintained (noncompliance requires repeating 6 weeks of splinting). Finally, an additional 6 weeks of splinting during the night and during high-risk activity allow for transitioning out of the splint full time.

○ **When should referral to an orthopedic surgeon be considered for mallet finger injuries?**

The lack of full passive extension may indicate an avulsion fracture or soft-tissue entrapment, which are best managed by an orthopedic surgeon. Avulsion fracture with more than 30% joint involvement also warrants referral.

○ **What is skier thumb or gamekeeper thumb?**

This is an injury to the ulnar collateral ligament of the thumb. Either may involve isolated ligamentous injury or bony avulsion.

○ **How does skier thumb manifest?**

The patient has tenderness at the ulnar aspect of the metacarpophalangeal joint of the thumb and may have laxity during stressing; however, before stress testing, radiographs of the thumb should be obtained to rule out partial avulsion fracture.

○ **What is the treatment for skier thumb?**

If the joint is stable, the thumb should be placed in a thumb spica splint for 6 weeks.

○ **When should referral to an orthopedic surgeon be considered for a patient with skier thumb?**

If the joint opens more than 30° to 40° compared with the contralateral side or if there is an avulsion fracture present, orthopedic referral is appropriate.

○ **What is turf toe?**

This is a sprain of the joint capsule and ligamentous complex of the hallux metatarsophalangeal joint caused by forced dorsiflexion of the hallux.

○ **How does turf toe present?**

The athlete has tenderness on the plantar aspect of the metatarsophalangeal joint of the hallux and discomfort with dorsiflexion of the hallux.

○ **What is the treatment for turf toe?**

Depending on the severity of the injury, treatment with NSAIDs, ice, taping, and use of a firm insole or walking boot to prevent dorsiflexion are appropriate.

○ **Which ligament is most commonly affected in low ankle sprains?**

The anterior talofibular ligament is most commonly affected in low ankle sprains, followed by the calcaneofibular ligament and the posterior talofibular ligament.

○ **Do ankle braces prevent recurrent ankle injuries?**

In patients with recurrent ankle sprains, rigid or lace-up ankle braces may be used to prevent recurrence.

○ **Can ankle sprains be prevented in athletes?**

Exercises focusing on ankle strengthening and proprioception (such as wobble-board or ankle disk exercises) can reduce the risk of ankle sprains.

○ **Which is more effective in treating ankle sprains: ice or heat?**

Ice appears to be superior to heat in recovery in grades 3 and 4 ankle sprains. No study results have shown a faster return to play with application of heat at any time in the recovery process.

○ **Are the Ottawa ankle rules effective in screening the need for radiography in acute ankle injuries?**

If the patient does not meet the criteria for the Ottawa ankle rules, fracture can be ruled out 99% of the time.

○ **What are the Ottawa ankle rules?**

The Ottawa ankle rules are a set of guidelines for assessing whether a foot radiography series is indicated in an acute ankle injury. Radiographic evaluation is indicated if there is any bony pain in the malleolar zone and any 1 of the following: (1) bony tenderness at the base of the fifth metatarsal, (2) bony tenderness at the navicular bone, or (3) the inability to bear weight both immediately and in the emergency department.

○ **What is a high ankle sprain?**

This is an injury to the tibiofibular syndesmosis. This may result in an unstable ankle, and orthopedic referral should be considered.

○ **What is the mechanism of a high ankle sprain?**

This injury is usually caused by dorsiflexion at the ankle with eversion of the foot and inversion of the tibia.

○ **What physical examination maneuver can be used to detect high ankle (syndesmosis) sprain?**

Pain in the superior portion of the ankle during cross-legged sitting with pressure applied to the medial aspect of the knee is suggestive of high ankle sprain.

○ **What is spondylosis?**

This is a degenerative condition of the spine resulting from age-related changes and intervertebral disk degeneration.

○ **What is spondylolisthesis?**

This is a slippage of the vertebral bodies, 1 over the other, in the anterior plane. Spondylolisthesis is graded 1 through 4 on the basis of percentage of slippage.

○ **What is the treatment for spondylolisthesis?**

If the displacement is less than 50% of the width of the vertebral body, treatment includes relative rest, NSAIDs, physical therapy, and possibly bracing. For higher grade instability, referral to a spine or orthopedic surgeon is appropriate.

○ **What is spondylolysis?**

This is a defect, such as a stress fracture, in the pars interarticularis of the posterior element of the spine.

○ **What are trigger points?**

Trigger points are focal areas of skeletal muscle that have become irritated and painful. They can cause pain locally and radiating to other areas.

○ **Should children be screened routinely for scoliosis?**

The US Preventive Services Task Force advises against general screening of pediatric patients for scoliosis.

○ **When should patients with scoliosis be referred for orthopedic treatment?**

If the patient has a Cobb angle of 20° or smaller, the patient can be observed with serial radiography every 6 months. Once the Cobb angle is greater than 20°, the patient should be referred for orthopedic evaluation.

○   **Can physical examination results, laboratory test findings, or severity of illness be used to predict splenic rupture in athletes with mononucleosis?**

All patients with mononucleosis should be considered at risk for splenic rupture because physical examination results, laboratory test findings, and severity of illness cannot be used to predict rupture accurately.

○   **How long should an athlete with mononucleosis be kept from rigorous physical exercise or contact sports?**

Athletes with confirmed mononucleosis should be kept from vigorous or contact exercises for 4 weeks, or longer, until they no longer have symptoms.

○   **What imaging modality is recommended for investigating possible stress fracture?**

Triple phase bone scanning has a higher sensitivity than does plain radiography in the identification of stress fracture, especially early in the course of the injury. Magnetic resonance imaging is better than plain radiography in the identification of stress fractures and is better for characterizing the injury than is bone scanning.

○   **What is the "dreaded black line?"**

This is a radiographic finding of lucency in the tibia that indicates a nonunion of tibial stress fracture. This is a highly morbid injury and often requires surgery and may take years to heal fully.

○   **What is the treatment for stress fracture?**

Initially, rest from all painful activities is the key to treatment. NSAIDs, ice, and physical therapy may also be helpful. Pain-free or nonweight bearing activities, such as swimming, may be started to maintain cardiovascular conditioning. A pneumatic air cast may help to speed recovery.

○   **What is a potential risk of conservative management of shoulder dislocation in athletes younger than 30 years?**

The risk of repeat dislocation in the general population is 50%, but for athletes, this risk is much higher (67%–97%). Surgical intervention reduces this risk in patients who are in high-demand physical activities and who are male. Evidence for other patient groups is lacking.

○   **Should athletes with first-time shoulder dislocation be treated conservatively or surgically?**

New evidence suggests that patients with first-time anterior shoulder dislocation with associated capsule or labral injuries had better patient satisfaction, fewer additional dislocations, and a more stable shoulder with surgical repair.

○   **What is the treatment for uncomplicated clavicular fracture that occurs in the middle third of the clavicle?**

Ice, analgesics and NSAIDs, and an arm sling for comfort are appropriate therapies. Traditionally, a figure-of-eight brace has been used, but this brace is uncomfortable, is associated with a higher complication rate, and does not improve outcomes.

○   **What findings suggest acromioclavicular sprain?**

The most common mechanism of injury is lateral force to an adducted shoulder. Patients often have tenderness at the acromioclavicular joint, separation (elevation of the distal clavicle relative to the acromion), and positive crossover test results.

○ **What is the treatment for acromioclavicular sprain?**

Types I and II (minimal acromioclavicular separation) are treated conservatively with immobilization for 2 weeks, followed by a graduated rehabilitation program.

○ **Define tennis elbow and golfer elbow.**

Tennis elbow is also known as "lateral epicondylitis" and golfer elbow is known as "medial epicondylitis of the elbow." These are tendinopathies at the insertion of the extensor and flexor groups of the forearm.

○ **What are effective treatments for lateral epicondylitis (tennis elbow)?**

Cortisone injection provides short-term relief (as long as 6 weeks) but does not offer long-term relief of symptoms. At 52 weeks, physiotherapy or simply watching and waiting are superior to cortisone injection.

○ **Which nerve is involved in carpal tunnel syndrome?**

In carpal tunnel syndrome, the median nerve is compressed at the wrist, resulting in paresthesias and weakness in the hand. Classically, it involves the thumb and the index and middle fingers.

○ **Are NSAIDs effective in treating carpal tunnel syndrome?**

NSAIDs are no more effective than placebo in treating carpal tunnel syndrome.

○ **Is corticosteroid injection an effective treatment for carpal tunnel syndrome?**

Corticosteroid injection is superior to placebo in treating carpal tunnel syndrome.

○ **What is a Colles fracture?**

A Colles fracture is a fracture of the distal radius with a dorsal displacement of the fractured bone.

○ **How is Colles fracture treated?**

If the fracture is nondisplaced, a short arm cast can be used. If the fracture has to be reduced, a long arm cast should be considered. Unstable fractures warrant referral to an orthopedic surgeon.

○ **What is osteochondritis dissecans?**

It is a localized area of subchondral bone necrosis. The femoral condyles, talar dome, and humeral head are most often affected.

○ **How is osteochondritis dissecans treated nonoperatively?**

The patient, depending on severity of symptoms, should refrain from competitive sports for approximately 6 to 8 weeks. The patient should participate only in pain-free activities of daily living and should bear weight only if pain free.

○ **What is the treatment for distal phalanx fractures?**

Uncomplicated, nondisplaced distal phalanx (or tuft) fractures can be treated by splinting of the DIP joint in extension for 3 to 4 weeks or until the finger is no longer sensitive to impact. If the fracture is angulated or transverse and displaced, orthopedic consultation is appropriate.

○   **What physical examination finding can help evaluate for rotation in a phalanx fracture?**

Examination of the semiflexed fingers should reveal fingernails in the same plane and all pointing toward the scaphoid bone. If there is overlap or the fingernails are out of alignment, then orthopedic consultation is appropriate.

○   **What is the treatment for dorsal proximal interphalangeal joint dislocation?**

This dislocation may be reduced at the sideline without radiography. Distal traction is applied to the distal phalanx, and volar pressure is applied to the middle phalanx. The digit should be splinted, and participation in the sport may continue. Close follow-up with radiography is required.

○   **What findings are suggestive of a meniscal tear in the knee?**

Twisting knee injury, locking sensation, effusion (gradual over 24 hours), joint line tenderness, or positive McMurray test results. Medial tear is more common than lateral tear.

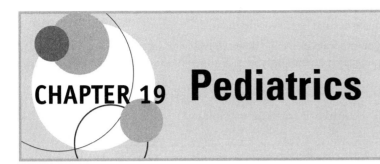

Susan Vanderberg-Dent, MD

○ **A child is born pink with blue extremities, limp, a heart rate of 80 beats per minute (bpm), slow irregular respirations, and a grimace. What is this infant's Apgar score?**

The Apgar score is 4.

Apgar Scores	0	1	2
Color	Blue, pale	Pink body, blue extremities	All pink
Muscle tone	Limp	Slight flexion	Active
Heart rate, bpm	0	Lower than 100	Higher than 100
Respirations	None	Slow, irregular	Strong, regular
Response to irritation	None	Some grimace	Strong grimace, cry

○ **What is the Moro reflex?**

An extension of the upper extremities at both shoulders and elbows in response to dropping an infant's head to a flat position from a 30° incline

○ **At what age does the Moro reflex disappear?**

6 months

○ **Touching the side of an infant's mouth or cheek causes the infant to turn its head toward the direction of the touch. What is this reflex called?**

The rooting reflex

○ **Which reflex has the earliest onset?**

The grasp reflex. It can be seen at 20 weeks of gestation.

○ **What are milia?**

Small, yellow-white papules, typically on the face of newborns. They are transient and are caused by retained sebum.

451

○ **What is the difference between cephalhematoma and caput succedaneum?**
- Cephalhematoma is a unilateral swelling on the scalp caused by subperiosteal hemorrhage.
- Caput succedaneum is a swelling on the scalp that extends beyond the suture lines and is caused by the pressure of labor and delivery.

○ **What do decreased femoral pulses during the newborn examination indicate?**

Coarctation of the aorta

○ **What is the importance of the red reflex during the newborn examination?**

A red reflex means that the infant does not have lens opacities or retinoblastoma.

○ **Why perform a back examination in a newborn?**

To look for signs of neural tube defects such as hairy tufts, hemangiomas, and lipomas

○ **What vitamin must all newborns receive within an hour of birth?**

Vitamin K1 oxide to prevent vitamin K–dependent hemorrhagic disease and other coagulation disorders

○ **What vaccination should be administered at birth?**

Hepatitis B

○ **Differentiate between Erb and Klumpke palsies.**

Both occur secondary to the trauma of birth. Newborns will have decreased or asymmetric arm movements.
- Erb palsy is an injury to the C5 and C6 nerve roots.
- Klumpke palsy is an injury to roots C7 through T2.

○ **Child development: At what ages are infants able to perform the following motor skills?**
1. Sit up
2. Walk
3. Crawl
4. Walk up stairs
5. Smile
6. Hold the head up
7. Roll over

Answers: (1) 5 to 7 months, (2) 11 to 16 months, (3) 9 to 10 months, (4) 14 to 22 months, (5) 2 months, (6) 2 to 4 months, and (7) 2 to 6 months

○ **At what age are infants capable of the following language skills?**
1. "Mama/dada" sounds
2. 1 word
3. Naming body parts
4. Combining words
5. Understandable speech

Answers: (1) 6 to 10 months, (2) 9 to 15 months, (3) 19 to 25 months, (4) 17 to 25 months, and (5) 2 to 4 years

○ **At what age is a child able to uncover a toy hidden by a scarf?**

9 to 10 months. This is called "object permanence," which is the understanding that an object one cannot see can still exist.

○ **A father comes to you distressed with his 3-year-old son and is concerned that his son cannot catch a ball. You reassure the father that children are not expected to perform that motor skill until they are older. At what age does this skill develop?**

5 to 6 years

○ **How many times a day should a healthy infant eat in the first 3 months of life?**

6 to 8 times, on average. The schedule should be dictated by the infant (ie, when he or she is hungry). By 8 months, meals are consumed only 3 to 4 times a day.

○ **At what age can a mother switch her child from breast milk or formula to whole cow milk?**

1 year. Skim or low-fat milk should not be used until the child is 2 years old. Nonpasteurized milk should never be used.

○ **What, if any, nutritional value does cow milk have over breast milk?**

Cow milk has a higher protein content than breast milk does. Both have the same caloric content (20 kcal/oz). Breast milk has a higher carbohydrate concentration and a greater amount of polyunsaturated fat and is easier for the infant to digest. For the obvious immunologic advantage, breast milk is best.

○ **A mother who is breastfeeding a 2-month-old baby complains of breast pain, swelling, fever, and a red coloration just above her left nipple. She wants to know if she can continue to breastfeed her infant. What do you tell her?**

She most likely has bacterial mastitis, which is most common in the first 2 months of breastfeeding. This is most frequently caused by *Staphylococcus aureus*. The mother should receive antibiotics and may continue breastfeeding if she chooses.

○ **At what age should solid foods be introduced?**

4 to 6 months. One food should be introduced at a time, with a 1- to 2-week interval before the introduction of the next new food. In this way, potential allergies can be defined.

○ **How much weight should an infant gain per day during the first 2 months of life?**

15 to 30 g/d. Newborns commonly lose 10% of their body weight during the first week of life because of a loss of extracellular water and a decrease in caloric intake. Healthy infants double their birth weight in 5 months and triple their weight in a year.

○ **When do infants begin teething?**

By age 6 months. They may become irritable, display decreased appetite, and drool excessively. Acetaminophen can be used to control the pain.

O   **What are the signs and symptoms of Reye syndrome?**

The patient is usually aged 6 to 11 years, with a prior viral illness and possible use of aspirin followed by intractable vomiting. The patient may be irritable, combative, or lethargic and may have right upper quadrant tenderness. Seizures may occur. Check for papilledema. Laboratory test findings include hypoglycemia and an elevated ammonia level (>20 times normal), but the bilirubin level is normal.

O   **Describe the stages of Reye syndrome.**

- Stage I: Vomiting, lethargy, and liver dysfunction
- Stage II: Disorientation, combativeness, delirium, hyperventilation, increased deep tendon reflexes, liver dysfunction, hyperexcitability, tachypnea, fever, tachycardia, sweating, and pupillary dilatation
- Stage III: Coma, decorticate rigidity, increased respiratory rate, and 50% mortality rate
- Stage IV: Coma, decerebrate posturing, no ocular reflexes, loss of corneal reflexes, and liver damage
- Stage V: Loss of deep tendon reflexes, seizures, flaccidity, respiratory arrest, and 95% mortality rate

O   **What is the treatment for Reye syndrome?**

- Stages I and II: Supportive
- Stages III to V: Intracranial pressure must be managed with elevation of the head of the bed, paralysis, intubation, furosemide, mannitol, dexamethasone, and pentobarbital coma

O   **What are the Wessel criteria for diagnosing infantile colic?**

3-3-3-3-3. Crying or irritability lasting longer than 3 hours a day, 3 days a week, or 3 weeks total, all in an infant younger than 3 months. Colic usually subsides after age 3 months.

O   **What percentage of infants develop colic?**

25%. The cause is unknown.

O   **Which standard infant immunization will most likely cause a reaction?**

The pertussis component of the diphtheria and tetanus toxoids and pertussis vaccine. Minor reactions (local induration and pain, mild fever) occur in 75% of children who receive the vaccine. This is the most common reaction, although reactions can be as severe as shock, encephalopathy, and convulsions. The acellular pertussis vaccine used now is less reactogenic than the older preparations were.

O   **When should toilet training be started?**

At about 18 months of age. The child must be neurodevelopmentally ready for training to be successful.

O   **When does physiologic jaundice occur in newborns?**

2 to 4 days after birth. Bilirubin levels may increase to 5 to 6 mg/dL.

O   **Name some causes of jaundice that occurs in the first day of life.**

- Sepsis
- Congenital infections
- ABO/Rh incompatibility

○ **When does jaundice caused by breastfeeding occur?**

By the seventh day of life. Bilirubin levels can reach 25 mg/dL.

○ **At what level of total serum bilirubin will scleral and facial jaundice be visible in the newborn?**

6 to 8 mg/dL. Jaundice of the shoulders and trunk occurs at levels of 8 to 10 mg/dL, and jaundice of the lower extremities is visible at levels of roughly 10 to 12 mg/dL.

○ **Can direct hyperbilirubinemia in a neonate be considered physiologic?**

No. It should be investigated thoroughly.

○ **What are some extrahepatic causes of direct hyperbilirubinemia with obstructive jaundice in the infant?**

Biliary atresia, common duct stenosis or stone, obstructive tumor, bile or mucous plug, or choledochal cyst

○ **What are some intrahepatic causes of direct hyperbilirubinemia with obstructive jaundice in the infant?**

Cytomegalovirus, toxoplasmosis, rubella, coxsackievirus, syphilis, hepatitis B, Epstein-Barr virus, urinary tract infection (UTI), cystic fibrosis, Gaucher disease, glycogen storage disease, hereditary fructose intolerance, α_1-antitrypsin deficiency, neonatal hepatitis, Zellweger syndrome, trisomy (17,18, or 21), and hepatic hemangiomatosis

○ **What are the most common causes of persistent direct hyperbilirubinemia in the neonate?**

Neonatal hepatitis and biliary atresia

○ **What is the treatment for biliary atresia?**

Surgery

○ **Which type of jaundice causes the highest levels of bilirubin elevation?**

A-O incompatibility

○ **What is kernicterus?**

A complex of neurologic symptoms caused by high levels of unconjugated bilirubin. This occurs when free bilirubin crosses the blood-brain barrier.

○ **What are some causes of hydrops fetalis?**
- Chronic anemia secondary to Rh incompatibility or homozygous α-thalassemia
- Intrauterine infection
- Cardiac disease
- Hypoproteinemia
- Chromosomal disorders

○ **What are some signs and symptoms of hydrops fetalis?**
- Ascites
- Congestive heart failure (CHF)
- Anasarca
- Pleural effusions
- Hepatosplenomegaly
- Pallor

○ **What is the normal heart rate, respiratory rate, and systolic blood pressure of newborns, 1-month-olds, 6-month-olds, 1-year-olds, 2- to 4-year olds, 5- to 8-year olds, 8- to 12-year olds, and children older than 12 years?**

Age	Heart Rate, bpm	Respiratory Rate, breaths per minute	Systolic Blood Pressure, mm Hg
Newborn	120–180	40–60	52–92
1 month	110–180	30–50	60–104
6 months to 1 year	120–140	25–35	65–125
2 to 4 years	100–110	20–30	80–95
5 to 8 years	90–100	4–20	90–100
8 to 12 years	60–110	12–20	100–110
Older than 12 years	60–105	12–16	100–120

○ **What are some signs and symptoms of dehydration?**

Sunken eyes, dry mucous membranes, sunken fontanelle, decreased tears, poor skin turgor, decreased urine output, lethargy, irritability, tachycardia, and hypotension

○ **What is a child's daily maintenance requirements for water, sodium, potassium, and chloride?**
- Water: 1500 mL/m^2
- Sodium: 2 to 3 mEq/kg
- Potassium: 2 to 3 mEq/kg
- Chloride: 2 to 3 mEq/kg

○ **When does colic most commonly occur?**

In the evenings. Colic is irritability, excessive inconsolable crying bouts, and fussiness in infants aged 1 to 4 months.

○ **What is the treatment for colic?**

Because the cause is not known, a specific treatment is not indicated. Reassurance to parents that the infant will outgrow this stage is appropriate. Rocking, carrying the infant, and vibrations (going for a car ride) may be helpful. It is important always to exclude other more serious problems that can cause inconsolable crying before diagnosing colic. Assess the parents' support system and risk factors for child abuse and neglect.

○ **Define sudden infant death syndrome (SIDS).**

SIDS is the unexpected death of a previously well infant whose death cannot be explained. SIDS pertains only to infants younger than 1 year.

○ **SIDS is the most common cause of death for infants in the first year of life. It occurs at a rate of 2 per 1000 (ie, 10,000 per year). What are 8 risk factors associated with SIDS?**

1. Prematurity with low birth weight
2. Previous episode of apnea or apparent life-threatening event
3. Mother is substance abuser
4. Family history of SIDS
5. Male sex
6. Low socioeconomic status
7. Prone sleeping position
8. Smoking during pregnancy

○ **In what season is the incidence of SIDS higher?**

In the winter

○ **Define failure to thrive (FTT).**

Infants who are below the third percentile in height or weight or whose weight is less than 80% of the ideal weight for their age. Almost all patients with FTT are younger than 5 years, and most of them are aged 6 to 12 months. Other disorders commonly confused with FTT include anorexia nervosa, bronchiectasis, cystic fibrosis, congenital heart disease, chronic renal disease, Down syndrome, hypothyroidism, inflammatory bowel disease, juvenile rheumatoid arthritis, human immunodeficiency virus, Hirschsprung disease, tuberculosis, malignancy, and Turner syndrome.

○ **What is the most common cause of FTT?**

Poor intake is responsible for 70% of FTT cases. One-third of these cases stem from poorly educated parents, ranging from inaccurate knowledge of what to feed a child to overdiluting formula in order to make it last longer. While in the hospital, patients are fed 150 to 200 kcal/kg per day (1.5 times their expected intake), which corrects environmental problems associated with poor feeding.

○ **What percentage of abused children brought to the emergency department will be killed by future abuse?**

About 5%

○ **Broken bones are found in 10% to 20% of abused children. What radiologic clues suggest child abuse?**

- Spiral fractures, especially before the onset of walking
- Scapula or sternal fractures
- Chip fractures or bucket-handle fractures
- Epiphyseal-metaphyseal posterior rib fractures in infants
- Several fractures in various stages of healing

○ **What other clinical findings would lead you to suspect child abuse?**

"Accident-prone" children, cigarette burns, retinal hemorrhages, subdural hematomas, head contusions in children who are preambulatory, back bruises in children who cannot climb, burns on the buttocks or in a stocking-glove distribution, and lesions in the shape of familiar objects (eg, belts and hands)

○ **What is the most common type of hypertension in children?**

Idiopathic or essential hypertension. One percent of pediatric patients and 3% of adolescent patients are hypertensive.

○ **What is the most common cause of secondary hypertension in children?**

Renal disease (polycystic kidney disease, infection, tumors, or congenital vascular abnormalities). Other causes are vascular, endocrine, neurologic, or pharmacologic in nature.

○ **How should you treat a newborn with cyanotic spells and great difficulty, breathing, especially during feeding?**

Surgery. This infant has choanal atresia. The septum between the nose and the pharynx is prohibiting the infant from breathing through the nose and must be removed surgically. Infants are obligate nasal breathers, as we all are, during feeding. The infant may have respiratory movement but no audible air entry into the lungs. Cyanosis is often relieved during crying bouts.

○ **What percentage of African Americans are heterozygous for the sickle cell gene?**

10%. Sickle cell is also common in Greek, Turkish, Arab, and Indian populations.

○ **What commonly precipitates aplastic crisis in a child with sickle cell disease?**

Viral infections, most commonly an infection with human parvovirus B19

○ **What does parvovirus B19 cause?**

Erythema infectiosum (Fifth disease)

○ **Between what ages will infants with sickle cell anemia show clinical manifestations of the disease?**

4 to 6 months. Before this, the infants are protected by leftover fetal hemoglobin. By age 4 to 6 months, they develop (1) anemia, (2) jaundice, (3) splenomegaly, and (4) hand-foot syndrome, in which the dorsal surfaces of the hands and feet swell and hurt because of infarction of the bone marrow of the metacarpal bones, metatarsal bones, and phalanges.

○ **What organism is most commonly implicated in childhood sickle cell infections?**

Streptococcus pneumoniae (60%). Daily doses of prophylactic penicillin are recommended for those least resistant to encapsulated bacteria. It is particularly important that these children are appropriately immunized against pneumococci, meningococci, and *Haemophilus influenzae* type B (Hib).

○ **Which organs are most commonly damaged in patients with sickle cell disease?**

Spleen, lung, liver, kidney, skeleton, and skin

○ **What is acute chest syndrome?**

Chest pain and hypoxemia and/or infiltrates at chest radiography in a patient with sickle cell disease

○ **What is the cause of acute chest syndrome?**

Pneumonia (most often caused by pneumococcal infection) or pulmonary infarct secondary to vasoocclusion

○ **How is acute chest syndrome treated?**

With early blood transfusion or exchange transfusion, hydration, oxygen, analgesics, and antibiotics

○ **A 1-hour-old, premature infant presents with tachypnea, grunting, chest wall retractions, nasal flaring, and cyanosis. What is a possible diagnosis?**

Hyaline membrane disease, also known as "infant respiratory distress syndrome." These patients have atelectasis, intrapulmonary shunting, hypoxemia, and cyanosis.

○ **What is the pathophysiology of hyaline membrane disease?**

The lungs are poorly compliant because of insufficient surfactant. These infants are generally preterm and have not developed chemically mature lungs.

○ **What does chest radiography in an infant with hyaline membrane disease look like?**

Atelectasis with diffuse, fine, granular areas of opacity.

○ **What is bronchopulmonary dysplasia?**

Residual chronic lung disease of infancy that persists secondary to neonatal lung disease. It can follow any illness that requires mechanical ventilation.

○ **On what does the incidence of bronchopulmonary dysplasia depend?**

Birth weight. The incidence is higher than 50% in neonates weighing less than 750 g and 40% in neonates weighing 750 to 1000 g.

○ **Describe the clinical features of bronchopulmonary dysplasia.**

Respiratory distress, tachypnea, reactive airways, hypoxia, hypercarbia, poor feeding, irritability, lethargy, increased oxygen requirement, and occasionally pulmonary edema and cor pulmonale.

○ **Patients with bronchopulmonary dysplasia may have chronic hypercarbia. Will administering oxygen diminish their respiratory drive?**

No.

○ **What are some causes of wheezing in an infant?**

Asthma, bronchiolitis, foreign body, bronchopulmonary dysplasia, pneumonia, cystic fibrosis, anaphylaxis, vascular rings, aspiration, mediastinal masses, and CHF

○ **What is the most common trigger for asthma?**

Viral infections

○ **How do you diagnose asthma in a small child?**

Clinically. The child will have recurrent episodes of wheezing or persistent cough and generally a family history of asthma, atopy, or allergies. Pulmonary function tests are useless until a child is about age 6 years, because younger children are not able to perform the tests.

○ **What are the indications for chest radiography in a patient with asthma?**

Suspicion of consolidation, effusion, pneumothorax, or impending respiratory failure. Findings at radiography are nonspecific and include hyperinflation, peribronchial cuffing, and atelectasis.

○ **Is extrinsic or intrinsic asthma more common in children?**

Extrinsic. This involves immunoglobulin E production in response to allergens.

○ **What percentage of children with asthma are likely to have symptoms persisting into adulthood?**

50%

○ **What is the most common cause of bronchiolitis?**

Respiratory syncytial virus (RSV). Other major causes are parainfluenza virus, influenza virus, mumps, echovirus, rhinovirus, *Mycoplasma*, and adenoviruses.

○ **What is bronchiolitis?**

An acute inflammation of the lower respiratory tract that results in obstruction of the small airways. Patients present with a prodrome of runny nose, low-grade fever, and decreased appetite, leading to increased respirations, retractions, and wheezing.

○ **What is the common age range for bronchiolitis?**

2 to 6 months, when maternal antibody to RSV is waning

○ **What is the most common cause of stridor in neonates?**

Congenital abnormalities, especially laryngotracheomalacia

○ **Can the type of stridor localize the level of the obstruction?**

Yes. Inspiratory stridor points to a site of obstruction above the vocal folds; expiratory stridor points to obstruction below the vocal folds.

○ **Define apnea.**

Apnea is a period of no respirations that lasts longer than 20 seconds.

○ **An 8-month-old infant is brought to your office. The mother says that she suddenly started having trouble breathing. She is afebrile and has no other symptoms. What do you do?**

Rule out foreign body with anteroposterior and lateral radiographs of the upper airway. Although this could be the manifestation of many respiratory problems, sudden onset of symptoms should pique your suspicion of a foreign body; 65% of deaths due to foreign body aspiration are in infants younger than 1 year.

○ **What is the most common cause of pneumonia in school-aged children?**

Mycoplasma pneumoniae. Other causes include *S pneumoniae*, parainfluenza virus, and influenza virus. These patients present with a persistent, dry, hacking cough. The chest may sound surprisingly clear, but chest radiography will reveal bilateral infiltrates. Treatment is with erythromycin or tetracycline, depending on patient age.

○ **A 3-day-old infant has a high fever and is coughing, grunting, and working hard to breathe. Chest radiography shows a reticulogranular pattern. The birth history is unremarkable. What is the probable diagnosis?**

Group B streptococcal pneumonia. The infant most likely contracted it while passing through an infected birth canal. The mortality rate can be as high as 40%, so early treatment with penicillin G is important. Other causes of pneumonia in newborns are *Listeria monocytogenes*, enteric gram-negative bacilli, chlamydia, rubella, cytomegalovirus, and herpes.

○ **Contrast pneumonia caused by *S pneumoniae* with pneumonia caused by *M pneumoniae*.**

Characteristic	S pneumoniae	M pneumoniae
Prodrome	Little	Mild fever, malaise, cough, hippocampal atrophy
Onset	Rapid	Gradual
Upper respiratory infection symptoms	Tachypnea, cough, occasional pleuritic pain	Little
Associated findings	High fever	Exanthem, arthritis, gastrointestinal (GI) complaints, neurologic complications
Pleural effusion	Occasional	Rare
Laboratory test results	Leukocytosis	White blood cell (WBC) count normal or slightly high
Treatment	Penicillin	Erythromycin

○ **What is the most common pneumonia in children younger than 5 years?**

RSV pneumonia. These children present with a nonproductive cough, rhonchi, rales, wheezing, and possibly fever and chills. Bilateral infiltrates, atelectasis, and air trapping are present at chest radiography. Other common viral pneumonias in this population are parainfluenza virus, adenovirus, and influenza B virus.

○ **What is the most common cause of bacterial pneumonia in pediatric patients?**

S pneumoniae. The child presents with productive cough, pleurisy, dyspnea, fever, and chills.

○ **True/False: Group A β-hemolytic *Streptococcus (Streptococcus pyogenes)* is a frequent cause of pharyngitis in patients younger than 3 years.**

False

○ **What is the most common cause of pharyngitis in children?**

Viruses. Most commonly, pharyngitis is caused by adenovirus, parainfluenza virus, rhinovirus, herpes simplex virus, RSV, Epstein-Barr virus, influenza virus, and Coxsackie virus.

○ **What is the most common bacterial cause of pharyngitis?**

In children older than 3 years the most common bacterial cause is group A β-hemolytic *Streptococcus*, though viruses are still the most common cause of pharyngitis overall.

○ **We know that the streptococcal antigen sampling tests for pharyngitis have a high false-negative rate (sensitivity is generally >50%). What is the false-negative rate for a single throat culture?**

10%

○ **How long should a school-aged child receive antibiotic treatment for streptococcal pharyngitis before returning to school?**

24 hours. The child with a true streptococcal infection is not infectious within a few hours after penicillin therapy is begun. The child may not feel well enough to return after 1 day but is not a risk to others.

○ **Rheumatic fever is preventable if antibiotic therapy is initiated before how many days after the start of streptococcal pharyngitis?**

9 days

○ **Is antibiotic therapy warranted for the prevention of poststreptococcal glomerulonephritis?**

No. Poststreptococcal glomerulonephritis is not preventable with antibiotic therapy.

○ **A 5-year-old boy is brought to your office by his father who tells you that he has had a 3-day history of fever, chills, and pain when swallowing. At examination, the boy has cervical lymphadenopathy, no cough, and erythematous tonsils with bilateral white exudates. What percentage of patients with this presentation will show group A β-hemolytic *Streptococcus* at throat culture?**

Twenty-five percent of patients with these symptoms and tonsillar exudates have positive culture results. Thirty percent of patients with streptococcal infection do not have tonsillar exudates. Fifteen percent to 20% of children have group A β-hemolytic *Streptococcus* as normal flora in their mouths.

○ **What is the most common cause of tonsillitis?**

Viral (75%). Only 25% of cases are due to group A β-hemolytic *Streptococcus*.

○ **What are the indications for tonsillectomy?**

Peritonsillar abscess; airway obstruction; 7 episodes of documented streptococcal tonsillitis within 1 year or 5 documented cases of streptococcal tonsillitis per year for 2 consecutive years; and unilateral enlargement of the tonsils, which may indicate malignancy.

○ **What is the usual age range for retropharyngeal abscess?**

6 months to 3 years

○ **What does "hot potato voice" suggest in a patient with sore throat?**

Peritonsillar abscess. Patients generally have ipsilateral otalgia, trismus, dysarthria, fever, drooling, and a muffled voice.

○ **What is the clinical presentation of a child with mononucleosis?**

Malaise, fever, headache, fatigue, sore throat, lymphadenopathy, and splenomegaly

○ **What virus causes mononucleosis?**

Epstein-Barr virus

○ **What age group is most commonly affected by mononucleosis?**

Adolescents and young adults in industrialized countries. Epstein-Barr viral infection generally occurs at a much earlier age in developing countries.

○ **What antibiotic should not be administered in patients with mononucleosis?**

Ampicillin. Almost all patients who have mononucleosis develop a generalized maculopapular rash with ampicillin administration.

○ **What is the treatment for mononucleosis?**

Rest. Do not use ampicillin. Patients are also counseled not to participate in contact sports because of the risk for splenic rupture. The illness can last weeks to months.

○ **What are the 3 stages of pertussis?**

1. Catarrhal stage: Rhinorrhea, cough, conjunctivitis (lasts 1 week)
2. Paroxysmal stage: Paroxysms of continuous coughing (lasts as long as 6 weeks)
3. Convalescent stage: Coughing decreases

○ **What is the treatment for pertussis?**

Patients and household contacts should be treated with azithromycin; erythromycin is less well tolerated, and the course of therapy is longer. Trimethoprim and sulfamethoxazole treatment is an alternative in children older than 2 months if macrolides are not tolerated. Immunizations should be appropriately updated; combined tetanus, diphtheria, acellular pertussis vaccine is now available for persons older than 7 years. Superinfective pneumonias can be serious and should be treated with broader coverage.

○ **Pertussis is most common in what age group?**

Infants younger than 6 months

○ **What is the classic triad in a child with cystic fibrosis?**

1. Chronic pulmonary disease
2. Malabsorption
3. Increased level of electrolytes in the sweat

○ **What are the most common pathogens infecting the lungs in a child with cystic fibrosis?**

S aureus and *Pseudomonas aeruginosa*

○ **What is the diagnostic test of choice in determining if a patient has cystic fibrosis?**

Quantitative pilocarpine iontophoresis sweat test (sweat chloride test)

○ **What would you expect the serum chloride level, sodium level, bicarbonate level, and pH in a patient with cystic fibrosis to be?**

Sodium and chloride levels will be low, representing renal compensation for the increased salt losses in the sweat. Bicarbonate level and pH are usually high.

○ **What might the chest radiograph in a patient with cystic fibrosis look like?**

Hyperinflated lungs, infiltrates, and peribronchial thickening

○ **How do most patients with cystic fibrosis die?**

They eventually die of respiratory failure complicated by cor pulmonale.

○ **What is the most common vasculitis in the pediatric population?**

Henoch-Schönlein purpura (HSP), which is a temporary allergic disorder of the blood vessels. Patients present with bruises over the lower extremities, abdomen, and buttocks. Bleeding from the GI and genitourinary tracts is also common. Associated arthritis occurs in 75% of cases.

○ **What is the typical rash of HSP?**

Palpable purpura measuring 1 to 2 mm in diameter, symmetrically distributed, generally located on the buttocks and thighs. The rash lasts 4 to 6 weeks.

○ **What other symptoms does a patient with HSP commonly have?**

Seventy-five percent have arthralgias or arthritis (typically of the feet and hands). Abdominal pain and microscopic hematuria are also common. Rarely, patients have central nervous system (CNS) involvement manifesting as seizures and coma.

○ **How can HSP be distinguished from idiopathic thrombocytopenic purpura (ITP)?**

The platelet count is normal in HSP. In HSP, the immune complex reacts with blood vessel walls causing capillary leakage. In ITP, immunoglobulin G antiplatelet antibodies develop and fix to normal platelets that are then destroyed.

○ **What is the most common thrombocytopenia in childhood?**

ITP. Platelet count and bone marrow examination can be used to confirm the diagnosis. Acute ITP generally follows an acute infection; 80% to 85% of cases resolve within 2 months. Acute ITP is most common in children aged 2 to 9 years.

○ **What other illnesses cause thrombocytopenia in children?**

Leukemia, lymphoma, myeloma, autoimmune collagen vascular disease, and drugs (thiazides, quinidine, and sulfa antibiotics).

○ **What is the treatment for ITP?**

Prednisone, intravenous (IV) gamma globulin, and supportive care. If the platelet count is below $50,000 \times 10^3/\mu L$, patients should be treated in the hospital. For severe cases, refractory to less aggressive treatment, splenectomy is performed.

○ **What is the most common cause of acquired acute renal failure in children?**

Hemolytic uremic syndrome (HUS)

○ **What is the classic triad of HUS?**

1. Microangiopathic hemolytic anemia
2. Thrombocytopenia
3. Acute renal failure

○ **What organs other than the kidney can be involved in HUS?**

The CNS, lungs, heart, and GI tract can all be involved. When systemic involvement occurs, it is difficult to distinguish HUS from thrombotic thrombocytopenic purpura.

○ **HUS is usually preceded by an infection, either viral or bacterial. What are the most common bacteria associated with HUS?**

Escherichia coli O157:H7

○ **What is the most common anemia in children?**

Iron-deficiency anemia. Most cases are caused by an inadequate intake of iron rather than loss through hemorrhage. It is most commonly seen in infants aged 6 to 12 months who are fed exclusively breast milk. The infant's rapid growth spurt puts a strain on iron stores. Other causes of anemia in children are lead poisoning and thalassemia.

○ **What are the signs and symptoms of iron-deficiency anemia?**

It can be asymptomatic, or there may be irritability, lethargy, fatigue, pallor, tachycardia, or even signs of CHF. Treatment for mild cases is oral iron 6 mg/kg per day. For severe cases, transfusions of packed red blood cells are indicated.

○ **Twenty percent of children with meningococcemia die. What is the major cause of death in these patients?**

Shock. Rapid administration of penicillin is the treatment of choice.

○ **What is the most common cause of cellulitis in the pediatric population?**

S aureus

○ **What are common causes of neonatal conjunctivitis?**

Chemical conjunctivitis due to silver nitrate drops, chlamydial conjunctivitis, and gonococcal conjunctivitis

○ **What are the most common causes of otitis media?**

Viral (35%), *S pneumoniae* (30%–35%), *H influenzae* (20%–25%), *Moraxella catarrhalis* (10%–15%), group A streptococci (2%), and *S aureus* (1%). In neonates, gram-negative bacilli account for 20% of cases, but these organisms are rare in older children.

○ **What are some risk factors for otitis media?**

Recent upper respiratory infection, white ethnicity, male sex, cleft palate, Down syndrome, bottle feeding, exposure to other young children, secondhand smoke, and family history of middle ear disease

○ **How common is otitis media?**

Very common. By age 6 months, 35% of children have had 1 episode of otitis media, and by age 7 years, 90% of children have had 1 or more bouts and 40% of children have had 6 or more episodes of acute otitis media. Otitis media most commonly affects children aged 5 to 24 months.

○ **When does recurrent otitis media most commonly occur?**

In the winter and early spring. A patient must have otitis media 3 or more times in a period of 6 months or 4 times within 1 year for the disease to be classified as recurrent otitis media. Children with the first episode of otitis media before age 1 year are considered otitis prone.

○ **What are the indications for placement of tympanostomy tubes?**

More than 3 months of bilateral otitis media with effusion (OME), more than 6 months of unilateral OME, hearing loss greater than 40 dB, or hearing loss greater than 20 dB with more than 4 months of OME. For recurrent acute otitis media, tympanostomy tubes are recommended if the patient experiences more than 3 bouts of acute otitis media over a 6-month period or 4 episodes within 1 year. Speech delay and symptoms of vestibular dysfunction may also be indications.

○ **Name the following condition: fluid collection in the middle ear that is usually painless, no sign of infection, and possible reduction in hearing acuity.**

OME, also known as serous or secretory otitis media. This is an underused diagnosis.

○ **How useful is the light reflex in evaluating for acute otitis media?**

It is useless. Tympanic membrane mobility (assessed by means of insufflation) is an appropriate diagnostic indicator of middle ear fluid.

○ **In what age groups will you most commonly see croup and epiglottitis?**

- Croup: 3 months to 3 years
- Epiglottitis: 2 to 7 years—classically, though with the Hib vaccine, it is becoming less common in young children

○ **What are the most common causes of croup?**

Most croup cases are caused by viruses, most commonly parainfluenza virus.

○ **What organism most commonly causes epiglottitis?**

Group A *Streptococcus* has now replaced Hib as the leading cause of epiglottitis, primarily because of the increased number of infants vaccinated with the Hib vaccine.

○ **What percentage of cases of stridor with fever are due to croup?**

90%

○ **When is croup most common?**

In the winter

○ **What is the presentation of a patient with epiglottitis?**

Acute onset of high fever, sore throat, dysphagia and respiratory distress, muffled voice, stridor, tripod sitting position, and drool. These children appear toxic.

○ **What is the manifestation of croup?**

A nonspecific upper respiratory infection followed gradually by a brassy or barking cough and inspiratory stridor with mild temperatures

○ **What is the treatment for epiglottitis?**

Oxygen; IV antibiotics for Hib, *S aureus*, *S pneumoniae*, and *S pyogenes*; intubation if necessary.

○ **What is the treatment for croup?**

Cool mist therapy for mild croup. Oxygen, cool mist, racemic epinephrine nebulizer, and corticosteroids for moderate and severe croup. Intubation and hospitalization are warranted for severe cases.

○ **What bone is most commonly fractured in newborns?**

Clavicle

○ **What is the most common cause of intoeing in children?**

Excessive femoral anteversion. Ninety percent to 95% of children will outgrow it with no treatment.

○ **A mother is concerned because her 18-month-old daughter has bowlegs and she does not want her stigmatized for wearing braces. What do you tell her?**

Bowlegs are caused by internal tibial torsion that spontaneously resolves by age 8 years in 95% of children. Her daughter will probably not have to wear braces, especially if she does a few simple leg exercises.

○ **What congenital foot deformity is associated with spina bifida or arthrogryposis?**

Congenital convex pes valgus (congenital vertical talus). This foot has a tightened heel cord, unlike the calcaneovalgus foot, and the sole has a rocker-bottom appearance. Fifty percent of children with this congenital malformation have spina bifida or arthrogryposis.

○ **A newborn you are examining has kidney-shaped soles and medial deviation of his heels. You are not able to dorsiflex his feet. What is the diagnosis?**

Clubfoot or what is medically known as "talipes equinovarus." Mild cases may be attributed to positioning in utero. More serious cases are due to anatomic abnormalities. Like congenital convex pes valgus, this anatomic abnormality may also be associated with spina bifida.

○ **What is the most common primary malignant bone tumor in the pediatric population?**

Osteogenic sarcoma

○ **In what pediatric population is osteogenic sarcoma most prevalent?**

Male adolescents

○ **Where do osteomas most frequently occur?**

At the metaphyseal ends of the long bones. Osteomas are most common in the distal femur, followed in order by the proximal tibia, proximal humerus, and proximal femur.

○ **The star of the local high school basketball team is brought into your office by his dad who says his son has been having pain just below his right knee for the past 2 weeks. The patient does not recall any trauma and says that the pain gets worse when he plays his games or when he walks down stairs. At examination, you notice a mild swelling just over the tibial tuberosity of his right knee. When you press there, the patient pulls away and says that is the spot. There is no effusion. What is your diagnosis?**

Osgood-Schlatter disease. This is a disease found in active adolescent boys. Pain and swelling are caused by detachment of cartilage over the tibial tuberosity that occurs with overuse of the quadriceps. Treatment is rest, ice, and nonsteroidal anti-inflammatory drugs (NSAIDs). Severe cases may require knee immobilization in extension, physical therapy, and no sports playing or excessive use. The disease is generally self-limiting.

○ **A 3-year-old girl is brought to your office. She is holding her right arm flexed at the elbow with her forearm pronated. She will not let you near it. What is your diagnosis?**

Subluxation of the radial head, commonly called "nursemaid elbow." This injury commonly occurs when an adult pulls or jerks a child up by the arm.

○ **What is the treatment for nursemaid elbow?**

Radial head subluxation (aka "nursemaid elbow") occurs with abrupt axial traction on an extended, pronated forearm. This can occur when caretakers lift a child up by the arm or if a child trips while holding an adult's hand. Relocation is performed by putting a finger over the radial head while supinating, then flexing, the elbow.

○ **A mother brings her 200-lb 14-year-old son to you, because he has been limping and complaining of knee pain for the past 2 weeks. What is your diagnosis?**

Slipped capital femoral epiphysis. Hip pain is commonly referred to the knee, most frequently the medial aspect of the knee. Patients may hold the hip in abduction and external rotation. Internal rotation is severely limited.

○ **What is the most serious complication of slipped capital femoral epiphysis?**

Avascular necrosis of the femoral head

○ **What is the treatment of slipped capital femoral epiphysis?**

In slipped capital femoral epiphysis, the epiphysis slips posteriorly on the femoral neck. Surgical pinning and immobilization are indicated. Some mild cases may be corrected with traction and internal rotation.

○ **What is the classic profile of a patient with a slipped capital femoral epiphysis?**

Slipped capital femoral epiphysis is most prevalent in obese boys aged 10 to 16 years at the peak of the growth spurt. Forty percent of patients presenting with this complaint are obese. African Americans are more commonly affected than are white Americans.

○ **How will a patient with slipped capital femoral epiphysis present?**

Patients usually complain of hip or knee pain and a limp sometimes secondary to trauma. At examination, they have limited medial rotation, flexion, extension, and abduction.

○ **A mother brings her 8-year-old boy in to see you because he has been complaining of pain in his legs intermittently for the past 2 weeks. He recalls no injury and says he only has the pain at nighttime or if he is playing really hard. Sometimes the pain even awaken him from sleep. What is a likely diagnosis?**

Growing pains. These pains usually occur in the lower limbs of growing children and are always bilateral. Treatment involves heat and massage.

○ **What is the most common site for osteochondritis dissecans?**

The lateral aspect of the medial femoral condyle. Other sites are the patella or the lateral condyle of the femur. Osteochondritis dissecans exists when a segment of articular or subchondral bone is separated from the surrounding bone, which manifests clinically as joint pain, stiffness, locking, clicking, and swelling. Theories about why osteochondritis dissecans occurs include repetitive trauma and disruption of vascular supply.

○ **There are 2 age peaks in the occurrence of osteochondritis dissecans. When are they?**

1. Children younger than 12 years
2. Young adults

This condition is more common in male patients than in female patients (3:1).

○ **A 3-year-old girl returns to your office with a limp and mild pain in her right hip. She was seen by you last week, and you sent her home with the diagnosis of viral syndrome and upper respiratory infection. The patient still has a mild fever (100.5°F). What is the diagnosis?**

Toxic synovitis. This is the most common nontraumatic cause of limp and hip pain in patients between aged 3 to 6 years. This is transient unilateral (95%) inflammatory arthritis that follows a viral illness within 3 to 6 days. Septic arthritis manifests with more severe symptoms, such as higher fever, guarding, malaise, and sharp pain.

○ **A father brings his 5-year-old son to you because he is limping and complaining of hip pain. At examination, you note that his quadriceps appears atrophied on the right side, his right leg is shorter than his left, and he has decreased motion at his hip joint, especially at internal rotation and abduction. He is otherwise healthy. What is the diagnosis?**

Legg-Calvé-Perthes disease. This disease is idiopathic, aseptic necrosis of the femoral head. It is most common in boys aged 4 to 8 years (male:female is 5:1). It is thought that Legg-Calvé-Perthes disease may be the result of an interruption in the blood flow to the femoral epiphysis because of trauma, synovitis, hyperviscosity, or coagulation abnormalities. The exact cause is unknown.

○ **What is the prognosis in a patient with Legg-Calvé-Perthes disease?**

After casting and braces for 1 to 2 years or surgery, 40% to 50% of patients still develop severe degenerative hip disease that requires hip replacement. Younger patients have a better prognosis.

○ **A 12-year-old forward on the local soccer team is brought in by her mother complaining of pain in the front of her knee. She denies any trauma or injuries and says that she feels like her knee is made of sandpaper because of a grating sensation when she runs or climbs stairs. This grating sensation is reproducible when you ask the patient to do a deep knee bend and is accompanied by some crepitus. Pressing down on the patella induces pain. What is the diagnosis?**

Chondromalacia patella, which is a breakdown of the cartilage. This disease generally manifests in prepubescent children.

○ **Differentiate between sprains and strains.**

- Sprains: Stretches or incomplete tears of a ligament
- Strains: Stretched tendons or muscles

○ **When is the peak incidence of scoliosis?**

Early adolescence. It is most commonly idiopathic in origin. Girls are more frequently affected than boys.

○ **Bowed legs, thinning of the skull, thickening of the costochondral junction, and prominences on the wrists and knees are suggestive of what disease?**

Rickets

○ **What will a radiograph of a child's knee who has rickets look like?**

There will be a widened space between the metaphysis and the epiphysis, and the ends of the metaphysis will be cupped and irregular.

○ **Rickets can be due to lack of sunlight or abnormal metabolism of what vitamin?**

Vitamin D

○ **What are the most common risk factors for inguinal hernia in the pediatric population?**

Male sex and prematurity

○ **Benign intracranial hypertension in the pediatric patient can be caused by an excess of what vitamin?**

Vitamin A. Children with vitamin A excess may present with headache, nausea, dizziness, irritability, stomach pain, insomnia, and possible changes in visual acuity.

○ **What are the most common complaints of children with Ewing sarcoma?**

Pain and swelling at the site. Systemic symptoms may also exist.

○ **Where in the body are you most likely to find osteogenic sarcoma?**

Fifty percent of cases occur in the knee joint and metastasize to the lungs.

○ **A white pupil or cat's-eye indicates what congenital malignancy?**

Retinoblastoma. This is a tumor arising from neural tissue of the retina. Treatment depends on the extent of the disease and can involve enucleation, radiation, and chemotherapy.

○ **What is the most common childhood malignancy?**

Acute lymphoblastic leukemia. Leukemia accounts for one-third of all cancers diagnosed in the pediatric population. Acute lymphoblastic leukemia accounts for 75% of all acute leukemias, and acute myelogenous leukemia accounts for 25%.

○ **What are some signs and symptoms of leukemia?**

Fatigue, petechia, bleeding, purpura, lymphadenopathy, hepatosplenomegaly, bone and joint pain, low-grade fever, and pallor

○ **What are the signs and symptoms of Hodgkin disease?**

Painless supraclavicular or cervical lymphadenopathy, hepatomegaly, splenomegaly, unexplained fever, and night sweats

○ **What are indications for lymph node biopsy?**

Nodes that continue to enlarge after 2 to 3 weeks, nodes that do not return to normal size after 5 to 6 weeks, or nodes associated with mediastinal enlargement at chest radiography

○ **How are childhood cases of non-Hodgkin lymphoma different from adult cases?**

They grow rapidly, are rarely nodular, and are as likely to be T-cell lymphomas as B-cell lymphomas.

○ **What is the most common tumor in a child's first year of life?**

Wilms tumor. Hepatoma is the second most common tumor at this age.

○ **One percent to 2% of patients with Wilms tumor develop secondary malignancies. Which types are most common?**

Hepatocellular carcinoma, leukemia, lymphoma, and soft-tissue sarcoma

○ **Wilms tumor is most commonly found in what age group?**

Children aged 1 to 3 years. Wilms tumors (nephroblastomas) are more common in girls (2:1) and generally manifest as a painless abdominal mass, with fever, decreased appetite, nausea, and vomiting. Forty percent are hereditary. Treatment is surgical resection and chemotherapy.

○ **What is the average age for pediatric patients to develop Wilms tumor?**

3 years old. Cure rates are as high as 90% in patients with no metastasis.

○ **What populations are most likely to have lead poisoning?**

Those living in the inner city, those of lower socioeconomic status, African Americans, and those living in housing built before 1960

○ **When patients have lead poisoning symptoms, what might you see?**

Lethargy, irritability, anorexia, constipation, abdominal pain, vomiting, clumsiness, regression in speech, and decreased hearing. If patients have levels over 70 μg/dL, they may have symptoms of lead encephalopathy, such as ataxia, seizures, and coma.

○ **What percentage of children with lead encephalopathy will develop permanent brain damage?**

70% to 80%

○ **What is the treatment for patients with blood lead levels of 25 to 44 μg/dL?**

If they have no symptoms, they can be treated with oral chelation therapy with succimer and removal of the lead source from the environment. With lower lead blood levels, environmental management and repeat screening are appropriate.

○ **What is the treatment for children without symptoms with blood lead levels of 45 to 69 μg/dL?**

Hospital admission for chelation therapy with calcium disodium versenate or dimercaptosuccinic acid (succimer)

○ **What is the treatment for children with symptoms with blood lead levels higher than 45 μg/dL or patients with blood lead levels higher than 70 μg/dL?**

British anti-Lewisite intramuscularly followed by calcium disodium versenate IV and hydration. Children with lead encephalopathy are also treated with fluid restriction, furosemide, and hyperventilation in an intensive care unit. The use of mannitol and dexamethasone are controversial.

○ **A child presents in diabetic ketoacidosis. On average, how dehydrated is this patient likely to be?**

125 mL/kg average fluid volume deficit

○ **You are treating a child in diabetic ketoacidosis. After an initial 20 mL/kg bolus of 0.9% normal saline and careful fluid replacement with 0.45% normal saline for maintenance and replacement, you are considering switching to dextrose 5% in 0.45% normal saline. At approximately what glucose level should this change in fluid selection occur?**

250 mg/dL

○ **What dose of insulin should be used for low-dose, continuous infusion therapy in a child?**

0.1 U/kg per hour of regular insulin

○ **A child with insulin-dependent diabetes mellitus presents unconscious. What is the correct amount of dextrose 50% in water (in milliliters per kilogram) to administer in this patient?**

0.5 mL/kg

○ **Are UTIs more common in boys or in girls?**

In the newborn period, they are twice as common in boys, but during childhood they are 10 times more common in girls.

○ **What is the most common organism causing UTIs in children?**

Fecal flora, most commonly *E coli*, which accounts for 80% of UTIs

○ **What is hypospadias?**

A defect in the penis in which the opening of the urethral meatus is on the ventral surface of the penis

○ **Why should boys with hypospadias not be circumcised?**

The treatment for hypospadias, if severe, is surgery. The foreskin of the penis is needed to reconstruct the urethra and should therefore not be removed.

○ **True/False: Cryptorchidism must be corrected by the age of 2 years to decrease the potential for testicular malignancy.**

False. The risk of malignancy exists regardless of correction. The risk of infertility is removed if the testes descend before the age of 2 years.

○ **What is the treatment for cryptorchidism?**

Medical treatment is with human chorionic gonadotropin. If unsuccessful, orchiopexy should be performed.

○ **A 15-year-old boy comes into your office complaining of 12 hours of a swollen, painful, red, testis, with associated nausea and vomiting. At examination, his affected testis is lying horizontally. The cremasteric reflex is absent, and elevating the testis causes more pain. What should you do?**

Call for a urologic consultation for presumed testicular torsion. While you are waiting, you may perform urinalysis to rule out infectious causes, try releasing the testis by turning it outward toward the thigh (much like opening a book), or sending the patient for Doppler ultrasonography. None of this should delay urologic consultation because this is a urologic emergency.

○ **What is Prehn sign?**

Elevation of the testis leads to improvement in testicular pain, which indicates epididymitis, though it is not diagnostic

○ **What are the 2 age peaks for incidence of testicular torsion?**

Perinatally and during puberty

○   **What is the eponym for congenital aganglionic megacolon?**

Hirschsprung disease. In this disease, a portion of the distal colon lacks ganglion cells, thus impairing the normal inhibitory innervation in the myenteric plexus. This impedes coordinated relaxation, which can, in turn, cause clinical symptoms of obstruction 85% of the time after the newborn period.

○   **Is Hirschsprung disease more common in boys or girls?**

Boys, by a ratio of 4:1

○   **What are the signs and symptoms of toxic megacolon in the first year?**

Decreased number of bowel movements, obstipation, sporadic abdominal distension, decreased appetite, FTT, vomiting, and bouts of nonbloody diarrhea

○   **How is toxic megacolon diagnosed?**

Abdominal radiographs showing a dilated colon, barium enema study showing dilated colon proximal to the lesion (with a cone-shaped transition zone between the 2), anorectal manometry, and biopsy of rectal tissue

○   **Acute enterocolitis with development of toxic megacolon is the life-threatening complication of Hirschsprung disease. Between what ages does this complication most frequently manifest?**

2 to 3 months. Treatment involves gastric decompression (rectal tube), nothing by mouth, IV fluids, and antibiotics.

○   **A 1-month-old infant frequently vomits directly after and as long as several hours after eating. The vomitus is never bloody or bilious, and the emesis is not forceful or projectile. It appears effortless, with small amounts of curdled milk drooling out of her mouth. The infant is in no apparent pain. What is a probable diagnosis?**

Gastroesophageal reflux disease (GERD)

○   **What percentage of infants have GERD?**

50%

○   **Do infants with GERD have high, low, or normal lower esophageal sphincter pressures?**

Unlike adults with GERD, who have lower esophageal sphincter pressures, infants generally have normal lower esophageal sphincter pressures. Their reflux may be caused by transient relaxation of the lower esophageal sphincter at inappropriate times or failure to increase lower esophageal sphincter pressure at times of increased gastric pressure. Other factors that cause GERD in infants are delayed gastric emptying, increased intragastric pressure, and impaired esophageal motility.

○   **What non-GI symptoms are seen with rotavirus?**

Patients may have fever and upper respiratory symptoms in addition to vomiting and diarrhea.

○   **What age group does rotavirus most commonly affect?**

6 months to 2 years. Rotavirus is most common in the fall and winter.

○   **What is a lasting sequela in 50% of infants affected with rotavirus?**

Lactose intolerance. It may last for several weeks after a rotavirus infection.

○ **What signs and symptoms tend to indicate a bacterial pathogen as the cause of diarrhea?**

Fever, acute onset of multiple bouts of diarrhea per day, and blood in the stool

○ **Which children with gastroenteritis should receive antibiotic treatment?**

Antibiotic therapy for gastroenteritis is generally reserved for children with high or prolonged fevers, those with inflammatory cells present in the stool, those with protracted diarrhea, and infants younger than 6 months

○ **What is the most common cause of intestinal obstruction in infants younger than 1 year?**

Intussusception. The classic patient presentation is vomiting, irritability, currant jelly stool, and a sausage-shaped mass in the right upper quadrant.

○ **Is intestinal intussusception associated with GI bleeding?**

Yes. However, the classic history of sudden onset of severe pain that often is relieved as quickly as it arose and is recurrent is more sensitive. The currant jelly stool associated with this disorder is present in only about half of the cases.

○ **What is the classic triad of symptoms associated with intussusception?**

1. Intermittent abdominal pain
2. Vomiting
3. Bloody stools

○ **A sausage-shaped mass is found in what percentage of patients with intussusception?**

60% to 95%

○ **About how old is the average patient who presents with intussusception?**

Sixty percent of cases occur in the first year, most commonly between the fifth and ninth months.

○ **How is intussusception treated?**

Either with air insufflation or barium enema. If these are unsuccessful, then surgical reduction is required.

○ **Is constipation more common in breastfed or formula-fed infants?**

Formula-fed infants. It is rare in breastfed infants.

○ **A new mother brings her 3-week-old infant to your office because he does not seem to be growing. He has constipation and intermittent vomiting with great force. What might you find at abdominal examination?**

This patient probably has pyloric stenosis. Expect a small, firm, mobile, olive-shaped mass in the right upper quadrant or epigastric area. If the stenotic pylorus cannot be palpated, then ultrasonography or radiography will reveal the defect. Treatment is pyloromyotomy.

○ **Pyloric stenosis is most common in what population?**

Male white Americans. The male:female ratio is 5:1, and the defect is 2.5 times as likely in white infants than African American infants.

○ **What is the average age for the onset of pyloric stenosis?**

4 weeks. The onset of pyloric stenosis is generally between the second and the fourth week of life. It is rarely diagnosed after the age of 5 months.

○ **Differentiate between omphalocele and gastroschisis.**
- Omphalocele is a herniation of the intestines into the umbilical cord.
- Gastroschisis is a herniation of the intestines through the abdominal wall because of a defective closure of the abdominal wall.

○ **What is summertime gastroenteritis in the pediatric population likely caused by?**

Enterovirus. Overall, the rotavirus is the most common cause of pediatric gastroenteritis; it is responsible for more than 50% of cases of acute diarrhea in this population. Rotavirus gastroenteritis generally is preceded by upper respiratory infection and is a self-limited disease that lasts 4 to 10 days. Other causes of gastroenteritis in children are parvoviruses, coxsackieviruses, echoviruses, adenoviruses, and caliciviruses, including *Norovirus*.

○ **What is the most common bacterial cause of gastroenteritis in the pediatric patient?**

Campylobacter jejuni. This, too, is a self-limited disease, lasting less than 1 week. These patients appear more sick than do those with viral syndromes. Fever, abdominal pain, copious diarrhea, vomiting, and malaise are common complaints. *C jejuni* is also the most common bacterial cause of gastroenteritis in the adult population.

○ **A family and their dog went on a summer vacation in the Grand Canyon. The trip was cut short because the whole family, including the dog, suddenly developed watery diarrhea and excessive gas in the abdomen. They have no fevers. What is the most likely parasitic cause?**

Giardia lamblia. This organism is commonly contracted from contaminated water or animal contact but can also be spread through person-to-person contact. It is diagnosed by means of microscopic examination of the stool. Treatment of the humans is rehydration and metronidazole; the dog's veterinarian should be consulted for canine treatment.

○ **What is the most common bacterial cause of pediatric mesenteric lymphadenitis?**

Yersinia enterocolitica

○ **A 2-week-old infant is brought to your office. The infant has acral distribution of an oval, maculopapular rash; thick, bloody nasal discharge; and hepatosplenomegaly. What is the most likely diagnosis?**

Congenital syphilis

○ **What is the association between prematurity and hyaline membrane disease?**

There is a positive correlation. With birth at 29 weeks of gestation, 60% of newborns have hyaline membrane disease. By 39 weeks of gestation, the incidence has decreased to near 0%. Treatment includes prevention of premature birth, glucocorticoid hormones for mothers who must deliver prematurely, and surfactant replacement.

○ **What is the most common cause of orbital cellulitis?**

Infection extended from the paranasal sinuses. The causative organisms are usually *H influenzae*, *S aureus*, group A β-hemolytic *Streptococcus*, and *S pneumoniae*. This is a serious condition because of the potential for infection to spread and cause meningitis, brain abscess, or cavernous sinus thrombosis.

○ **What is the most common cause of conjunctivitis in the pediatric population?**

Adenovirus

○ **What is the most common cause of seasonal allergic pediatric rhinitis?**

Ragweed pollen. It is otherwise known as "hay fever." The most common perennial allergens are house dust and house-dust mites, followed by feathers, dander, and mold spores. Removal of the allergen, if possible, is the best treatment. Treat the patient with intranasal cromolyn sodium or corticosteroids.

○ **What is allergic shiner?**

Bluish purple rings under the eyes associated with allergies. They result from decreased or obstructed periorbital venous drainage.

○ **How can you clinically distinguish orbital cellulitis from periorbital cellulitis?**

Only orbital cellulitis will manifest with proptosis and limited extraocular movements, but both will have fever, eyelid swelling, erythema, and leukocytosis.

○ **Which type of brain tumor occurs most frequently in pediatric patients?**

Medulloblastoma

○ **A 7-year-old girl presents with joint pain everywhere, fever, and hard bumps on her elbows and forearm. Three weeks ago she had strep throat. What is the diagnosis?**

Rheumatic fever. Rheumatic fever is most common in children aged 5 to 15 years. It is always preceded by infection with group A *Streptococcus*. The Jones criteria are used to make the diagnosis. Patients must meet either 2 major criteria or 1 major and 2 minor criteria.

Major criteria

- Polyarthritis
- Carditis
- Erythema marginatum
- Subcutaneous nodules
- Chorea

Minor criteria

- Fever
- Arthralgia
- Prior rheumatic heart disease
- Elevated sedimentation rate
- Elevated C-reactive protein level
- Prolonged P-R interval

○ **What does a high-pitched holosystolic, blowing, apical murmur that radiates to the axilla suggest?**

Mitral valve regurgitation. This is the valve most commonly affected by rheumatic heart disease.

○ **What is the treatment for rheumatic fever?**

Bed rest, NSAIDs, penicillin, and hospitalization. Patients must have long-term follow-up of the ensuing valvular disease, as well as checkups for recurrence.

○ **What heart defect is associated with trisomy 18 syndrome?**

Ventricular septal defect

○ **What heart defect is associated with rubella syndrome?**

Patent ductus arteriosus

○ **What percentage of children has heart murmurs?**

50%. Only 10% of children with heart murmurs have pathologic heart murmurs.

○ **What is the most common innocent heart murmur?**

Still murmur, a vibratory murmur heard only in systole. Other innocent heart murmurs are venous hum, pulmonary flow murmur, and neonatal pulmonary artery branch murmur.

○ **What are the common characteristics of an innocent heart murmur?**

The patient is otherwise physically healthy, with no signs of cyanosis, shortness of breath, or lethargy. The murmur is low frequency; does not radiate; has no associated thrill; is located in the mid-to-lower sternal border (as opposed to higher up); is systolic; and is accentuated by sitting up, exercise, fever, anxiety, or crying.

○ **A normal-looking term neonate presents with tachypnea, cyanosis, and CHF. What is the likely disease?**

Congenital cardiac disease, such as severe coarctation of the aorta and hypoplastic left heart syndrome

○ **What is the most common congenital heart disorder?**

Ventricular septal defects. These defects account for approximately 38% of all congenital heart disorders. Other disorders include atrial septal defects (18%), pulmonary valve stenosis (13%), pulmonary artery stenosis (7%), aortic valve stenosis (4%), patent ductus arteriosus (4%), and mitral valve prolapse (4%).

○ **What is the most common congenital heart disease associated with Down syndrome?**

Septal defects, most commonly endocardial cushion defects. These are inflow ventricular septal defects that have associated abnormalities of the tricuspid and mitral valves.

○ **Name several clinical presentations of pediatric heart disease.**
  • Cyanosis
  • Squatting
  • CHF
  • Pathologic murmur
  • Cardiogenic shock
  • Hypertension
  • Tachyarrhythmias
  • Abnormal pulses
  • Syncope

○ **True/False: During childhood, symptoms of aortic stenosis are common.**

False. Even if severe, the left ventricle has the ability to hypertrophy in childhood, compensating for many years.

○ **What radiographic findings are often seen in coarctation of the aorta?**

The 3 sign, made up of the aortic knob and the dilated postcoarctation segment of the descending aorta. The E sign is the same thing seen in a negative image on a barium esophagram.

○ **Name 4 congenital heart lesions with a right-sided aortic arch.**

1. Truncus arteriosus
2. Transposition of the great vessels
3. Tetralogy of Fallot
4. Tricuspid atresia

○ **Supraventricular tachycardia (SVT) in adults usually occurs with a ventricular rate of about 150 to 200 bpm. What is the range of ventricular rates in children?**

220 to 360 bpm

○ **What is the treatment for a pediatric patient with SVT?**

Adenosine at 0.1 mg/kg

○ **Verapamil should not be used to treat infants younger than what age?**

2 years. It can lead to asystole.

○ **If cardioversion is necessary to treat an infant with unstable SVT, what is the appropriate amount of joules to use?**

0.25 to 1 J/kg

○ **What congenital heart defect classically is associated with precordial thrill and high-pitched, harsh pansystolic murmur best heard on the left sternal border?**

Ventricular septal defect. Prognosis for ventricular septal defect is good: 50% will close spontaneously within the first year of life.

○ **A newborn with a systolic ejection murmur and widely split S2 probably has which congenital heart malformation?**

Atrial septal defect, which is caused by a patent foramen ovale that allows blood to be shunted back from the left atrium to the right. This results in increased blood flow through the pulmonary artery and delay in the closure of the pulmonic valve, which causes the split S2.

○ **Coarctation of the aorta is associated with narrowing of the aortic arch. Where is the narrowing located?**

Just distal to the origin of the left subclavian artery. The narrowing causes hypertensive upper extremities and normotensive lower extremities.

○ **Match the congenital heart defect with the direction of the shunt (ie, right-to-left or left-to-right).**

  1. Ventricular septal defect

  2. Patent ductus arteriosus

  3. Transposition of the great vessels

  4. Tetralogy of Fallot

  5. Atrial septal defect

  6. Pulmonary stenosis

  Answers: (1) L to R, (2) R to L, (3) L to R, (4) R to L, (5) L to R, and (6) R to L

○ **A premature newborn with bounding pulse, precordial thrill, and continuous machinelike murmur heard best just under the left clavicle most likely has what congenital heart defect?**

  Patent ductus arteriosus. This heart defect should be treated with an injection of indomethacin, which produces closure within a few days. If patency persists, surgery is necessary.

○ **What is atrioventricular canal defect?**

  A result of an endocardial cushion defect in which a 2-chambered heart is produced. The 2 atria are connected by an atrial septal defect, and the 2 ventricles are connected by a ventricular septal defect.

○ **By what age does a child reach half of her or his adult height?**

  2 years. However, by this time the child will have attained only 20% of his or her adult weight.

○ **How is short stature due to heredity and short stature due to constitutional delay in growth differentiated?**

  Bone age determination. In children with familial short stature, bone age is normal. In children with constitutional growth delay, bone age is delayed, as is sexual maturation.

○ **When is menarche in relation to the female growth spurt?**

  Girls have menarche just after their peak growth spurt. This is just the opposite of boys, who are well on their way through puberty before they hit their peak growth spurt.

○ **What are the first signs of puberty in boys?**

  Growth of the testes, followed by thinning and pigmentation of the scrotum, growth of the penis, and development of pubic hair.

○ **A 15-year-old boy has developed small breasts. His parents want this situation corrected surgically. What do you recommend?**

  Surgery is a consideration if the physical abnormality is causing severe psychological pain or if the breasts have persisted for a long time. Surgery is not recommended because gynecomastia in adolescents generally lasts only 1 to 2 years. Gynecomastia occurs in 36% to 64% of pubertal boys.

○ **What drugs can cause gynecomastia?**

  Marijuana, hormones, digitalis, spironolactone, cimetidine, ketoconazole, antihypertensives, antidepressants, and amphetamines

○ **A 5-month-old infant appears lethargic yet flinches at every little noise. At physical examination, you note a cherry red spot on the macula. What are the diagnosis and prognosis?**

Tay-Sachs disease. This is an autosomal recessive disorder affecting the gray matter. Myoclonic and akinetic seizures begin 1 to 3 months after the initial symptoms of decreased alertness and hyperacusis (excessive reaction to noise). Patients usually do not survive past age 4 years.

○ **You are examining a 5-year-old, and you notice 8 café au lait spots ranging from 6 to 9 mm in diameter, freckles in the axillary region, and a Lisch nodule (pigmented hamartoma of the iris). What disease are you worried about?**

Neurofibromatosis (von Recklinghausen disease). Neurofibromatosis should be investigated in any child with more than 5 café au lait spots larger than 5 mm. For adolescents, the spots must be larger than 15 mm. Neurofibromatosis is an autosomal dominant disease that affects the nervous system, integument, bone, muscle, and several other organs.

○ **List 3 other diseases that affect both the skin and the CNS.**

1. Bourneville disease (tuberous sclerosis): Ash-leaf skin lesions, seizures, and mental retardation
2. Sturge-Weber syndrome: Port wine stain in trigeminal distribution, glaucoma, and possible seizures
3. Ataxia-telangiectasia (Louis-Bar syndrome): Progressive ataxia, telangiectasis most noticeably on the conjunctiva and ears, lung infections, and malignant lymphomas

○ **A mother brings her 5-month-old infant to your office because the infant is weak and lethargic; has a fixed gaze; and will not eat, even his favorite treat, honey on the pacifier. The infant has no fever. What is the diagnosis?**

Infant botulism. "Honey" is the key word. Botulism spores can lay dormant in honey and are not killed by pasteurization. Once ingested, these spores germinate and produce a toxin that causes the illness. Adult botulism is generally from ingestion of the toxin, not the spores, in foods. Treatment is supportive. Infants younger than 1 year should not be fed honey.

○ **A pediatric patient who sustained head trauma 1 week ago now has a seizure. What is the risk that this patient will have another seizure in the future?**

75%. Patients with posttraumatic epilepsy have a high rate of recurrent seizures and should therefore receive long-term anticonvulsant treatment.

○ **A 4-year-old boy has red cheeks, low-grade fever, and maculopapular rash in a lacy reticular pattern that began on his arms and spread to his trunk and legs. The rash has come and gone for the past 2 weeks. What is the diagnosis?**

Erythema infectiosum, also known as "Fifth disease" or "slapped cheek syndrome." The patient may also have constitutional symptoms, such as pharyngitis, headache, myalgia, coryza, or GI problems.

○ **What is the treatment for Fifth disease?**

None. It is self-limited. Pregnant women in contact with infected children should be tested because Fifth disease during pregnancy is associated with fetal death and red cell aplasia with fetal hydrops.

○ **A patient is brought in by her father and has had a high fever for 4 days that was then followed by maculopapular rash that began on her trunk and spread to her arms and legs. She has no other complaints. What are the diagnosis and prognosis?**

This patient has roseola infantum (exanthem subitum). This is a self-limited disease caused by human herpesvirus 6 with no treatment and few complications.

○ **An 11-year-old is brought in by his mother who says he has a fever, sore throat, and rash that feels like sandpaper. What is a likely diagnosis?**

Scarlet fever (scarlatina). This illness usually results from a pharyngeal infection with group A streptococcal strains that produce erythrogenic toxin. The rash is erythematous and finely punctuated, and it begins on the trunk and spreads to the extremities. The skin feels like sandpaper. Patients also have Pastia lines and strawberry tongue. The rash lasts about a week, and then the skin desquamates for several more weeks.

○ **What is the treatment for the patient with scarlatina?**

Penicillin for 10 days. If the child is allergic to penicillin, a macrolide can be used.

○ **What are Pastia lines?**

Areas of increased erythema in the folds of the skin

○ **What other childhood rash may manifest with strawberry tongue?**

Kawasaki disease

○ **What is the most common cause of stomatitis in children aged 1 to 3 years?**

Acute herpetic gingivostomatitis caused by herpes simplex virus

○ **Six days ago, a 5-year-old girl had malaise, cough, coryza, photophobia, conjunctivitis, and mild fever. Four days ago, she had small grayish white dots the size of sand grains on her buccal mucosa. Two days ago, her fever climbed to 102°F, and she developed a morbilliform rash that began on the head and has now spread to the rest of her body. Her history indicates that she has not received her childhood immunizations. What is the diagnosis?**

Measles

○ **Where are Koplik spots most commonly found?**

Opposite the lower molars on the buccal mucosa. They can be as small as grains of sand and are commonly grayish white with a red areola and may occasionally bleed. Remember: "Kops" catch "weasels," which rhymes with "measles."

○ **Describe the rash of measles.**

A maculopapular rash that begins at the hairline and spreads to the rest of the body. Lesions are initially individual but become confluent over time. The rash starts 2 weeks after initial exposure to infection.

○ **What is the treatment for measles?**

Treatment of symptoms

○ **What are the 3 stages of measles, and what are the associated signs and symptoms?**

1. Incubation stage (10–12 days), which has no signs or symptoms
2. Prodromal (or catarrhal) stage, which is characterized by Koplik spots, low-grade fever, coryza, and cough
3. Final stage, which consists of the classic rash and high fever

○ **When is the child with measles infectious?**

During the prodromal phase until 5 days after the rash has begun

○ **What are some complications of measles?**

Photosensitivity, pharyngitis, encephalitis, subacute sclerosing panencephalitis, and disseminated intravascular coagulation

○ **What is the most characteristic sign of rubella?**

Adenopathy, most notably in the retroauricular, postoccipital, and posterior cervical chains. The adenopathy usually appears before the rash.

○ **What are some common complications of mumps?**

• Orchitis or epididymitis
• Meningoencephalomyelitis
• Mild pancreatitis
• Unilateral deafness

○ **What rash is associated with a herald patch?**

Pityriasis rosea. A herald patch is a single round or oval lesion that heralds the impending maculopapular rash called "pityriasis rosea." The second rash to appear is on the trunk. Small crops of mildly itchy, oval scaly patches create a Christmas tree pattern. Sometimes the rash is associated with pharyngitis and malaise.

○ **What is the treatment for pityriasis rosea?**

None. The secondary patches fade in several weeks. Sunlight may hasten the disappearance of the rash.

○ **An 11-year-old unimmunized boy is brought to your office by his pregnant mother. He has a 4-day history of fever, cough, and coryza. A pruritic, confluent, and flushing maculopapular rash began on his face 2 days ago and then spread to the rest of his body. At examination, you notice he has posterior auricular, along with cervical and suboccipital, lymphadenopathy. What is the diagnosis?**

Rubella (German measles)

○ **The mother in the above case is 2 months pregnant. What should you do?**

Check the mother for serologic evidence of immunity to rubella, even if she has documented receipt of rubella vaccine in the past. If she is not immune, counsel her on the associated risks of congenital defects. If she chooses to carry the fetus to term, advise her to stay away from her infected son because there is a prolonged shedding of the virus. In addition, she should receive some passive protection; 0.25 to 0.50 mL/kg immune serum globulin should be administered intramuscularly within the first week of exposure. Do not administer rubella vaccine in a pregnant woman, but if she is not immune, administer the vaccine immediately after birth or termination.

○ **When is the risk of congenital defects due to maternal rubella infection greatest?**

In the first few months of gestation. During months 1 to 3, there is a 30% to 60% risk of congenital defects. By the fourth month, the risk is only 10%. By 5 to 9 months, there is a rare chance that the child will have a defect. Congenital rubella can cause deafness, glaucoma, cataracts, retardation, and congenital heart defects.

○ **Describe the look and timing of the rubella rash.**

It is a maculopapular to confluent rash that appears and spreads quickly, sometimes over 24 hours.

○ **Aside from the rash, what are some concomitant findings with rubella?**

Rubella can manifest concomitantly with polyarthritis, splenomegaly, and low-grade fever.

○ **When is the child with rubella infectious?**

1 week before and 1 week after the rash

○ **Of the many types of diaper rash, how is candidal diaper dermatitis distinguished?**

Babies with candidal dermatitis will have satellite lesions away from the groin area. Otherwise, this rash presents as a large, red confluent vesiculopustular plaque with a clearly demarcated border. Treatment is with topical antifungals.

○ **What causes Rocky Mountain spotted fever (RMSF)?**

Rickettsia rickettsii. Characteristic spots result from rickettsial invasion of endothelial cells in small blood vessels, including arterioles. *Dermacentor andersoni*, a wood tick, is the vector.

○ **Why is RMSF of concern in pediatric patients?**

Two-thirds of RMSF patients are children younger than 15 years.

○ **Describe the rash of RMSF.**

The rash begins as erythematous blanching macules on the wrists, hands, ankles, and feet that spread to the whole body and that appear 3 to 5 days after the onset of fever, headache, and chills. As the illness progresses, the rash becomes papular and even purpuric. Conjunctivitis, photophobia, and even signs of meningoencephalitis can occur.

○ **What is the treatment for RMSF?**

Chloramphenicol, which has the risk of causing rare aplastic anemia, or doxycycline. In young children, the risk of dental staining with doxycycline use is low, and the risk of using less effective therapy is high.

○ **Kawasaki disease is most common in what age group?**

0 to 2 years. Eighty percent of patients with Kawasaki are younger than 4 years.

○ **What are the diagnostic criteria for Kawasaki disease?**

Fever for at least 5 days plus 4 of the following:

- Polymorphous exanthem on the trunk
- Bilateral conjunctivitis
- Lesions in the oral cavity
- Cervical lymphadenopathy
- Peripheral extremity rashes (erythematous initially, then desquamating during the convalescent phase)

○ **What is the most serious complication of Kawasaki disease?**

The formation of coronary artery aneurysms that can rupture or thrombose. Cardiac involvement occurs in 10% to 40% of children within the first 2 weeks of the disease. Kawasaki disease is also known as "mucocutaneous lymph node syndrome" or "infantile polyarteritis."

○ **How long does the fever of Kawasaki disease last?**

2 weeks

○ **What is the treatment for Kawasaki disease?**

High doses of aspirin for the acute phase, low doses once the child is afebrile, and IV gamma globulin

○ **A 3-month-old presents to your office with flaky grayish white plaques on the buccal mucosa, lips, gingiva, and tongue and decreased appetite. How do you treat this patient?**

Nystatin oral suspension, anesthetic gel before feeding, and cool liquids for discomfort. This patient has oral thrush (candidiasis).

○ **When is thrush most common?**

Candidal gingivostomatitis is most common during the first 3 months.

○ **What is the most common skin infection among pediatric patients in the emergency department?**

Nonbullous impetigo, a bacterial infection of the dermis, caused by group A β-hemolytic *Streptococcus* and *S aureus*

○ **Describe the rash of impetigo.**

Lesions are either vesicopustular or bullous. Vesicopustular lesions begin as small pustules with an erythematous rim. The pustules rupture and leave a honeylike exudate that then crusts over. Bullous impetigo begins as red macules that grow to become large fluid-filled lesions with erythematous bases. The bullae then rupture and leave a clear coat over the desquamated area.

○ **How does impetigo spread?**

By means of direct contact

○   **What is the recommended treatment for impetigo?**

Dicloxacillin, cephalexin, or clindamycin. Mupirocin, a topical therapy, can be used for mild cases without bullae.

○   **Erysipelas (St Anthony fire) is another pediatric exanthem caused by primary bacterial infection. What organism causes this uncommon cellulitis, usually characterized by pain at the affected site, along with malaise and fever?**

Erysipelas is also caused by group A β-hemolytic *Streptococcus*. Mild cases may be treated with oral antibiotics, but more severe cases require parenteral antibiotic therapy. Recurrences are common and can lead to irreversible lymphedema (elephantiasis nostras).

○   **A 10-year-old boy is brought to your office because his mother has noticed red, scaly blistering on the top of the child's feet and toes. What is the diagnosis?**

This is probably a case of contact dermatitis caused by new shoes. It is most frequent in preadolescent patients. Tinea pedis, or athlete's foot, is more commonly seen between the toes.

○   **What rash is associated with rheumatic fever?**

Erythema marginatum. This is a pink, nonpruritic, evanescent rash that covers the trunk and inner surfaces of the arms and legs. It spreads in wavy lines and rings with clear-cut margins. Subcutaneous nodules over bony prominences are also noted.

○   **How are head lice treated?**

Treatment is with permethrin shampoo. Malathion and lindane may also be used but not with infants. A second shampooing should be applied 1 week after the initial treatment.

○   **How are lice spread?**

By direct contact. They do not live long on inanimate objects. Outbreaks are more common in the winter.

○   **A mother brings her 5-month-old infant to your office because she noticed small raised papules between the webbing of his fingers. She says he has been scratching there at nighttime. What is the treatment?**

This child most likely has scabies. Treatment is with a single application of permethrin cream. All close contacts should also be treated because scabies is spread through direct contact.

○   **How is pinworm diagnosed?**

The female pinworm deposits her eggs in the perianal region at nighttime, hence the intense anal pruritus associated with pinworm infestation. Eggs can be detected by pressing tape to the perianal area. Sometimes the worms themselves can be seen directly.

○   **How is pinworm infestation treated?**

Oral mebendazole or albendazole

○ **A 3-week-old infant presents with greasy scales and yellow crusts in his scalp, under his arms, and in the folds of his neck and groin. These lesions have been present since birth. What is the diagnosis?**

Seborrheic dermatitis. This is an inflammatory disorder of the sebaceous glands that is common in the first month of life and is generally characterized by the diffuse scaling in the scalp known as "cradle cap." Treatment for infants is shampooing and topical hydrocortisone cream.

○ **What is the major cause of fever in infants aged 0 to 3 months?**

Virus (95%)

○ **What are the most common causes of meningitis in neonates?**

Group B streptococci and *E coli*

○ **What are the most common causes of meningitis in infants and children?**

S pneumoniae, Neisseria meningitidis, and Hib

○ **What is the Brudzinski sign?**

A sign of meningeal irritation. Passive neck flexion causes involuntary leg flexion.

○ **What is the Kernig sign?**

Neck pain is elicited with passive knee extension in a leg that is flexed 90° at the hip. This is also a sign of meningeal irritation.

○ **What are some signs and symptoms of meningitis?**

Headache, lethargy, stiff neck, irritability, confusion, vomiting, bulging fontanelle, poor feeding, and petechiae

○ **Describe the CSF features of bacterial versus viral meningitis.**

CSF Feature	Bacterial	Viral
Opening pressure	Increased	Increased
WBCs	100 to 10,000/μL	10 to 500/μL
Protein level	Increased	Mildly increased
Glucose level	Decreased	Normal
Gram stain or culture result	Positive for bacteria	No bacteria

○ **What are the contraindications for lumbar puncture?**

Increased intracranial pressure, shock, cellulitis or abscess over lumbar vertebrae, respiratory failure, or bleeding diathesis

○   **What is spina bifida cystica?**

Herniation of the meninges and/or spinal cord through a defect in the lumbar vertebrae

○   **What are some causes of obstructive hydrocephalus?**

Congenital aqueductal stenosis, myelomeningoceles, Dandy-Walker malformation, Arnold-Chiari malformation, intraventricular hemorrhage, and meningitis

○   **What is the most common congenital anomaly of the nervous system?**

Myelomeningocele. This occurs when the neural tube fails to close. It is frequently associated with hydrocephalus or Arnold-Chiari malformation.

○   **How might you recognize an infant with fetal alcohol syndrome?**

Small eyes and midface, long smooth philtrum, mild ptosis, flat nasal bridge, short nose, thin upper lip, epicanthal folds, joint contractures, and kidney malformations

○   **If a pregnant woman drinks 4 to 6 alcoholic drinks per day through pregnancy, what is the likelihood that her infant will have fetal alcohol syndrome?**

30% to 45%

○   **What is the typical body habitus of a child with homocystinuria?**

Long thin limbs and fingers, scoliosis, osteoporosis, and sternal deformities

○   **What other features are common to homocystinuria?**

Mild mental retardation, strokes, myocardial infarctions, and dislocated lenses

○   **What is PKU?**

Phenylketonuria is an enzyme deficiency that prevents the conversion of phenylalanine to tyrosine, which results in the toxic buildup of phenylacetic acid and phenyllactic acid. Patients with PKU have mental retardation, hypopigmentation, hypertonicity, tremors, and behavior disorders.

○   **Is it possible to prevent retardation in PKU?**

Yes. Newborn screening can be used to detect PKU early enough to be able to start a diet with no phenylalanine.

○   **What is the most common chromosomal anomaly in Down syndrome?**

Ninety-five percent of Down syndrome patients have trisomy 21. The remaining 5% have either translocation or mosaicism.

○   **What are the characteristic features of a child with Down syndrome?**

Epicanthal folds; flat nasal bridge; small nose, mouth, chin and palpebral fissures; hypotonia, endocardial cushion and septal defects; GI abnormalities; and low mental capacity.

○ **What birth defects are associated with trisomy 13?**

Microcephaly with open lesions of the scalp, holoprosencephaly, microphthalmos, coloboma, omphalocele, ambiguous genitalia, severe retardation, congenital heart disease, and cleft lip and/or palate. Ninety percent of infants with trisomy 13 die before age 1 year.

○ **What birth defects are associated with trisomy 18?**

Neural tube defects, congenital heart disease, dislocated hips, rocker-bottom feet, overlapping fingers, intrauterine growth retardation, microcephaly, prominent occiput, micrognathia, severe mental retardation, and various CNS malformations. As with infants with trisomy 13, 90% of infants with trisomy 18 die before age 1 year.

○ **When do the symptoms of Duchenne muscular dystrophy begin?**

Between the ages of 2 and 4 years. Children experience proximal muscle weakness and have delayed walking.

○ **What do most children with Duchenne muscular dystrophy usually die of?**

CHF or pneumonia. Children with this disease do not generally live more than 25 years.

○ **What is the Gower sign?**

A maneuver used to reach a standing position from a prone position in patients with Duchenne muscular dystrophy. First, the child pushes off the floor creating an arch (hands and feet on the floor, buttocks in the air), the patient then puts his or her hands on his or her knees 1 by 1 and walks the hands up the thighs until able to stand. This maneuver indicates weak back and pelvic girdle muscles.

○ **Febrile seizures occur when the patient's temperature does what?**

Increases rapidly. Febrile seizures are more closely related to rapid increase in temperature than to the highest temperature reached. These seizures occur in children aged 6 months to 6 years and are within the context of febrile illness, are less than 15 minutes in duration, and are tonic-clonic generalized and simple. By definition, febrile seizures must be associated with no focal neurologic defects and be present in a patient with no prior neurologic disorders.

○ **What is the risk for recurrent febrile seizures after an episode of febrile seizure?**

30% to 35%. Control of fevers with acetaminophen and tepid baths is the recommended treatment.

○ **What is the risk of developing epilepsy after febrile seizure?**

1%

○ **Phenobarbital is probably the most effective drug used to treat febrile seizures. Should all patients with a febrile seizure receive phenobarbital as prophylaxis against future similar seizures?**

Although its use may be warranted in patients who are particularly ill, who have had repeated febrile seizures, or who have underlying neurologic disease, phenobarbital is not recommended as prophylactic treatment.

○ **Neonatal seizures have a broad range of manifestations. What are the 2 most frequent causes of neonatal myoclonic seizures?**

1. Metabolic disorders

2. Hypoxia

○ **Infantile spasms usually occur in children younger than 6 months. Is it true that these patients have a high rate of developmental disorders?**

Yes. Eighty-five percent of these patients have developmental disorders.

○ **Are infantile spasms a form of seizures?**

Yes. Infantile spasms are attacks in which an infant lying on his or her back suddenly bends the arms, straightens the legs, and arches the neck and back. Such spasms last a few seconds. These spasms may develop into other forms of seizures in adulthood.

○ **Infantile spasms represent a significant disorder and require aggressive evaluation. In addition to anticonvulsants, what hormone plays a role in their management?**

Corticotropin

○ **How long must a continuous seizure last to be defined as status epilepticus?**

At least 20 minutes

○ **What is a neuroblastoma?**

A malignant tumor arising from the sympathetic neuroblasts in the sympathetic chain and adrenal medulla. Two-thirds of the tumors occur in the abdomen and pelvis. The other third occurs in the posterior mediastinum and neck. Symptoms generally are related to impingement on local structures (eg, bowel obstruction, hypertension, radiculopathy).

○ **When do neuroblastomas most commonly occur?**

Before age 4 years

○ **Which 3 organisms most commonly cause bacteremia in both immunized and unimmunized children?**

1. *S pneumoniae*
2. *N meningitidis*
3. Hib

○ **Which 2 organisms most commonly cause sepsis in the neonate?**

1. *Group B Streptococcus*
2. *E coli*

○ **Which 3 organisms most commonly cause sepsis after the newborn period?**

1. Hib
2. *N meningitidis*
3. *S pneumoniae*

○ **Differentiate sepsis from bacteremia.**

● Bacteremia is the symptom of fever with positive blood culture results.
● Sepsis is bacteremia with focal findings.

○ **What condition is most commonly associated with occult bacteremia in children?**

Otitis media. Other associated conditions are bacterial pneumonia; streptococcal pharyngitis; and, most importantly, meningitis.

○ **What is the appropriate fluid bolus for a pediatric patient in shock?**

20 mL/kg

○ **At what rate should the urine output of a pediatric patient be maintained?**

1 to 2 mL/kg per hour

○ **What drug can be administered in pediatric patients with meningitis to decrease sequelae, especially deafness?**

Dexamethasone

○ **Which is a more common cause of dysuria among female pediatric patients: UTI or vulvovaginitis?**

Vulvovaginitis

○ **What cytomegalovirus infection route of transmission is most serious for a newborn?**

Transfusion. Transfusing blood containing cytomegalovirus can be deadly for newborns who are not protected by maternal antibodies. Other transmission routes are via the birth canal, breast milk, and the home environment. These infections appear benign and generally result in only minor respiratory infections.

○ **What is the usual presentation of a child with ventricular septal defect?**

Most of these children are totally without symptoms, and the defect usually is not diagnosed until they are school age.

○ **Is wheezing an integral part of asthma?**

No. Thirty-three percent of children with asthma will have only cough variant asthma with no wheezing.

○ **What are the most common extrinsic allergens that affect children with asthma?**

Dust and dust mites

○ **Which condition must be ruled out when childhood nasal polyps are found?**

Cystic fibrosis

○ **What is the incidence of meconium ileus in newborn infants with cystic fibrosis?**

Meconium ileus is most commonly seen in infants with cystic fibrosis, but fewer than 10% of infants with cystic fibrosis have meconium ileus.

○ **What are the McConnochie criteria for diagnosing bronchiolitis?**
- Acute expiratory wheezing
- Age 6 months or younger
- Signs of viral illness, such as fever or coryza
- With or without pneumonia or atopy
- The first such episode

○ **Foreign body aspiration occurs most commonly in which age group?**

1- to 3-year-old children

○ **What is the most common cause of cardiac arrest in children?**

Hypoxia

○ **What are the most common arrhythmias in pediatric patients?**

Sinus bradycardia and asystole

○ **Is Graves disease more common in boys or girls?**

Girls are affected 5 times more than boys are.

○ **What are the classic signs and symptoms of Graves disease?**

Emotional lability, autonomic hyperactivity, exophthalmos, tremor, increased appetite with no weight gain or weight loss, diarrhea, and goiter in nearly all affected individuals

○ **What is the definition of precocious puberty?**

The onset of secondary sexual characteristics before age 8 years in girls and 9 years in boys

○ **How much water should a newborn baby receive in addition to infant formula or breastfeeding?**

In normal situations, newborns need no additional free water. In fact, excess free water is the major cause for water intoxication in infancy and the development of subsequent hyponatremic seizures.

○ **What are common causes of delayed puberty?**

Constitutional growth delay, inadequate nutrition or being underweight, and chronic illness

○ **What percentage of teenage girls has an eating disorder?**

20%

○ **What is the most common breast tumor in adolescence?**

Fibroadenoma (>90%)

○ **What endocrine abnormalities can lead to galactorrhea in a teenage girl?**

Hypothyroidism and an increased prolactin level (ie, from pituitary adenoma)

○ **How common are varicoceles?**

Dilation of the veins of the spermatic cords occurs in about 15% of adolescent boys (usually on the left side).

○ **What is the most common solid tumor in adolescent boys?**

Testicular seminoma

○ **What should you suspect in a child who presents with tender and swollen pectoral nodes?**

Cat-scratch disease

○ **What is thought to be the mode of inoculation in cat-scratch disease?**

Rubbing the eye after contact with a cat

○ **What 4 classes of contact with a patient with meningococcal disease require prophylaxis?**

1. People who live in the same household
2. Attendees of the same child-care facility or school in the previous 7 days
3. Those who have been directly exposed to the index case's secretions, such as by kissing or sharing of food
4. Health care providers whose mucous membranes were unprotected during resuscitation or intubation of the patient

○ **What is the most effective treatment of allergic rhinitis?**

Topical use of a corticosteroid, such as beclomethasone nasal spray

○ **What is the most common congenital anomaly of the penis?**

Hypospadias

○ **What is the treatment for testicular torsion?**

Prompt surgical exploration. If the testis is explored within 6 hours of torsion, 90% of gonads will survive after detorsion and fixation.

○ **What are the complications of circumcision?**

Hemorrhage, infection, dehiscence, denudation of the shaft, glandular injury, and urinary retention

○ **A 6-year-old boy is treated for intussusception. What tumor is associated with this?**

After age 5 years, it would be unusual to have intussusception without a lead point. The most likely malignancy would be non-Hodgkin lymphoma.

○ **How does cryptorchidism affect the risk of testicular malignancy?**

The risk is 30 to 50 times greater than in a normal testicle. About one-eighth of testicular tumors develop in cryptorchid testes.

○ **What is the most common cause of bowel obstruction in children?**

Hernia

○ **What is Osler-Weber-Rendu syndrome?**

Hereditary hemorrhagic telangiectasias in the small intestine

○ **What is osteochondrosis?**

It refers to pathologic changes in a secondary growth center (either epiphysis or apophysis) involving infarction, revascularization, reabsorption, and replacement of affected bone. It may also be seen after traction on bone.

○ **What findings comprise shaken baby syndrome?**

Retinal hemorrhage, subdural hematoma, and rib fractures

○ **What are some causes (according to age) of painful limping?**

- 1 to 3 years: Infection, occult trauma, or neoplasm
- 4 to 10 years: Infection, transient synovitis of the hip, Legg-Calvé-Perthes disease, rheumatologic disorder, trauma, or neoplasm
- 11 years or older: Slipped capital femoral epiphysis, rheumatologic disorder, or trauma

○ **What is the Ortolani maneuver?**

Gentle abduction with the hip in flexion while lifting up on the greater trochanter, which results in reduction of a dislocated hip with a palpable clunk as the femoral head slips over the posterior rim of the acetabulum. Asymmetry of the legs and/or irregular thigh and gluteal folds also indicate developmental dysplasia of the hip.

○ **What is the treatment for scoliosis?**

Treatment is based on cause of the scoliosis, degree of deformity, degree of skeletal maturity, and curve progression. Observation is indicated for mild, idiopathic curve (less than 20°) with clinical examination and radiography every 6 months. Bracing is indicated for those in whom the curve is considered acceptable at diagnosis but whose curve is likely to progress. Surgical correction is usually indicated for curves greater than 30° to 40° or those with significant cosmetic deformity.

○ **What are the adverse effects of methylphenidate?**

Methylphenidate is a psychostimulant used to treat attention-deficit/hyperactivity disorder. Adverse effects include depression, headache, hypertension, insomnia, poor weight gain, and abdominal pain.

○ **You see a child with recurrent episodes of otitis media and cough. What environmental exposure history should you elicit?**

Exposure to cigarette smoke in the household

○ **What organism is the most common cause of septic joints in children?**

S aureus

○ **What organism is the most common cause of septic joints in adolescents?**

Neisseria gonorrhoeae

○ **What is the Samter triad?**

1. Asthma

2. Nasal polyps

3. Aspirin allergy

○ **What is the best single predictor of the presence of pneumonia in children?**

Tachypnea

○ **What is the normal IV maintenance amount for a 25-kg child?**

1600 mL/d or 65 mL/h. The formula is as follows: 4 mL/kg per hour or 100 mL/kg per day for the first 10 kg; 2 mL/kg per hour or 50 mL/kg per day for the second 10 kg; and 1 mL/kg per hour or 20 mL/kg per day for all further weight

○ **What are the daily sodium requirements of premature and full-term newborns?**

Premature: 3 to 4 mEq/kg per day

Full term: 1 to 2 mEq/kg per day

○ **What is the definition of apnea in an infant?**

Apnea is cessation of breathing either for more than 20 seconds or for a shorter period associated with cyanosis or bradycardia.

○ **What is ALTE?**

Apparent life-threatening event. It is apnea associated with color change (cyanosis or redness), loss of muscle tone, and choking or gagging.

○ **Compared with an otherwise healthy infant, how much more likely is a child with a history of ALTE to have SIDS?**

About 3 to 5 times more likely

○ **What is the correct workup in an infant aged 16 days with a temperature of 38°C who appears well?**

Do not let looks deceive you at this age. A full septic workup, antibiotics, and admission are indicated.

○ **In what percentage of patients with ITP is there an antecedent viral illness?**

Roughly 70%. The interval between infection and onset of purpura is usually about 2 weeks.

○ **What is the test of choice for serologic diagnosis of ITP?**

No specific test exists. Platelet count is usually low ($<20,000 \times 10^3/\mu L$), with megathrombocytes. The WBC and red blood cell counts are usually normal.

○ **Describe a patient with intussusception.**

Patients are most likely young; 70% of patients have intussusception within the first year of life. In children, the cause is thought to be secondary to lymphoid tissue at the ileocecal valve; in adults, it is thought to be caused by local lesions, Meckel diverticulum, or tumor. At examination, bowel sounds are usually normal. Intussusception typically involves the terminal ileum. Meckel diverticulum is the single most common intrinsic bowel lesion involved.

○ **A child is born to a hepatitis B surface antigen–negative mother. Which vaccine should the child receive?**

Hepatitis B vaccine (recombinant) (2.5 μg) or hepatitis B vaccine (10 μg). The second dose should be administered at least 1 month after the first, and the third dose at least 2 months later, but not before age 6 months.

○ **An unvaccinated 13-year-old boy comes to your office. Should he receive hepatitis B vaccine if there are no known carriers in his family?**

Yes

○ **When is the measles, mumps, and rubella vaccine administered?**

The first is administered at age 12 to 15 months and the second at 4 to 6 years.

○ **How common is vaccine-associated paralytic polio?**

1 in 2.4 million cases

○ **Which polio vaccine can induce secondary transmission of vaccine virus?**

Oral polio vaccine. This vaccine is no longer recommended in the United States.

○ **What is a complication of central sleep apnea in children?**

SIDS

○ **Where in the airway are foreign bodies usually lodged in children older than 1 year?**

In the lower airway

○ **At what age do most children most commonly present with intestinal malrotation? Also, what are common complications, signs, and symptoms?**

Malrotation usually occurs in children younger than 12 months. Volvulus is a common complication. Signs and symptoms include vomiting, blood-streaked stools, and abdominal pain.

○ **Describe the rash associated with exanthem subitum (roseola).**

The rash is usually found on the trunk and the neck and is maculopapular.

○ **What is the most common cause of death among children aged 1 to 12 months?**

SIDS

○   **Which is the most common type of hernia in children?**

Indirect

○   **What conditions produce cardiac syncope in pediatric patients?**

Aortic stenosis and tetralogy of Fallot

○   **What are 2 unique clinical findings of tetralogy of Fallot?**

1. Boot-shaped heart at radiography

2. Exercise intolerance that is relieved by squatting

○   **What is the most common cause of CHF in the second week of life?**

Coarctation of the aorta

○   **What is the most common cause of pediatric bacteremia?**

S pneumonia

○   **A patient has staccato cough and history of conjunctivitis in the first few weeks after birth. What type of pneumonia is likely?**

Chlamydia

○   **What 2 viral illnesses are associated with Reye syndrome?**

1. Varicella (chicken pox)

2. Influenza B

○   **What are the signs and symptoms of Reye syndrome?**

Irritability, combativeness, lethargy, right upper quadrant tenderness, history of influenza B or recent chicken pox, papilledema, hypoglycemia, and seizures. Laboratory test results reveal hypoglycemia, an ammonia level 20 times greater than normal, and a normal bilirubin level.

○   **What are the first, second, and third drugs of choice for the treatment of seizures in children?**

1. Phenobarbital

2. Phenytoin

3. Carbamazepine

○   **Why is diazepam avoided in neonatal seizures?**

It may cause hyperbilirubinemia by uncoupling the bilirubin-albumin complex.

○   **What is the most common cause of painless lower GI bleeding in an infant or child?**

Meckel diverticulum.

○ **A 16-month-old presents with bilious vomiting, a distended abdomen, and blood in the stool. What is the diagnosis?**

Malrotation of the midgut

○ **A child presents with periodic abdominal cramps, currant jelly stools, and a sausage-like tumor in the right lower quadrant. Contrast material–enhanced radiography shows a coil spring sign. What is the diagnosis?**

Intussusception

○ **In the pediatric esophagus, where is a foreign body most commonly lodged?**

In the cricopharyngeal narrowing

○ **A baby is brought to the emergency department because of vomiting and persistent crying. At examination, a testicle is tender and enlarged. What is the diagnosis?**

Testicular torsion

○ **A child presents with bluish discoloration of the gingiva. What is the probable diagnosis?**

Chronic lead poisoning. Expect the erythrocyte protoporphyrin level to be elevated with this condition.

○ **What is the most common dysrhythmia in a child?**

Paroxysmal atrial tachycardia

○ **How many days after administration of measles vaccine do fever and rash usually develop?**

7 to 10 days

○ **What is the most common suppurative complication of acute otitis media?**

Tympanic membrane perforation. Other complications include mastoiditis, cholesteatoma, and intracranial infections.

○ **Compare the rashes and the corresponding symptoms and signs of roseola and measles.**

- Roseola usually causes a fever as high as 104°F that lasts 3 to 5 days. The child does not appear particularly ill, although adenopathy may be noted. As the fever decreases, the child may develop maculopapular rash, which will last from a few hours to a few days.
- Measles usually begins with 3 to 4 days of fever, conjunctivitis, and upper respiratory tract symptoms. The characteristic rash is also maculopapular and confluent, but it distinctively begins on the face and moves down the body. Koplik spots are diagnostic.

○ **What is the little bone behind the tympanic membrane?**

The malleus

○ **Describe the signs and symptoms of varicella (chicken pox).**

Onset of varicella rash occurs 1 to 2 days after prodromal symptoms of slight malaise, anorexia, and fever. The rash begins on the trunk and scalp, appearing as faint macules and later becoming vesicles.

○ **How does a patient older than 12 months present with sickle cell disease?**

Pain in the joints, bones, and abdomen. The child may have abdominal tenderness and even rigidity. Mild icterus and anemia may be present.

○ **How does a child present with erythema infectiosum (Fifth disease or slapped cheek syndrome)?**

There are no prodromal symptoms. The illness usually begins with the sudden appearance of erythema of the cheeks, followed by a maculopapular rash on the trunk and extremities that evolves into a lacy pattern.

○ **What is the initial antibiotic treatment for a child with epiglottitis?**

Treat with a parenteral third-generation cephalosporin. The most likely cause of this condition is Hib.

With the widespread use of the Hib vaccine, streptococci are becoming a relatively more common cause. The number of cases is decreasing.

○ **What is the most common growth plate (Salter class) injury?**

Salter II fracture

○ **What is the most common cause of abdominal pain in children?**

Constipation

○ **In a child, does coarctation of the aorta typically cause cyanosis?**

No, unless it is severe

○ **What are the 8 common clinical presentations of pediatric heart disease?**

1. Cyanosis
2. Pathologic murmur
3. Abnormal pulses
4. CHF
5. Hypertension
6. Cardiogenic shock
7. Syncope
8. Tachyarrhythmias

○ **What are the classic findings of shaken baby syndrome?**

- FTT
- Lethargy
- Seizures
- Retinal hemorrhages
- Subarachnoid hemorrhage or subdural hematoma from torn bridging veins visible at computed tomography

○ **True/False: High fever in neonates with bacterial pneumonia usually follows a period of general fussiness and decreased feeding.**

True

○ **Conjunctivitis is an associated finding in about what percentage of neonates with *Chlamydophila pneumoniae*?**

About 50%

○ **How many days after birth should newborns stop losing weight?**

About 6 days

○ **True/False: A neonate's stool color can be an important sign.**

False. Unless blood is evident, stool color is insignificant.

○ **What is the difference between vomiting and regurgitation?**

- Vomiting is caused by forceful diaphragmatic and abdominal muscle contraction.
- Regurgitation occurs without effort.

○ **Is regurgitation dangerous in an otherwise thriving neonate?**

No. However, it can be dangerous for newborns with FTT or respiratory problems, and it may be associated with chronic aspiration.

○ **True/False: Bacterial and parasitic causes of diarrhea in the neonate are rare.**

True

○ **What are some entities in the differential diagnosis of bloody diarrhea in the neonate?**

Necrotizing enterocolitis, bacterial enteritis, allergic reactions to milk, and iatrogenic causes secondary to antibiotics

○ **What are some of the signs of sepsis to look for in babies with necrotizing enterocolitis?**

Poor feeding, lethargy, fever, jaundice, abdominal distension, and poor color

○ **What should be considered in the case of a neonate who has never passed stool?**

Meconium ileus or plug, Hirschsprung disease, intestinal stenosis or atresia, and imperforate anus

○ **Anal stenosis, hypothyroidism, and Hirschsprung disease can all manifest with what clinical sign?**

Constipation that was not present at birth but that began before the infant was aged 1 month

○ **Why are quinolones contraindicated for children?**

Quinolones impair cartilage growth.

○ **A young boy is presented for evaluation after being bitten by a coral snake. He appears to be fine. What is appropriate management?**

Admit to the intensive care unit and be ready for respiratory arrest. Coral snake venom is neurotoxic.

○ **What are some common entities in the differential diagnosis of a limp or gait abnormality in a child?**

Legg-Calvé-Perthes disease (avascular necrosis of the femoral head), Osgood-Schlatter disease (avulsion of the tibial tubercle), infection, toxic transient tenosynovitis, patellofemoral subluxation, chondromalacia patella, slipped capital femoral epiphysis, septic arthritis, limb length inequality, metatarsal fracture, proximal stress fracture, and toddler fracture (spiral tibia fracture)

○ **In the evaluation of retropharyngeal abscess, what is the usual age of the patients, how do they present, what diagnostic tests are used in their evaluation, and what treatment modalities are recommended?**

Retropharyngeal abscess is most commonly seen in children younger than 4 years. The usual patient presentation is with dysphagia, a muffled voice, stridor, and the sensation of a lump in the throat. Patients usually prefer to lie supine. Diagnosis is made with soft-tissue lateral neck radiography, which may demonstrate edema and air-fluid levels. Computed tomography may be useful. Treatment includes airway opening, IV antibiotics, and admission to the intensive care unit. Intubation may rupture the abscess.

○ **What are the most common causes of epiglottitis?**

Hib is most common. *Pneumococcus*, *Staphylococcus*, and *Branhamella* may also be causes. Presentation is most common among children around age 5 years.

○ **What is the usual cause of facial cellulitis in children younger than 3 years?**

H influenzae

○ **A 2-year-old girl has jammed a pencil into the lateral portion of her soft palate. What complication might develop?**

Ischemic stroke that results in contralateral hemiparesis is a potential complication of soft-palate pencil injuries.

○ **What is normal systolic blood pressure in a newborn?**

60 mm Hg

○ **Discuss infantile spasms.**

Onset is by age 3 to 9 months. A spasm typically lasts seconds and may occur in single episodes or bursts. Electroencephalographic results are often abnormal, and 85% of these patients will be mentally handicapped.

○ **What is the most likely cause of CHF in a premature infant?**

Patent ductus arteriosus

○ **What is the most likely cause of CHF during the first 3 days of life?**

Transposition of the great vessels that leads to cyanosis and failure

○   **What is the most likely cause of CHF during the first week of life?**

Hypoplastic left ventricle

○   **What is the most likely cause of CHF during the second week of life?**

Coarctation of the aorta

○   **What is the most common cause of painless upper GI bleeding in an infant or child?**

Varices from portal hypertension

○   **What are the signs and symptoms of aortic stenosis in a child?**

Exercise intolerance, chest pain, and a systolic ejection click with a crescendo-decrescendo murmur radiating to the neck with a suprasternal thrill. No cyanosis.

○   **What are the "7 deadly sins of childhood?"**

1. Colic
2. Awakening at night
3. Separation anxiety
4. Normal exploratory behavior
5. Normal negativism
6. Normal poor appetite
7. Toilet training resistance

○   **What is their significance?**

These behaviors, although normal at certain developmental stages, can be difficult for parents and can predispose the child to being abused.

○   **Who should receive meningococcal conjugate vaccine?**

All healthy children aged 11 to 12 years, as well as those aged 13 to 18 years and college freshmen residing in a dormitory who are previously unvaccinated, should receive the vaccine. Children at high risk for meningococcal disease may be vaccinated as early as 24 months and may require revaccination every 5 years.

○   **What is the recommendation for human papillomavirus immunization?**

All girls aged 11 to 12 years should receive the first dose of the vaccine, with the subsequent doses to be administered in 2 and 6 months.

○   **A child presents at age 6 months having received only the birth dose of hepatitis B vaccine. Does the child need to restart the 3-dose series now?**

No. Children who are behind on vaccinations do not need to restart a series regardless of how much time has passed between doses. This child should receive dose 2 of hepatitis B vaccine today and dose 3 after an interval of at least 8 weeks.

○ **Which children should receive influenza vaccine?**

All children older than 6 months should receive yearly influenza vaccine.

○ **How does the administration of influenza vaccine in children differ from that in adults?**

Children younger that 9 years should receive 2 doses at least 4 weeks apart the first time they are vaccinated. Children younger than 3 years should receive 0.25 mL of vaccine, which is half the dose administered in adults and older children.

○ **Which children can receive the live attenuated influenza vaccine?**

The live vaccine may be used in healthy children aged at least 2 years.

○ **Who should receive hepatitis A vaccine?**

All children aged 1 year or older should receive 2 doses a minimum of 6 months apart.

○ **Can persons older than 7 years be immunized against pertussis?**

Yes. They should be immunized to decrease the risk of infecting vulnerable infants. The combined tetanus, diphtheria, acellular pertussis vaccine contains a lower dose of acellular pertussis vaccine and is recommended for administration as a booster in all children aged 11 or 12 years and in those aged 13 to 18 years if not previously received (generally no sooner than 5 years after the last tetanus, diphtheria vaccine).

○ **What is the most important early intervention to prevent infection in an animal bite wound?**

Irrigation with saline to remove debris and decrease the bacterial inoculum

○ **Which is more likely to become infected: a dog bite or a cat bite?**

Cat bites are more likely to become infected because the long, sharp teeth of a cat produce deeper puncture wounds that are less amenable to irrigation and cleansing.

○ **What group of bacteria is a common cause of infection in dog or cat bites?**

Pasteurella species, notably *P multocida*

○ **What agents are effective for treating *Pasteurella* species?**

Amoxicillin and clavulanate, trimethoprim and sulfamethoxazole, and azithromycin. Fluoroquinolones, although effective, are not indicated in children.

○ **What newer macrolide antibiotic is indicated for use in children younger than 6 months?**

Azithromycin

○ **Why are tetracycline and similar drugs not recommended for children younger than 8 years?**

This class of drugs can cause staining of developing dental enamel. They should generally be avoided in children whose adult dentition is still developing (younger than 8 years).

○   **Why should aspirin be avoided in children with influenza or varicella?**

It is associated with the development of Reye syndrome.

○   **What are the most common food allergies in children?**

Egg, milk, soy, wheat, and peanuts (in order of prevalence)

○   **What are common coexisting conditions in children with attention-deficit/hyperactivity disorder?**

Anxiety disorder, conduct disorder, developmental disorder, mood disorder, oppositional defiant disorder, substance abuse, and tic.

○   **Drug holidays are often used with methylphenidate to decrease adverse effects. Should drug holidays also be used with atomoxetine?**

No. Atomoxetine must be administered every day for it to be effective.

○   **What are the indications to feed an infant soy-based formula?**

Galactosemia, congenital lactase deficiency, or vegan parents who wish to avoid all foods of animal origin. Healthy infants with gastroenteritis should return to breast milk or milk-based formula after their dehydration has been corrected. Soy formula should be avoided in preterm infants.

○   **What is the caloric density of breast milk, regular infant formula, enriched formula, and formula for premature infants?**

- Breast milk: 20 kcal/oz
- Regular infant formula: 20 kcal/oz
- Enriched formula: 22 kcal/oz
- Formula for premature infants: 24 kcal/oz

○   **Should an infant with milk protein allergy be fed soy-based formula?**

No. These children are often sensitive to soy protein and should instead receive hypoallergenic (hydrolyzed protein-based) or nonallergenic (amino acid–based) formula.

○   **How does the presentation of depressed adolescents differ from that of depressed adults?**

Adolescents are more often irritable and may demonstrate different moods, depending on the surroundings or setting. Other common presentations include school avoidance and underperformance, substance use, and frequent arguments.

○   **Which adolescents should be screened for depression?**

The US Preventive Services Task Force recommends that all patients between the ages of 12 and 18 years be screened for major depressive disorder.

○   **At what age should infants begin to be screened for autism spectrum disorders?**

9 months. Eye contact, speech development, and social behaviors should be evaluated.

○ **What are the salient characteristics that suggest a child may have autism?**

Failure to demonstrate babbling, pointing, or other communicative gestures by age 12 months; no use of single words by age 16 months; no use of novel 2-word phrases by age 24 months; regression of language or social skills at any age

○ **How intelligible should a small child's speech be to someone who does not know the child well?**

By age 36 months, a child's speech should be at least 50% intelligible, and by age 48 months, it should be at least 75% intelligible.

○ **A 2-year-old girl's mother reports that the family flew from Detroit to Chicago earlier today and that the child has not stopped crying since landing. She had a mild cold last week but is otherwise well. She is afebrile. At otoscopic examination, her tympanic membranes show evidence of hemorrhage. What is the likely diagnosis?**

This is likely barotrauma from the changing air pressures encountered during the flight. Preexisting eustachian tube dysfunction from a cold or allergy can increase the likelihood of barotrauma.

○ **What is cholesteatoma?**

It is a slowly enlarging epithelial cyst that develops in a retraction pocket or perforation in the superior aspect of the tympanic membrane. Although not malignant in the histologic sense, cholesteatoma can result in erosion of the ossicles, inner ear structures, and facial nerve canal.

○ **What are potential risks and complications of pacifier use?**

Because pacifier use may be associated with early weaning, it is best postponed until the mother-infant dyad has established successful breastfeeding. Use after age 6 months may increase the risk of otitis media. Use after age 2 years may increase risk of dental malocclusion.

○ **What are potential benefits of pacifier use?**

Pacifiers are effective in improving pain relief for infants undergoing minor procedures. They may be useful in transitioning preterm infants from enteral feeding to bottle feeding. Pacifier use at bedtime in infants from 1 to 6 months may reduce the risk of SIDS.

○ **Consistent results from randomized controlled trials (strength of recommendation "A") have demonstrated the effectiveness of what first-line intervention in the management of childhood eczema?**

Topical emollients, which provide increased hydration to the skin and also have a steroid-sparing effect

○ **The recommendation to place infants in the supine position for sleep has resulted in a significant decrease in SIDS incidence. What complication of supine sleeping has become more common?**

Deformational plagiocephaly, or occipital flattening

○ **What can be done to reduce the risk of such skull deformity?**

Infants need to spend supervised time in the prone position ("tummy time") and alternate which side of the occiput is placed downward when the infant is put to bed.

○ **What are salient characteristics indicating Munchausen syndrome by proxy?**

Recurrent ALTEs, especially if these occur with a lone caregiver; children older than 6 months, unexplained death of 2 or more siblings, or simultaneous death of twins

○ **What are some measures that may be taken to decrease the risk of injury to young baseball players?**

Use of batting helmets with face shields, mouth guards, reduced-impact baseballs, and breakaway bases

○ **What defines secondary enuresis?**

The child develops enuresis after at least 6 months of urinary continence.

○ **What are some diagnostic considerations in a previously toilet-trained young child who begins to wet the bed again?**

UTI, sexual abuse, diabetes mellitus, family stressor (eg, divorce, new sibling, moving), constipation, seizure disorder, obstructive sleep apnea

○ **Which treatment modality for enuresis is supported by the best evidence?**

An enuresis alarm that senses wetness and awakens the child. A disadvantage is sleep disruption of the child and other family members.

○ **How is midparental height calculated?**

For boys: [father's height in cm + (mother's height in cm +13 cm)]/2
For girls: [(father's height in cm −13 cm) + mother's height in cm]/2

○ **How is this calculation useful?**

It can be used to estimate a child's adult height potential, which will generally be within 5 cm on either side of this value.

○ **Other than having tall parents, what is the most common cause of stature exceeding the 95th percentile?**

Obesity, which can cause mildly advanced bone age, growth velocity, and pubertal status

○ **What is the best approach for a breastfed infant who is consistently above the 95th percentile in weight?**

Although this infant would be considered overweight, it is not recommended that the mother restrict feedings of breast milk. Helpful advice includes feeding when the child is hungry and using cuddling as a response to other crying and/or distress. Breastfeeding is protective against obesity in later life. As the child's diet increases, sound advice includes encouragement of activity and restriction of juice intake.

○ **What is the difference between strabismus and amblyopia?**

Strabismus refers to a disorder of ocular alignment, whereas amblyopia refers to a loss of visual acuity because of disuse of the eye during a key period of development. Untreated strabismus can lead to amblyopia.

○ **What is pseudostrabismus?**

A child with a broad nasal bridge or epicanthal folds may appear to have esotropia but normal ocular alignment is found at examination.

○ **What is the difference between esotropia and esophoria and between exotropia and exophoria?**

"Eso" refers to the eye deviating nasally relative to the fixating eye, and "exo" refers to the eye deviating temporally. "Tropia" refers to strabismus that is apparent without interruption of visual fixation, and "phoria" refers to strabismus that is elicited only with interruption of visual fixation.

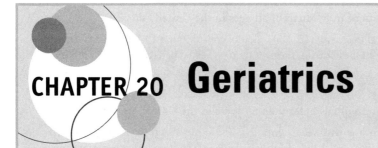

CHAPTER 20 Geriatrics

Raj C. Shah, MD

○ **What is the average life expectancy from birth for men and women in the United States?**
For all persons, 77 years; for men, 75 years and for women, 80 years

○ **What is the number of years someone in the United States will live if he or she is currently aged 65 years?**
For all persons, 18 years; for men, 17 years and for women, 20 years

○ **What is the number of years someone in the United States will live if he or she is currently aged 75 years?**
For all persons, 12 years; for men, 11 years and for women, 13 years

○ **What is the number of years someone in the United States will live if he or she is currently aged 85 years?**
For all persons, 7 years; for men, 6 years and for women, 7 years

○ **What is the number of years someone in the United States will live if he or she is currently aged 100 years?**
For all persons, 3 years; for men, 2 years and for women, 3 years

○ **How many people currently are older than 65 years in the United States?**
Approximately 30 million

○ **How many people will be older than 65 years in the United States in 2030?**
Approximately 70 million

○ **What percentage of the elderly are ambulatory?**
90%

○ **What percentage of the elderly live in nursing homes?**
10%

○ **What are the leading actual causes of death of individuals of all ages in the United States?**

Tobacco use (18.1%), poor diet and physical inactivity (15.2%), ethanol consumption (3.5%), microbial agents (3.1%), toxic agents (2.3%), motor vehicle crashes (1.8%), firearms (1.2%), sexual behavior (0.8%), and illicit drug use (0.7%)

○ **What are the leading causes of death of individuals older than 65 years in the United States?**

Heart disease, malignant neoplasms, cerebrovascular disease, chronic lower respiratory tract disease, influenza and pneumonia, Alzheimer disease, diabetes mellitus, nephritis, nephritic syndrome and nephrosis, unintentional injuries, and septicemia

○ **What is the recommendation for screening for abdominal aortic aneurysm in older persons?**

Onetime ultrasonographic screening recommended at age 65 years

○ **At what age can cervical cancer screening be stopped?**

Age 65 years, if the woman has a history of normal screening results

○ **At what age can breast cancer screening be stopped?**

Approximately age 75 to 80 years, if the woman is at average risk and has average overall health status

○ **At what age can colon cancer screening be stopped?**

Approximately age 75 years for men and 80 years for women, after life expectancy and comorbidities are taken into consideration

○ **At what age can prostate cancer screening be stopped?**

If conducted at all, it may be stopped at age 75 years or when life expectancy is less than 10 years

○ **Does the use of antioxidant supplements decrease mortality?**

In randomized controlled primary and secondary prevention trials, vitamins A and E and beta-carotene supplementation increased mortality. Vitamin C and selenium supplementation had no significant effect on mortality. This does not rule out the effects of other antioxidants and deals with supplementation rather than dietary sources only.

○ **What age group benefits the most from reduction in mortality with aspirin prophylaxis?**

Individuals aged between 70 and 84 years at highest risk for coronary heart disease

○ **How many additional years of life expectancy are gained if an individual in the United States quits smoking at age 65 years?**

1.4 to 2.0 years for men and 2.7 to 3.7 years for women

○ **How is fatigue different from sleepiness?**

Persons who are sleepy are temporarily aroused with activity, whereas fatigue is intensified by activity in the short term. Persons with sleepiness feel better after a nap, but those with fatigue have lack of energy, mental exhaustion, and nonrestorative sleep.

○ **How is fatigue different from depression?**

Fatigue is associated with lack of energy or stamina to complete specific tasks, whereas grief and depression are more associated with being unable to do anything.

○ **What age group is at the highest risk for suicide in the United States?**

White men older than 65 years

○ **Is the incidence of epidural and subdural hematomas higher or lower in elderly patients?**

Epidural hematomas are less common, and subdural hematomas are more common.

○ **What are nonpharmacologic interventions to reduce the risk of delirium in hospitalized patients?**

Regular daily activities that are cognitively stimulating; correction of dehydration; early mobilization (bedside range-of-motion exercises if the patient is bedridden); minimization of unnecessary noise and stimuli; promotion of good sleep hygiene; removal of urinary catheters and physical restraints, when indicated; repeated reorientation; and the use of eyeglasses or a magnifying lens. These interventions reduce the risk of developing delirium in older hospitalized patients by as much as 3%.

○ **What is the most common complication in older hospitalized persons?**

Delirium. It affects about 20% of individuals older than 65 years.

○ **What are 4 items associated with increased risk for delirium in older hospitalized persons?**

1. Vision impairment
2. Cognitive impairment
3. Severe illness (Acute Physiology and Chronic Health Evaluation score >16 or nurse rating of severe)
4. Elevated ratio of serum urea nitrogen to serum creatinine (>18)
   - 0 items: 10% increased risk for delirium
   - 1 or 2 items: 25% increased risk for delirium
   - 3 or 4 items: 80% increased risk for delirium

○ **What are the outcomes associated with delirium in older hospitalized persons?**

Length of hospitalization increased by 8 days. Mortality rate is twice as high. Physical and cognitive recovery at 6 months and 12 months are significantly worse than in age-matched hospitalized patients without delirium.

○ **What is the most common subtype of delirium in hospitalized older persons?**

Hypoactive. The subtypes of delirium are hyperactive (agitated, anxious, disoriented, or delusional), hypoactive (subdued, lethargic, stuporous, or comatose), or mixed.

○ **What are 4 features associated with the diagnosis of delirium?**

1. Acute onset

2. Fluctuating course

3. Presence of inattention

4. Either disorganized thinking or altered level of consciousness

○ **Which pharmacologic agents have been approved to treat the symptoms of Alzheimer disease?**

Tacrine, donepezil, rivastigmine, galantamine, and memantine. The first 4 agents are acetylcholinesterase inhibitors. By blocking the enzyme that breaks down acetylcholine in the brain, more acetylcholine is available as a neurotransmitter. Tacrine was the first acetylcholinesterase agent approved but is no longer used clinically because it required dosing 4 times a day and had associated liver toxicity. Memantine is a partial antagonist of the N-methyl-d-aspartate receptor and blocks the effects of glutamate toxicity. Donepezil, rivastigmine, and galantamine have been approved by the US Food and Drug Administration for use in mild-to-moderate Alzheimer disease. Donepezil and memantine (alone or in combination) have been approved for use in moderate-to-severe Alzheimer disease.

○ **Giant cell arteritis is a chronic inflammation of the large blood vessels. What arteries are most commonly involved?**

The carotid and the cranial arteries. Blindness may result in 20% of afflicted patients. Treat with high-dose corticosteroids.

○ **What are the common neurologic signs and symptoms of giant cell arteritis?**

Amaurosis fugax, deafness, depression, and paralysis. Amaurosis fugax is the most dangerous because it can lead to permanent monocular or binocular blindness.

○ **What is the most common cause of hearing loss in the elderly?**

Presbycusis. Other causes include neoplasms, noise exposure, ototoxic drugs, and otosclerosis.

○ **Presbycusis is a hearing loss at which end of the audible range?**

The high end (4000 to 8000 Hz)

○ **What is the most common cause of cataract development?**

Old age. Cataracts occur congenitally, from medication, or from trauma. Slitlamp examination may show absent red reflex and gray clouding of the lens.

○ **What is the most common cause of blindness in the elderly?**

Senile macular degeneration. Patients experience a gradual loss of central vision. The macula appears hemorrhagic or pigmented because of atrophic degeneration of the retinal vessels that results in leaking vessels, fibrosis, and scarring of the retina.

○ **What age group accounts for the most cases of visual impairment?**

Adults older than 80 years. Although adults older than 80 years are about 8% of the population in the United States, 70% of cases of severe visual impairment exist in this group.

○ **What are common morbidities associated with vision loss in older persons?**

Depression, social withdrawal, isolation, falls, institutionalization, and self-administered medication errors

○ **At what age should periodic screening for vision problems begin?**

Age 65 years. How often older adults should be screened is not well determined. Most screening for visual acuity should be performed with a Snellen chart.

○ **Is universal glaucoma screening recommended in older adults?**

According to the US Preventive Services Task Force, there is no recommendation for or against routine screening for glaucoma in older adults. However, some subgroups at higher risk, such as African Americans, may benefit from periodic screening.

○ **What tool is commonly used to screen for age-related macular degeneration?**

The Amsler grid. The patient is asked to look at the grid and report any way in which lines or areas are missing or distorted. The specificity and sensitivity of the Amsler grid for detection of age-related macular degeneration in primary practices are not known.

○ **What condition accounts for nearly 60% of blindness in persons of European descent older than 65 years?**

Age-related macular degeneration

○ **What are the 2 types of age-related macular degeneration?**

1. Wet (neovascular or exudative)
2. Dry (nonneovascular or nonexudative)

○ **What is the recommended interval for screening for retinopathy in older persons with newly diagnosed diabetes?**

A dilated examination should be conducted within 1 year after diabetes is diagnosed. Examinations should be conducted at least annually thereafter for individuals without retinopathy or with minimal nonproliferative retinopathy. Examinations should be conducted every 6 to 12 months in individuals with diabetes and stable nonproliferative retinopathy. For persons with diabetes and unstable proliferative retinopathy or macular edema, dilated eye examination every 2 to 4 months is recommended.

○ **What intervention has the best evidence of preventing vision loss in older persons, especially those with diabetes?**

Sustained blood pressure control. In the UK Prospective Diabetes Study, lowering blood pressure below 150/85 mm Hg in persons with diabetes reduced the risk of progressive diabetic retinopathy, irrespective of hemoglobin A_{1c} level. A decrease of 10 mm Hg in systolic blood pressure provided an 11% relative risk reduction in the incidence of photocoagulation or vitreous hemorrhage.

○ **Does supplementation with antioxidants and zinc, alone or in combination, prevent or delay onset of macular degeneration?**

No. However, antioxidant and zinc supplementation may delay progression of age-related macular degeneration in some persons with advanced disease as shown in the Age-Related Eye Disease Study.

○   **Compared with the incidence in individuals aged 30 years, what is the incidence of dental root caries in individuals older than 60 years?**

The incidence is twice as high in all individuals older than age 60. It rises to 64% in persons older than 80 years, and as many as 96% of individuals older than 80 years have coronal caries.

○   **What are risk factors for development of dental caries in older persons?**

Decreased salivary flow rate, history of caries, institutionalization, lack of routine dental care, low socioeconomic status, nonfluoridated community water supply, and poor oral hygiene

○   **What percentage of older persons have xerostomia?**

Xerostomia is the subjective sensation of dry mouth caused by decreased saliva production. It affects 29% to 57% of older persons.

○   **What are risk factors for xerostomia in older persons?**

Head or neck irradiation, human immunodeficiency virus, medication use (angiotensin-converting enzyme [ACE] inhibitors, α- and β-blockers, analgesics, anticholinergics, antidepressants, antihistamines, antipsychotics, anxiolytics, calcium-channel blockers, diuretics, muscle relaxants, or sedatives), salivary gland aplasia, Sjögren syndrome, and smoking

○   **What are treatments for xerostomia in older persons?**

Stopping medications known to decrease salivary flow, increasing intake of water, avoiding alcohol, decreasing intake of caffeinated or sugary foods or drinks, using sugarless chewing gum or candy, and using over-the-counter salivary substitutes

○   **What is the cause of denture stomatitis?**

Oral candidiasis. It can be treated with topical antifungals and repair of ill-fitting dentures.

○   **An elderly patient with chronic chronic obstructive pulmonary disease is most likely to contract what kind of pneumonia?**

Haemophilus influenzae pneumonia. Ampicillin is the drug of choice. This population is at risk and should be vaccinated.

○   **What is helpful in controlling the symptoms of dyspnea in advanced lung disease or terminal cancer?**

Oral morphine. Nebulized morphine does not provide additional benefits when compared to oral opioids.

○   **What is the most common cause of community-acquired pneumonia in the elderly?**

Streptococcus pneumoniae

○   **In the elderly, what is the most common cause of death resulting from community-acquired infections: institutional or nosocomial?**

In the community and in institutions, it is bacterial pneumonia; in hospitals, it is urinary tract infection (UTI).

○ **What are the most common sources of sepsis in the elderly?**

Respiratory, urinary, and intraabdominal, in order of importance

○ **What percentage of elderly patients with sepsis do not present with a fever?**

25%

○ **What is the second most common cause of infection in nursing home residents?**

Pneumonia

○ **What are the most common causes of viral pneumonia in nursing home residents?**

- Influenza
- Respiratory syncytial virus

○ **What is the most common cause of bacterial pneumonia in nursing home residents?**

S pneumoniae. However, in severe cases of nursing home–acquired pneumonia requiring hospitalization and mechanical ventilation, *Staphylococcus aureus* and enteric gram-negative organisms appear to exceed *S pneumoniae*.

○ **Does aspiration pneumonitis require antibiotic treatment?**

Aspiration pneumonitis is caused by inflammation of the lung parenchyma because of inadvertent aspiration of gastric contents, which may be common in older and especially frail adults. Antibiotic treatment is not needed if signs of lung inflammation are transient (<24 hours).

○ **Aspiration pneumonitis with what risk factors requires antibiotic treatment?**

- Stroke
- Dementia
- Gastroesophageal reflux disease
- Tube feeding

○ **A 65-year-old African American patient has hypertension and gout. What medications should be prescribed?**

Although diuretics are the most effective drugs for the treatment of hypertension in African American patients, this patient has gout, which will be exacerbated by the use of diuretics. ACE inhibitors or calcium-channel blockers are better choices for this patient.

○ **An elderly woman presents with high blood pressure and a history of congestive heart failure. What is the antihypertensive drug of choice?**

ACE inhibitors. They will reduce both preload and afterload.

○ **An elderly man presents with high blood pressure and a history of noninsulin-dependent diabetes mellitus. What is the antihypertensive drug of choice?**

ACE inhibitors. They have renal protective properties.

○ **An elderly African American man presents with high blood pressure and a history of angina. What is the antihypertensive drug of choice?**

Calcium-channel blockers

○ **What percentage of adults older than 65 years are affected by aortic stenosis?**

3%. Aortic stenosis leads to greater morbidity and mortality than do other cardiac valve diseases.

○ **What is the prognosis in patients with asymptomatic aortic stenosis?**

The same as for age- and sex-matched control patients

○ **What is the prognosis in patients with symptomatic aortic stenosis?**

2 to 3 years of life. Symptoms include the triad of syncope, angina, and dyspnea.

○ **What is the major risk of tricyclic antidepressants in the elderly?**

Orthostatic hypotension because it can lead to falls

○ **What is the incidence of morbidity and mortality in patients older than 60 years who present with syncope?**

One in 5 will have significant morbidity or mortality within 6 months.

○ **What are some of the most common causes of dysphagia in the elderly population?**
- Hiatal hernia
- Reflux esophagitis
- Webs and rings
- Cancer

○ **What geriatric ethnic population is at greatest risk for esophageal cancer?**

Elderly African American patients have a risk 4 times that of elderly white Americans. Other populations at risk include those who are Chinese, Iranian, or South African.

○ **What is the most common cause of abdominal pain in the elderly?**

Constipation

○ **What is the most common cause of acute abdominal pain in the elderly?**

Acute cholecystitis. Approximately 50% of patients older than 65 years have gallstones.

○ **Describe the clinical features of appendicitis in the elderly.**

Anorexia and vomiting are less common, and migration of the pain to the right lower quadrant is absent in as many as 60% of elderly patients. The elderly account for 50% of deaths due to appendicitis. Half of elderly patients with appendicitis have normal white blood cell counts at presentation.

○ **Who has a higher rupture rate in appendicitis: the very young or the very old?**

The very old. The rupture rate for geriatric patients is 65% to 90%, with an associated mortality rate of 15%. The pediatric population has a rupture rate of 15% to 50%, with an associated mortality rate of 3%.

○ **What is the most common cause of large-bowel obstruction in the elderly?**

Fecal impaction. Other causes are stenosing diverticula, neoplasms, and volvulus. Adhesions are rarely a cause of obstruction in the large bowel.

○ **In the elderly, what is a common adverse effect of verapamil?**

Constipation

○ **Why is it unsafe to administer digoxin and furosemide in a geriatric patient?**

Hypokalemia and digoxin toxicity may result.

○ **What is the most common form of incontinence in the elderly?**

Urge incontinence. It is more common in women and is due to detrusor hyperreflexia or decreased sensory capabilities.

○ **Strokes, Parkinson disease, and Alzheimer disease are most commonly associated with which type of incontinence?**

Urge incontinence

○ **What drugs are used to treat stress incontinence?**

α-Adrenergic agonists and estrogen

○ **What is the prevalence of benign prostatic hypertrophy in older men?**

90% in men older than 70 years

○ **What symptoms are commonly associated with benign prostatic hypertrophy?**

- Hesitancy
- Weak stream
- Nocturia
- Incontinence

○ **In what situation are 5-α reductase inhibitors, such as finasteride and dutasteride, most effective for treatment of benign prostatic hypertrophy?**

When prostate volume is greater than 40 mL (normal prostate volume is 20 to 30 mL)

○ **What works better for treatment of benign prostatic hypertrophy: doxazosin, finasteride, or both?**

Both. For finasteride alone, the number needed to treat (NNT) (in 4 years) to reduce risk of acute urinary retention was 26 and for surgical intervention was 18. For doxazosin alone, the NNT to reduce clinical progression of symptoms was 14 over 4 years. The combination of finasteride and doxazosin was better than either agent alone.

○ **What is the most common obstructive cause of acute urinary retention in older men?**

Benign prostatic hypertrophy. Men in their 70s have a 10% chance of having acute urinary retention; men in their 80s have more than a 30% chance.

○ **What is the most common cause of UTIs in noncatheterized elderly patients?**

Escherichia coli

○ **What is the most common cause of relapsing UTIs in elderly patients?**

Chronic bacterial prostatitis, caused by *E coli*, *Proteus*, *Klebsiella pneumoniae*, and enterococci.

○ **What may result from the administration of an aminoglycoside or cephalosporin in an elderly patient who is dehydrated?**

Acute renal failure secondary to tubulointerstitial injury. This may also occur if an aminoglycoside or cephalosporin is administered in an elderly patient who is receiving furosemide or who has preexisting renal disease.

○ **What are risk factors for drug-induced nephropathy?**

- Age older than 60 years
- Baseline renal insufficiency (glomerular filtration rate <60 mL/min/1.73 m^2)
- Volume depletion
- Multiple exposures to nephrotoxins
- Diabetes
- Heart failure
- Sepsis

○ **What percentage of community- and hospital-acquired episodes of acute renal failure are due to drug-induced nephropathy?**

20%

○ **What is the Trendelenburg test for varicose veins?**

Raise the leg above the heart, then quickly lower it. If the leg veins become distended immediately after this test, there is valvular incompetency.

○ **What percentage of adults older than 60 years have osteoarthritis of the knee?**

10%

○ **What is the mortality rate for geriatric patients who have sustained a hip fracture?**

Twenty-five percent will die in the first year after the fracture.

○ **What is an effective treatment to prevent vertebral fractures in postmenopausal women?**

Bisphosphonates. Alendronate has been studied the most. A 10-mg daily dose of alendronate is effective for secondary (NNT = 16) and primary (NNT = 50) prevention of vertebral fractures. It is also effective for secondary prevention of nonvertebral fractures, including hip or wrist fractures (NNT = 100), but not for primary prevention of nonvertebral fractures.

○ **What are common risk factors for osteoporosis in white men?**

- Age older than 70 years
- Low body weight (body mass index $<20–25$ kg/m^2)
- Weight loss of more than 10%
- Physical inactivity
- Use of oral corticosteroids
- Previous fragility fracture

Androgen deprivation is a strong predictor of osteoporosis and fracture. Ethanol use increases risk of fracture but is not associated with decreased body mineral density. Cigarette smoking and low intake of dietary calcium are moderate predictors of an increased risk for low bone mass.

○ **How do you differentiate clinically between polymyalgia rheumatica and polymyositis?**

In polymyositis, there are proximal muscle pain, weakness, and tenderness and elevated muscle enzyme levels. In contrast, polymyalgia rheumatica manifests with an elevated sedimentation rate, which is also seen in giant cell arteritis, which is associated with polymyalgia rheumatica.

○ **What percentage of pressure ulcers occur in individuals older than 65 years?**

70%

○ **What are the most common sites for pressure ulcers?**

- Sacrum
- Heels
- Ischial tuberosities
- Greater trochanters
- Lateral malleoli

○ **What causes pressure ulcers?**

Unrelieved pressure (greater than the arterial capillary pressure) that results in blood-flow impediment and deprivation of oxygen and nutrients to tissue

○ **What are intrinsic and extrinsic risk factors for pressure ulcers?**

- Intrinsic risk factors include limited mobility, poor nutrition, comorbidities (eg, diabetes mellitus, depression, collagen vascular disorders, peripheral vascular disease, decreased pain sensation, immunodeficiency, congestive heart failure, malignancies, end-stage renal disease, chronic obstructive pulmonary disease, and dementia), and aging skin.
- Extrinsic risk factors include pressure from any hard surface, friction and shear from involuntary muscle movements, and moisture (eg, incontinence, perspiration, and wound drainage).

○ **What are the stages for pressure ulcers?**

According to the National Pressure Ulcer Advisory Panel

- Stage I: Intact skin with nonblanching redness
- Stage II: Sallow, open ulcer with red-pink wound bed
- Stage III: Full-thickness tissue loss with visible subcutaneous fat
- Stage IV: Full-thickness tissue loss with exposed muscle and bone

○   **How often should a bedridden patient be repositioned to try to prevent development of pressure ulcers?**

According to the Agency for Health Care Policy and Research, every 2 hours

○   **What are examples of static pressure-reducing devices and dynamic pressure-reducing devices?**

Static devices include foam, water, gel, and air mattresses or mattress overlays. Dynamic devices are alternating-pressure devices and low-air-loss and air-fluidized surfaces that use a power source to redistribute localized pressure. The benefit of dynamic versus static devices is unclear.

○   **What are the basic components of pressure ulcer management?**
- Pressure reduction and relief for the skin
- Necrotic tissue debridement
- Wound cleansing
- Bacterial load and colonization management
- Wound dressing selection

○   **What is the most common complication of a pressure ulcer?**

Sepsis

○   **What is the most common primary bone malignancy in older persons?**

Multiple myeloma. The median age at diagnosis is 70 years.

○   **What is the initial manifestation of multiple myeloma?**

Unexplained backache or bone pain in the long bones, ribs, skull, and pelvis; pathologic fracture; and peripheral neuropathy. Anorexia, nausea, somnolence, and polydipsia may be associated with hypercalcemia in multiple myeloma. Weakness and malaise are associated with anemia. Recurrent infections can be caused by impaired antibodies or leukopenia. Patients may lose weight. Thirty-four percent of patients present with incidental findings concerning total protein, creatinine, calcium, or hemoglobin levels.

○   **What is the most common peripheral neuropathy of multiple myeloma?**

Carpal tunnel syndrome

○   **What is the most common region for pathologic fracture in multiple myeloma?**

Vertebral compression fracture. Pathologic fracture is the presenting symptom in 26% to 34% of patients.

○   **What are the criteria for smoldering (asymptomatic) multiple myeloma?**
- Serum M protein level of 3 g/dL or more
- 10% or more bone marrow plasma cells
- Nonrelated organ or tissue impairment or symptoms

○   **Which group of individuals with multiple myeloma should not be treated?**

Those with smoldering or asymptomatic multiple myeloma. Early treatment has no effect on mortality and may increase the risk of acute leukemia. They should receive close follow-up with laboratory testing every 3 to 4 months.

○ **Which treatment is beneficial in decreasing morbidity with multiple myeloma?**

Bisphosphonates decrease vertebral fractures and pain but not mortality. Intravenous bisphosphonates (pamidronate and zoledronic acid) have been approved for use in multiple myeloma, but oral bisphosphonates are not effective.

○ **What immunizations should a person with multiple myeloma receive?**

- Influenza
- *S pneumoniae*
- *H influenzae* type B

○ **What is hospice?**

Hospice is a philosophy that the dying patient has physical, psychological, social, and spiritual aspects, and it uses an interdisciplinary team to provide a wide range of services to support the primary caregiver of the dying patient. To be eligible for hospice in the United States, a patient must have a terminal illness and have an estimated prognosis of less than 6 months to live.

CHAPTER 21 Behavioral Science

Lorna H. London, PhD

○ **What are the components of the multiaxial diagnostic system?**

- Axis I: Symptoms and syndromes comprising a mental disorder, including substance abuse or addiction
- Axis II: Personality and developmental disorders underlying the Axis I diagnosis
- Axis III: Physical medical problems or conditions that may or may not contribute to the Axis I diagnosis
- Axis IV: Psychosocial factors
- Axis V: Global Assessment of Functioning (scale of 0–100) adaptive ability or disability

○ **Is violence more likely between family members or nonfamily members?**

Family members. Twenty percent to 50% of the murders in the United States are committed by family members. The rate of spousal abuse is as high as 16% in the United States.

○ **In what percentage of child sexual abuse cases is the abuser known by the child?**

90%. In 50% of such cases, the mother is also abused.

○ **What is the epidemiology of domestic violence?**

Ninety-five percent of the abused are women. An estimated 4 million women are battered each year. Domestic abuse is the number 1 cause of injuries to women between the ages of 15 and 44 years. More than half of all women murdered in the United States are killed by an intimate partner. Abuse often escalates when a woman attempts to leave the relationship. According to the US Department of Health and Human Services, root causes for domestic violence include the following: (1) power and control, (2) growing up in a cycle of violence, and (3) distorted concept of manhood.

○ **What are the clinical clues for domestic violence?**

- Any evidence of injury during pregnancy or late entry into prenatal care
- Patients presenting with injuries after significant delay or in various stages of healing, especially to the head, neck, breasts, abdomen, or in areas suggesting a defensive posture, such as bruises on the forearms
- Vague complaints or unusual injuries, such as bites, scratches, burns, or rope marks

○ **Define alcoholism and discuss the prevalence of alcoholism in the United States.**

Alcoholism is clinically referred to as "ethanol dependence" and is characterized by a pattern of tolerance and withdrawal. According to the National Institute on Alcohol Abuse and Alcoholism, 1 in 13 American adults abuse ethanol, and 10% to 15% is the lifetime prevalence for alcoholism; 10% of men and 3.5% of women are alcoholic.

○ **What age range has the highest prevalence of drinking problems?**

18- to 29-year-old adults

○ **What laboratory test result changes are suggestive of alcoholism?**

Look for an increase in levels of alanine aminotransferase, aspartate aminotransferase, alkaline phosphatase, amylase, bilirubin, cholesterol, gamma-glutamyltransferase, lactate dehydrogenase, triglycerides, and uric acid and in mean corpuscular volume and prothrombin time and a decrease in levels of serum urea nitrogen, calcium, hematocrit, magnesium, phosphorus, and protein and in coagulation time and platelet count.

○ **Describe the symptoms of ethanol withdrawal and their temporal relations.**

- Autonomic hyperactivity: Tachycardia, hypertension, tremors, anxiety, and agitation occur 6 to 8 hours after the patient's last drink.
- Hallucinations: Auditory, visual, and tactile hallucinations occur 24 hours after the patient's last drink.
- Global confusion: Confusion occurs 1 to 3 days after the patient's last drink.

○ **What is the difference in treatment methods between ethanol withdrawal and sedative hypnotic withdrawal?**

- Ethanol withdrawal is treated with benzodiazepine, carbamazepine, or paraldehyde.
- Sedative hypnotic withdrawal is treated with the substitution of a long-acting barbiturate.

○ **What is the prevalence of mental illness in the United States?**

Approximately 57.7 million (26.2%) American adults older than 18 years have a diagnosable mental disorder in a given year.

○ **Discuss the important factors in understanding suicide.**

More than 90% of people who commit suicide have a diagnosable mental disorder, most commonly a depressive disorder or a substance abuse disorder. The highest suicide rates are in white men older than 85 years. According to 2008 statistics from the National Institute of Mental Health, 4 times as many men as women die by suicide; however, women attempt suicide 2 to 3 times more often than men do.

○ **A patient presents with tearing eyes, a runny nose, tachycardia, hair on end, abdominal pains, nausea, vomiting, diarrhea, insomnia, pupillary dilatation, and leukocytosis. What is the diagnosis?**

Opiate and/or opioid withdrawal. Treat with methadone. Clonidine may blunt some of the adverse effects.

○ **What is the most effective long-term treatment program for alcoholism?**

Alcoholics Anonymous

○ **What is the difference between a malingering and a factitious disorder?**

A malingerer's incentive is external, such as workers' compensation. The goal of someone with a factitious disorder is to enter into the sick role. Both involve feigning illness.

○ **What is the difference between methadone and heroin?**

Methadone causes analgesia but does not cause euphoria. Habituation occurs with both drugs. The withdrawal symptoms of methadone are less severe, but they last longer.

○ **What are the 2 most common behavior problems seen by general practitioners?**

  1. Anxiety

  2. Depression

○ **Describe a patient with generalized anxiety disorder.**

Patients with this disorder appear apprehensive, restless, and irritable and are easily distracted. Patients can also experience muscle tension and fatigue, as well as various autonomic symptoms, such as palpitations, shortness of breath, chest tightness, nausea, or diffuse weakness and numbness.

○ **Name a few substances that might mimic generalized anxiety when ingested.**

Nicotine, caffeine, amphetamines, cocaine, and anticholinergics. Ethanol and sedative withdrawal can also mimic this disorder.

○ **What are 8 common medical causes of anxiety or anxiety attacks?**

  1. Ethanol withdrawal

  2. Thyrotoxicosis

  3. Caffeine

  4. Stroke

  5. Cardiopulmonary emergencies

  6. Hypoglycemia

  7. Psychosensory or psychomotor epilepsy

  8. Pheochromocytoma

○ **Match the aphasia with the anatomy involved.**

  1. Broca aphasia   **a.** Superior temporal gyrus, posterior third

  2. Global aphasia   **b.** Arcuate fasciculus near the dominant parietal lobe

  3. Wernicke aphasia   **c.** Middle cerebral artery occlusion

  4. Conduction aphasia   **d.** Left frontal lobe, posterior inferior region

  Answers: (1) d, (2) c, (3) a, and (4) b

○ **What accounts for the most referrals to child psychiatrists?**

Attention-deficit/hyperactivity disorder, which accounts for 30% to 50% of child psychiatric outpatient cases

○ **What chromosomal abnormality do autistic patients commonly have?**

Fragile X syndrome (8%)

○ **What percentage of patients with autism are mute?**

50%

○ **Bereavement generally lasts how long?**

6 months. Full melancholic syndrome, hallucinations, and suicidal ideation are not common in bereavement.

○ **Which has an earlier onset: bipolar disorder or unipolar disorder?**

Bipolar. Onset of bipolar disorder is usually in the patient's 20s or 30s; onset of unipolar disorder is usually between ages 35 and 50 years.

○ **Differentiate between bipolar I, bipolar II, and hypomania.**

- Bipolar I: Mania and major depression
- Bipolar II: Hypomania and major depression
- Hypomania: Mania without severe impairment or psychotic features

○ **Are most patients with affective disorder bipolar or unipolar?**

Unipolar (80%)

○ **Which is most commonly the first episode of bipolar disease: mania or depression?**

Mania. Depression is rarely the first symptom. In fact, only 5% to 10% of patients who develop depression first have manic episodes later.

○ **Other than classic mania, what can lithium be used to treat?**

Bulimia, anorexia nervosa, alcoholism in patients with mood disorders, leukocytosis in patients receiving antineoplastic medication, cluster headaches, and migraine headaches

○ **Postural tremor is a major adverse effect of lithium. How is this adverse effect controlled?**

Minimize the dose during the workday and administer small doses of β-blockers.

○ **Should people who are physically active have the lithium dosage increased or decreased?**

Increased. Lithium, a salt, is excreted more than sodium in sweat.

○ **True/False: A patient starting lithium will be expected to gain weight.**

True. All psychotropic medications cause weight gain, hence lithium's usefulness in combating anorexia nervosa.

○ **What is the potential complication associated with treating manic depression and congestive heart failure simultaneously?**

Lithium toxicity. A low-salt diet and/or sodium-losing diuretics can cause lithium retention and toxicity.

○ **At what level does lithium toxicity begin?**

14 mg/L. Above this level, nausea, diarrhea, vomiting, rigidity, tremor, ataxia, seizures, delirium, coma, and death can occur.

○ **What is the clinical presentation of a patient with borderline personality disorder?**

This person will likely experience chronic feelings of emptiness or boredom, severe mood swings, volatile and unstable relationships, continuous and uncontrollable anger, and impulsivity.

○ **What findings in a female patient who presents with parotid gland swelling and eroding tooth enamel might you expect?**

Bulimia, which is associated with elevated levels of serum amylase and hypokalemia

○ **List some common laboratory test findings associated with eating disorders.**

Hyponatremia; hypokalemia; hypocalcemia; hypophosphatemia; anemia; hypoglycemia; starvation ketoacidosis; abnormal glucose tolerance; hypothyroidism due to low triiodothyronine levels; persistently elevated cortisol levels due to starvation; low levels of follicle-stimulating hormone, luteinizing hormone, and estrogens; and elevated levels of growth hormone

○ **What are criteria A through D for the diagnosis of catatonic disorder?**

- A: Manifestations of any of the following: echolalia, echopraxia, excessive purposeless motor activity, motor immobility, extreme negativism, resistance to external instruction or movement, or peculiar involuntary movements such as bizarre posturing or grimacing
- B: Evidence from history, examination, and laboratory findings that the catatonia is a result of a medical condition
- C: Criterion A actions not attributable to another mental condition
- D: Criterion A actions not occurring only during a bout of delirium

○ **The pleasurable effects of cocaine are due to its effect on what?**

Dopamine 2 receptors

○ **What is the treatment for cocaine toxicity?**

Acidify the urine and administer neuroleptics and phentolamine

○ **In infancy, simple repetitive reactions like nail-biting, thumb-sucking, masturbation, or temper tantrums are manifestations of what psychological reaction?**

Adjustment reactions. These are responses to separation from the caregiver and are often associated with developmental delay.

○ **What is the prevalence of conduct disorder?**

10%. It is more common in boys, and it is hereditary.

○ **If untreated, children with conduct disorders may be predisposed to developing what adult disorder?**

Antisocial personality disorder. About 40% of these children will exhibit some disease as adults.

○ **What is conversion disorder?**

An internal psychological conflict that manifests itself through somatic symptoms. Voluntary motor or sensory functions are affected. Examples include weakness, imbalance, dysphagia, and changes in vision, hearing, or sensation. These symptoms are not feigned or intentionally produced. They are also not fully explained by medical conditions.

○ **Delirium is most likely to occur in patients with which types of conditions?**

Those with multiple medical problems, decreased renal function, and a high white blood cell count and in those who use anticholinergics, propranolol, scopolamine, or flurazepam

○ **Describe dementia.**

Disturbed cognitive function that results in impaired memory, personality, judgment, and/or language. Dementia has an insidious onset, or it may manifest as acute worsened mental state when the patient is facing other physical or environmental stressors.

○ **Describe delirium.**

Clouding of consciousness that results in disorientation, decreased alertness, and impaired cognitive function. Acute onset, visual hallucinosis, and fluctuating psychomotor activity are all commonly seen. These symptoms are variable and may change within hours.

○ **Delirium versus dementia: who is more likely to die within a month of onset, and who is more likely to fully recover after onset?**

Patients with delirium are 15% to 30% more likely to die within a month of the onset. They are also more likely to fully recover from their delirium than are patients with dementia.

○ **What are 2 major causes of dementia?**

1. Alzheimer disease
2. Multi-infarction

○ **Name some over-the-counter and street drugs that may produce delirium or acute psychosis.**

Salicylates, antihistamines, anticholinergics, ethanol, phencyclidine, lysergic acid diethylamide (LSD), mescaline, cocaine, and amphetamines

○ **What are 8 common medical causes of depression?**

1. Stroke
2. Viral syndromes
3. Corticosteroids
4. Cushing disease
5. Antihypertensive medication
6. Systemic lupus erythematosus
7. Multiple sclerosis
8. Subcortical dementias, such as Huntington and Parkinson diseases and human immunodeficiency virus encephalopathy

○ **Name some vegetative symptoms.**

Loss of appetite, lack of concentration, chronic fatigue, agitation, restlessness, inability to sleep, and weight loss

○ **What is dysthymia?**

Dysthymia is a chronic mood disorder that last for more than 2 years. The severe symptoms that sometimes accompany depression, such as delusions and hallucinations, are absent. Patients with dysthymia have some good days; they react to their environment, and they have no vegetative signs. Ten percent of patients with dysthymia develop major depression.

○ **Name some symptoms of major depression.**

Remember "IN SAD CAGES."

Interest

Sleep

Appetite

Depressed mood

Concentration

Activity

Guilt

Energy

Suicide

○ **Wild and abundant dreams may result from the withdrawal of what drugs?**

Antidepressants. Other adverse effects of withdrawal are anxiety, akathisia, bradykinesia, mania, and malaise.

○ **What is a dystonic reaction?**

A common adverse effect of neuroleptics seen in the emergency department. It involves muscle spasms of the tongue, face, neck, and back. Severe laryngospasm and extraocular muscle spasms may also occur. Patients may bite their tongues, leading to an inability to open the mouth, tongue edema, or hemorrhage.

○ **How are dystonic reactions treated?**

Diphenhydramine, 25 to 50 mg intramuscularly (IM) or intravenously (IV), or benztropine, 1 to 2 mg IV or by mouth. Remember that dystonias can recur acutely.

○ **What are the 5 Kübler-Ross stages of dying?**

1. Denial
2. Anger
3. Bargaining
4. Depression
5. Acceptance

Patients may undergo all, or only a few, of these stages. Not every person goes through these stages in the same order. These stages may also be experienced by people going through other catastrophic personal losses.

○ **Define the following dyspraxias: ideomotor, kinesthetic, and constructional.**

- Ideomotor: Patient is unable to perform simple motor tasks despite adequate understanding and sensory and motor strength
- Kinesthetic: Patient is unable to position his or her extremities on command despite adequate understanding and sensory and motor strength
- Constructional: Patient cannot copy simple shapes despite adequate understanding and sensory and motor strength

○ **What psychiatric disease is the most hereditary?**

Idiopathic enuresis. If 1 parent has enuresis, there is a 44% chance that the child will also have the disease. If both parents have it, the likelihood increases to 77%.

○ **By what age do most children stop wetting their beds?**

4 years. Thirty percent of 4-year-olds and 10% of 6-year-olds still wet their beds.

○ **What is the medical treatment for idiopathic enuresis?**

Desmopressin nose drops or imipramine. Most cases eventually resolve spontaneously.

○ **What is folie à deux?**

An induced psychotic disorder. A patient who has a close relationship with another patient begins forming the same delusions as that patient.

○ **How should a 12-year-old child who snorts and shouts obscenities be treated?**

With neuroleptics. Gilles de la Tourette syndrome develops in childhood with facial twitches, uncontrollable arm movements, and tics. The condition worsens with adolescence.

○ **A 24-year-old man presents complaining of pleuritic pain, palpitations, dyspnea, dizziness, and tingling in his arms, legs, and lips. What is the diagnosis?**

Hyperventilation syndrome, which is frequently associated with anxiety. The tingling is caused by decreased carbonate levels in the blood. This should always be a diagnosis of exclusion.

○ **A 20-year-old man is brought to your office by a concerned friend. It appears the patient sleeps excessively, has been eating excessively, and is getting into fights at bars whenever he goes out. He also has been hypersexual. What is the diagnosis?**

Kleine-Levin syndrome. It can be treated with stimulants.

○ **Hallucinogens affect what neurotransmitter?**

Serotonin

○ **Olfactory hallucinations are associated with lesions in what areas of the brain?**

The periuncal or the inferior and medial surfaces of the temporal lobe

○ **What does a previously healthy patient most likely have when he becomes suddenly and intensely excited, goes into a delirious mania, develops catatonic features, and develops a high fever?**

Lethal catatonia. Such patients have a 50% death rate without treatment. Treat these patients with electroconvulsive therapy.

○ **How is lethal catatonia differentiated from neuroleptic malignant syndrome?**

By the timing of the hyperthermia. In lethal catatonia, severe hyperthermia occurs during the excitement phase before catatonic features develop. In neuroleptic malignant syndrome, hyperthermia develops later in the course of the disease with the onset of stupor.

○ **What is the treatment for a "bad trip" on LSD?**

Constantly remind patients that their perceptions are only distortions due to the drug. This is called "talking down." Chlorpromazine can be used IM for severe or uncontrollable anxiety.

○ **Who is at a greater risk for mood disorders: men or women?**

Women. The ratio is 7:3.

○ **What state is associated with akinetic mutism?**

Abulic state, which is like coma vigil. Patients seem awake and may have their eyes open. They respond to questions slowly. The cause is typically depressed frontal lobe function.

○ **What is an extreme case of factitious disorder?**

Munchausen syndrome. These patients may actually try to cause harm to themselves (eg, by injecting feces into their veins) and are accepting or seeking of invasive procedures. Munchausen by proxy is another example. In this disease, the patient seeks medical care for another, usually a child.

○ **What laboratory test results would you expect to be elevated in a patient with neuroleptic malignant syndrome?**

Creatine kinase level is usually elevated, which correlates to a higher risk of fatality due to myoglobinuria. Serum alkaline phosphatase and serum aminotransferase levels are elevated. Leukocytosis with a left shift, hyponatremia, and hypokalemia are also present. Treatment for neuroleptic malignant syndrome is with dopaminergic agents, muscle relaxants, discontinuation of neuroleptics, and supportive therapy. The mortality rate is 20%.

○ **Differentiate between low-potency, medium-potency, and high-potency neuroleptics and give examples of drugs in each category.**

Low-potency neuroleptics have greater sedative, postural hypotensive, and anticholinergic effects. High-potency neuroleptics have greater extrapyramidal effects.
- Low potency: Chlorpromazine
- Medium potency: Perphenazine
- High potency: Haloperidol, droperidol, thiothixene, fluphenazine, and trifluoperazine

○ **Why should 600 mg/d of thioridazine not be exceeded?**

Exceeding this dosage causes retinitis pigmentosa. Thioridazine is a piperidine phenothiazine with a low frequency of extrapyramidal effects.

○ **Why is haloperidol 1 of the preferred neuroleptics?**

It can be used IM in emergencies and has few adverse effects. It does, however, have a high frequency of extrapyramidal effects.

○ **What psychiatric disorder is associated with carcinoma of the pancreas?**

Depression

○ **What is the only neuroleptic with tardive dyskinesia as an adverse effect?**

Clozapine. Patients receiving clozapine can develop agranulocytosis and are at higher risk for seizures than are patients receiving other neuroleptics. Other adverse effects include hypotension, anticholinergic symptoms, and oversedation.

○ **You are considering chemical restraint. List your options.**

Benzodiazepines

- Lorazepam, 1 to 2 mg IV, or 2 to 6 mg orally every 30 minutes
- Midazolam, 2 to 4 mg IV every 30 minutes
- Diazepam, 5 mg IV or orally every 30 minutes

Sedative hypnotics

- Haloperidol, 1 to 5 mg IM or IV, titrate to clinical response
- Droperidol, 1 to 2 mg IV every 30 minutes

Benzodiazepines may be administered in combination with the sedative hypnotics to both hasten and potentiate their effect. Titrate to effect and monitor appropriately.

○ **A patient has ingested a phenothiazine and arrives hypotensive. What interventions may be considered?**

IV crystalloid boluses usually suffice. Severe cases are best managed with norepinephrine or metaraminol. These pressors stimulate α-adrenergic receptors preferentially. β-Agonists, such as isoproterenol, are contraindicated owing to the risks of β-receptor-stimulated vasodilatation.

○ **What happens when ethanol is combined with an anxiolytic (eg, benzodiazepine)?**

Death can occur because of their combined respiratory depressive effects.

○ **Name another contraindication to benzodiazepine use.**

Known hypersensitivity, acute narrow-angle glaucoma, and pregnancy (especially in the first trimester)

○ **What should be used to treat a hypertensive crisis caused by the combination of monoamine oxidase inhibitors with a known toxin?**

An α- and β-adrenergic antagonist, such as labetalol. Also consider nifedipine or nitroglycerin. If unsuccessful, consider IV phentolamine or sodium nitroprusside.

○ **Name some drugs contraindicated in a patient receiving monoamine oxidase inhibitors.**

Meperidine and dextromethorphan can cause toxic reactions, such as excitation and hyperpyrexia. The effects of indirect-acting adrenergic drugs are potentiated, including ephedrine, sympathomimetic amines in cold remedies, amphetamines, cocaine, and methylphenidate.

○ **Name the 3 common monoamine oxidase inhibitors (ie, chemical name).**

1. Phenelzine
2. Isocarboxazid
3. Tranylcypromine

○ **Obsessive-compulsive disorders generally begin before what age?**

25 years

○ **What are some common obsessions?**

Dirt and contamination, order and symmetry, religion and philosophy, daily decisions. Compulsion does not relieve the anxiety of the obsession. Serotonin reuptake inhibitors and exposure therapy can be helpful.

○ **A 6-year-old boy consistently wets his pants. You tell his mother to reward the child with treats and praise during dry periods because this will help reinforce the desired behavior. What is this type of conditioning?**

Positive operant conditioning. The basic principles were defined by Ivan Pavlov.

○ **What is organic brain syndrome?**

A reversible or irreversible mental condition believed to be caused by either disease or the use of a substance that interrupts normal anatomic, physiologic, or biochemical brain functions.

○ **A 20-year-old woman complains of sudden episodes of palpitations, diaphoresis, light-headedness, a fear of losing control, a sense of being choked, tremors, and paresthesias. What is the diagnosis?**

Panic disorder. Panic disorders need not be linked to any events, although they are commonly associated with agoraphobia, social phobia, mitral prolapse, and late nonmelancholic depression.

○ **Which is the most common type of paraphilia?**

Pedophilia

○ **Paresis without clonus or anesthesia to midline are examples of what conversion disorder?**

Pseudoneurologic disorder. The findings do not match the medical neuropathophysiology.

○ **What brain system does phencyclidine (PCP) most commonly affect?**

The vestibulocerebellar system. This has a positive analgesic effect. However, the adverse effects, including dizziness, muscular incoordination, nystagmus, delirium, anxiety, irritability, and catalepsy, weigh heavily against any positive effect.

○ **How is a patient with PCP overdose treated?**

Acidify the urine with cranberry juice or ammonium chloride, administer benzodiazepine, and restrain the patient.

○ **Cite an example for each of the following perceptual disturbances: illusion, complete auditory hallucination, functional hallucination, and extracampine hallucination.**

- Illusion: A kitten is perceived as a dragon. (The patient misinterprets reality.)
- Complete auditory hallucination: The patient claims to hear people talking when no one is around. (Clear voices are reportedly heard. They are perceived as being external to the patient.)
- Functional hallucination: The patient hears voices only when cars honk their horns. (Hallucinations occur only after sensory stimulus in the same category as the hallucination.)
- Extracampine hallucination: The patient can see people waving from the top of the Eiffel Tower, even though she is in Chicago. (Hallucinations are external to the patient's normal range of senses.)

○   **What is the most common phobia in men?**

Social phobia

○   **What is the most common specific phobia in children?**

Animal phobia

○   **At what age will a child understand concrete operations as defined by Piaget?**

6 to 12 years. By this age, a child is able to distinguish that a line of 5 pennies all touching is equal to those same 5 pennies spread out into a longer line.

○   **Can a person acquire posttraumatic stress disorder (PTSD) if he or she did not actually witness a disturbing event?**

Yes. According to the *Diagnostic and Statistical Manual of Mental Disorders, Fourth Edition*, one can experience PTSD if an event, such as a violent personal assault, a serious accident, or the serious injury of a close friend or family member, is learned of indirectly. PTSD can also occur after a person hears of a life-threatening disease affecting a friend or family member.

○   **A 28-year-old woman who was raped 6 months ago has been psychologically sound thus far. She now suddenly develops recurrent flashbacks of the rape, nightmares, intense fear, avoidance of all men, a diminished memory of the rape, and an exaggerated startle response. Is this woman experiencing PTSD?**

Yes. This is delayed-onset PTSD. The onset of symptoms occurs at least 6 months after the provoking event.

○   **What are the 5 criteria for brief reactive psychosis?**

1. Precipitating stressful event
2. Rapid onset of the psychosis
3. Affective lability and mood intensity
4. Symptoms that match the stressful event
5. Resolution of symptoms once the stressor is removed, generally within 2 weeks

○   **What brain lesions sites are most commonly associated with psychosis?**

Temporolimbic system, caudate nucleus, and frontal lobes

○   **List some life-threatening causes of acute psychosis.**

Remember "WHHHIMP."

Wernicke encephalopathy

Hypoxia

Hypoglycemia

Hypertensive encephalopathy

Intracerebral hemorrhage

Meningitis or encephalitis

Poisoning

○ **What signs and symptoms suggest an organic source for psychosis.**

Acute onset; disorientation; visual or tactile hallucinations; age younger than 10 years or older than 60 years; and any evidence suggesting overdose, such as abnormal vital signs, pupil size and reactivity, or nystagmus

○ **When are women at the greatest risk for psychiatric illness?**

The first few weeks post partum. A psychiatric illness most often occurs in patients who are primiparous, have poor social support, or have a history of depression.

○ **When does postpartum psychosis begin?**

Within a week to 10 days after childbirth. A second, smaller peak occurs 5 to 7 months later, correlating with the first menses post partum. The risk of psychosis is lowest during pregnancy.

○ **What is the difference between schizophrenia and schizophreniform disorder?**

Schizophreniform disorder has the same signs and symptoms as schizophrenia, but these symptoms have been present for less than 6 months. The impaired functioning in schizophreniform disorder is not consistent. Schizophreniform disorder is generally a provisional diagnosis, with schizophrenia following.

○ **What are some characteristics of schizophrenia?**

Delusional disorder, hallucinations (usually auditory), disorganized thinking, loosening of associations, disheveled appearance, and the inability to realize thoughts and behavior are abnormal

○ **What are the 5 first-rank symptoms of Schneider?**

1. Experiences of influence
2. Thought broadcasting
3. Experiences of alienation
4. Complete auditory hallucinations
5. Delusional perceptions

First-rank symptoms occur in 60% to 75% of patients with schizophrenia. They also develop in patients with affective disorder, more commonly during manic stages.

○ **What are the 5 criteria for diagnosing schizophrenia?**

1. Psychosis
2. Emotional blunting
3. Absence of affective features or episodes
4. Clear consciousness
5. Absence of coarse brain disease, systemic illness, and drug abuse

○ **By what age does the onset of schizophrenia generally occur?**

Eighty percent of patients with schizophrenia develop the disease before their early 20s. The disease is rare after age 40 years.

○ **What are 5 causes of schizophrenia?**

1. Viral infection in the central nervous system
2. Problem during pregnancy that affects neuronal development
3. Head injury
4. Seizure disorder
5. Street drugs

○ **When is the average onset of separation anxiety?**

Age 9 years. Children with separation anxiety fear leaving home, going to sleep, being alone, going to school, and losing their parents; 75% develop somatic complaints to avoid attending school.

○ **Name 8 drugs that decrease sexual desire.**

1. Antidepressants
2. Antihypertensives
3. Anticonvulsants
4. Neuroleptics
5. Digitalis
6. Cimetidine
7. Clofibrate
8. High doses or long-term ingestion of ethanol or street drugs

○ **What sexual orientation will a child reared by a homosexual couple most likely have?**

Heterosexual

○ **How does the insomnia of patients with melancholia differ from that of patients with dysthymia?**

Patients with melancholia have difficulty staying asleep; this is often associated with early morning wakefulness. Patients with dysthymia have trouble falling asleep and have a tendency to oversleep.

○ **Which populations have the greatest incidence of insomnia?**

Women and the elderly. Insomnia can involve trouble falling asleep or trouble staying asleep. It is generally initiated by a stressor in the patient's life.

○ **In which stage of sleep do we spend the most time?**

Stage 2 accounts for 50% of our sleep. This stage is characterized by sleep spindles and K complexes on electroencephalograms. Rapid eye movement (REM) sleep accounts for only 25% of our sleep.

○ **Is somnambulism more common in children or adults?**

Fifteen percent to 30% of children sleepwalk, whereas only 1% of adults do. Sleepwalking begins around age 4 years and generally resolves by age 15 years.

○ **Sleepwalking and pavor nocturnus (night terrors) are disturbances of which stage of sleep?**

Stage 4. A stage 4 sleep depressant, such as a long-acting benzodiazepine, is effective in curbing this behavior.

○ **Narcolepsy is a disorder of which sleep cycle?**

REM sleep. Attacks of sleep, dreams, and paralysis last anywhere from 10 minutes to 1 hour. Amphetamines and planned naps throughout the day can help.

○ **A 30-year-old woman complains of calf pain, a headache, shooting pain when flexing her right wrist, random epigastric pain, bloating, and irregular menses, all of which cannot be explained after medical examination. What is the diagnosis?**

Somatization disorder—many unexplained medical symptoms involving multiple systems. To diagnose somatization disorder, one must have 4 or more unexplained pain symptoms. Symptoms generally begin in childhood and are fully developed by age 30 years. Somatization disorder is more common in women than men.

○ **Major depression and bipolar affective disorder account for what percentage of suicides?**

50%. Another 25% are due to substance abuse, and another 10% are attributed to schizophrenia.

○ **What percentage of patients with melancholia attempt suicide?**

15%

○ **Give examples of the following thought disorders: perseveration, non sequiturs, derailment, tangential speech, neologism, private word usage, and verbigeration.**

- Perseveration: "I've been wondering if the mechanical mechanisms of this machine are mechanically sound. Mechanically speaking, I must understand the mechanisms." (A repetition of certain words or phrases is found in the natural flow of speech.)
- Non sequiturs: Q: "Are you nervous about the upcoming boards?" A: "Why no, the king of France is an excellent king." (The patient's answers are unrelated to the questions asked.)
- Derailment: "I first became interested in the study of medicine after mom bought me a toy ambulance. Toys can be very dangerous, especially if they are very small and can be swallowed. I've been having difficulty swallowing lately." (The patient suddenly switches lines of thought, though the second follows the first.)
- Tangential speech: A: "Those are nice clothes you're wearing today." B: "Of course I'm wearing clothes today." A: "I mean, I like the outfit you have on." B: "I think everyone should wear clothes, except on Friday, because Friday is casual day at my office." (Conversations are on the right subject matter; but the responses are inappropriate to the previous questions or comments.)
- Neologism: "I'm going to explaphrase (explain by paraphrasing) the meaning of agnonoctaudiophobia (things that go bump in the night)." (Neologisms are meaningless combinations of 2 or more words to invent a new word.)
- Private word usage: "I can't believe the loquacious way he is formicating those tripods." (Words and or phrases used in unique ways.)
- Verbigeration: "I have been studying, have been studying, have been studying, for hours for hours hours hours." (The patient repeats words, especially at the end of a thought.)

○ **Define the following: akathisia, echolalia, catalepsy, waxy flexibility, stereotypy, gegenhalten.**

- Akathisia: Internal restlessness. Patients feel as if they are jumping out of their skin.
- Echolalia: Meaningless automatic repetition of someone else's words. This may occur immediately or even months after hearing the words.
- Catalepsy: Patients maintain the same posture for a long time.
- Waxy flexibility: Patients resist changing position, then gradually allow themselves to be moved, much like a clay figure.
- Stereotypy: Patients go through repetitive motions that have no purpose.
- Gegenhalten: Patients resist external manipulation with the same force as that applied.

○ **What psychiatric problems are associated with violence?**

Acute schizophrenia, paranoid ideation, catatonic excitation, mania, borderline and antisocial personality disorders, delusional depression, PTSD, and decompensated obsessive-compulsive disorder

○ **What are the prodromes of violent behavior?**

- Anxiety
- Defensiveness
- Volatility
- Physical aggression

○ **Match the following:**

1. Hypomania	a. 1 or more hypomanias plus 1 or more major depressive symptoms
2. Melancholia	b. A mild manic episode
3. Bipolar II	c. Deep depression and vegetative characteristics
4. Unipolar mania	d. Manic episodes only
5. Cyclothymia	e. Many mild episodes of hypomania and depression

Answers: (1) b, (2) c, (3) a, (4) d, and (5) e

○ **A 27-year-old man arrives somnolent with a pulse of 130 beats per minute, respiration of 26 breaths per minute, blood pressure of 170/80 mm Hg, and temperature 105°F. You note diffuse muscular rigidity and intermittent focal muscle twitching and/or jerking that lasts for 1 to 2 seconds. As you examine the patient, the nurse returns from the waiting area with news from the family that the patient has had a progressive decline in mental status for the last 2 days after seeing his psychiatrist. The patient has had a history of psychosis for almost a year. What process should be included in the differential diagnosis at this time?**

Neuroleptic malignant syndrome

○ **For patients who are experiencing hypertension, what behavioral and lifestyle modifications can help them manage their symptoms?**

The recommended lifestyle modifications for patients with hypertension include the following:

- Regular aerobic exercise
- Weight loss, if overweight
- Limiting ethanol intake to less than 1 oz/d
- Maintaining adequate amounts of dietary calcium, magnesium, and potassium
- Reducing saturated fats and cholesterol in the diet
- Reducing sodium intake to approximately 110 mg/d

○ **True/False: Risk factors for coronary heart disease can include psychological stress and type A behavior pattern.**

True. In addition to known risk factors, such as hypertension, a diet high in fat and cholesterol, diabetes, obesity, and a sedentary lifestyle, emotional stress and the anger and hostility often associated with a type A behavior pattern are considered possible risk factors for coronary heart disease.

○ **What accounts for more than 80% of all physician visits, affecting more than 50 million Americans, and costing more than $70 billion annually in health care costs?**

Pain. The Joint Commission requires that physicians consider pain a fifth vital sign when evaluating patients. In the assessment of the cause of pain, it is important for the physician to understand patient's beliefs, attitudes, and coping styles to effectively manage the patient's pain.

○ **Describe the most common types of headaches and discuss the role that mind-body therapies play in the management of these headaches.**

Migraine and tension-type headaches are commonly experienced by patients seeking care from family physicians. Effective treatment of these headaches includes a combination of medications and alternative therapies. Mind-body therapies, such as biofeedback, hypnosis, cognitive-behavioral therapy, and stress management and relaxation training, significantly reduce the symptoms of these types of headaches.

○ **A mother comes to your office for her 6-week examination after the birth of her first child. She is tearful, appears frustrated, and claims that she does not know why she had the baby. She feels unable to care for the baby and explains that she becomes tense when the baby cries. Explain what the mother is experiencing, what may have contributed to her situation, and what you can do to help her.**

It is likely that she is experiencing postpartum depression (PPD) or major depressive disorder, with postpartum onset. PPD occurs in approximately 10% to 20% of women within a few months after delivery. Symptoms associated with PPD include depressed mood, tearfulness, sleep and appetite problems, feelings of inadequacy, suicidal thoughts, and difficulties with concentration. Risk factors for PPD include hormonal changes, mental illness before pregnancy, marital stress, financial pressures, and limited social support. Some antidepressants, such as sertraline, can be used safely in breastfeeding mothers to help manage the depression. Individual and group psychotherapy are also effective and are often recommended alongside pharmacotherapy for effective treatment.

○ **A patient recently returned from military combat and is showing signs of PTSD. You refer him to a psychologist, who proposes to implement components of cognitive-behavioral therapy. Which of the following aspects of cognitive-behavioral therapy would be the most effective: relaxation training, education about trauma response, assertiveness training, in vivo exposure, or conjoint therapy with a loved one?**

In vivo exposure. With in vivo exposure, the patient is exposed to traumatic memories, cues, and recollections of a traumatic event. When recounting the event, the patient is seeking to reduce emotional and behavioral avoidance and to reestablish a sense of effective coping strategies.

○   **A patient is brought in because she believes butterflies are landing all around her. The butterflies talk to her and tell her to love everyone. She denies suicidal ideation and any desire to harm herself or others. She has no record of harming people in the past. Can this person be institutionalized against her will?**

No. Unless the patient is a danger to herself or others, she cannot be confined to an institution despite questionable mental status.

○   **Hypoactive sexual desire disorder is caused by 1 or more factors from a key triad. What is this triad?**

1. Relationship problems
2. Performance anxiety
3. Fear of the consequences (eg, STDs or pregnancy)

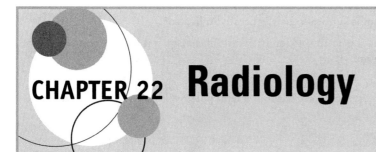

CHAPTER 22 Radiology

William A. Schwer, MD

○ **What is the purpose of ultrasonography (US) gel?**

It displaces air and provides a medium for coupling the probe to the skin surface without impedance mismatching.

○ **What 2 features does duplex US combine?**

1. High-resolution image
2. Doppler capability

○ **When using Doppler US, what audible characteristics differentiate arterial from venous flow?**

Arterial flow is characterized by sharp, brisk changes in pitch throughout the cardiac cycle—higher pitched during peak systole and lower pitched during diastole (ie, multiphasic). Venous flow varies with the respiratory cycle, and venous signals are lower pitched and more consistent throughout the cardiac cycle (ie, monophasic).

○ **What is the diagnostic test of choice for documenting deep vein thrombosis (DVT)?**

Duplex US provides the most accurate radiographic diagnosis of DVT. The accuracy of physical examination for DVT is generally considered 50%.

○ **List some of the advantages and disadvantages of diagnostic peritoneal lavage (DPL), computed tomography (CT), and US for assessing trauma.**

Assessment Procedure	Advantages	Disadvantages
DPL	Low complication rate, performed at bedside	Invasive, time-consuming, cannot show retroperitoneal injury, significant false-positive rate
CT	Shows location and extent of injury, including the retroperitoneum	Expensive, time-consuming, requires travel and interpretation expertise, requires the patient be moved out of the ER, so patient monitoring is not optimal, and interpretation requires radiological expertise
US	Fast, inexpensive, performed at bedside, good for hemoperitoneum	Operator-dependent, not good for identifying specific organ injury

○   **In what size of abdominal aortic aneurysm is surgical repair generally indicated?**

Larger than 4 cm. US is extremely sensitive for detecting abdominal aortic aneurysm, but it is not sensitive for the detecting ruptured abdominal aortic aneurysm.

○   **With what structure can an intrauterine gestational sac without a fetal pole, yolk sac, or cardiac activity be confused?**

The pseudosac of an ectopic pregnancy

○   **What is the primary use of US in women with positive human chorionic gonadotropin test results who present with abdominal pain and/or vaginal bleeding?**

Verification of intrauterine pregnancy. The incidence of simultaneous intrauterine and extrauterine pregnancies is about 1 in 30,000. US may not be able to help verify that ectopic pregnancy exists.

○   **What is the only true diagnostic sign of ectopic pregnancy at US?**

A fetus with cardiac activity outside the uterus. Complex masses and fluid in the cul-de-sac can be seen with other conditions (eg, pelvic abscess and ruptured ovarian cysts).

○   **What is the role of US in detecting placenta previa and placenta abruptio?**

US cannot be used to detect placenta abruptio but can be used to rule out placenta previa in the third trimester.

○   **What is the incidence of allergic reaction to intravenous (IV) contrast materials?**

Severe allergic reactions occur in approximately 1 in 14,000 patients; fatal reactions occur in about 1 in 40,000.

○   **True/False : Oral contrast material should be avoided in patients with marginal renal function.**

False. Little iodine is absorbed when administered in oral contrast material, so any nephrotoxic effect is minimized. Barium is inert and not absorbed at all.

○   **What are contraindications to the use of oral iodine or barium contrast material?**

Barium cannot be administered when complete colon obstruction exists or intestinal perforation is suspected. Severe allergy to iodine is the only contraindication to oral iodine-containing preparations.

○   **True/False: IV contrast material is contraindicated in chronic renal failure.**

False. Contrast material can be removed by means of dialysis, and the kidney is already maximally impaired.

○   **The standard unit for measuring absorbed radiation is the gray (1 J/kg). How many rad are equivalent to 1 Gy?**

100 rad equal 1 Gy

○ **Describe the typical shape and vessel origin of subdural hematoma and epidural hematoma at CT.**
- Subdural hematoma is typically crescent shaped. It can be arterial in origin but is most often caused by the tearing of bridging veins. Acute subdural hematoma is hyperattenuated relative to the brain and becomes isoattenuated to the brain in 1 to 3 weeks.
- Epidural hematoma is biconvex (lenticular) and usually arterial in origin. Epidural hematoma does not cross intact skull sutures but can cross the tentorium and the midline.

○ **What percentage of subdural hematomas are bilateral?**
About 25%

○ **Why does the performance DPL make the evaluation of subsequent CT scans more difficult?**
Air and fluid are introduced during DPL.

○ **What is the test of choice for evaluating and staging renal trauma?**
IV contrast material–enhanced CT. CT is more accurate than intravenous pyelography because intravenous pyelography is not sensitive for renal injuries.

○ **In what circumstances might the magnetic field of magnetic resonance (MR) imaging be detrimental to patients?**
Patients who have any ferrous metal or electrical equipment in their body the function of which can be disrupted by strong magnetic fields. Examples include pacemakers, metal foreign bodies in the eye (eg, welders), ferromagnetic intracerebral aneurysm clips (unless they are made of nonmagnetic steel), and cochlear implants. Relative contraindications for MR imaging include certain prosthetic heart valves, implantable defibrillators, bone growth, and neurostimulators. One might also include patients who are claustrophobic.

○ **Although bone scans are useful for detecting subtle fractures missed at radiography, why is it not always useful for recent fractures?**
Bone scans may not show the increased bone turnover until hours or days after trauma because skeletal uptake depends on blood flow and osteoblastic activity. Positive scan results demonstrate asymmetric skeletal uptake.

○ **Are radionucleotide studies most helpful in determining the bleeding site in upper or lower gastrointestinal bleeding?**
Lower

○ **What 2 studies can depict testicular torsion and differentiate it from epididymitis, orchitis, or torsion of the appendix testis?**
1. Technetium 99m nuclear studies
2. Duplex US

○ **What is the silhouette sign?**
The silhouette sign describes the loss of a normal interface between lung and soft tissue (ie, silhouette) caused by any disease that either replaces or displaces normal air-filled lung. This sign is commonly applied to the heart, mediastinum, chest wall, and diaphragm. The greater the difference in attenuation between 2 adjacent structures, the sharper the distinction will be between them.

○   **Using the silhouette sign, what will be obscured in consolidated right lower lobe pneumonia?**

You will not be able to differentiate the right hemidiaphragm, but the border of the right side of the heart will be seen through the consolidation because the right middle lobe is entirely anterior as is the heart.

○   **How is osteoporosis defined?**

Osteoporosis is defined as bone mineral density greater than 2.5 standard deviations from the young adult mean.

○   **Does systemic hypertension increase the risk of vascular complications from arteriography?**

Yes. At withdrawal of the catheter, compression above the arterial systolic pressure is required to affect hemostasis. Systemic hypertension, particularly in the obese patient, makes bleeding at the puncture site more likely.

○   **Do ultrasound waves travel more quickly in fat or in watery soft tissue?**

Ultrasound waves travel approximately 20% more slowly in fat. This makes the depth of echoes that are deep to large fatty regions appear further from the probe than they actually are.

○   **During what period of development is the fetus most sensitive to irradiation?**

Gestation at 8 to 15 weeks is when the rate of proliferation of DNA is at a maximum, making the fetus most sensitive to radiation.

○   **How long after iodine 131 scanning are women advised to avoid pregnancy?**

The recommended delay is 4 months.

○   **How frequently do pleural effusions coincide with cases of pulmonary embolism?**

Pleural effusions occur in 25% to 50% of pulmonary emboli.

○   **What is the most common chest wall tumor seen at radiography?**

Lipoma

○   **What is the most common malignant rib tumor?**

The most common malignant rib tumors are from metastatic disease or multiple myeloma.

○   **What is the most common type of pleural neoplasm?**

The pleural space is a common site of metastasis for adenocarcinomas of the ovary, stomach, breast, and lung.

○   **Which hemidiaphragm is higher at chest radiography in most people?**

The right hemidiaphragm is higher by 15 to 30 mm in 90% of people, most likely due to elevation by the liver.

○   **What characteristic feature at chest radiography indicates *Klebsiella pneumoniae* infection?**

Lobar expansion at chest radiography is considered a characteristic feature of *K pneumoniae* infection.

○ **What does chest radiography reveal in cases of tuberculosis?**

Cavitation of the right upper lobe. Lower lung infiltrates, hilar adenopathy, atelectasis, and pleural effusion are also common, although as many as 5% of patients may have normal results at chest radiography.

○ **What is the characteristic finding of *Mycoplasma pneumoniae* at chest radiography?**

Consolidation of 1 lobe is common, and bilateral or multilobular involvement frequently is observed with pneumonia caused by *M pneumoniae*.

○ **Is panlobular or centrilobular emphysema associated with α₁-antitrypsin deficiency?**

Panlobular emphysema is classically associated with α_1-antitrypsin deficiency and is most severe in the lower lobes.

○ **What is the most sensitive radiographic test for the detection of lymph node invasion in bronchogenic carcinoma?**

The sensitivity and specificity of positron emission tomography for the detection of lymph node invasion in bronchogenic carcinoma exceeds 80%, considerably better than either CT or MR imaging.

○ **What are the causes of an enlarged left atrium?**
- Left atrial myxoma
- Atrial septal defect
- Mitral regurgitation
- Patent ductus arteriosus
- Hypertrophic obstructive cardiomyopathy

○ **Which of the following does not cause an enlarged right ventricle: pulmonary regurgitation, pulmonary arteriovenous malformations, right-to-left shunt, left-sided heart failure, or chronic pulmonary emboli?**

All except right-to-left shunt cause right ventricular hypertrophy.

○ **What are the recognized causes of pancreatic calcification?**

Insulinoma
Hyperparathyroidism
Cavernous lymphangioma
Acute pancreatitis

○ **Which radiographic test is best for identifying a normal appendix?**

The normal appendix is seen more frequently at CT, which is the key advantage of CT over US.

○ **What percentage of gallstones is visible on a plain abdominal radiograph?**

Only as many as 20% of gallstones contain enough calcium to be visible on a plain abdominal radiograph.

○ **What percentage of renal calculi is visible on a plain abdominal radiograph of the kidneys, ureter, and bladder?**

Eighty percent of renal calculi contain calcium, making them radiopaque at plain radiography.

○ **What are some of the causes of contrast medium nephrotoxicity?**

- Dehydration
- High osmolality of the contrast material
- Diabetic nephropathy
- Myeloma

○ **At CT or MR imaging, where in the brain are the most common sites of hemorrhage due to hypertension?**

The most common sites of bleeding from hypertension occur in the basal ganglia, thalamus, and pons.

○ **What organism is the most common cause of brain abscess?**

Streptococcus

○ **During examination of a lateral radiograph of an adult cervical spine, the predental space looks particularly wide. What width is normal for an adult?**

2.5 to 3 mm. If the space is greater than 3 mm, consider that the transverse ligament has ruptured or is at least lax.

○ **When evaluating a radiograph of a pediatric cervical spine, what are the normal values?**

The predental space in a child is smaller than 5 mm. The posterior cervical line attaching the base of the spinous process of C1 to C3 should be considered. If the base of the C2 spinous process lies more than 2 mm behind the posterior cervical line, a hangman fracture should be suspected. The distance from the anterior border of C2 to the posterior wall of the fornix is less than 7 mm. Finally, the distance from the anterior border of C6 to the posterior wall of the trachea is 14 mm in children younger than 15 years; it is less than 22 mm in an adult.

○ **How is laryngeal fracture diagnosed at plain radiography?**

On a lateral soft-tissue radiograph of the cervical spine, check for retropharyngeal air and elevation of the hyoid bone. The hyoid bone is usually at the level of C3 if there is no evidence of a laryngeal fracture. Elevation of the hyoid bone above C3 suggests a laryngeal fracture.

○ **What is the best view of the zygomatic arch on a face radiograph?**

The modified basal view. This is also called the "jug-handle," "submental-occipital," or "submental-vertical" view.

○ **What is the differential diagnosis of a ring lesion at CT?**

Toxoplasmosis, lymphoma, fungal infection, tuberculosis, cytomegalovirus, Kaposi sarcoma, or hemorrhage

○ **An anteroposterior radiograph of the hand shows a triangular lunate bone. What is the diagnosis?**

Dislocation of the lunate bone. Lateral radiographs reveal what resembles a cup spilling water.

○ **What radiographic view is required to diagnose perilunate dislocation?**

Lateral view

○ **In a boxers fracture, how much angulation of the fifth metacarpal neck is acceptable?**

No more than 50°

○ **Posterior dislocation of the shoulder is often missed with a standard radiographic shoulder series. What radiographic view aids in this diagnosis?**

The scapular Y view

○ **At radiography of the elbow, you find a posterior fat pad sign. What is the diagnosis?**

Occult fracture, such as a supracondylar fracture of the humerus. Posterior fat pad seen on a lateral radiograph of the flexed elbow is usually due to hemarthrosis caused by a fracture.

○ **What are the most common findings of osteomyelitis at radiography?**

- Periosteal elevation
- Demineralization

○ **What are the radiographic findings in ischemic bowel disease?**

Thumbprinting at plain radiography, with a ground-glass appearance and absence of bowel gas

○ **Describe Kerley A and B lines.**

- Kerley A lines are straight, nonbranching lines in the upper lung fields.
- Kerley B lines are horizontal, nonbranching lines at the periphery of the lower lung fields.

○ **What is the order of appearance of congestive heart failure at chest radiography?**

Initially, cephalization and the redistribution of blood flow is observed, with the subsequent appearance of interstitial edema with evident Kerley B lines, as well as perihilar haze. These findings are followed by alveolar infiltrates in the typical butterfly appearance. Finally, flagrant pulmonary edema and effusions become evident.

○ **On an upright chest radiograph, what is the earliest sign of left ventricular failure?**

Apical redistribution of the pulmonary vasculature

○ **What contrast material–enhanced radiographic findings are associated with Crohn disease?**

Segmental involvement of the colon with an abnormal mucosal pattern and fistulas, often without involvement of the rectum. Narrowing of the small intestine may also be visible.

○ **How does chronic pericardial effusion appear at chest radiography?**

Gradual pericardial sac distension results in a water bottle appearance of the heart

○ **What common finding on a sinus radiograph suggests basilar skull fracture?**

Blood in the sphenoid sinus

○ **Describe a hangman fracture.**

It is a C2 bilateral pedicle fracture.

CHAPTER 23

Preventive Medicine and Biostatistics

Steven K. Rothschild, MD

O **What conditions must exist for screening programs to be appropriate?**

- The disease must have a significant effect on quality and/or duration of life.
- The disease must have a long asymptomatic period in which it can be discovered before the individual becomes sick.
- The screening test must be acceptable to the population.
- The screening test must have relatively low risk.
- Further workup after positive screening test results must have acceptable risk, given the number of false-positive test results.
- Treatment during the asymptomatic period must lead to better morbidity and mortality than waiting for symptoms to develop.

O **How is the prevalence of a disease determined?**

A cohort study is needed in which a population sample is selected and the number of people within that cohort who have the disease at a given point or period in time is determined. Repeated measures are not necessary because that would be used to identify new cases, or incidence.

O **Differentiate between type I and type II errors.**

Type I error is the likelihood of a false-positive result for a study, meaning that the study suggests that 1 treatment is better than another when no real difference exists. If 1 treatment really is better than another, but the study failed to detect that difference, it is a type II error.

When a statement indicates $P <.05$, this is another way of saying that the likelihood that a measured difference is due to random chance is less than 5% or that the likelihood of type I error is less than 5%.

O **What is the difference between Medicaid and Medicare?**

- Medicaid is a means-tested insurance program administered by the states. Each state determines its own qualifications for Medicaid, but in general Medicaid is available only to low-income individuals who also fit into a specific eligibility group recognized by state and federal law. Such groups include children, pregnant women, the disabled or blind, and the elderly.
- Medicare is not means tested. Every adult older than 65 years receives Medicare regardless of income or health status. Adults with end-stage renal disease and certain disabilities also qualify. Medicare is administered by the federal government.

○ **What is the difference between Medicare Parts A, B, and D?**

- Medicare part A is hospital insurance that begins when an individual reaches the age of 65 years. Most people do not pay a premium for part A because they or their spouse paid into the Medicare system through payroll taxes. In addition to hospital inpatient care, part A will pay for short-term rehabilitation stays in a skilled nursing facility, hospice care, and some home health services.
- Medicare part B is medical insurance. This requires paying an additional monthly premium. Part B pays for doctor bills and other outpatient care when they are medically necessary. Under the law, individuals who do not purchase part B coverage when it first becomes available to them may pay a premium if they wish to buy it later in life.
- Medicare part D is prescription drug coverage, a new feature that began in 2006. Individuals must pay a monthly premium and select from any private insurance company that provides coverage. Under the law, individuals who do not purchase part D coverage when it first becomes available to them may pay a premium if they wish to buy it later in life.

○ **What is the difference between a deductible and a copayment?**

- A deductible is the amount of health care cost that the individual must pay each year before the insurance, whether private or public, begins to pay for medical care bills. Once the deductible is reached, the insurance may not pay for 100% of all costs.
- A copayment is that portion of a medical bill that the individual must pay for and may be set as either a flat rate (eg, $20 for all outpatient appointments) or a percentage of charges.

○ **What are the 3 components of the epidemiologic triad?**

- Agent: The fundamental cause of the disease (eg, *Streptococcus* in pneumonia or asbestos in mesothelioma)
- Host: The individual (ie, each person has varying levels of susceptibility to illness, so 2 individuals exposed to the same agent may not develop the same illness)
- Environment: Factors, such as temperature, crowding, or access to resources, that can increase or decrease susceptibility to illness

○ **From 2000 to 2007, 8 people per 1000 had a diagnosis of disease X each year. Starting in 2008, 12 people per 1000 had the diagnosis. List 3 possible reasons for this apparent increase in the incidence of disease X.**

1. There was an outbreak of the disease.

2. A new test was developed that allowed the disease to be diagnosed in more people.

3. Scientists developed new criteria for the diagnosis of X that included more patients.

○ **A disease is considered an epidemic when it occurs at a higher rate than usual in a population. When is a disease considered endemic?**

When it is typically present at a high rate in a population. For example, some might consider overweight and obesity to be endemic in the US population at present.

○ **For death certificates, distinguish the following terms: manner of death, immediate cause of death, and underlying cause of death.**

- The manner of death is the immediate context of the death (eg, natural causes, accident, suicide, or homicide). Typically, the medical examiner must certify deaths deemed not to be of natural causes.
- The immediate cause of death is the final diagnosis leading to the individual's death, listed as specifically as possible. Note that physicians can no longer list "cardiac arrest" or "old age" as a cause of death.
- The underlying cause of death is the underlying disease that ultimately resulted in death. For example, for a patient who died of gangrene (the immediate cause), diabetes mellitus might be the underlying cause of death.

○ **List the top 10 causes of death in the United States today.**

Ranking	Cause	Percentage of all Deaths (%)
1	Heart disease	27.2
2	Cancer	23.1
3	Cerebrovascular disease	6.3
4	Chronic lower respiratory diseases	5.1
5	Accidents (unintentional injury)	4.7
6	Diabetes mellitus	3.1
7	Alzheimer disease	2.8
8	Influenza and pneumonia	2.5
9	Nephritis, nephrotic syndrome, and nephrosis	1.8
10	Septicemia	1.4

○ **According to the US Centers for Disease Control and Prevention (CDC), what are the major actual causes of death (ie, the external, modifiable, nongenetic factors that contribute to death) in the United States?**

Ranking	Cause	Percentage of all Deaths (%)*
1	Tobacco	18.1
2	Poor diet and physical inactivity	16.6
3	Ethanol consumption	3.5
4	Microbial agents	3.1
5	Toxic agents	2.3
6	Motor vehicles	1.8
7	Firearms	1.2
8	Sexual behavior	0.8
9	Illicit drug use	0.7

*Note that these modifiable risk factors account for approximately 48.1% of all US deaths.

○   **Why is it necessary for death rates to be age adjusted?**

It is necessary to adjust for age because the incidence of many diseases increases with advanced age. A larger percentage of men in Florida might die from prostate cancer than in Utah in any given year, but with a median age of 39.3 years, men in Florida are, on average, more than 11 years older than men in Utah, where the median age is 28 years. If the death rate is adjusted so that the rate mathematically recalculated as though the age distribution in both states were the same as the death rate in the United States as a whole, Utah's age-adjusted death rate appears higher: 169.4 deaths per 100,000 lives versus Florida's 127.0 deaths per 100,000 lives.

○   **A town in the United States has a population of 10,000 people. Fifty people have a diagnosis of active tuberculosis, and in the last year, 5 people died of tuberculosis. If possible, calculate prevalence, incidence, mortality rate, and case-fatality rate by using these data.**

Prevalence: 0.5%   (50 cases divided by a population of 10,000)
Mortality rate: 0.05%   (5 deaths per 10,000)
Case-fatality rate: 10%   (5 deaths per 50 people with the disease)
Incidence cannot be calculated with these data.

○   **What is the difference between absolute risk reduction and relative risk reduction?**

Assume that for men older than 50 years with uncontrolled blood pressure, there is a 12% chance of having a myocardial infarction (MI) in the next 10 years. If the blood pressure is lowered below 130/80 mm Hg, the 10-year risk is reduced to 8%. The absolute risk reduction is 4%, and the relative risk reduction is 33%.

○   **In the preceding example, what is the number needed to treat?**

The number needed to treat is the number of patients who would have to have their blood pressure lowered to prevent just 1 heart attack in the next 10 years. In the example above, one would need to lower the blood pressure of 25 men to prevent 1 heart attack (ie, the number needed to treat is 25). This is calculated as the reciprocal of the absolute risk reduction, or 1 divided by 0.04.

○   **What does a κ statistic tell you, and how is it calculated?**

A κ statistic is a way to express interrater reliability or the likelihood that 2 observers or tests would reach the same conclusion. It is calculated as follows:

$$\frac{(\text{percent agreement observed}) - (\text{percent agreement expected by chance})}{100\% - (\text{percent agreement expected by chance})}$$

○   **A newly developed test is said to help detect colorectal polyps with a sensitivity of 95% and specificity of 90%. Approximately 10% of adults older than 50 years have such polyps. What are the positive predictive value and the negative predictive value of this new test?**

The positive predictive value is 51.3%.
The negative predictive value is 99.3%.

○ **Men with prostate cancer detected by means of positive prostate-specific antigen (PSA) test results live longer after receiving the diagnosis than do men who have prostate cancer detected by means of digital rectal examination. Results from 2 recent randomized clinical trials of the PSA test failed to show any difference in survival for men who underwent PSA testing and those who did not. How can this failure of the PSA test be explained?**

This is an example of lead-time bias. Lead-time bias occurs when survival from the time of diagnosis increases without the patient actually living longer.

Think of lead-time bias this way. Two cars are next to each other at a red light, and both drivers are looking for a gas station because their gas tanks are on empty. One sees the sign for the gas station up ahead, and it takes her 5 minutes to drive there. The driver next to her is driving the exact same speed, but he does not see the gas station sign until 2 minutes later, so once he sees the station it only takes him 3 minutes to get there. The distance was the same for both drivers, but for the first 1 it was 5 minutes away, and for the second 1 it was 3 minutes away.

○ **What is the difference between lead-time bias and length-biased sampling?**

In lead-time bias, screening appears to increase survival time but in reality only increases the amount of time someone knows he or she has a disease. In length-biased sampling, the disease detected with screening is typically less aggressive than the disease detected without screening. A slow-growing tumor will exist for much longer—and will be more likely to be discovered at screening—than will a rapidly growing tumor.

○ **What is the recommended maximum amount of sodium an adult should consume daily?**

Current guidelines suggest that healthy adults should consume no more than 2300 mg/d. This is approximately 1 teaspoon of salt per day.

However, it is important to recognize that more than two-thirds of adults are in a category in which restrictions are greater. The CDC recommends that adults older than 40 years, African Americans, and anyone with hypertension should limit sodium to no more than 1500 mg/d.

○ **What is the DASH diet?**

"DASH" stands for "Dietary Approaches to Stop Hypertension" and has been promoted by the National Heart Lung and Blood Institute of the US National Institutes of Health to control hypertension. Besides limitation of sodium intake, the diet recommends consumption of whole grains, fruits and vegetables, fish and chicken, low-fat dairy products, beans, and nuts. The diet limits consumption of red meats, sugar, fast foods, and processed foods.

○ **Approximately how many calories a day does a moderately active 45-year-old man need to maintain current weight: 1800–2000, 2100–2300, 2400–2600, 2700–2900, or 3000–3200?**

2400–2600 calories a day. For a woman of the same age, and a comparable activity level, maintenance caloric intake is about 2000 calories a day.

○ **What are the recommended blood pressure and lipid targets for persons with type 2 diabetes mellitus?**

Patients with diabetes should be treated to achieve blood pressure below 130/80 mm Hg, low-density lipoprotein cholesterol level below 100 mg/dL, high-density lipoprotein cholesterol level above 50 mg/dL, and triglyceride level below 150 mg/dL.

○ **What vaccines are contraindicated in immunocompromised persons, such as HIV-positive persons with cluster of differentiation 4 cell counts below 200?**

Live virus vaccines should be avoided in persons with immunocompromising conditions. These include measles-mumps-rubella, varicella, and zoster vaccines.

○ **What immunizations are recommended for persons with cochlear implants?**

Because of findings of increased risk of meningitis due to *Streptococcus pneumoniae* among children with cochlear implants, the CDC recommends immunization with 7-valent pneumococcal conjugate and 23-valent pneumococcal polysaccharide vaccines.

Additional vaccines can protect against other bacterial causes of meningitis: *Haemophilus influenzae* type b conjugate and meningococcal tetravalent vaccines.

○ **What are the documented risks and benefits associated with hormone replacement therapy in postmenopausal women?**

According to the findings of the Women's Health Initiative, a group of clinical trials and observational studies conducted in more than 161,000 women, estrogen plus progestin therapy (compared to placebo therapy) was associated with increased risk of heart attack, increased risk of stroke, increased risk of blood clots, and increased risk of breast cancer. Benefits of estrogen plus progestin therapy included reduced risk of colorectal cancer and fewer fractures.

Compared with placebo, estrogen therapy alone resulted in increased risk of stroke and increased risk of blood clots. There was no difference in the risk for heart attack or colorectal cancer. The effect on breast cancer risk was uncertain. Benefits of estrogen therapy alone included a reduced risk of fracture.

○ **What percentage of the US population is homeless?**

It is difficult to determine consistent statistics because the population varies over time. The period prevalence, meaning the number of people who are likely to experience homelessness during a defined period, is a more useful statistic. The most reliable study results suggest that 3.5 million Americans are likely to experience homelessness in a given year, making up approximately 1% of the US population.

○ **What percentage of the US homeless population is composed of families?**

Families with children constitute approximately one-third of the homeless population. They are thought by many to be the most rapidly growing population among the homeless.

○ **What vaccines should be considered in persons older than 65 years?**
- Pneumococcal polysaccharide (1 time)
- Zoster (1 time)
- Tetanus-diphtheria (every 10 years)
- Influenza (annually)

○ **Which of the following statements about the US Vaccine Adverse Event Reporting System (VAERS) is true?**

1. **All adverse events should be independently verified by local health authorities before reporting to the CDC.**
2. **It is appropriate to report mild uncomplicated events such as low-grade fever or rashes.**
3. **Events should only be reported to VAERS if it is reasonably certain that they were caused by a vaccine.**
4. **Vaccine-related injuries and compensation are not defined by the VAERS system.**

2. VAERS provides definitions of events that must be reported by law. However, any provider or patient can report any suspected event to VAERS. The system defines events that qualify for compensation under the no-fault Vaccine Injury Compensation Program.

○　**Smoking cigarettes doubles the incidence of coronary artery disease (CAD). How long does it take after someone quits smoking before the relative risk of CAD decreases to that of nonsmokers?**

The relative risk decreases to that of nonsmokers within 3 years.

○　**True/False: All adults without symptoms who are older than 50 years should be screened at least once for type 2 diabetes.**

False. Screening for diabetes is recommended only in adults without symptoms with sustained blood pressures higher than 135/80 mm Hg. For these patients, a new diagnosis of diabetes would result in more intensive treatment to reduce the risk of heart disease.

○　**What are the components of metabolic syndrome?**

Several definitions exist at present. The American Heart Association definition says a person has metabolic syndrome when at least 3 of the following 5 conditions are present:

1. Elevated waist circumference: In men, 40 in (102 cm) or larger; in women, 35 in (88 cm) or larger

2. Elevated triglyceride levels: 150 mg/dL or higher

3. Low levels of high-density lipoprotein ("good") cholesterol: In men, lower than 40 mg/dL; in women, lower than 50 mg/dL

4. Elevated blood pressure: 130/85 mm Hg or higher

5. Elevated fasting glucose levels: 100 mg/dL or higher

○　**How much does metabolic syndrome increase the risk of CAD?**

Metabolic syndrome is present in about 20% of the US population and is estimated to double the risk of cardiovascular events. Persons with metabolic syndrome have approximately 5 times the risk of developing type 2 diabetes.

○　**In 1950, the age-adjusted death rate for heart disease in the United States was 586.8 per 100,000 residents. In 2005, the rate was only 211.1 per 100,000 residents. What are the major causes of this reduction?**

Although improvements in the treatment of CAD have contributed somewhat to the reduction, the major causes are reduction in the prevalence of smoking, increased physical activity, and improved dietary habits. Treatment of hypertension and high cholesterol have also contributed.

○　**True/False: Fewer than 6% of teenage girls have eating disorders.**

False. In the Youth Risk Behavior Surveillance System (YRBSS), 18.8% of girls in 9th through 12th grades reported fasting at least 24 hours to try to control their weight; 10.9% reported use of diet pills, and 7.5% used vomiting or laxatives.

○　**For a child or adult with sickle cell anemia, which of the following is not a recommended precaution?**
1. **Lizards would be poor pets because of the risk of salmonella exposure.**
2. **Do not drink raw milk or other unpasteurized dairy products.**
3. **Physical activity at high altitude should be avoided.**
4. **Avoid regular use of antibiotics because this may lead to resistance.**

Daily use of penicillin is recommended between the ages of 2 months and 5 years to reduce the risk of infections.

○ **Which age group is at highest risk of developing rheumatic fever as a result of group A β-hemolytic streptococcal infections: infants younger than 3 months, children aged 3 to 18 years, adults aged 19 to 65 years, or adults older than 65 years?**

Children aged 3 to 18 years. Rheumatic fever is rare in infants in the United States. Initial attacks of rheumatic fever are uncommon in adults, but there can be recurrences in those with a history of it.

○ **What medication is the best treatment for preventing nephropathy in diabetic patients?**

Angiotensin-converting enzyme inhibitors or angiotensin II receptor blockers. They reduce the onset of end-stage renal disease, dialysis, and transplants by 50%.

○ **A nonsmoking 56-year-old woman with no symptoms and no significant risk factors who is in a mutually monogamous relationship seeks primary care. What preventive services are recommended?**

- Screening for obesity, high blood pressure, lipid levels, depression, and ethanol misuse
- Mammographic screening for breast cancer by and screening for colonic cancer
- Recommendation of using of aspirin to prevent cardiovascular disease
- Behavioral counseling regarding ethanol and healthy diet

○ **What are the known risks of long-term exposure to secondhand cigarette smoke?**

According to the CDC, nonsmokers who are exposed to secondhand smoke at home or work increase their heart disease risk by 25% to 30%. Lung cancer risk is increased by an estimated 20% to 30%. Children exposed to secondhand smoke have increased risk of sudden infant death syndrome, acute respiratory infections, ear problems, and more frequent and severe asthma attacks.

○ **Which of the following statements about smoking relapse among untreated smokers (those who try to quit on their own) is true?**

1. **Most relapses occur between 30 and 60 days after quitting.**
2. **Approximately 20% will continue abstinence 6 months after quitting.**
3. **Fifty percent of all smokers will at some point in their lives quit smoking successfully.**
4. **Fewer than 10% of all smokers attempt to quit on their own each year.**

3. 41% of smokers try to quit each year, and 72% of those attempts are without assistance from physicians or other treatment. Most will relapse within 8 days. Among ever smokers (those who have smoked at least 100 cigarettes in their lives), however, more than 50% will ultimately become nonsmokers.

○ **Which of the following statements about adolescent sexuality in the United States is false?**

1. **Approximately 1 in 10 sexually active teens contracts a sexually transmitted infection each year.**
2. **A total of 47.8% of high school students report having ever engaged in sexual activity.**
3. **Between 1991 and 2007, the percentage of adolescents who report having ever engaged in sexual activity decreased.**
4. **More than 85% of adolescents report receiving information about HIV and AIDS in school.**

1. An estimated 1 in 4 sexually active adolescents contracts a sexually transmitted infection each year.

○ **What antibiotics should be prescribed for a child who is a close contact (household contact or playmate) of a child with meningococcal meningitis?**

Rifampin, ciprofloxacin, and ceftriaxone are approved for use as chemoprophylaxis for close contacts.

○   **What population is at greatest risk of contracting meningococcal meningitis?**

1. **Children aged 3 to 5 years in day-care settings**

2. **College freshmen living in dormitories**

3. **Adults aged 21 to 50 years working in health care**

4. **Adults older than 80 years living in nursing homes**

2. College freshmen in dormitories have a rate of 5.1 per 100,000; students should be immunized before leaving for college.

○   **The CDC travel Web site recommends malaria prophylaxis with primaquine for travelers going to rural Limón province in Costa Rica. What are the contraindications to using this medication?**

Primaquine cannot be used by women who are pregnant or breastfeeding. It cannot be used in patients who have known glucose-6-phosphate dehydrogenase (G6PD) deficiency or those who have not yet been tested for G6PD deficiency. Testing is mandatory before prescribing primaquine.

○   **What preventive measures would you recommend to a patient planning a trip to Mexico that included Mexico City, as well as hiking and camping in rural areas along the border with Guatemala?**

- Immunizations: Hepatitis A, hepatitis B, typhoid, and rabies
- Pack: Sunblock, antibacterial hand sanitizer, insect repellant, bed nets treated with permethrin, bismuth subsalicylate, and over-the-counter antidiarrheal agents
- Chemoprophylaxis against malaria: Consult the CDC Web site to determine local resistance patterns.
- Water: Drink only bottled, boiled, or carbonated water. If this is not possible, use iodine tablets or portable water filters to purify tater. Avoid tap water, fountain drinks, and ice cubes.

○   **A friend is headed to Benin on the west coast of Africa. What immunizations and prophylactic treatments must she receive before departing?**

In addition to confirming that she is current with routine adult vaccinations (measles-mumps-rubella, diphtheria-pertussis-tetanus), she should receive the following:

- Hepatitis A vaccine
- Hepatitis B vaccine
- Inactivated or oral polio vaccine
- Typhoid vaccine
- Rabies vaccine
- Yellow fever vaccine
- Meningococcal vaccine
- Malaria chemoprophylaxis (not chloroquine)

○   **How is *Norovirus* spread?**

Norovirus (formerly known as the "Norwalk agent") can be spread person to person via the fecal-oral route or through contaminated airborne droplets, food, water, environmental surfaces, and fomites.

○   **What percentage of American adults are obese?**

26.7%. Another 36.5% are considered overweight, with a body mass index (BMI) of 25.0 to 29.9 kg/m^2. Currently, only 1 state (Colorado) has a prevalence of obesity lower than 20%.

○ **Under what conditions could BMI higher than 30 kg/m² be considered normal or healthy?**

BMI is an unreliable tool in body builders and in pregnant women. Also, paradoxically prolonged survival rates among obese persons have been found in some with congestive heart failure or peripheral arterial disease or those undergoing hemodialysis. This finding, however, may be artifactual because patients tend to lose weight as these illnesses progress and their health deteriorates.

○ **Which medications can cause weight gain?**

Treatments for diabetes, including insulin, sulfonylureas, and thiazolidinediones; certain psychiatric medications, including antipsychotics, lithium, and tricyclic antidepressants; corticosteroids; some anticonvulsants (phenytoin and valproate); and hormonal contraceptives

○ **Obesity is a risk factor for what common diseases?**

CAD, type 2 diabetes, hypertension, left ventricular hypertrophy, sleep apnea, cholelithiasis, pulmonary emboli, and osteoarthritis

○ **What is a 26-year-old's estimated target heart rate during exercise?**

Between 126 and 175 beats per minute. The target heart rate is 65% to 90% of the maximal heart rate. Maximal heart rate is 220 minus age.

○ **For an adult at an increased risk for coronary heart disease (CHD) events, such as MI, the US Preventive Services Task Force recommends which of the following screenings?**

1. **Annual resting echocardiogram**
2. **Exercise treadmill stress test every 3 to 5 years**
3. **Transthoracic echocardiogram every 5 to 10 years**
4. **Electron beam CT for coronary calcium every 10 years**
5. **The Task Force does not recommend for or against any routine screening for CHD.**

5. The Task Force does not recommend for or against any routine screening for CHD. The US Preventive Services Task Force finds insufficient evidence to recommend for or against any of the currently available screening methods for the prediction of risk in adults at high risk of CHD. For adults at low risk, the Task Force found evidence to recommend against screening.

○ **Which immunizations do healthy adults older than 65 years need?**

Tetanus booster every 10 years, influenza vaccination every year, and onetime immunizations with zoster (shingles) vaccine and pneumococcal vaccine

○ **How much aspirin should be taken daily to reduce the risk of CHD or stroke?**

The optimal dose has not been definitively established, but current recommendations call for 75 mg daily or 325 mg every other day. For men, aspirin is associated with a 32% relative risk reduction for MI, but with no effect on strokes or all-cause mortality. In contrast, for women, aspirin is associated with a 17% reduction in relative risk of stroke but has no effect on MI or all-cause mortality. The US Preventive Services Task Force recommends aspirin for healthy men aged 45 to 79 years and healthy women aged 55 to 79 years.

○ **Besides aspirin use, what actions can be taken to prevent stroke in patients with increased risk factors?**

- Control of blood pressure
- Control of diabetes
- Control of cholesterol levels
- Not smoking cigarettes
- Treating atrial fibrillation, either by means of cardioversion to sinus rhythm or long-term anticoagulation with warfarin
- Engaging in moderate physical activity at least 30 minutes on most days
- Adhering to a diet low in sodium and saturated fats
- Maintaining a healthy weight

○ **Of the currently available antiviral medications effective against *Influenzavirus*, which are effective in the treatment of both *Influenzavirus A* and *Influenzavirus B*?**

Oseltamivir and zanamivir are both approved to treat *Influenzavirus A* and *Influenzavirus B* infection. Oseltamivir can be used in people aged 1 year or older, whereas zanamivir is approved for treatment in people aged 7 years or older. Amantadine and rimantadine are approved only against *Influenzavirus A*.

○ **When should the influenza vaccine be administered?**

In September, or as soon as vaccine becomes available. Seasonal outbreaks typically peak around January but can occur as early as October.

○ **What is a contraindication to the use of the nasal-spray influenza vaccine?**

The nasal-spray flu vaccine is a live attenuated virus. It is approved for any healthy person between the ages of 2 and 49 years. It should not be administered in anyone who is pregnant or anyone who takes care of a person who is immunocompromised.

○ **How many milligrams of folic acid should a pregnant woman, or one who is planning to become pregnant, take on a daily basis?**

400 to 800 μg daily to reduce the risk of neural tube defects

○ **When should Rho(D) immune globulin (anti-Rh immunoglobulin) be used during pregnancy?**

In Rh-negative women at 28 weeks of gestation and again within 3 days after birth if the child is Rh positive. It should also be used in the event of any mixing of fetal and maternal blood, as might occur during a spontaneous miscarriage.

○ **What conditions should be routinely screened for in all newborns?**

- Hypothyroidism
- Phenylketonuria
- Sickle cell anemia

○ **What findings at preparticipation sports physical examination should alert the physician to the possibility of hypertrophic obstructive cardiomyopathy? Why is this important?**

Hypertrophic obstructive cardiomyopathy is 1 of the most common causes of sudden cardiac death in young athletes. Physicians should inquire about family history of hypertrophic obstructive cardiomyopathy or any history of dyspnea, angina, or syncope in the child. Although cardiac examination results are often completely normal, the physician should examine for harsh midsystolic murmur, typically located at the fourth intercostal space at the left sternal margin. Hypertrophic obstructive cardiomyopathy must be suspected if the murmur increases in intensity with bearing down for the Valsalva maneuver or when the child stands up or exercises. Squatting may diminish the murmur.

○ **What interventions reduce the risk of developing type 2 diabetes in patients at risk?**

In the Diabetes Prevention Program trial, increasing moderate physical activity to 150 minutes per week and achieving 7% weight loss reduced the risk of developing diabetes by more than 58%. The benefit was greatest among adults older than 60 years who reduced their risk by more than 70%.

○ **Matching:**

1. Sensitivity	**a.** Actual number of positive results divided by total number of positive test results
2. Specificity	**b.** Actual number of positive results divided by total number with the disease
3. Positive predictive value	**c.** Actual number of negative results divided by total number without the disease
4. Negative predictive value	**d.** Actual number of negative results divided by total number of negative test results

Answers: (1) b, (2) c, (3) a, and (4) d

○ **If your results on the board examinations are 2 standard deviations above the mean, you will have done better than what percentage of physicians or residents taking the test with you?**

97.5%. If your results are 1 standard deviation above the mean, you will have done better than 84% of your fellow medical students. A total of 64.26% of all values lie within 1 standard deviation of the mean, 95.44% of all values lie within 2 standard deviations of the mean, and 99.72% of all values lie within 3 standard deviations of the mean.

○ **Three hundred hypertensive patients are randomly assigned to 3 groups. Each group is given a separate treatment plan, and the results are recorded. What statistical analysis method is appropriate?**

Analysis of variance (appropriate for comparing 2 or more sample means)

○ **Fifty obese individuals are randomly divided into 2 groups. One group follows diet A for 3 months; the other group follows diet B. What statistical method would you use to compare the results?**

The *t* test is the appropriate method to use when comparing group means of 2 separate samples. It is also appropriate when dealing with small sample sizes.

○ **Why would you use a correlation coefficient?**

To measure the degree of linear relationship between 2 variables

○ **Match the prevention with the example that fits.**

   1. Primary prevention   **a.** Tetanus booster shots every 10 years

   2. Secondary prevention   **b.** Controlling blood sugar with appropriate diet and insulin

   3. Tertiary prevention   **c.** Identifying and treating a patient with asymptomatic diabetes mellitus

   Answers: (1) a, (2) c, and (3) b

   - Primary prevention prevents a disease from ever occurring.
   - Secondary prevention prevents future problems if actions are taken during an asymptomatic period.
   - Tertiary prevention prevents further complications in a disease that is already present.

○ **True/False: Patients with hypertension are at a greater risk for CAD and stroke than are healthy persons.**

   True. Hypertensive patients have a 3 to 4 times greater risk of CAD and a 7 times greater risk of stroke.

○ **People with elevated serum cholesterol levels have a greater risk for cardiovascular disease. Decreasing one's cholesterol by 1% reduces the risk of death due to heart disease by what percentage?**

   2%

○ **What percentage of deaths due to CHD can be attributed to smoking?**

   25%. Smokers with CHD have a 70% higher incidence of MI and death than do nonsmokers with CHD.

○ **What percentage of people older than 65 years live independently?**

   80%. By age 85 years, only 54% of men and 38% of women still live independently at home.

○ **What must be checked in a patient with Down syndrome before medical clearance can be given for participation in sports?**

   Atlantoaxial instability must be ruled out by means of cervical radiography. Ten percent to 20% of children with Down syndrome have unstable atlantoaxial joints.

○ **When should you first check a child's blood lead level?**

   Age 1 to 2 years. By this age, children are mobile and can easily find paint chips and other lead-based objects.

○ **How much does the average teenager grow during adolescence?**

   Teenagers generally increase their height by 15% to 20% and double their weight.

○ **According to the CDC, what are 6 health behaviors in adolescents that are modifiable and will decrease their risk of morbidity and mortality?**

   1. Using seat belts

   2. Not drinking and driving

   3. Using condoms if having sex

   4. Not smoking

   5. Eating low-fat diets

   6. Doing aerobic exercise

○ **How many prescriptions does the average 65-year-old have?**

3 to 5. More than 80% of senior citizens have at least 1 chronic illness.

○ **What can elderly patients do to prevent falls?**

- Remove clutter from house
- Remove throw rugs
- Ensure good lighting
- Put nonslip patches in bathtub

○ **At what age can routine Papanicolaou (Pap) smears be discontinued?**

Age 70 years, if the patient has had several negative examination results. Cervical cancer reaches a plateau by this age, so further screening is not necessary.

○ **Geographically, where is multiple sclerosis most prevalent?**

In the northern United States. Migration to warmer climates does not seem to affect the disease. People born in the north will still have a higher incidence of the disease.

○ **Should pregnant women abstain from intercourse?**

There is no risk to the mother or the fetus if the mother engages in sex with orgasm during the first 2 trimesters. In the third trimester, anorgasmic intercourse is safe until the 34th week. Intercourse should be avoided if there is bleeding.

○ **What percentage of lung cancer is related to smoking?**

80%

○ **What types of cancer are more common in farmers?**

Cancer of the lip, Hodgkin disease, leukemia, malignant melanoma, multiple myeloma, and prostate cancer

○ **What cancer causes the most deaths in women?**

- Lung cancer
- Breast cancer
- Colorectal cancer

○ **What are the 4 most common cancers in men?**

1. Skin cancer
2. Lung cancer
3. Colorectal cancer
4. Prostate cancer

○ **What cancer causes the most deaths in men?**

- Lung cancer
- Colorectal cancer
- Prostate cancer

○ **Overall, cancer deaths have increased 7% between 1971 and 1991. What cancers have actually shown a decrease in death rates?**

Cancer of the bladder, colon, cervix, larynx, mouth, pharynx, stomach, testes, thyroid, and uterus and Hodgkin disease

○ **At what concentration is ozone damaging to your health?**

10 ppm. Initial effects are tearing, pulmonary edema, and pain in the trachea.

○ **What is the incubation period of the Epstein-Barr virus?**

30 to 50 days

○ **What is the biggest risk factor for prostate cancer?**

Age. The median age for diagnosis of prostate cancer is 72 years.

○ **Name 7 risk factors for malignant melanoma.**

1. Fair skin
2. Sensitivity to sunlight
3. Excessive exposure to the sun
4. Dysplastic moles
5. 6 or more moles larger than 0.5 cm
6. Prior basal or squamous cell carcinoma
7. Parental history of skin cancer

○ **What percentage of melanomas occur in sun-exposed areas?**

Only 65%. A good screening of all surface areas is important. In African American, Hispanic, and Asian patients, acral lentiginous melanomas are more common. Careful examination of subungual, palmar, and plantar surfaces is important in these populations.

○ **Which malignancies are more common in obese individuals?**

Endometrial cancer, breast cancer (postmenopausal), gallbladder cancer, biliary cancer, prostate cancer, and colorectal cancer

○ **For what common diseases is obesity is a risk factor?**

CAD, noninsulin-dependent diabetes mellitus, hypertension, left ventricular hypertrophy, sleep apnea, cholelithiasis, pulmonary emboli, and osteoarthritis

○ **What is the risk of sudden death in morbidly obese patients compared with that in patients with normal BMI?**

15 to 30 times higher

○ **How much blood must be lost to the gastrointestinal system to be detected at hemoccult testing?**

20 mL/d. Healthy patients normally lose 0.5 to 2.0 mL/d.

○ **A patient comes in for vaccinations and has an upper respiratory infection and a fever of 37.5°C. Can you administer vaccines in this patient?**

Yes. Upper respiratory infection or gastrointestinal illness are not contraindications to vaccination. Fever may be as high as 38°C and the vaccine can still be administered. Likewise, use of antibiotics or recent exposure to illness is not a reason to delay vaccination.

○ **When administering the Mantoux skin test in a person with HIV, what level of induration indicates a positive reaction?**

Greater than 5 mm. In individuals with risk factors for tuberculosis, induration must be greater than10 mm. For those with no risk factors, induration must be greater than 15 mm.

○ **What is a contraindication to the administration of influenza vaccine?**

A history of anaphylactic hypersensitivity to eggs or their products

○ **Which routine screenings should be performed in pregnant women?**

- Hepatitis B
- Syphilis
- Rubella
- Gonorrhea
- Other sexually transmitted diseases (STDs)

Women in high-risk categories should also be screened for HIV.

○ **In which ethnic group is diabetes is most common?**

Hispanics. The prevalence in Hispanics is 1.7 to 2.4 times higher than in non-Hispanics; the death rate is also twice as high. Reasons for the high rate of disease in this group are attributed to increased incidence of obesity and hyperinsulinemia.

○ **What diet is recommended to reduce the risk of colon cancer?**

Decrease fat, especially saturated fat; increase fiber; increase cruciferous vegetables; decrease ethanol; and decrease smoked, salted, or nitrate-based foods

○ **What are the risk factors for colon cancer?**

- Age older than 50 years
- Familial polyposis (100%)
- Ulcerative colitis
- Crohn disease
- Radiation exposure
- Benign adenomas
- Previous history of colon cancer

○ **What percentage of patients with gonococcal genital infections have concomitant *Chlamydia trichomatis* infections?**

45%. This is why treatment for gonorrhea includes ceftriaxone and doxycycline to cover both infections.

○ **A woman with condyloma acuminatum is how many times more likely to develop cervical cancer than is a woman without this lesion?**

4 times more likely. These women should have yearly Pap smears and be screened for other STDs.

○ **Patients with cirrhosis or chronic active hepatitis should have what routine testing to screen for hepatoma?**

α-Fetoprotein should be measured every 6 months, and ultrasonography should be performed at the same time. These patients are at a higher risk for developing liver cancer.

○ **How can gallstone formation be prevented in patients undergoing rapid weight loss?**

10 mg/kg per day of ursodeoxycholic acid

○ **How can gallstone formation be prevented in patients receiving total parenteral nutrition for more than a month?**

Daily ingestion of 100 kcal or injection of cholecystokinin

○ **According to the Holmes and Rahe Stress Scale, what are life's top 10 most stressful events?**

1. Death of spouse or child
2. Divorce
3. Separation
4. Institutional detention
5. Death of close family member
6. Major personal injury or illness
7. Marriage
8. Job loss
9. Marital reconciliation
10. Retirement

○ **What is the number 1 cause of death for African American boys and men between the ages of 10 and 24 years?**

Firearm injury. The overall homicide rate for young men in the United States is more than 7 times that of the next developed country.

○ **Do intentional or unintentional causes account for more firearm-related deaths?**

Intentional causes account for 94% of firearm deaths, suicide for 48%, and homicide for 46%. Unintentional firearm injuries account for about 4%. Only 1% of firearm deaths occur as a result of legal intervention. The number of firearm-related fatalities has more than doubled in the last 30 years.

○ **What are risk factors for homicide?**

Most homicide victims are killed by someone they know, someone of the same race, and usually during an argument or fight. Drugs and alcohol are important cofactors, as is the presence of a handgun.

○ **What are the relative risks for suicide and homicide if a gun is kept in the home?**

Suicide is 5 times more likely. Homicide is 3 times more likely. The victim is 43% more likely to be a member of the family than an intruder. In the case of domestic violence, a gun at home increases the risk of homicide 20-fold.

○   **In addition to the history, physical examination, laboratory tests, and collection of physical evidence, what needs to be done in cases of child sexual abuse?**

- File a report with child protective services and law enforcement agencies.
- Provide emotional support to the child and family.
- Schedule a return appointment for follow-up of STD cultures and testing for pregnancy, HIV, or syphilis, as indicated.
- Ensure follow-up for psychological counseling by connecting the child and family to the appropriate services in your area.

○   **What is the standard of care for survivors of domestic violence currently recommended by the Joint Commission, American Medical Association, and CDC?**

- Establish a confidential system to identify domestic violence survivors.
- Document the abuse.
- Collect physical evidence.
- Evaluate safety issues and potential for lethality or suicide.
- Formulate a safety plan with the victim.
- Advise the patient of all his or her options and resources.
- Refer for counseling and other services, including legal assistance.
- Coordinate with law enforcement.
- Transport to a shelter if desired or needed.
- Follow-up with a domestic violence advocate.

BIBLIOGRAPHY

Abbasi NR, Shaw HM, Rigel DS, et al. Early diagnosis of cutaneous melanoma: revisiting the ABCD criteria. *JAMA*. 2004;292 (22):2771–2776.

ACIP provisional recommendations from the Advisory Committee on Immunization Practices for the prevention of human rabies. www.cdc.gov/VACCINES/pubs/ACIP-list.htm. Accessed October 5, 2009.

Adams SM, Good MW, Defranco GM. Sudden infant death syndrome. *Am Fam Physician*. 2009;79(10):870–874.

Agostini R. *Medical and Orthopedic Issues of Active and Athletic Women*. Philadelphia, PA: Hanley and Belfus; 1994.

Agur AMR, Dalley AF. *Grant's Atlas of Anatomy*. 12th ed. Philadelphia, PA: Lippincott Williams & Wilkins; 2009.

Albert RH, Clark MM. Cancer screening in the older patient. *Am Fam Physician*. 2008;78(12):1369–1374, 1376.

Alvarez DJ, Rockwell PG. Trigger points: diagnosis and management. *Am Fam Physician*. 2002;65(4):653–660.

American Academy of Pediatrics Committee on Sports Medicine. Atlantoaxial instability in Down syndrome. *Pediatrics*. 1984;74:152–154.

American Academy of Sleep Medicine. *International Classification of Sleep Disorders: Diagnostic and Coding Manual*. 2nd ed. Westchester, IL: American Academy of Sleep Medicine; 2005.

American College of Obstetricians and Gynecologists. Exercise during pregnancy and the postpartum period. ACOG Technical Bulletin 189. Washington, DC: American College of Obstetricians and Gynecologists; 1994.

American Heart Association. *Textbook of Pediatric Advanced Life Support*. Dallas, TX: American Heart Association; 2002.

American Psychiatric Association. *Diagnostic and Statistical Manual of Mental Disorders*. 4th ed. Washington, DC: American Psychiatric Publishing, Inc. 2000:83.

Andersen K, Jensen PO, Lauritzen J. Treatment of clavicular fractures: figure-of-eight bandage versus a simple sling. *Acta Orthop Scand*. 1987;58:71–74.

Anderson BJ. Skin infections in Minnesota high school state tournament wrestlers: 1997–2006. *Clin J Sport Med*. 2007;17(6):478–480.

Angevaren M, Aufdemkampe G, Verhaar HJ, Aleman A, Vanhees L. Physical activity and enhanced fitness to improve cognitive function in older people without known cognitive impairment. *Cochrane Database Syst Rev*. 2008;(2):CD005381.

Arias E. United States life tables, 2003. *Natl Vital Stat Rep*. 2006;54(14):1–40.

Armstrong C. ACP guidelines on screening for osteoporosis in men. *Am Fam Physician*. 2008;78(7):882.

Asgari MM, Begos DG. Spontaneous splenic rupture in infectious mononucleosis: a review. *Yale J Biol Med*. 1997;70:175–182.

Auerbach PS. *Wilderness Medicine: Management of Wilderness and Environmental Emergencies*. 5th ed. St Louis, MO: Mosby; 2007.

Bach AW. Finger joint injuries in active patients: pointers for acute and late-phase management. *Phys Sportsmed*. 1999;27:89–104.

Bachmann LM, Kolb E, Koller MT, Steurer J, ter Riet G. Accuracy of Ottawa Ankle Rules to exclude fractures of the ankle and mid-foot: systematic review. *BMJ*. 2003;326:417.

Bahn RS, Burch HS, Cooper DS, et al. The Role of Propylthiouracil in the Management of Graves' Disease in Adults: report of a meeting jointly sponsored by the American Thyroid Association and the Food and Drug Administration. *Thyroid*. 2009;19:673–674.

Barahmani N, Schabath MB, Duvic M. History of atopy or autoimmunity increases risk of alopecia areata. *J Am Acad Dermatol*. 2009;61:581.

Barker LR, Fiebach NH, et al. *Principles of Ambulatory Medicine*. Philadelphia, PA: Lippincott Williams & Wilkins; 2007.

Barua M, Cil O, Paterson AD, et al. Family history of renal disease severity predicts the mutated gene in ADPKD. *J Am Soc Nephrol*. 2009;20:1833.

Bellamy N, Campbell J, Robinson V, Gee T, Bourne R, Wells G. Intraarticular corticosteroid for treatment of osteoarthritis of the knee. *Cochrane Database Syst Rev*. 2006;(2):CD005328.

Bellamy N, Campbell J, Robinson V, Gee T, Bourne R, Wells G. Viscosupplementation for the treatment of osteoarthritis of the knee. *Cochrane Database Syst Rev*. 2006;(2):CD005321.

Benjamin HJ, Briner WW Jr. Little league elbow. *Clin J Sport Med*. 2005;15:37–40.

Bhatnagar V, Kaplan RM. Treatment options for prostate cancer: evaluating the evidence. *Am Fam Physician*. 2005;71(10):1915–1922.

Bigosinski K, Mjaanes J. Return to play decisions in athletes with skin conditions. *Illinois Pediatrician*. 2008;4:18–19.

Bishop J, Kaeding C. Treatment of the acute traumatic acromioclavicular separation. *Sports Med Arthrosc*. 2006;14(4):237–245.

Bluestein D, Javaheri A. Pressure ulcers: prevention, evaluation, and management. *Am Fam Physician.* 2008;78(10):1186–1194.

Bohmer E, Hoffmann P, Abdelnoor M, Arnesen H, Halvorsen S. Efficacy and safety of immediate angioplasty versus ischemia-guided management after thrombolysis in acute myocardial infarction in areas with very long transfer distances results of the NORDISTEMI (NORwegian study on DIstrict treatment of ST-elevation myocardial infarction). *J Am Coll Cardiol.* 2010;55(2):102–110.

Bonow RO, Carabello BA, Chatterjee K, et al. 2008 Focused Update Incorporated Into the ACC/AHA 2006 Guidelines for the Management of Patients With Valvular Heart Disease: A Report of the American College of Cardiology/American Heart Association Task Force on Practice Guidelines (Writing Committee to Revise the 1998 Guidelines for the Management of Patients With Valvular Heart Disease): Endorsed by the Society of Cardiovascular Anesthesiologists, Society for Cardiovascular Angiography and Interventions, and Society of Thoracic Surgeons. *Circulation.* 2008;118:e523–e661.

Bottoni CR, Wilckens JH, DeBerardino TM, et al. A prospective, randomized evaluation of arthroscopic stabilization versus nonoperative treatment in patients with acute, traumatic, first-time shoulder dislocations. *Am J Sports Med.* 2002;30:576–580.

Bradley WG, Daroff RB, Fenichel G, Jankovic J. *Neurology in Clinical Practice e-dition.* 5th ed. Butterworth-Heinemann; 2008.

British Committee for Standards in Haematology, Blood Transfusion Task Force. Guidelines for the use of platelet transfusions. *Br J Haematol.* 2003;122(1):10–23.

Brukner P. Concussion. *Aust Fam Physician.* 1996;25:1445–1448.

Brukner P. Exercise-related lower leg pain: bone. *Med Sci Sports Exerc.* 2000;32(3 suppl):S15–S26.

Burroughs KE. Athletes resuming activity after infectious mononucleosis. *Arch Fam Med.* 2000;9:1122–1123.

Buist DSM, Anderson ML, Reed SD, et al. Short-term hormone therapy suspension and mammography recall: a randomized trial. *Ann Intern Med.* 2009;150:752.

Calbresi PA. Diagnosis and management of multiple sclerosis. *Am Fam Physician.* 2004;70(10):1935–1944.

Cantor WJ, Fitchett D, Borgundvaag B, et al. Routine early angioplasty after fibrinolysis for acute myocardial infarction. *N Engl J Med.* 2009;360:2705.

Cassas KJ, Cassettari-Wayhs A. Childhood and adolescent sports-related overuse injuries. *Am Fam Physician.* 2006;73(6):1014–1022.

Cattran DC, Coppo R, Cook HT, et al. The Oxford classification of IgA nephropathy: rationale, clinicopathological correlations, and classification. *Kidney Int.* 2009;76:534.

Centers for Disease Control and Prevention. Recommended immunization schedule for persons aged 0 through 18 years—United States, 2009. http://www.cdc.gov/mmwr/preview/mmwrhtml/mm5751a5.htm. Accessed January 26, 2010.

Centers for Disease Control and Prevention (CDC). Updated recommendation from the Advisory Committee on Immunization Practices (ACIP) for revaccination of persons at prolonged increased risk for meningococcal disease. *MMWR Morb Mortal Wkly Rep.* 2009;58(37):1042–1043.

Chern K, ed. *Emergency Ophthalmology—A Rapid Treatment Guide.* New York, NY: McGraw-Hill Professional; 2003.

Cheung A, Ewigman B, Zuckerbrot RA, Jensen PS. Adolescent depression: is your young patient suffering in silence? *J Fam Psychol.* 2009;58(4):187–192.

Chiarelli AM, Majpruz V, Brown P, et al. The contribution of clinical breast examination to the accuracy of breast screening. *J Natl Cancer Inst.* 2009;101:1236.

Chou R, Baisden J, Carragee EJ, et al. Surgery for low back pain: a review of the evidence for an American Pain Society Clinical Practice Guideline. *Spine (Phila Pa 1976).* 2009;34:1094.

Chou R, Loeser JD, Owens DK, et al. Interventional therapies, surgery, and interdisciplinary rehabilitation for low back pain: an evidence-based clinical practice guideline from the American Pain Society. *Spine (Phila Pa 1976).* 2009;34:1066.

Chou R, Qaseen A, Snow V, et al. Diagnosis and treatment of low back pain: a joint clinical practice guideline from the American College of Physicians and the American Pain Society. *Ann Intern Med.* 2007;147:478–491.

Coats DK, Paysse EA, Bleiberg J, et al. Duration of cognitive impairment after sports concussion. *Neurosurgery.* 2004;54:1073–1080.

Corey BA. Diagnosis and treatment of streptococcal pharyngitis. *Am Fam Physician.* 2009;79(5):383–390.

Coutinho JM, Ferro JM, Canhao P, et al. Cerebral venous and sinus thrombosis in women. *Stroke.* 2009;40:2356.

Davis MD, el-Azhary RA, Farmer SA. Results of patch testing to a corticosteroid series: a retrospective review of 1188 patients during 6 years at Mayo Clinic. *J Am Acad Dermatol.* 2007;56:921.

Davy AR, Drew SJ. Management of shoulder dislocation: are we doing enough to reduce the risk of recurrence? *Injury.* 2002;33:775–779.

Dawson B, Trapp RG. *Basic & Clinical Biostatistics.* 4th ed. New York, NY: McGraw-Hill; 2004.

DeLee J, Drez D. *Orthopedic Sports Medicine: Principles and Practice.* Philadelphia, PA: Saunders; 2003.

Delgado Almandoz JE, Yoo AJ, Stone MJ, et al. Systematic characterization of the computed tomography angiography spot sign in primary intracerebral hemorrhage identifies patients at highest risk for hematoma expansion: the spot sign score. *Stroke.* 2009;40:2994.

Deschaintre Y, Richard F, Leys D, Pasquier F. Treatment of vascular risk factors is associated with slower decline in Alzheimer disease. *Neurology.* 2009;73:674.

Diaz J, Leblank K. Common spider bites. *Am Fam Physician.* 2007;75(6):869–873.

Dodge WF, West EF, Smith EH, Harvey B 3rd. Proteinuria and hematuria in schoolchildren: epidemiology and early natural history. *J Pediatr.* 1976;88:327–347.

Doyle LW, Crowther CA, Middleton P, Marret S, Rouse D. Magnesium sulphate for women at risk of preterm birth for neuroprotection of the fetus. *Cochrane Database Syst Rev.* 2009;(1):CD004661.

Driscol C, Pope ET. *The Family Practice Desk Reference.* 4th ed. Chicago, IL: American Medical Association; 2003.

Dumont L, Mardirosoff C, Tramer MR. Efficacy and harm of pharmacological prevention of acute mountain sickness: quantitative systematic review. *BMJ.* 2000;321:267–272.

Ebell MH. Brief screening instruments for dementia in primary care. *Am Fam Physician.* 2009;79(5):497.

Edwards JL. Diagnosis and management of benign prostatic hyperplasia. *Am Fam Physician.* 2008;77(10):1403–1410.

Ehlers JP, Shah CP, eds. *The Wills Eye Manual: Office and Emergency Room Diagnosis and Treatment of Eye Disease.* 5th ed. Philadelphia, PA: Lippincott Williams & Wilkins; 2008.

Eiff MP, Hatch RL, Calmbach WL. *Fracture Management for Primary Care.* 2nd ed. Philadelphia, PA: Saunders; 2003.

El Ghissassi F, Baan R, Straif K, et al. A review of human carcinogens—part D: radiation. *Lancet Oncol.* 2009;10:751.

Ely JW, Hansen MR, Clark EC. Diagnosis of ear pain. *Am Fam Physician.* 2008;77(5):621–628.

Erickson T, Hryhorczuk DO, Lipscomb J, Burda A, Greenberg B. Brown recluse spider bites in an urban wilderness. *J Wilderness Med.* 1990;1(4):258–264.

Erqou S, Kaptoge S, Perry PL, et al. Lipoprotein(a) concentration and the risk of coronary heart disease, stroke, and nonvascular mortality. *JAMA.* 2009;302:412.

Esposito K, Maiorino MI, Ciotola M, et al. Effects of a Mediterranean-style diet on the need for antihyperglycemic drug therapy in patients with newly diagnosed type 2 diabetes: a randomized trial. *Ann Intern Med.* 2009;151:306.

Farley DR, Zietlow SP, Bannon MP, Farnell MB. Spontaneous rupture of the spleen due to infectious mononucleosis. *Mayo Clin Proc.* 1992;67:846–853.

Federman DG, Kirsner RS. The patient with skin disease: an approach for nondermatologists. *Ostomy Wound Manage.* 2002;48:22.

Feinstein RA, LaRussa J, Wang-Dohlman A, Bartolucci AA. Screening adolescent athletes for exercise-induced asthma. *Clin J Sport Med.* 1996;6(2):119–123.

Finckh A, Zufferey P, Schurch MA, Balagué F, Waldburger M, So AK. Short-term efficacy of intravenous pulse glucocorticoids in acute discogenic sciatica: a randomized controlled trial. *Spine (Phila Pa 1976).* 2006;31(4):377–381.

Fisher DR, DeSmet AA. Radiologic analysis of osteochondritis dissecans and related osteochondral lesions. *Contemp Diag Rad.* 1993;16:1–5.

Flaherty JD, Bax JJ, De Luca L, et al. Acute heart failure syndromes in patients with coronary artery disease early assessment and treatment. *J Am Coll Cardiol.* 2009;53:254.

Fleischer AB Jr, Feldman SR, McConnell RC. The most common dermatologic problems identified by family physicians, 1990–1994. *Fam Med.* 1997;29:648.

Food and Drug Administration. Public Health Alert: Heparin: Change in reference standard. www.fda.gov/Safety/MedWatch/SafetyInformation/SafetyAlertsforHumanMedicalProducts/ucm184687.htm. Accessed October 7, 2009.

Food and Drug Administration. Stimulant medications used in children with attention-deficit/hyperactivity disorder: communication about an ongoing safety review. http://www.fda.gov/Safety/MedWatch/SafetyInformation/SafetyAlertsforHumanMedicalProducts/ucm166667.htm. Accessed June 15, 2009.

Ford ES, Bergmann MM, Kroger J, et al. Healthy living is the best revenge: findings from the European Prospective Investigation into Cancer and Nutrition—Potsdam Study. *Arch Intern Med.* 2009;169:1355.

Fortuna RJ, Robbins BW, Halterman JS. Ambulatory care among young adults in the United States. *Ann Intern Med.* 2009;151:379.

French SD, Cameron MC, Walker BF, Reggars JW, Esterman AJ. Superficial heat or cold for low back pain. *Cochrane Database Syst Rev.* 2006;(1):CD004750.

Fuccio L, Zagari RM, Eusebi LH, et al. Meta-analysis: can Helicobacter pylori eradication treatment reduce the risk for gastric cancer? *Ann Intern Med.* 2009;151:121.

Furlan AD, Imamura M, Dryden T, Irvin E. Massage for low-back pain. *Cochrane Database Syst Rev.* 2008;(4):CD001929.

Gabrielli A, Layon AJ, Civetta YM. *Kirby's Critical Care.* 4th ed. Philadelphia, PA: Lippincott Williams & Wilkins; 2008.

Galioto NJ. Peritonsillar abscess. *Am Fam Physician.* 2008;77(2):199–202.

Garbutt JM, Goldstein M, Gellman E, et al. A randomized, placebo-controlled trial of antimicrobial treatment for children with clinically diagnosed acute sinusitis. *Pediatrics.* 2001;107:619.

Gardner DG, Shoback D. *Greenspan's Basic & Clinical Endocrinology.* 8th ed. New York, NY: McGraw-Hill; 2007.

Gartlehner G, Gaynes BN, Hansen RA, et al. Comparative benefits and harms of second-generation antidepressants: background paper for the American College of Physicians. *Ann Intern Med.* 2008;149:734.

Gerritsen AA, de Krom MC, Struijs MA, Scholten RJ, de Vet HC, Bouter LM. Conservative treatment options for carpal tunnel syndrome: a systematic review of randomised controlled trials. *J Neurol.* 2002;249:272–280.

Gibson JNA, Waddell G. Surgical interventions for lumbar disc prolapse. *Cochrane Database Syst Rev.* 2007;(2):CD001350.

Gillespie WJ, Grant I. Interventions for preventing and treating stress fractures and stress reactions of bone of the lower limbs in young adults. *Cochrane Database Syst Rev.* 2000;(2):CD000450.

Girardet RG, Lahoti S, Howard LA, et al. Epidemiology of sexually transmitted infections in suspected child victims of sexual assault. *Pediatrics.* 2009;124:79.

Glass C. Role of the primary care physician in Hodgkin lymphoma. *Am Fam Physician.* 2008;78(5):616–622.

Goldberg B, Saraniti A, Witman P, et al. Preparticipation sports assessment: an objective evaluation. *Pediatrics.* 1980;66:736–745.

Goldberger A. *Clinical Electrocardiography: A Simplified Approach.* 7th ed. Philadelphia, PA: Elsevier; 2006.

Gomez JE, Landry GL, Bernhardt DT. Critical evaluation of the 2-minute orthopedic screening examination. *Am J Dis Child.* 1993; 147:1109–1113.

Gonsalves WC, Chi AC, Neville BW. Common oral lesions: part II, masses and neoplasia. *Am Fam Physician.* 2007;75(4):509–512

Gonsalves WC, Wrightson AS, Henry RG. Common oral conditions in older persons. *Am Fam Physician.* 2008;78(7):845–852.

Graber M, Jones J, Wilbur J. *The Family Medicine Handbook.* 5th ed. Iowa City, IA: University of Iowa; 2009.

Graham L. AAFP and ACP release guideline on dementia treatment. *Am Fam Physician.* 2008;77(8):1173–1175.

Greenberg PL, Sun Z, Miller KB, et al. Treatment of myelodysplastic syndrome patients with erythropoietin with or without granulocyte colony-stimulating factor: results of a prospective randomized phase 3 trial by the Eastern Cooperative Oncology Group (E1996). *Blood.* 2009;114:2393.

Gregory DS, Seto CK, Wortley GC, Shugart CM. Acute lumbar disk pain: navigating evaluation and treatment choices. *Am Fam Physician.* 2008;78(7):835–842.

Grimard BH, Larson JM. Aortic stenosis: diagnosis and treatment. *Am Fam Physician.* 2008;78(6):717–724.

Habif TB. *Clinical Dermatology.* 5th ed. St Louis, MO: Mosby; 2009.

Hagen KB, Hilde G, Jamtvedt G, Winnem M. Bed rest for acute low-back pain and sciatica. *Cochrane Database Syst Rev.* 2004;(4): CD001254.

Hak AE, Karlson EW, Feskanich D, et al. Systemic lupus erythematosus and the risk of cardiovascular disease: results from the nurses' health study. *Arthritis Rheum.* 2009;61:1396.

Handoll HH, Vaghela MV. Interventions for treating mallet finger injuries. *Cochrane Database Syst Rev.* 2004;(3):CD004574.

Hankin FM, Peel SM. Sport-related fractures and dislocations in the hand. *Hand Clin.* 1990;6:429–453.

Hanley ME, Welsh CH. *Current Diagnosis and Treatment in Pulmonary Medicine.* New York, NY: McGraw-Hill; 2003.

Harsora P, Kessman J. Nonpharmacologic management of chronic insomnia. *Am Fam Physician.* 2009;79(2):125.

Harrison TR. *Principles of Internal Medicine.* 16th ed. New York, NY: McGraw-Hill; 2004.

Hayden J, van Tulder MW, Malmivaara A, Koes BW. Exercise therapy for treatment of non-specific low back pain. *Cochrane Database Syst Rev.* 2005;(3):CD000335.

He W, Sengupta M, Velkoff VA, DeBarros KA. 65+ in the United States: 2005. Current population reports: special studies. Washington, DC: US Census Bureau (P23–209), US Government Printing Office; 2005. http://www.census.gov/prod/2006pubs/p23–209.pdf. Accessed May 27, 2008.

Hebert AA, Friedlander SF, Allen DB. Topical fluticasone propionate lotion does not cause HPA axis suppression. *J Pediatr.* 2006;149:378.

Heidelbaugh JJ, Gill AS, Van Harrison R, Nostrant TT. Atypical presentations of gastroesophageal reflux disease. *Am Fam Physician.* 2008;78(4):483–488.

Hermanns-Lê T, Scheen A, Piérard GE. Acanthosis nigricans associated with insulin resistance: pathophysiology and management. *Am J Clin Dermatol.* 2004;5(3):199–203.

Hoff G, Grotmol T, Skovlund E, Bretthauer M. Norwegian Colorectal Cancer Prevention Study Group. Risk of colorectal cancer seven years after flexible sigmoidoscopy screening: randomised controlled trial. *BMJ.* 2009;338:b1846.

Holder KK, Kerley SS. Alendronate for fracture prevention in postmenopause. *Am Fam Physician.* 2008;78(5):579.

Hopkinson WJ, St. Pierre P, Ryan JB, Wheeler JH. Syndesmosis sprains of the ankle. *Foot Ankle.* 1990;10:325–330.

Hunt SA, Abraham WT, Chin MH, et al. 2009 focused update incorporated into the ACC/AHA 2005 Guidelines for the Diagnosis and Management of Heart Failure in Adults: a report of the American College of Cardiology Foundation/American Heart Association Task Force on Practice Guidelines: developed in collaboration with the International Society for Heart and Lung Transplantation. *Circulation.* 2009;119(14):e391–e479.

Huntzinger A. ACP releases recommendations for palliative care at the end of life. *Am Fam Physician.* 2008;78(9):1093.

Hussain A, Hagroo GA. Osgood-Schlatter disease. *Sports Exer Injury.* 1996;2:202–206.

Infante M, Cavuto S, Lutman FR, et al. A randomized study of lung cancer screening with spiral computed tomography: three-year results from the DANTE trial. *Am J Respir Crit Care Med.* 2009;180:445.

Inouye SK, Bogardus ST Jr, Charpentier PA, et al. A multicomponent intervention to prevent delirium in hospitalized older patients. *N Engl J Med.* 1999;340(9):669–676.

International Expert Committee report on the role of the A1C assay in the diagnosis of diabetes. *Diabetes Care.* 2009;32:1327.

Jackson JL, O'Malley PG, Kroenke K. Evaluation of acute knee pain in primary care. *Ann Intern Med.* 2003;139:575–588.

Jakobsen BW, Johannsen HV, Suder P, Sojbjerg JO. Primary repair versus conservative treatment of first-time traumatic anterior dislocation of the shoulder: a randomized study with 10-year follow-up. *Arthroscopy.* 2007;23:118–123.

Jarvik JG, Comstock BA, Kliot M, et al. Surgery versus non-surgical therapy for carpal tunnel syndrome: a randomised parallel-group trial. *Lancet.* 2009;374:1074.

Jemal A, Siegel R, Ward E, et al. Cancer statistics, 2009. *CA Cancer J Clin.* 2009;59:225.

Jenik AG, Vain NE, Gorestein AN, Jacobi NE. Does the recommendation to use a pacifier influence the prevalence of breastfeeding? *J Pediatr.* 2009;155:350.

Jenkinson DM, Harbert AJ. Supplements and sports. *Am Fam Physician.* 2008;78(9):1039–1046.

Joint National Committee of Prevention. The Seventh Report of the Joint National Committee on Prevention, Detection, Evaluation, and Treatment of High Blood Pressure (JNC 7). http://www.nhlbi.nih.gov/guidelines/hypertension/. Accessed January 26, 2010.

Joy E, Van Hala S, Cooper L. Health-related concerns of the female athlete: a lifespan approach. *Am Fam Physician.* 2009;79(6):489–495.

Kaplan BJ, Sadock VA, Pedro R. *Kaplan and Sadock's Comprehensive Textbook of Psychiatry.* 9th ed. Philadelphia, PA: Lippincott Williams & Wilkins, 2009.

Katz VL, Lentz GM, Lobo RA, Gershenson DM. *Comprehensive Gynecology.* 5th ed. Philadelphia, PA: Mosby Elsevier; 2007.

Katzung BG, Masters SB, Trevor AJ. *Basic and Clinical Pharmacology.* 11th ed. New York, NY: McGraw-Hill; 2009.

KDIGO clinical practice guidelines for the diagnosis, evaluation, prevention, and treatment of chronic kidney disease-mineral and bone disorder (CKD-MBD). *Kidney Int.* 2009;76(suppl 113):S1.

Khakoo G, Sofianou-Katsoulis A, Perkin MR, Lack G. Clinical features and natural history of physical urticaria in children. *Pediatr Allergy Immunol.* 2008;19:363.

Kilip S, Bennett J, Chambers MD. Iron deficiency anemia. *Am Fam Physician.* 2007;75:671–678.

Kinkade S. Evaluation and treatment of acute low back pain. *Am Fam Physician.* 2007;75(8):1190–1192.

Kirkley A, Birmingham TB, Litchfield RB, et al. A randomized trial of arthroscopic surgery for osteoarthritis of the knee. *N Engl J Med.* 2008;359:1097–1107.

Kiter E, Bozkurt M. The crossed-leg test for examination of ankle syndesmosis injuries. *Foot Ankle Int.* 2005;26:187–188.

Kloos RT, Eng C, Evans DB, et al. Medullary thyroid cancer: management guidelines of the American Thyroid Association. *Thyroid.* 2009; 19:565.

Klossner D, ed. *2008–09 NCAA Sports Medicine Handbook.* 19th ed. Indianapolis, IN: The National Collegiate Athletic Association; 2008.

Koes B, van Tulder M. Low back pain (acute). *Clin Evid.* 2006;15:416–418.

Koopmans CM, Bijlenga D, Groen H, et al. Induction of labour versus expectant monitoring for gestational hypertension or mild pre-eclampsia after 36 weeks' gestation (HYPITAT): a multicentre, open-label randomised controlled trial. *Lancet.* 2009;374:979.

Krengel S, Hauschild A, Schafer T. Melanoma risk in congenital melanocytic naevi: a systematic review. *Br J Dermatol.* 2006;155:1–8.

Kripke C. Aerobic activity for cognitive function: Cochrane for clinicians. *Am Fam Physician.* 2009;79(7):560.

Kuhn J. Treating the initial anterior shoulder dislocation—an evidence-based medicine approach. *Sports Med Arthrosc.* 2006;14:192–198.

Kujala UM, Kvist M, Heinonen O. Osgood-Schlatter's disease in adolescent athletes: retrospective study of incidence and duration. *Am J Sports Med.* 1985;13:236–241.

Kuppermann N, Holmes JF, Dayan PS, et al. Identification of children at very low risk of clinically-important brain injuries after head trauma: a prospective cohort study. *Lancet.* 2009;374:1160.

Kurowski K, Boxer R. Food allergies: detection and management. *Am Fam Physician.* 2008;77(12):1678–1686.

Kurth T, Tzourio C. Migraine and cerebral infarct-like lesions on MRI: an observation, not a disease. *JAMA*. 2009;301:2594.

Landon MB, Spong CY, Thom E, et al. A multicenter, randomized trial of treatment for mild gestational diabetes. *N Engl J Med*. 2009; 361:1339.

Lateef H, Patel D. What is the role of imaging in acute low back pain. *Curr Rev Musculoskelet Med*. 2009;2(2):69–73.

Lawson BR, Comstock RD, Smith GA. Baseball-related injuries to children treated in hospital emergency departments in the United States 1994–2006. *Pediatrics*. 2009;123(6):1028–1034.

Layke JC, Lopez P. Gastric cancer: diagnosis and treatment options. *Am Fam Physician*. 2004;69:1133–1140, 1145–1146.

LeBlond R, Brown D, DeGowin RL. *DeGowin's Diagnostic Examination*. 9th ed. New York, NY: McGraw-Hill; 2008.

Leggit JC, Meko CJ. Acute finger injuries: part I, tendons and ligaments. *Am Fam Physician*. 2006;73(5):810–816, 823.

Leggit JC, Meko CJ. Acute finger injuries: part II, fractures, dislocations, and thumb injuries. *Am Fam Physician*. 2006;73(5): 827–834.

Lindor KD, Gershwin ME, Poupon R, et al. Primary biliary cirrhosis. *Hepatology*. 2009;50:291.

Lok AS, McMahon BJ. Chronic hepatitis B: update 2009. *Hepatology*. 2009;50:661.

Lonstein JE, Carlson JM. The prediction of curve progression in untreated idiopathic scoliosis during growth. *J Bone Joint Surg Am*. 1984; 66:1061–1071.

Loudon J, Bell S, Johnson J. *The Clinical Orthopedic Assessment Guide*. 2nd ed. Champaign, IL: Human Kinetics Publishers; 2009.

Maitra RS, Johnson DL. Stress fractures: clinical history and physical examination. *Clin Sports Med*. 1997;16:259–274.

Manore MM. Dietary recommendations and athletic menstrual dysfunction. *Sports Med*. 2002;32:887–901.

Maron BJ, Thompson PD, Ackerman MJ, et al. Recommendations and considerations related to preparticipation screening for cardiovascular abnormalities in competitive athletes: 2007 update: a scientific statement from the American Heart Association Council on Nutrition, Physical Activity, and Metabolism: endorsed by the American College of Cardiology Foundation. *Circulation*. 2007; 115(12):1643–1455.

Maron BJ, Thompson PD, Puffer JC, et al. Cardiovascular pre-participation screening of competitive athletes A statement for health professions form the Sudden Death Committee (clinical cardiology) and Congenital Defects Committee (Cardiovascular Disease in the Young), American Heart Association. *Circulation*. 1996;94:850.

Marshall S, Tardif G, Ashworth N. Local corticosteroid injection for carpal tunnel syndrome (Cochrane Review). *Cochrane Database Syst Rev*. 2002;(4):CD001554.

Marx JA. *Rosen's Emergency Medicine*. 7th ed. St Louis, MO: Mosby; 2009.

McCrea M, Guskiewicz KM, Marshall SW, et al. Acute effects and recovery time following concussion in collegiate football players: the NCAA Concussion Study. *JAMA*. 2003;290:2556–2563.

McCrory P, Meeuwisse W, Johnston K, et al. Consensus Statement on Concussion in Sport: the 3rd International Conference on Concussion in sport held in Zurich, November 2008. *Br J Sports Med*. 2009;43(Suppl 1):i76–i84.

Menter A, Korman NJ, Elmets CA, et al. Guidelines of care for the management of psoriasis and psoriatic arthritis: section 4—guidelines of care for the management and treatment of psoriasis with traditional systemic agents. *J Am Acad Dermatol*. 2009;61:451.

Micheli LJ, Ireland ML. Prevention and management of calcaneal apophysitis in children: an overuse syndrome. *J Pediatr Orthop*. 1987;7: 34–38.

Miller MO. Evaluation and management of delirium in hospitalized older patients. *Am Fam Physician*. 2008;78(11):1265–1270.

Mills K, Nelson AC, Winslow BT, Springer KL. Treatment of nursing-home acquired pneumonia. *Am Fam Physician*. 2009;79(11):976–982.

Monteleone GP Jr. Stress fractures in the athlete. *Orthop Clin North Am*. 1995;26:423–432.

Monto AS, Ohmit SE, Petrie JG, et al. Comparative efficacy of inactivated and live attenuated influenza vaccines. *N Engl J Med*. 2009; 361:1260.

Moseley JB, O'Malley K, Petersen NJ, et al. A controlled trial of arthroscopic surgery for osteoarthritis of the knee. *N Engl J Med*. 2002; 347:81–88.

Murad SD, Plessier A, Hernandez-Guerra M, et al. Etiology, management, and outcome of the Budd-Chiari syndrome. *Ann Intern Med*. 2009;151:167.

Nau KC, Lewis WD. Multiple myeloma: diagnosis and treatment. *Am Fam Physician*. 2008;78(7):853–859.

Naughton CA. Drug-induced nephrotoxicity. *Am Fam Physician*. 2008;78(6):743–750.

NCAA Committee on Competitive Safeguards and Medical Aspects of Sports. Concussion and second-impact syndrome. In: *NCAA Sports Medicine Handbook*. Overland Park, KS: NCAA; 1994.

Nelson WE. *Textbook of Pediatrics*. 17th ed. Philadelphia, PA: Saunders; 2004.

New York Heart Association. What are blood pressure and hypertension? http://www.nhlbi.nih.gov/hbp/hbp/whathbp.htm. Accessed January 26, 2010.

Nwosu B, Lee MM. Evaluation of short and tall stature in children. *Am Fam Physician*. 2008;78(5):597–604.

Obedian RS, Grelsamer RP. Osteochondritis dissecans of the distal femur and patella. *Clin Sports Med*. 1997;16:157–174.

O'Brien SM, Shahian DM, Filardo G, et al. The Society of Thoracic Surgeons 2008 cardiac surgery risk models: part 2, isolated valve surgery. *Ann Thorac Surg*. 2009;88:S23.

O'Connor NR. Infant formula. *Am Fam Physician*. 2009;79(7):565–570.

Orava S, Malinen L, Karpakka JJ, et al. Results of surgical treatment of unresolved Osgood-Schlatter lesion. *Ann Chir Gynaecol*. 2000;89:298–302.

Osguthorpe JD, Nielsen DR. Otitis externa: review and clinical update. *Am Fam Physician*. 2006;74(9):1510–1515.

Otis CL, Drinkwater B, Johnson M, Loucks A, Wilmore J. American College of Sports Medicine position stand: the female athlete triad. *Med Sci Sports Exerc*. 1997;29:i–ix.

Pacific Primary Care. Clinical orthopedics. http://www.clinicalmedconsult.com. Published June 2008.

Pagel JF. Excessive daytime sleepiness. *Am Fam Physician*. 2009;79(5):391–396.

Park MK. *Pediatric Cardiology for Practitioners*. St Louis, MO: Mosby; 2002.

Park MK, Smith PC, Wanserski G, Neher JO. Aspirin in patients with acute ischemic stroke. *Am Fam Physician*. 2009;79(3):226.

Peggs JF, Reinhardt RW, O'Brien JM. Proteinuria in adolescent sports physical examinations. *J Fam Pract*. 1986;22:80–81.

Pelletier AL, Thomas J. Vision loss in older persons. *Am Fam Physician*. 2009;79(11): 963–970.

Pipe A, Ayotte C. Nutritional supplements and doping. *Clin J Sport Med*. 2002;12(4):245–249.

Preston J, Cucuzella M, Jamieson B. Clinical inquiries: what best prevents exercise-induced bronchoconstriction for a child with asthma? *J Fam Pract*. 2006;55(7):631–633.

Rader R, McCauley L, Callen EC. Current strategies in the diagnosis and treatment of childhood attention-deficit/hyperactivity disorder. *Am Fam Physician*. 2009;79(8):657–665.

Rakel RE. *Textbook of Family Medicine*. 7th ed. Philadelphia, PA: Saunders; 2007.

Ramakrishnan K. Evaluation and treatment of enuresis. *Am Fam Physician*. 2008;78(4):489–496.

Ramakrishnan K, Sparks RA, Berryhill WE. Diagnosis and treatment of otitis media. *Am Fam Physician*. 2007;76(11):1650–1658.

Ranucci M, Castelvecchio S, Menicanti L, et al. Risk of assessing mortality risk in elective cardiac operations: age, creatinine, ejection fraction, and the law of parsimony. *Circulation*. 2009;119:3053.

Ratcliffe S. *Family Medicine Obstetrics*. 3rd ed. St Louis, MO: Mosby; 2008.

Reamy BV, Slakey JB. Adolescent idiopathic scoliosis: review and current concepts. *Am Fam Physician*. 2001;64(1):111–116.

Renko M, Salo E, Putto-Laurila A, et al. A randomized, controlled trial of tonsillectomy in periodic fever, aphthous stomatitis, pharyngitis, and adenitis syndrome. *J Pediatr*. 2007;151:289.

Retraction—Combination treatment of angiotensin-II receptor blocker and angiotensin-converting-enzyme inhibitor in non-diabetic renal disease (COOPERATE): a randomised controlled trial. *Lancet*. 2009;374(9697):1226.

Roberts IS, Cook HT, Troyanov S, et al. The Oxford classification of IgA nephropathy: pathology definitions, correlations, and reproducibility. *Kidney Int*. 2009;76:546.

Roberts JR, Hedges J. *Clinical Procedures in Emergency Medicine*. 5th ed. Saunders Elsevier; 2008.

Robertson DJ, Burke CA, Welch HG, et al. Using the results of a baseline and a surveillance colonoscopy to predict recurrent adenomas with high-risk characteristics. *Ann Intern Med*. 2009;151:103.

Rosenstock J, Fonseca V, McGill JB, et al. Similar progression of diabetic retinopathy with insulin glargine and neutral protamine Hagedorn (NPH) insulin in patients with type 2 diabetes: a long-term, randomised, open-label study. *Diabetologia*. 2009;52:1778.

Rudy DR, Zdon MJ. Update on colorectal cancer. *Am Fam Physician*. 2000;61:1759–1770, 1773–1774.

Rupp NT, Brudno DS, Guill MF. The value of screening for risk of exercise-induced asthma in high school athletes. *Ann Allergy*. 1993; 70:339–342.

Sambrook AM, Cooper KG, Campbell MK, Cook JA. Clinical outcomes from a randomised comparison of microwave endometrial ablation with thermal balloon endometrial ablation for the treatment of heavy menstrual bleeding. *BJOG*. 2009;116:1038.

Sandercock P, Gubitz G, Foley P, Counsell C. Antiplatelet therapy for acute ischaemic stroke. *Cochrane Database Syst Rev*. 2003;(2): CD000029.

Sartori C, Allemann Y, Duplain H, et al. Salmeterol for the prevention of high-altitude pulmonary edema. *N Engl J Med*. 2002;346:1631–1636.

Scarmeas N, Luchsinger JA, Schupf N, et al. Physical activity, diet, and risk of Alzheimer disease. *JAMA*. 2009;302:627.

Schuetz P, Christ-Crain M, Thomann R, et al. Effect of procalcitonin-based guidelines vs standard guidelines on antibiotic use in lower respiratory tract infections: the ProHOSP randomized controlled trial. *JAMA*. 2009;302:1059.

Scott D, Kowalczyk A. Clinical evidence concise: osteoarthritis of the knee. *Am Fam Physician*. 2008;77(8):1149.

Selius BA, Subedi R. Urinary retention in adults: diagnosis and initial management. *Am Fam Physician*. 2008;77(5):643–650.

Sexton S, Ruby N. Risks and benefits of pacifiers. *Am Fam Physician*. 2009;79(8):681–685.

Shahian DM, O'Brien SM, Filardo G, et al. The Society of Thoracic Surgeons 2008 cardiac surgery risk models: part 1, coronary artery bypass grafting surgery. *Ann Thorac Surg*. 2009;88:S2.

Shannon MH, Borron SW, Burns M. *Haddad and Winchester's Clinical Management of Poisoning and Drug Overdose*. 4th ed. Philadelphia, PA: Saunders; 2007.

Sharp HM, Hillenbrand K. Speech and language development and disorders in children. *Pediatr Clin North Am*. 2008;55(5):1159–1173, viii.

Shoene R. Illness at high altitude. *Chest*. 2008;134:402–416.

Silk H, Douglass AB, Douglass JM, Silk L. Oral health during pregnancy. *Am Fam Physician*. 2008;77(8):1139–1144.

Silver JM, McAllister TW, Yudofsky, SC. *Textbook of Traumatic Brain Injuries*. Arlington, VA: American Psychiatric Publishing; 2005.

Simon RP, Greenberg DA, Aminoff MJ. *Clinical Neurology*. 7th ed. New York, NY: McGraw-Hill; 2009.

Singer DE, Chang Y, Fang MC, et al. The net clinical benefit of warfarin anticoagulation in atrial fibrillation. *Ann Intern Med*. 2009; 151:297.

Sinha T, David A. Recognition and management of exercise-induced bronchospasm. *Am Fam Physician*. 2003;67:769–774, 776.

Slade BA, Leidel L, Vellozzi C, et al. Postlicensure safety surveillance for quadrivalent human papillomavirus recombinant vaccine. *JAMA*. 2009;302:750.

Sloan JP, Hain R, Pownall R. Clinical benefits of early cold therapy in accident and emergency following ankle sprain. *Arch Emerg Med*. 1989;6:1–6.

Smidt N, van der Windt DA, Assendelft WJ, et al. Corticosteroid injections, physiotherapy, or a wait-and-see policy for lateral epicondylitis: a randomised controlled trial. *Lancet*. 2002;359:657–662.

Smith PC, Schmidt SM, Allensworth-Davies D, Saitz R. Primary care validation of a single-question alcohol screening test. *J Gen Intern Med*. 2009;24:783.

Smith SC , Allen J, Blair SN, et al. AHA/ACC guidelines for secondary prevention for patients with coronary and other atherosclerotic vascular disease: 2006 update endorsed by the National Heart, Lung, and Blood Institute. *J Am Coll Cardiol*. 2006;47:2130.

Spalding MC, Sebesta SC. Geriatric screening and preventive care. *Am Fam Physician*. 2008;78(2):206–215.

Spooner CH, Spooner GR, Rowe BH. Mast-cell stabilizing agents to prevent exercise-induced bronchoconstriction. *Cochrane Database Syst Rev*. 2003;(4):CD002307.

Stevens A, Wrightson RM. Universal newborn hearing screening. *Am Fam Physician*. 2007;75(9):1349–1352.

Stevens LA, Nolin TD, Richardson MM, et al. Comparison of drug dosing recommendations based on measured GFR and kidney function estimating equations. *Am J Kidney Dis*. 2009;54:33.

Stessman J, Hammerman-Rozenberg R, Cohen A, et al. Physical activity, function, and longevity among the very old. *Arch Intern Med*. 2009;169:1476.

Taylor EN, Fung TT, Curhan GC. DASH-style diet associates with reduced risk for kidney stones. *J Am Soc Nephrol*. 2009;20:2253.

Tong TC, Schneir AB, Clark RF. Arthropod bites and stings. In: Erickson TB, Ahrens WR, Aks SE, Baum CR, Ling LJ, eds. *Pediatric Toxicology: Diagnosis and Management of the Poisoned Child*. New York, NY: McGraw-Hill; 2005:556–566.

Towheed TE, Maxwell L, Anastassiades TP, et al. Glucosamine therapy for treating osteoarthritis. *Cochrane Database Syst Rev*. 2005; (2):CD002946.

US Preventive Services Task Force. Recommendation statement: screening of infants for hyperbilirubinemia to prevent chronic bilirubin encephalopathy. *Pediatrics*. 2009;124:1172.

US Preventive Services Task Force. Screening for adolescent idiopathic scoliosis: policy statement. *JAMA*. 1993;269:2664–2666.

US Preventive Services Task Force. Screening for carotid artery stenosis: US Preventive Services Task Force recommendation statement [published correction appears in *Ann Intern Med*. 2008;148(3):248]. *Ann Intern Med*. 2007;147(12):854–859.

van Tulder MW, Touray T, Furlan AD, Solway S, Bouter LM. Muscle relaxants for non-specific low-back pain. *Cochrane Database Syst Rev*. 2003;(4):CD004252.

Verdecchia P, Staessen JA, Angeli F, et al. Usual versus tight control of systolic blood pressure in non-diabetic patients with hypertension (Cardio-Sis): an open-label randomised trial. *Lancet*. 2009;374:525.

Verhagen E, van der Beek A, Twisk J, Bouter L, Bahr R, van Mechelen W. The effect of a proprioceptive balance board training program for the prevention of ankle sprains: a prospective controlled trial. *Am J Sports Med.* 2004;32:1385–1393.

Waikar SS, Mount DB, Curhan GC. Mortality after hospitalization with mild, moderate, and severe hyponatremia. *Am J Med.* 2009; 122:857.

Wald ER, Nash D, Eickhoff J. Effectiveness of amoxicillin/clavulanate potassium in the treatment of acute bacterial sinusitis in children. *Pediatrics.* 2009;124:9.

Walker C. Antioxidant supplements do not improve mortality and may cause harm. *Am Fam Physician.* 2008;78(9):1079.

Warren MP, Miller KK, Olson WH, et al. Effects of an oral contraceptive (norgestimate/ethinyl estradiol) on bone mineral density in women with hypothalamic amenorrhea and osteopenia: an open-label extension of a double-blind, placebo-controlled study. *Contraception.* 2005;72:206–211.

Watson NF, Buchwald D, Goldberg J, et al. Neurologic signs and symptoms in fibromyalgia. *Arthritis Rheum.* 2009;60:2839.

Weckmann MT. The role of the family physician in the referral and management of hospice patients. *Am Fam Physician.* 2008;77(6):807–812.

Wein AJ, Kavoussi LR, Novick AC, Partin AW, Peters CA. *Campbell-Walsh Urology.* 9th ed. Philadelphia, PA: Elsevier; 2010.

Weiner DS. *Pediatric Orthopedics for Primary Care Physicians.* 2nd ed. Cambridge, England: Cambridge University Press; 2004.

Welch HG, Albertsen PC. Prostate cancer diagnosis and treatment after the introduction of prostate-specific antigen screening: 1986–2005. *J Natl Cancer Inst.* 2009;101:1325.

Welker MJ, Orlov D. Thyroid nodules. *Am Fam Physician.* 2003;67(3):559–566.

Wolff K, Johnson RA. *Fitzpatrick's Color Atlas and Synopsis of Clinical Dermatology.* 6th ed. New York, NY: McGraw-Hill's AccessMedicine; 2009.

Wolfson AB, Hendey GW, Hendry PL, Linden CH, Rosen CL, eds. *Harwood-Nuss' Clinical Practice of Emergency Medicine.* Philadelphia, PA: Lippincott Williams & Wilkins; 2010.

Wong DM. Guidelines for the use of antibiotics in acute upper respiratory tract infections. *Am Fam Physician.* 2006;74(6):956–966.

Wong GL, Wong VW, Chan Y, et al. High incidence of mortality and recurrent bleeding in patients with Helicobacter pylori-negative idiopathic bleeding ulcers. *Gastroenterology.* 2009;137:525.

Yamada T, Alpers DH, Kalloo AN, Kaplowitz N, Owyang C, Powell DW. *Textbook of Gastroenterology.* 5th ed. Hoboken, NJ: Wiley-Blackwell; 2008.

Yates JE, Pfifer JB, Flake D. Do nonmedicated topicals relieve childhood eczema? *J Fam Psychol.* 2009;58(5):280–281.

Yosipovitch G, Greaves MW, Schmelz M. Itch. *Lancet.* 2003;361:690.

Young T, Evans L, Finn L, Palta M. Estimation of the clinically diagnosed proportion of sleep apnea syndrome in middle-aged men and women. *Sleep.* 1997;20(9):705–706.

Zhang W, Moskowitz RW, Nuki G, et al. OARSI recommendations for the management of hip and knee osteoarthritis: part II, OARSI evidence-based, expert consensus guidelines. *Osteoarthr Cartil.* 2008;16:137–162.

Zuber TJ, Mayeaux TJ. *Atlas of Primary Care Procedures.* Philadelphia, PA: Lippincott Williams & Wilkins; 2009.